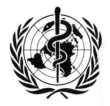

D0118117

World Health Organization Classification of Tumours

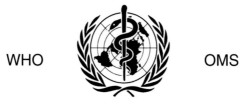

WHO   OMS

International Agency for Research on Cancer (IARC)

Pathology and Genetics of Tumours of the Lung, Pleura, Thymus and Heart

Edited by

William D. Travis

Elisabeth Brambilla

H. Konrad Müller-Hermelink

Curtis C. Harris

IARC*Press*

Lyon, 2004

World Health Organization Classification of Tumours

Series Editors   Paul Kleihues, M.D.
                  Leslie H. Sobin, M.D.

Pathology and Genetics of Tumours of the Lung, Pleura, Thymus and Heart

Editors   William D. Travis, M.D.
           Elisabeth Brambilla, M.D.
           H. Konrad Müller-Hermelink, M.D.
           Curtis C. Harris, M.D.

Coordinating Editors   Wojciech Biernat, M.D.
                        Janice Sych, Ph.D.

Editorial Assistants   Stéphane Sivadier
                        Agnès Meneghel
                        Voichita Meyronein

Layout   Vanessa Meister
          Marlen Grassinger
          Sibylle Söring

Illustrations   Thomas Odin

Printed by   Team Rush
              69603 Villeurbanne, France

Publisher   IARCPress
             International Agency for
             Research on Cancer (IARC)
             69008 Lyon, France

This volume was produced in collaboration with the

International Academy of Pathology (IAP)

and the

International Association for the Study of Lung Cancer (IASLC)

The WHO Classification of Tumours of the Lung, Pleura, Thymus and Heart presented in this book reflects the views of a Working Group that convened for an Editorial and Consensus Conference in Lyon, France, March 12-16, 2003.

Members of the Working Group are indicated in the List of Contributors on page 289.

Published by IARC Press, International Agency for Research on Cancer,
150 cours Albert Thomas, F-69008 Lyon, France

Format for bibliographic citations:
Travis W.D., Brambilla E., Muller-Hermelink H.K., Harris C.C. (Eds.): World Health
Organization Classification of Tumours. Pathology and Genetics of Tumours of the
Lung, Pleura, Thymus and Heart. IARC Press: Lyon 2004

IARC Library Cataloguing in Publication Data

Pathology and genetics of tumours of the lung, pleura, thymus and heart /
 editors W.D. Travis... [et al.]

 (World Health Organization classification of tumours ; 7)

 1. Lung neoplasms - genetics 2. Lung neoplasms - pathology
 3. Pleura neoplasms - genetics 4. Pleura neoplasms, - pathology
 5. Thymus neoplasms - genetics 6. Thymus neoplasms - pathology
 7. Heart neoplasms – genetics 8. Heart neoplasms - pathology
 I. Travis William D. II. Series

ISBN 92 832 2418 3   (NLM Classification: WJ 160)

Contents

CHAPTER 1

Tumours of the Lung

With more than 1.1 million deaths annually worldwide, lung cancer is the most frequent and one of the most deadly cancer types. In men, 85-90% of cases can be attributed to tobacco smoking. Some Western countries in which the smoking habit took off about 100 years ago, tobacco control programmes have led to a significant decline in mortality. Unfortunately, the habit has now spread to many newly industrialized countries, particularly in Asia, and in Europe, there is a worrying trend of increasing smoking prevalence in young women. The prognosis of lung cancer is still poor, with 5-years survival rates of approximately 10% in most countries. Thus, primary prevention by not starting or by stopping smoking remains the most promising approach.

The association between smoking and lung cancer is not solely based on epidemiological studies. Lung tumours of smokers frequently contain a typical, though not specific, molecular fingerprint in the form of G:C > T:A mutations in the TP53 gene which are probably caused by benzo[a]pyrene, one of the many carcinogens in tobacco smoke.

WHO histological classification of tumours of the lung

Malignant epithelial tumours

Squamous cell carcinoma	8070/3
Papillary	8052/3
Clear cell	8084/3
Small cell	8073/3
Basaloid	8083/3
Small cell carcinoma	8041/3
Combined small cell carcinoma	8045/3
Adenocarcinoma	8140/3
Adenocarcinoma, mixed subtype	8255/3
Acinar adenocarcinoma	8550/3
Papillary adenocarcinoma	8260/3
Bronchioloalveolar carcinoma	8250/3
Nonmucinous	8252/3
Mucinous	8253/3
Mixed nonmucinous and mucinous or indeterminate	8254/3
Solid adenocarcinoma with mucin production	8230/3
Fetal adenocarcinoma	8333/3
Mucinous ("colloid") carcinoma	8480/3
Mucinous cystadenocarcinoma	8470/3
Signet ring adenocarcinoma	8490/3
Clear cell adenocarcinoma	8310/3
Large cell carcinoma	8012/3
Large cell neuroendocrine carcinoma	8013/3
Combined large cell neuroendocrine carcinoma	8013/3
Basaloid carcinoma	8123/3
Lymphoepithelioma-like carcinoma	8082/3
Clear cell carcinoma	8310/3
Large cell carcinoma with rhabdoid phenotype	8014/3
Adenosquamous carcinoma	8560/3
Sarcomatoid carcinoma	8033/3
Pleomorphic carcinoma	8022/3
Spindle cell carcinoma	8032/3
Giant cell carcinoma	8031/3
Carcinosarcoma	8980/3
Pulmonary blastoma	8972/3
Carcinoid tumour	8240/3
Typical carcinoid	8240/3
Atypical carcinoid	8249/3
Salivary gland tumours	
Mucoepidermoid carcinoma	8430/3
Adenoid cystic carcinoma	8200/3
Epithelial-myoepithelial carcinoma	8562/3
Preinvasive lesions	
Squamous carcinoma *in situ*	8070/2
Atypical adenomatous hyperplasia	
Diffuse idiopathic pulmonary neuroendocrine cell hyperplasia	

Mesenchymal tumours

Epithelioid haemangioendothelioma	9133/1
Angiosarcoma	9120/3
Pleuropulmonary blastoma	8973/3
Chondroma	9220/0
Congenial peribronchial myofibroblastic tumour	8827/1
Diffuse pulmonary lymphangiomatosis	
Inflammatory myofibroblastic tumour	8825/1
Lymphangioleiomyomatosis	9174/1
Synovial sarcoma	9040/3
Monophasic	9041/3
Biphasic	9043/3
Pulmonary artery sarcoma	8800/3
Pulmonary vein sarcoma	8800/3

Benign epithelial tumours

Papillomas	
Squamous cell papilloma	8052/0
Exophytic	8052/0
Inverted	8053/0
Glandular papilloma	8260/0
Mixed squamous cell and glandular papilloma	8560/0
Adenomas	
Alveolar adenoma	8251/0
Papillary adenoma	8260/0
Adenomas of the salivary gland type	
Mucous gland adenoma	8140/0
Pleomorphic adenoma	8940/0
Others	
Mucinous cystadenoma	8470/0

Lymphoproliferative tumours

Marginal zone B-cell lymphoma of the MALT type	9699/3
Diffuse large B-cell lymphoma	9680/3
Lymphomatoid granulomatosis	9766/1
Langerhans cell histiocytosis	9751/1

Miscellaneous tumours

Harmatoma	
Sclerosing hemangioma	8832/0
Clear cell tumour	8005/0
Germ cell tumours	
Teratoma, mature	9080/0
Immature	9080/3
Other germ cell tumours	
Intrapulmonary thymoma	8580/1
Melanoma	8720/3

Metastatic tumours

---

[1] Morphology code of the International Classification of Diseases for Oncology (ICD-O) {6} and the Systematized Nomenclature of Medicine (http://snomed.org). Behaviour is coded /0 for benign tumours, /3 for malignant tumours, and /1 for borderline or uncertain behaviour.

TNM classification of the lung

TNM classification of carcinomas of the lung {738,2045}

T – Primary Tumour

TX   Primary tumour cannot be assessed, or tumour proven by the presence of malignant cells in sputum or bronchial washings but not visualized by imaging or bronchoscopy

T0   No evidence of primary tumour

Tis   Carcinoma in situ

T1   Tumour 3 cm or less in greatest dimension, surrounded by lung or visceral pleura, without bronchoscopic evidence of invasion more proximal than the lobar bronchus, i.e., not in the main bronchus (1)

T2   Tumour with any of the following features of size or extent:
- More than 3 cm in greatest dimension
- Involves main bronchus, 2 cm or more distal to the carina
- Invades visceral pleura
- Associated with atelectasis or obstructive pneumonitis that extends to the hilar region but does not involve the entire lung

T3   Tumour of any size that directly invades any of the following: chest wall (including superior sulcus tumours), diaphragm, mediastinal pleura, parietal pericardium; or tumour in the main bronchus less than 2 cm distal to the carina1 but without involvement of the carina; or associated atelectasis or obstructive pneumonitis of the entire lung

T4   Tumour of any size that invades any of the following: mediastinum, heart, great vessels, trachea, oesophagus, vertebral body, carina; separate tumour nodule(s) in the same lobe; tumour with malignant pleural effusion (2)

Notes: 1. The uncommon superficial spreading tumour of any size with its invasive component limited to the bronchial wall, which may extend proximal to the main bronchus, is also classified as T1.
2. Most pleural effusions with lung cancer are due to tumour. In a few patients, however, multiple cytopathological examinations of pleural fluid are negative for tumour, and the fluid is non-bloody and is not an exudate. Where these elements and clinical judgment dictate that the effusion is not related to the tumour, the effusion should be excluded as a staging element and the patient should be classified as T1, T2, or T3.

N – Regional Lymph Nodes[#]

NX   Regional lymph nodes cannot be assessed

N0   No regional lymph node metastasis

N1   Metastasis in ipsilateral peribronchial and/or ipsilateral hilar lymph nodes and intrapulmonary nodes, including involvement by direct extension

N2   Metastasis in ipsilateral mediastinal and/or subcarinal lymph node(s)

N3   Metastasis in contralateral mediastinal, contralateral hilar, ipsilateral or contralateral scalene, or supraclavicular lymph node(s)

M – Distant Metastasis

MX   Distant metastasis cannot be assessed

M0   No distant metastasis

M1   Distant metastasis, includes separate tumour nodule(s) in a different lobe (ipsilateral or contralateral)

Stage Grouping

Occult carcinoma	TX	N0	M0
Stage 0	Tis	N0	M0
Stage IA	T1	N0	M0
Stage IB	T2	N0	M0
Stage IIA	T1	N1	M0
Stage IIB	T2	N1	M0
	T3	N0	M0
Stage IIIA	T1, T2	N2	M0
	T3	N1, N2	M0
Stage IIIB	Any T	N3	M0
	T4	Any N	M0
Stage IV	Any T	Any N	M1

A help desk for specific questions about the TNM classification is available at http://www.uicc.org/tnm/
[#]The regional lymph nodes are the intrathoracic, scalene, and supraclavicular nodes.

Lung cancer epidemiology and etiology

M. Parkin
J.E. Tyczynski
P. Boffetta

J. Samet
P. Shields
N. Caporaso

Geographical differences

Lung cancer is the most common cancer in the world today (12.6% of all new cancers, 17.8% of cancer deaths). There were an estimated 1.2 million new cases and 1.1 million deaths in 2000; the sex ratio (M:F) is 2.7. Lung cancer is relatively more important in the developed than developing countries as it accounts for 22% versus 14.6% of cancer deaths, respectively. In developed countries, geographic patterns are very much a reflection of past exposure to tobacco smoking {505}.

In men, the areas with the highest incidence and mortality are Europe (especially Eastern Europe), North America, Australia/New Zealand, and South America. The rates in China, Japan and South East Asia are moderately high, while the lowest rates are found in southern Asia (India, Pakistan), and sub-Saharan Africa. In certain population subgroups (e.g. US blacks, New Zealand Maoris), incidence is even higher, and with current incidence rates, men in these two groups have about a 13% chance of developing a lung cancer before the age of 75.

In women, the geographic pattern is somewhat different, chiefly reflecting different historical patterns of tobacco smoking. Thus, the highest incidence rates are observed in North America and North West Europe (U.K., Iceland, Denmark) with moderate incidence rates in Australia, New Zealand and China.

Differences by histology

Almost all lung cancers are carcinomas (other histologies comprise well under 1%). In the combined data from the series published in Cancer Incidence in Five Continents {1554}, small cell carcinomas comprise about 20% of cases and large cell /undifferentiated carcinomas about 9%. But for the other histological types, the proportions differ by sex: squamous cell carcinomas comprise 44% of lung cancers in men, and 25% in women, while adenocarcinomas comprise 28% cases in men and 42% in women. Incidence rates, and the estimated rates by histological subtype have been reported for 30 populations for which a relatively high proportion of cases had a clear morphological diagnosis {1554}. Figure 2 shows overall incidence rates, and the estimated rates by histological subtype for 30 populations for which a relatively high proportion of cases had a clear morphological diagnosis {1554}. Among men, only in certain Asian populations (Chinese, Japanese) and in North America (USA, Canada) does the incidence of adenocarcinoma exceed that of squamous cell carcinoma. In women, however, adenocarcinoma is the dominant histological type almost everywhere, except for Poland and England where squamous cell carcinomas predominate, and Scotland where small cell carcinoma is the most frequent subtype {1554}. Adenocarcinomas are particularly predominant in Asian females (72% cancers in Japan, 65% in Korea, 61% in Singapore Chinese). The differences in histological profiles are strongly influenced by the evolution of the epidemic of smoking-related lung cancer over time (see below).

Time trends

Because tobacco smoking is such a powerful determinant of risk, trends in lung cancer incidence and mortality are a reflection of population-level changes in smoking behaviour, including dose, duration, and type of tobacco used {685, 1206}. Study of time trends in lung cancer incidence or mortality by age group shows that the level of risk is closely related to birth cohort; in the U.K. and U.S. cohort-specific incidence is related to the smoking habits of the same generation {228,1152}. Thus, in men, the countries where smoking was first established were first to see a diminution in smoking prevalence, followed, in the same generations of men, by a decline in risk. Changes are first seen among younger age groups {1396}, and as these generations of men reach the older age groups, where lung cancer is most common, a decline in overall incidence and mortality is seen. The U.K. was the first to show this incidence/mortality falling since 1970-74, followed by Finland, Australia, The Netherlands, New Zealand, the U.S.A., Singapore and, more recently, Denmark, Germany, Italy and Sweden {221}. In

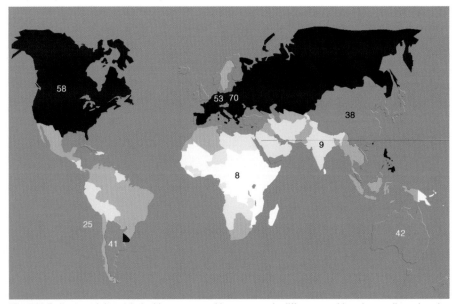

Fig. 1.01 Estimates of the male incidence rates of lung cancer in different world regions, adjusted to the world standard age distribution (ASR). From Globocan 2000 {572A}.

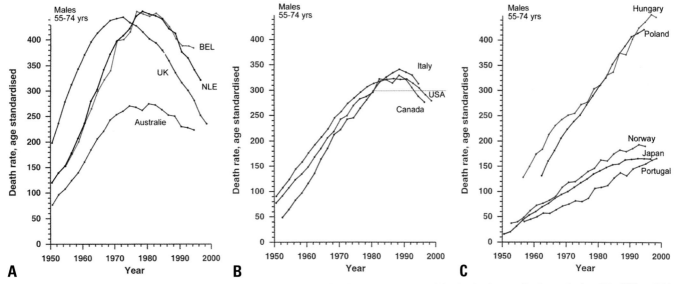

Fig. 1.02 Trends in male lung cancer mortality. **A** In some countries with early, high rates, a substantial reduction in mortality began in the 1970s (UK) or 1980s (Belgium, Netherlands, Australia). **B** In other countries (Italy, USA, Canada), the decline started in the 1990s. **C** Failure to achieve a significant reduction in tobacco consumption until recently has in some countries caused rising lung cancer mortality without apparent levelling off in males at ages 55-74. From R. Peto et al. {1589A}.

most other countries there is a continuing rise in rates, and this is most dramatic in some countries of Eastern and Southern Europe (i.e. Hungary, Spain) {223,2042}. In women, the tobacco habit has usually been acquired recently, or not at all. Thus, the most common picture in western populations is of rising rates, while in many developing countries (where female smoking generally remains rare), lung cancer rates remain very low. A few countries, where prevalence of smoking in women is declining, already show decreasing rates in younger women; in the U.K., where this trend is longest established, there is already a decline in overall incidence and mortality since about 1990 {221,2042}.

There are, however, clear differences in time trends by histological type. In the U.S. {487,2027} squamous cell carcinoma reached maximum incidence in men in 1981, but the incidence of adenocarcinoma continued to rise (until about 1987 in black males, around 1991 in whites). As a result, adenocarcinoma is now the most frequent form of lung cancer in men in USA, while it had only constituted a small minority of cases (around 5%) in the 1950s {2027,2029}. In contrast, the incidence of both histological types has continued to increase in females, though there is a sug-

gestion that the incidence of squamous cell carcinomas had reached its maximum by 1990. These changes were related to specific birth cohorts, with maximum incidence in men in the 1925-29 cohort for squamous cell carcinomas and 1935-39 for adenocarcinomas, and in women some 10-20 years later {487,2241}. Somewhat similar observations (increasing adenocarcinoma and decreasing squamous cell carcinoma) have been reported from the Netherlands {923}, Japan {1843} and the U.K. {779}. While part of this differential trend may be due to artefact (changes in classification and coding, improved diagnostic methods for peripheral tumours), the

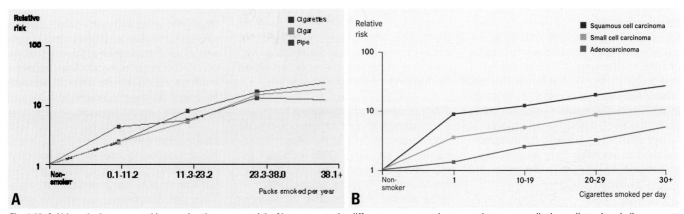

Fig. 1.03 A Although cigarette smoking carries the greatest risk of lung cancer, the differences among tobacco products are small when adjusted to similar amounts of tobacco consumption. Adapted from Boffetta et al. {191}. **B** All lung carcinomas are strongly associated with tobacco smoking, the risk being highest for squamous cell carcinoma, followed by small cell carcinoma and adenocarcinoma. Adapted from J.H. Lubin and W.J. Blot {1211} and {2250}.

incidence of adenocarcinomas is truly rising. In part, it may be due to an ever-increasing proportion of ex-smokers in the population, since the decline in risk of lung cancer on smoking cessation is faster for squamous cell tumours than for small cell carcinomas and adenocarcinomas {927, 1211}. It seems probable, too, that changes in cigarette composition, to low tar, low nicotine, filtered cigarettes, are also responsible, as switching to these "safer" brands results (in addicted smokers) to more intense smoking (more puffs, deeper inhalation), and hence greater exposure to these carcinogens in the peripheral lung where adenocarcinomas are more common {336,2177}.

Tobacco smoking

There is overwhelming evidence that tobacco smoking is the major cause of lung cancer in most human populations {884}. The smoke inhaled by smokers of cigarettes and other tobacco products contains numerous carcinogens, as well as agents that cause inflammation.

An increased risk of lung cancer in smokers has been demonstrated in epidemiological studies conducted during the 1950s in the United States {2176} and United Kingdom {504}, and the causal role of smoking has been recognized by public health and regulatory authorities since the mid-1960s. The geographical and temporal patterns of lung cancer today largely reflect tobacco consumption dating from two or three decades back. Because of the strong carcinogenic potency of tobacco smoke, a major reduction in tobacco consumption would result in the prevention of a large fraction of human cancers, including lung cancer {2155}.

Relative risk (RR)

The risk among smokers relative to the risk among never-smokers is in the order of 8-15 in men and 3-10 in women. For those who smoke without quitting, recent relative risk estimates are as high as 20 to 30. The overall relative risk reflects the contribution of the different aspects of tobacco smoking: average consumption, duration of smoking, time since quitting, age at start, type of tobacco product and inhalation pattern {192}.

Risk attributed to tobacco smoking

The proportion of lung cancer cases due to tobacco smoking has been estimated

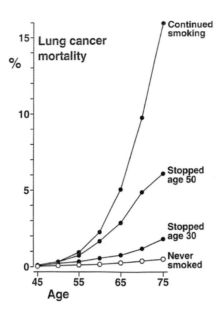

Fig. 1.04 The effects of stopping smoking at different ages on the cumulative risk (%) of death from lung cancer up to age 75. From R. Peto et al. {1588A}.

by comparing incidence (or mortality) rates in different areas, with the rates in non-smokers observed in large cohort studies {1553,1589}. Based on the worldwide incidence rates estimated for 2000. Worldwide, 85% of lung cancer in men and 47% of lung cancer in women is estimated as being the consequence of tobacco smoking.

Dose and duration

Several large cohort and case-control studies have provided detailed information on the relative contribution of duration and amount of cigarette smoking in excess lung cancer risk. Duration of smoking is the strongest determinant of risk, but this also increases in proportion to the number of cigarettes smoked {884}. The strong role of duration of smoking explains the observation that early age of starting is associated with a morbid lung cancer risk later in life.

Effect of cessation of smoking

An important aspect of tobacco-related lung carcinogenesis is the effect of cessation of smoking. The excess risk sharply decreases in ex-smokers after approximately 5 years since quitting; in some studies the risk after 20 or more years since cessation approaches that of never-smokers. However an excess risk throughout life likely persists even in

long-term quitters {884}. Thus, smoking cessation is beneficial at all ages.

Type of cigarettes and inhalation

Some studies show a lower lung cancer risk among smokers of low-tar and low-nicotine cigarettes than among other smokers {192}, but recent evidence suggests that low tar cigarettes are not less harmfull, and may be worse. A similar effect has been observed among long-term smokers of filtered cigarettes, or compared to smokers of unfiltered cigarettes. Smokers of black (air-cured) tobacco cigarettes are at two- to three-fold higher relative risk of lung cancer than smokers of blond (flue-cured) tobacco cigarettes. Tar content, presence of filter and type of tobacco are interdependent; high-tar cigarettes tend to be unfiltered and, in regions where black and blond tobacco are used, more frequently made of black tobacco.

A 1.5- to 3-fold difference in relative risk of lung cancer has been observed in several studies between smokers who deeply inhale cigarette smoke and smokers of comparable amounts who do not inhale or inhale slightly.

Type of tobacco products

Although cigarettes are the main tobacco product smoked in western countries, a dose-response relationship with lung cancer risk has been shown also for cigars, cigarillos and pipe, with a similar carcinogenic effect of these products {191}. A stronger carcinogenic effect of cigarettes than of cigars and pipe in some studies might arise due to different inhalation patterns or composition of cigars {902}.

An increased risk of lung cancer has also been shown with the bidis widely smoked in India and water pipes in China {884}. Adequate epidemiological data are not available on lung cancer risk following consumption of other tobacco products, such as narghile in western Asia and northern Africa, and hooka in India.

Lung cancer type

Tobacco smoking increases the risk of all major histological types of lung cancer, but appears to be strongest for squamous cell carcinoma, followed by small cell carcinoma and adenocarcinomama. The association between adenocarcinoma and smoking has become stronger over time, and adenocarcinoma has become the most common type in many Western countries.

Impact of sex and ethnicity
Whilst earlier studies have suggested a difference in risk of lung cancer between men and women who have smoked a comparable amount of tobacco, more recent evidence does not support this notion: the carcinogenic effect of smoking on the lung appears to be similar in men and women.

The higher rate of lung cancer among Blacks in the United States as compared to other ethnic groups is likely explained by higher tobacco consumption {486}. Indeed, there is no clear evidence of ethnic differences in susceptibility to lung carcinogenesis from tobacco.

Involuntary smoking

The collective epidemiologic evidence and biologic plausibility lead to the conclusion of a causal association between involuntary tobacco smoking and lung cancer risk in non-smokers {884}. This evidence has been challenged on the basis of possible confounding by active smoking, diet or other factors, and of possible reporting bias. However, when these factors were taken into account, the association was confirmed {884}. Several large-scale studies and meta-analyses consistently reported an increased risk of lung cancer in the order of 20–25% {190,603,754}.

Additional evidence of a carcinogenic effect of involuntary smoking comes from the identification in people exposed to involuntary smoking of nicotine-derived carcinogenic nitrosamines such as NNK, of haemoglobin adducts of 4-amino-byphenyl, a carcinogen in tobacco smoke and of albumin adducts of polycyclic aromatic hydrocarbons {884}. The comparison of levels of cotinine, the main metabolite of nicotine, suggests that exposure to involuntary smoking entails

Table 1.01
Occupational agents and exposure circumstances classified by the IARC Monographs Programme (http://monographs.iarc.fr), as carcinogenic to humans, with the lung as target organ.

Agents, mixture, circumstance	Main industry, use
Arsenic and arsenic compounds	Glass, metals, pesticides
Asbestos	Insulation, filters, textiles
Beryllium and beryllium compounds	Aerospace
Bis(chloromethyl)ether and	
Chloromethyl methyl ether	Chemical intermediate
Cadmium and cadmium compounds	Dye/pigment
Chromium[VI] compounds	Metal plating, dye/pigment
Dioxin (TCDD)	Chemical industry
Nickel compounds	Metallurgy, alloy, catalyst
Plutonium-239	Nuclear
Radon-222 and its decay products	Mining
Silica, crystalline	Stone cutting, mining, glass, paper
Talc containing asbestiform fibers	Paper, paints
X- and gamma-radiation	Medical, nuclear
Coal-tar pitches	Construction, electrodes
Coal-tars	Fuel
Soots	Pigments
Exposure circumstances	
Aluminum production	
Coal gasification	
Coke production	
Haematite mining (underground) with exposure to radon	
Iron and steel founding	
Painter (occupational exposure)	

an exposure equivalent of 0.1-1.0 cigarettes per day: the extrapolation of the relative risk found in light smokers is consistent with the relative risk detected in people exposed to involuntary tobacco smoking.

Occupational exposure

The important role of specific occupational exposures in lung cancer etiology is well established in reports dating back to the 1950s {192}. The table lists the occupational agents recognized as lung carcinogens by the International Agency for Research on Cancer (IARC). The most important occupational lung carcinogens include asbestos, crystalline silica, radon, mixtures of polycyclic aromatic hydrocarbons and heavy metals.

Welding and painting were consistently associated with increased risk of lung cancer. However, the exact agent(s) in these jobs have not yet been identified. Although their contribution to the global burden of lung cancer is relatively small, occupational carcinogens are responsible for an important proportion of tumours among exposed workers. For most known occupational carcinogens, some synergism has been shown with tobacco smoking.

Clinical features and staging

F.R. Hirsch
B. Corrin
T.V. Colby

Signs and symptoms

Patients with lung cancer present with progressive shortness of breath, cough, chest pain/oppression, hoarseness or loss of voice, haemoptysis (mostly with squamous cell carcinoma). Pneumonia (often recidivant) is the presenting feature in many patients. Relative to other forms of non small cell lung cancer, adenocarcinoma is more often asymptomatic, being more frequently identified in screening studies or as an incidental radiologic finding {5,391}. Patients with small cell lung cancer (SCLC) differ in many ways from those with non-small cell lung cancer (NSCLC), in that they often present with symptoms referable to distant metastases (see below). About 10% of patients with SCLC present with superior vena cava syndrome. Stridor and haemoptysis are rare symptoms in patients with SCLC. Symptoms related to disseminated disease include weight loss, abdominal pain due to involvement of the liver, adrenals and pancreas, and pain due to bone (marrow) metastases. At presentation brain metastases are identified in 5-10% of patients with SCLC and neurological symptoms occur, but CNS involvement develops during the course of the disease in many patients and multiple lesions are usually found in autopsy in patients with CNS involvement {848,1048,1493}.

Paraneoplastic symptoms

Paraneoplastic symptoms are common in lung cancer. Endocrine and paraneoplastic syndromes are less common in adenocarcinoma than in other histologic types of lung cancer. SCLC is characterized by neuroendocrine activity and some of the peptides secreted by the tumour mimic the activity of pituitary hormones. About 10% have abnormal ACTH like activity. Latent diabetes may become symptomatic but a Cushing syndrome is rare, probably because of short latency. Some SCLCs (15%) produce antidiuretic hormone (ADH) (Inappropriate ADH syndrome, Schwartz-Bartter syndrome) leading to water retention with oedema. The patients feel clumsy, tired and weak, and the plasma sodium is low. This is associated with an inferior prognosis {1523,1849}. Cerebrospinal metastases or meningeal seeding may cause neurological symptoms. Neurological symptoms may also be a paraneoplastic phenomenon, which might include sensory, sensorimotor, and autoimmune neuropathies and encephalomyelitis. The

Table 1.02
Signs and symptoms of lung carcinoma. Approximately 5-20% of cases are clinically occult. Modified, from T.V. Colby et al. {391}

Systemic symptoms Weight loss, loss of appetite, malaise, fever **Local /direct effects** From endobronchial growth and/or invasion of adjacent structures including chest wall and vertebral column Cough, dyspnoea, wheeze, stridor, haemoptysis Chest pain/back pain Obstructive pneumonia (+/- cavitation) Pleural effusion **Extension to mediastinal structures** Nerve entrapment : recurrent laryngeal nerve (hoarseness), phrenic nerve (diaphragmatic paralysis), sympathetic system (Horner syndrome), brachial plexopathy from "superior sulcus" tumours Vena cava obstruction: superior vena cava syndrome Pericardium: effusion, tamponade Myocardium: arrythmia, heart failure Oesophagus: dysphagia, bronchoesophageal fistula Mediastinal lymph nodes: pleural effusion **Metastatic disease** Direct effects related to the organ(s) involved **Paraneoplastic syndromes** Dermatomyositis/polymyositis Clubbing Hypertrophic pulmonary osteoarthropath Encephalopathy Peripheral neuropathies Myasthenic syndromes (including Lambert-Eaton) Transverse myelitis Progressive multifocal leukoencephalopathy	**Endocrine syndromes** Parathormone-like substance: hypercalcemia Inappropriate antidiuretic hormone: hyponatremia ACTH: Cushing syndrome, hyperpigmentation Serotonin: carcinoid syndrome Gonadotropins: gynecomastia Melanocyte-stimulating hormone: increased pigmentation Hypoglycemia, hyperglycemia Hypercalcitonemia Elevated growth hormone Prolactinemia Hypersecretion of vasoactive intestinal polypeptide (VIP): diarrhea **Hematologic/coagulation defects** Disseminated intravascular coagulation Recurrent venous thromboses Nonbacterial thrombotic (marantic) endocarditis Anemia Dysproteinemia Granulocytosis Eosinophilia Hypoalbuminemia Leukoerythroblastosis Marrow plasmacytosis Thrombocytopenia **Miscellaneous (very rare)** Henoch-Schönlein purpura Glomerulonephritis, Nephrotic syndrome Hypouricemia, Hyperamylasemia Amyloidosis Lactic acidosis Systemic lupus erythematosus

symptoms may precede the primary diagnosis by many months, and might in some cases be the presenting complaint. They may also be the initial sign of relapse from remission. A specific example is the Lambert-Eaton myasthenic syndrome resulting in proximal muscular weakness that improves with continued use and hypoflexia and dysautonomy. Characteristic electromyographic findings confirm the diagnosis. This syndrome may also occur months before the tumour is disclosed {1497}. The weakness will often improve when the tumour respond on therapy. Hypercalcemia is rare in SCLC, and almost pathognomic for squamous cell carcinoma.

Relevant diagnostic procedures
Fiberoptic bronchoscopy allows macroscopic examination of the respiratory tree up to most of the subsegmental bronchi and biopsies associated to bronchial aspiration and brushing. Biopsies of bone, liver, lymph node (mediastinoscopy), skin and adrenal gland may also be used for diagnosis if they are metastatically involved. Pulmonary function tests are performed if surgery seems possible. Serum tumour markers are not routinely recommended. Because of its central location squamous cell carcinoma is readily diagnosed by bronchoscopic biopsy and/or brush and/or sputum cytology {532}. Fluorescence bronchoscopy may be useful for assessing the extent of associated intraepithelial neoplasia. For peripheral lesions transthoracic CT guided fine needle aspiration biopsy is now generally preferred.

Due to common central location, small cell carcinoma is often diagnosed via bronchoscopically retrieved histologic and cytologic samples and to a lesser extent sputum cytology.

Small peripheral lesions are often subjected to fine needle aspiration biopsy, transbronchial biopsy, or sometimes wedge resection for initial diagnosis.

Staging of NSCLC
The internationally accepted TNM staging system is recommended. The stage of the disease is important for prognosis and treatment planning. Pathologic staging is based on the pathologic evaluation of sampled tissues according to the TNM system. For patients in whom surgical resection is attempted, there are surgical protocols for sampling the lymph node stations, including superior mediastinal nodes (numbered 1-4), aortic nodes (numbered 5 and 6), inferior mediastinal nodes (numbered 7-9) and nodes associated with the lobectomy specimen labeled "N1" nodes (numbered 10-14).

Staging of SCLC
The TNM staging classification is generally not utilized in SCLC, as it does not predict well for survival. SCLC is usually staged as either limited or extensive disease. The consensus report of the International Association for the Study of Lung Cancer (IASLC) modified the older VALG classification in accordance with the revised TNM system:

Limited disease
Disease restricted to one hemithorax with regional lymph node metastases including:

Table 1.03
Tumour markers found in the serum of patients with lung carcinoma. From refs {5,13,391}.

Hormones
Adrenocorticotropic hormone (ACTH)
Melanocyte-stimulating hormone (MSH)
Human chorionic gonadotropin (hCG)
Human placental lactogen (HPL)
Human growth hormone (HGH)
Parathyroid hormone (PTH)
Calcitonin
Antidiuretic hormone (ADH)
Prolactin
Bombesin (gastrin-releasing peptide)
5-Hydroxytryptophan (serotonin)
Oestradiol
Hypoglycemic factor
Renin, Erythropoietin
Glucagon, Insulin
Neuron-specific enolase (NSE)
ß-Endorphin, Gastrin, Secretin
Serum proteins
Alpha fetoprotein (AFP)
Carcinoembryonic antigen (CEA)
Placental alkaline phosphatase (PAP)
Histaminase
L-dopa decarboxylase
Anti-Purkinje cell antibodies
Antineuronal nuclear antibodies (ANNA)
Ferritin

Table 1.04
Imaging techniques in lung cancer staging.
From T.V. Colby et al. {391}.

Conventional radiographs	Primary detection/characterization of parenchymal tumour Assessment of main bronchi/tracheal involvement Detection of chest wall invasion Assessment of hilar and mediastinal invasion/adenopathy Detection of obstructive atelectasis/pneumonitis Detection of pleural effusion
CT	Assessment of main bronchi/tracheal involvement Detection of chest wall invasion Assessment of hilar and mediastinal invasion/adenopathy Detection of liver, adrenal, brain metastases
MRI	Detection of chest wall invasion (particularly superior sulcus [tumours]) Detection of mediastinal or spinal canal invasion Assessment of hilar and mediastinal adenopathy in patients with equivocal CT examinations or contraindications to intravenous contrast media Characterization of isolated adrenal masses
Ultrasound	Detection of pleural effusion/guidance for thoracentesis Guidance for biopsy of peripheral lung or mediastinal mass
Gallium-67 scan	Detection of hilar and mediastinal adenopathy Detection of distal metastases
Pulmonary angiography	Evaluation of central pulmonary artery invasion

Table 1.05
Chest radiographic findings at presentation according to histologic type of lung carcinoma. From ref {391}.

Radiographic Feature	Squamous Cell Carcinoma	Adeno-carcinoma	Small Cell Carcinoma	Large Cell Carcinoma
Nodule <or= 4 cm	14%	46%	21%	18%
Peripheral location	29%	65%	26%	61%
Central location	64%	5%	74%	42%
Hilar/perihilar mass	40%	17%	78%	32%
Cavitation	5%	3%	0%	4%
Pleural/chest wall involvement	3%	14%	5%	2%
Hilar adenopathy	38%	19%	61%	32%
Mediastinal adenopathy	5%	9%	14%	10%

Table 1.07
Stage and survival in NSCLC*. Modified, from {232}.

Stage	Survival (%)	
	3 yr	5 yr
Clinical stage		
cIA (n = 687)	71	61
cIB (n = 1189)	46	38
cIIA (n = 29)	38	34
cIIB (n = 357)	33	24
cIIIA (n = 511)	18	13
cIIIB (n = 1,030)	7	5
cIV (n = 1,427)	2	1
Pathologic stage		
pIA (n = 511)	80	67
pIB (n = 549)	67	57
pIIA (n = 76)	66	55
pIIB (n = 375)	46	39
pIIIA (n = 399)	32	23

> Hiliar ipsilateral and contralateral
> Mediastinal ipsilateral and contralateral
> Supraclavicular ipsilateral and contralateral
> Ipsilateral pleural effusion (independent of cytology)

Limited disease is equivalent to stage I-III of the TNM system.

Extensive disease

All patients with sites of disease beyond the definition of limited disease, equivalent to stage IV in the TNM system.

Staging Procedures

The staging procedures have the primary goal to distuingish patients who are candidate for surgery, those with loco-regional disease, and those with metastatic disease.

Standard procedures include chest X-ray, general physical examination, bronchoscopy and blood samples. If findings at these procedures do not preclude surgery or radiotherapy, staging proceeds with a CT-scan of chest and upper abdomen. Staging stops here if the CT scan shows definitive signs of inoperable disease such as tumour invasion of the mediastinum or distant metastases to the liver or the adrenals. If, however, surgery seems possible, lymph nodes in the mediastinum must be examined for metastatic deposits. If none of the lymph nodes are enlarged (greatest diameter >1.5 cm) and the tumour is proven to be of the squamous cell type, lymph node biopsies can be omitted; otherwise a preoperative mediastinoscopy with biopsies is recommended. In recent years this invasive procedure has been enhanced by PET scan, although the accuracy (diagnostic sensitivity and specificity) of this imaging procedure has not yet been fully validated in lung cancer. If PET is not available, ultrasonography is still a very helpful procedure and allows fine needle biopsies from suspect lesions in abdominal sites plus other deeply located structures such as axil-lary lymph nodes and the thyroid gland. SCLC is characterized by a rapid dissemination to extrathoracic organs. Autopsy studies performed 1 month after surgical resection showed that 63% (12 of 19 patients) with SCLC had distant metastases compared to 14-40% of patients with NSCLC {848}.

Staging of SCLC includes bronchoscopy, chest X-ray, chest CT scan, upper abdominal CT scan or ultrasonography plus a bone marrow examination and/or a bone scintigram. Bone scintigrams are still used but this procedure will probably be left with the increasing availability of PET scanners. Finally, magnetic resonance imaging (MRI) scans are useful if bone metastases or central nervous system metastases are suspected. Patients with neurological symptoms should have a cranial CT or MR scan.

Staging of SCLC will prove extensive stage disease in about 65% of the patients due to metastases to one or more of the following sites: the contralateral lung (10%), skin or distant lymph nodes (10%), brain (10%), liver (25%), adrenals (15%), bone marrow (20%), retroperitoneal lymph nodes (5%), or pancreas (5%). Osteolytic bone metastases and hypercalcaemia are rarely seen, but are almost pathognomonic for squamous cell carcinoma. Enlarged adrenals might represent metastases but can also be a glandular hypertrophy due to ectopic ACTH secretion from the tumour, which is observed in about 10% of patients with SCLC {780,847,887, 1849}.

Table 1.06
Stage of lung carcinoma at presentation by histologic subtype. SEER data 1983-1987.
Modified, from reference {192}.

Stage	Squamous	Adenocarcinoma	Small cell	Large cell
Localized	21.5%	22.2%	8.2%	15.2%
Regional	38.5%	33.1%	26.1%	31.5%
Distant	25.2%	35.9%	52.8%	40.3%
Unstaged	14.8%	8.8%	12.8%	12.9%

Tissue collection and interpretation

Optimal tissue collection is important for a precise classification of lung tumours. Several diagnostic approaches are available, including sputum cytology, bronchoalveolar lavage, bronchoscopic biopsy, brushing and washing, thoracoscopic biopsy, resected surgical material and needle biopsies as well as pleural cytology.

Rapid fixation and minimal trauma are important. Small specimens may not show differentiation when the tumour is excised; it is, therefore, advisable to limit categorization to SCLC and NSCLC. The current classification is largely based on standard H&E sections. Some lung carcinomas remain unclassified. They usually fall into the "non-small cell carcinoma" category or are cases where small biopsy or cytology specimens preclude definitive histologic typing.

Histologic heterogeneity

Lung cancers frequently show histologic heterogeneity, with variation in appearance and differentiation from microscopic field to field and from one histologic section to the next {1676}. Almost 50% of lung carcinomas exhibit more than one of the major histologic types. This fact has important implications for lung tumour classification and must be kept in mind, especially when interpreting small biopsies.

The designation of a minimum requirement such as 10% for the adenocarcinoma and squamous cell carcinoma components of adenosquamous carcinoma or the spindle and/or giant cell carcinoma component of pleomorphic carcinomas set in the 1999 WHO classification are maintained in this classification, recognizing that they are an arbitrary criterion since the extent of histologic sampling will influence classification of such tumours {584,2024}. Although these tumours may be suspected on small specimens such as bronchoscopic or needle biopsies, a definitive diagnosis requires a resected specimen. If this problem arises in a resected tumour, additional histologic sections may be helpful. Nevertheless, defining a specific percentage for a histologic component can be a useful criterion for entities such as adenosquamous carcinoma and pleomorphic carcinoma.

The concept of pulmonary neuroendocrine tumours

W.D. Travis

Tumours with neuroendocrine morphology

Neuroendocrine tumours of the lung are a distinct subset of tumours, which share morphologic, ultrastructural, immunohistochemical and molecular characteristics and although these tumours are classified into different morphologic categories within the WHO classification, certain concepts relating specifically to neuroendocrine tumours merit discussion. The major categories of morphologically identifiable neuroendocrine tumours are small cell carcinoma (SCLC), large cell neuroendocrine carcinoma (LCNEC), typical carcinoid (TC), and atypical carcinoid (AC). Historical terms such as well-differentiated neuroendocrine carcinoma, neuroendocrine carcinoma (grade 1-3), intermediate cell neuroendocrine carcinoma, malignant carcinoid and peripheral small cell carcinoma resembling carcinoid, should be avoided {1999}.

With regard to nomenclature, the terms typical and atypical carcinoid are preferred for a number of reasons. Clinicians are familiar with these diagnostic terms and the tumours share a distinctive basic microscopic appearance, resembling carcinoids found at other body sites. Spindle cell, oncocytic and melanocytic patterns and stromal ossification occur in both typical and atypical carcinoids. Patients with typical and atypical carcinoids are also significantly younger than those with SCLC and LCNEC. Within the high-grade neuroendocrine tumours, LCNEC and SCLC are morphologically distinct and it has not been proven that chemotherapy used for SCLC is effective for patients with LCNEC.

With regard to distinguishing the four main types of neuroendocrine tumours, all show varying degrees of neuroendocrine morphologic features by light microscopy including organoid nesting, palisading, a trabecular pattern, and rosette-like structures, with the cardinal distinguishing features being mitotic activity and the presence or absence of necrosis. For mitotic activity, Arrigoni, et al. {75} originally proposed that atypical carcinoids had between 5-10 mitoses per 10 high power fields. However, the mitotic range for atypical carcinoid was recently modified to 2-10 mitoses per 2 mm^2 (10 high power fields – see below for mitosis counting method) {2028}. The presence of necrosis also distinguishes atypical from typical carcinoid. Cytologic atypia is unreliable as a diagnostic feature.

A mitotic count of 11 or more mitoses per 2 mm^2 (10 high power fields) is the main criterion for separating LCNEC and SCLC from atypical carcinoid {2028}. LCNEC and SCLC usually have very high mitotic rates, with an average of 70-80 per 2 mm^2 (10 high power fields in some microscope models). LCNEC and SCLC also generally have more extensive necrosis than atypical carcinoid. LCNEC are separated from SCLC using a constellation of criteria, which include larger cell size, abundant cytoplasm, prominent nucleoli, vesicular or coarse chromatin, polygonal rather than fusiform shape, less prominent nuclear molding and less conspicuous deposition of hematoxylin-stained material (DNA) in blood vessel walls. LCNEC cells more closely resemble those of a large cell carcinoma than a carcinoid tumour. Mitoses should be counted in the areas of highest mitotic activity and the fields counted should be filled with as many viable tumour cells as possible. Since the area viewed in a high power field varies considerably depending on the microscope model, we define the mitotic range based on the area of viable tumour examined. These criteria were established on a microscope with a 40X objective, an eyepiece field of view number of 20 and with no magnification changing devices. With this approach the area viewed in one high power field is 0.2 mm^2 and 10 high power fields = 2 mm2. If microscopes with other objective and eyepiece field of view numbers are used, the area in a high power field should be measured to allow calibration to cover a 2 mm^2 area.

There is substantial reproducibility (kappa statistic of .70) for this subclassification scheme. The greatest reproducibility is seen with SCLC and typical carcinoid. The most common disagreements involve LCNEC vs SCLC, followed by typical carcinoid vs atypical carcinoid, and atypical carcinoid vs LCNEC. Additional research on atypical carcinoid and LCNEC is needed to better define their clinical characteristics and optimal therapy.

Interestingly, despite separation into four main groups, there is increasing evidence that TC and AC are more closely associated to each other than to LCNEC and SCLC. Clinically, approximately 20-40% of patients with both typical and atypical carcinoids are non-smokers while virtually all patients with SCLC and LCNEC are cigarette smokers. In contrast to SCLC and LCNEC, both typical and atypical carcinoids can occur in patients with Multiple Endocrine Neoplasia (MEN) type I {464}. In addition, neuroendocrine cell hyperplasia with or without tumourlets is relatively frequent in both typical and atypical carcinoids but not in LCNEC or SCLC. Histologic heterogeneity with other major histologic types of lung carcinoma (squamous cell carcinoma, adenocarcinoma, etc.) occurs with both SCLC and LCNEC but not with typical or atypical carcinoids {2024}. In contrast to large cell neuroendocrine carcinoma, most typical and atypical carcinoids are readily diagnosed by light microscopy without the need for immunohistochemistry or electron microscopy. There are also genetic data indicating that SCLC is closer to LCNEC than to the TC and AC, in that abnormalities in many genetic markers such as p53 {1516,1622}, bcl2/bax {217}, cyclin D1 {746}, RB loss and LOH at 3p {726} are seen in a high percentage of both SCLC and LCNEC with minimal and intermediate percentages of TC and AC showing abnormalities, respectively (see below).

Non-small cell carcinomas with neuroendocrine differentiation

Some lung carcinomas, which do not show neuroendocrine morphology by light microscopy, demonstrate immunohistochemical and/or ultrastructural evidence of neuroendocrine differentiation. Neuroendocrine differentiation can be shown by immunohistochemistry in 10-20% of squamous cell carcinomas, adenocarcinomas, and large cell carcinomas. It is seen most often in adenocarcinomas. These tumours are collectively referred to as NSCLC with neuroendocrine differentiation (NSCLC-ND). While this issue has drawn much interest, there is controversy over whether these tumours have worse or better survival and whether they are more or less responsive to chemotherapy than NSCLC lacking neuroendocrine differentiation. Therefore these tumours require further study before they are included as a separate category in a histologic classification. They should be classified according to the conventional typing herein, with neuroendocrine differentiation noted {2024}.

Table 1.08
Criteria for diagnosis of neuroendocrine tumours.
From W.D. Travis et al. {2024}

Typical carcinoid
A tumour with carcinoid morphology and less than 2 mitoses per 2 mm^2 (10 HPF), lacking necrosis and 0.5 cm or larger

Atypical carcinoid
A tumour with carcinoid morphology with 2-10 mitoses per 2 mm^2 (10 HPF) OR necrosis (often punctate)

Large cell neuroendocrine carcinoma
1. A tumour with a neuroendocrine morphology (organoid nesting, palisading, rosettes, trabeculae)
2. High mitotic rate: 11 or greater per 2 mm^2 (10 HPF), median of 70 per 2 mm^2 (10 HPF)
3. Necrosis (often large zones)
4. Cytologic features of a non-small cell carcinoma (NSCLC): large cell size, low nuclear to cytoplasmic ratio, vesicular, coarse or fine chromatin, and/or frequent nucleoli. Some tumours have fine nuclear chromatin and lack nucleoli, but qualify as NSCLC because of large cell size and abundant cytoplasm.
5. Positive immunohistochemical staining for one or more NE markers (other than neuron specific enolase) and/or NE granules by electron microscopy.

Small cell carcinoma
Small size (generally less than the diameter of 3 small resting lymphocytes)
1. Scant cytoplasm
2. Nuclei: finely granular nuclear chromatin, absent or faint nucleoli
3. High mitotic rate (11 or greater per 2 mm^2 (10 HPF), median of 80 per 2 mm^2 (10 HPF)
4. Frequent necrosis often in large zones

Table 1.09
The spectrum of neuroendocrine (NE) proliferations and neoplasms. From W.D. Travis et al. {2024}

Neuroendocrine cell hyperplasia and tumourlets
NE cell hyperplasia
NE cell hyperplasia with fibrosis and/or inflammation
NE cell hyperplasia adjacent to carcinoid tumours
Diffuse idiopathic NE cell hyperplasia with or without airway fibrosis
Tumourlets

Tumours with NE morphology
Typical carcinoid
Atypical carcinoid
Large cell neuroendocrine carcinoma
Small cell carcinoma

Non-small cell carcinomas with NE differentiation

Other tumours with NE properties
Pulmonary blastoma
Primitive neuroectodermal tumour
Desmoplastic round cell tumour
Carcinomas with rhabdoid phenotype
Paraganglioma

Genetic and molecular alterations

A. Gazdar
W.A. Franklin
E. Brambilla
P. Hainaut
J. Yokota
C.C. Harris

Molecular and pathological diversity of lung cancers

Lung cancers result from complex, genetic and epigenetic changes characterized by stepwise malignant progression of cancer cells in association with accumulation of genetic alterations. This process, referrred to as multistep carcinogenesis, develops through the clonal evolution of initiated lung cells. Initiation consists in the acquisition of defined genetic alterations in a small number of genes that confer a proliferative advantage that facilitates progression towards invasive carcinoma. Many environmental carcinogens present in tobacco smoke or in industrial pollutants can act as initiators for bronchial or bronchiolar-alveolar epithelial cells {807,2145}. These carcinogens often have a global effect on the entire bronchial tree, resulting in the frequent occurrence of several primary lesions within the same, exposed organ. This observation has led to the concept of field carcinogenesis.

Over the past 25 years, evidence has accumulated for stepwise accumulation of genetic changes in all major histological types of lung cancers. These changes include allelelic losses (LOH), chromosomal instability and imbalance, mutations in oncogenes and tumor suppressor genes, epigenetic gene silencing through promoter hypermethylation and aberrant of expression of genes involved in the control of cell proliferation {564,687,1235,1323,2209}. Although many of these genetic changes occur independently of histological type, their frequency and timing of occurrence with respect to cancer progression is different in small cell lung carcinomas (SCLC), that may originate from epithelial cells with neuro-endocrine features, and non-small cell lung carcinomas (NSCLC), that originate from bronchial or alveolar epithelial cells. Furthermore, a number of genetic and epigenetic differences have been identified between squamous cell carcinoma (SCC), that arises from bronchial epithelial cells through a squamous metaplasia/dysplasia process),

and adenocarcinoma (ADC), that derives from alveolar or bronchiolar epithelial cells {2017,2209}.

Genetic changes frequent in all major histological types

Invasive lung carcinoma display multiple genetic alterations, such as LOH at many different loci including 3p14-23 {220, 1210,1446}, 8q21-23 {2159}, 9p21 {670,1299}, 13q, 17q, 18q and 22p {687, 1268,1996,2209}. However, three frequent aberrations emerge as common changes in all histological types of lung cancers.

TP53 mutations

The most frequent one is mutation in the tumor suppressor gene TP53, encoding the p53 protein that plays multiple, antiproliferative roles, in particular in response to genotoxic stress {881,1947}. Inactivating TP53 mutations (mostly missense mutations) are detected in up 50% of NSCLC and in over 70% of SCLC {1591}. In both SCC and ADC, there is evidence that mutation can occur very early in cancer progression and that their prevalence increases from primary, in situ lesions to advanced, metastatic carcinomas.

Retinoblastoma pathway

The second most common alteration is inactivation of the pathway controlling RB1 (retinoblastoma gene, 13q11), a suppressor gene encoding the Rb protein that acts as a "gatekeeper" for the G1 to S transition of cell cycle {215, 2209}. The most common mechanisms for inactivation of this pathway are loss of RB1 expression, silencing of INK4 (also termed CDKN2a, encoding p16) through LOH (9p21) and promoter hypermethylation, and overexpression of CCND1 (encoding cyclin D1), sometimes consecutive to gene amplification (11q13) {189,215}. These three genes act in a sequential manner within the signalling cascade that controls Rb inactivation by phosphorylation. There is a constant inverse correlation between loss of Rb

protein, inactivation of p16 and overexpression of cyclin D1, consistent with the notion that these events have essentially similar functional consequences {215}. Interestingly, the mechanism by which this pathway is altered differs between NSCLC and SCLC. Loss of Rb protein expression is detectable in over 80-100% of high grade neurorendocrine tumors, most of them retaining normal p16 and cyclin D1 expression {189,670}. In contrast, loss of Rb protein is less common in NSCLC (15%) but inactivation of INK4 is present in up to 70% of the cases, whereas amplification of CCDN1 is detectable in a significant proportion of SCC (10%) {215,2209}. It should also be noted that the INK4 gene locus contains a reading frame encoding another protein, p14arf, which is different from p16 but also plays roles in growth suppression. Initial studies suggested that the expression of p14arf is often lost in SCLC, suggesting that alterations of the INK4 locus may have functional consequences other than deregulation of the cascade controlling RB1 {669}. Recent reports indicate that p14arf methylation does not play a role of in the development of SCLC and NSCLC {1550,1746}.

LOH 3p

The third common genetic event that occurs in all lung cancers irrespective of their histological type is LOH on chromosome 3p, detectable in up to 80% of NSCLC as well as SCLC {220,1210, 1446}. This region encompasses several potential tumor suppressor genes, including FHIT, RASSF1 and SEMA3B {1167,1183,2209}. The FHIT gene (Fragile Histidine Triad) is located in a highly fragile chromosomal site where it is particularly prone to partial deletion as a result of direct DNA damage by carcinogens present in tobacco smoke {895}. FHIT encodes a protein with ADP hydrosylase activity that has been proposed to have various intracellular functions, including regulation of DNA replication and signalling stress responses {112}. RASSF1 encodes a protein involved in the control of the activity of members of the RAS family of oncogenes. SEMA3B encodes semaphorin 3B, a member of a family of genes encoding secreted proteins with critical roles in development of neuronal and epithelial tissues. The contributions of these genes to the development of lung cancers is still poorly under-

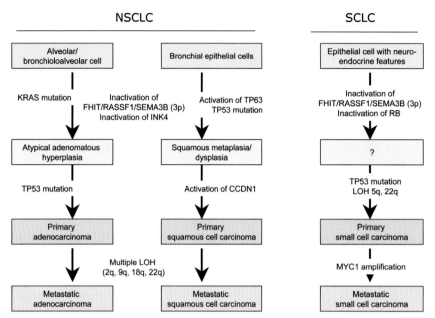

NSCLC

Alveolar/bronchioloalveolar cell
→ KRAS mutation →
Atypical adenomatous hyperplasia
→ TP53 mutation →
Primary adenocarcinoma
→ Multiple LOH (2q, 9q, 18q, 22q) →
Metastatic adenocarcinoma

Bronchial epithelial cells
→ Activation of TP63 / TP53 mutation →
Squamous metaplasia/dysplasia
→ Activation of CCDN1 →
Primary squamous cell carcinoma
→
Metastatic squamous cell carcinoma

Inactivation of FHIT/RASSF1/SEMA3B (3p) / Inactivation of INK4

SCLC

Epithelial cell with neuro-endocrine features
→ Inactivation of FHIT/RASSF1/SEMA3B (3p) / Inactivation of RB →
?
→ TP53 mutation / LOH 5q, 22q →
Primary small cell carcinoma
→ MYC1 amplification →
Metastatic small cell carcinoma

Fig. 1.05 Genetic models for the development non-small cell lung carcinomas (NSCLC) and of small cell lung carcinoma (SCLC). From J. Yokota and T. Kohno {2209}.

stood. Their expression is frequently lost in tumors, despite the presence of residual, apparently intact alleles. This observation has led to the hypothesis that several genes in chromosome 3p are common targets for epigenetic abnormalities through mechanisms that are not yet fully elucidated {560}.

Genetic changes in histological types of lung cancer

Among the less common changes observed in lung cancers, some appear to be more frequent in specific histological types. For example, mutations at codon 12 in KRAS are found in 30 to 40% of ADC but are extremely rare in other forms of NSCLC or in SCLC {402,1669}. KRAS mutation is detected in a significant proportion of atypical alveolar hyperplasias, indicating that this lesion is a potential pre-invasive lesion for ADC {2126}. In contrast, mutational activation of the beta-catenin gene is rare {1502} but has been identified in different histological types of lung cancer {1801,1904}. Mutations of the APC gene, another component of the Wnt pathway, have been identified in up to 5% of squamous cell and small cell lung cancer {1502}. Amplifications of MYC (8q21-23) are found only in a minority of advanced NSCLC (less than 10%) but are common in pre-invasive stages SCLC (30%). Similarly, LOH on chromosome 5q are

frequent at early stages of SCLC but are infrequent in non-metastatic NSCLC {2209}. The target gene on chromosome 5q is still not identified.

The gradual increase of molecular abnormalities along the spectrum of neuroendocrine lung tumours strongly supports the grading concept of typical carcinoid as low grade, atypical carcinoid as intermediate grade and large cell neuroendocrine carcinoma and small cell lung carcinoma as high-grade neuroendocrine lung tumours. MEN1 gene mutation and LOH at the MEN1 gene locus 11q13 was recently demonstrated in 65% of sporadic atypical carcinoids {463} and was not found in high grade neuroendocrine tumours {464}.

Although epigenetic silencing of genes, mainly through promoter hypermethylation, is widespread in all forms of lung cancers, the methylation profile of tumors varies with histological type. SCLC, carcinoids, SCC and ADC have unique profiles of aberrantly methylated genes. In particular, the methylation rates of APC, CDH13 and RARb are significantly higher in ADC than in SCC {2017}.

Several striking differences also exist at the level of gene expression. The p63 protein, encoded by TP63, a member of the TP53 gene family located on chromosome 3q, is highly expressed and sometimes amplified in SCC but not in other histological types {826}. This protein

plays a role in squamous differentiation and its presence may be required for the development of SCC. As there is no squamous epithelium in the normal lung, deregulation of p63 expression may be a fundamental event in the pathogenesis of the metaplasia that precedes SCC.

DNA adducts and mutagen fingerprints

About 90% of lung cancers in Western countries, and a rapidly growing number of cancers in non-western countries, are caused by smoking. Tobacco smoke is a mixture of over 4800 chemicals, including over 60 that were classified as carcinogens by the International Agency for Research on Cancer. They belong to various classes of chemicals, including polycyclic aromatic hydrocarbons (PAH), aza-arenes, N-nitrosamines, aromatic amines, heterocyclic aromatic amines, aldehydes, volatile hydrocarbons, nitro compounds, miscellaneous organic compounds, and metals and other inorganic compounds {807,1591}. Although the dose of each carcinogen per cigarette is quite small, the cumulative dose in a lifetime of smoking can be considerable. In target cells, most of these carcinogens are converted to intermediates compounds by Cytochrome P450 enzymes, which catalyze the addition of an oxygen to the carcinogen, increasing its water solubility. The resulting metabolites are readily converted to excretable soluble forms by glutathione S-transferase, providing an efficient detoxification mechanism. However, during this process, electrophilic (electron-deficient) intermediates are formed, that are highly reactive with DNA, resulting in the formation of DNA adducts {2145}.

Cells are equipped with elaborate systems to eliminate DNA adducts from the genome, including the nucleotide excision repair pathway (NER, that preferentially eliminates so-called bulky DNA adducts consisting of large chemical groups covalently attached to DNA), the base excision repair systems (BER), that removes DNA bases altered by attachment of small chemical groups or fragmented by ionizing radiation or oxidation, as well as a specialized, direct repair system that acts through the enzyme O^6-methylguanine DNA methyltransferase (O^6MGMT), which repairs the miscoding methylated base O^6-methylguanine. Many of these enzymes are polymorphic in the human population. Thus, the balance between metabolic activation, detoxification and repair varies among individuals and is likely to affect cancer risk {1570,1970}.

Carcinogens can damage DNA in specific ways depending upon their chemical nature {881}. TP53 mutations are more frequent in lung cancers of smokers than in non-smokers {1591,2058}. Studies of data compiled in the IARC TP53 mutation database (see www.iarc.fr) have shown that the pattern of TP53 mutations in lung cancers of smokers is unique, with an excess of transversions at G bases (G to T, 30%) that are uncommon in non-tobacco-related cancers (9%). In lung cancers of non-smokers, the overall prevalence of G to T transversions is 13%. In subjects with the highest reported exposure to tobacco, G to T transversions represent almost 50% of all mutations. These transversions preferentially occur at a limited number of codons (157, 158, 245, 248, 273) that have been experimentally identified as sites of adduction for metabolites of benzo(a)pyrene, one of the major PAH in tobacco smoke {477,1591}. Mutations at these codons can be found in histologically normal lung tissues adjacent to cancers in smokers, as well as in lung tissues of smokers without lung cancers {880}. This observation provides direct evidence that some tobacco compounds can act as carcinogens in lung cells. Comparisons between histological types reveal an excess of G to T transversions for all histological types in smokers, implying a general, causal effect of tobacco carcinogens {1591}. However, there are considerable differences in TP53 mutation patterns according to histological type and, significantly, gender. Interestingly, the vast majority of lung cancers with TP53 mutations in non-smokers are adenocarcinomas occurring in women {1588,2020}. Thus, the difference in G to T transversions between smokers and non-smokers is mainly due to female non-smokers having a low frequency of these transversions compared to female smokers.

Several other genes also show different rates of alterations in smokers and non-smokers. These genes include mutations in KRAS, that are more frequent in smokers (30%) than in non-smokers (5%), as well as hypermethylation of INK4 and FHIT genes {1236, 2017,2058, 2162}.

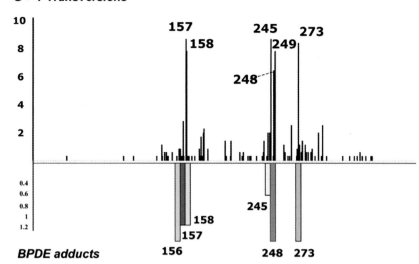

Fig. 1.06 Mutational hotspots for G to T transversions in lung cancers of smokers: concordance with positions of DNA adducts in the TP53 gene in primary bronchial cells exposed to benzo(a)pyrene in vitro. Codon numbers are indicated. Adapted from G.P. Pfeifer et al. {1591}.

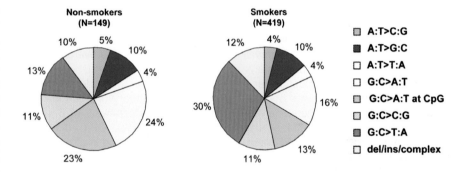

Fig. 1.07 Pattern of TP53 mutations in lung carcinomas. Note the high frequency of G:C>T:A mutations in tumours of smokers, probably due to benzo(a)pyrene or related tobacco carcinogens. Adapted from G.P. Pfeifer et al {1591}.

Impact of genetic studies on lung cancer therapy

Despite accumulating knowledge on the specificity of the genetic pathways leading to different histological types of lung cancers, there is still little understanding of how these events cooperate with each other in cancer progression. One of the main challenges remains the identification of events that are predictive of the rate of progression towards metastatic cancer. However, the identification of a limited number of genes that are often altered at early stages of lung cancers (such as methylation of INK4 or of genes on 3p, mutations in TP53 and in KRAS) represent an interesting opportunity for developing approaches for early detection, for example using material from bronchial lavages and expectorations {1322}. In the future, many of these alterations may provide interesting targets for designing new, alternative therapeutic strategies.

Genetic susceptibility

H. Bartsch
A. Haugen
A. Risch
P. Shields
P. Vineis

The risk of lung cancer in subjects with a family history of this tumour is about 2.5 {1781}. Given the strong link between exposure to carcinogens (mostly tobacco smoke) and lung cancer, the study of genetic polymorphisms as possible risk modifiers has focused on enzymes involved in Phase I/II-xenobiotic metabolism, DNA-repair and the effects on nicotine addiction.

Phase I

CYP1A1 bioactivates polycyclic aromatic hydrocarbons (PAH). Several variant alleles are known (http://www.imm.ki.se/CYPalleles/cyp1a1.htm). Two closely linked polymorphisms, MspI at 6235 nt and I462V, have been extensively studied in relation to lung cancer, yielding inconsistent results. In a pooled analysis an OR of 2.36 (95% confidence interval (CI) 1.16 - 4.81) for the MspI homozygous variant genotype in Caucasians was found {2086}. The OR was not significant for this variant in a meta-analysis including both Caucasians and Asians {870}. The frequencies of CYP1A1 allelic variants are substantially lower in Caucasians than in Asians and the functional significance has not been convincingly shown. PAH-exposed individuals with variant CYP1A1 alleles had higher levels of PAH-DNA adducts in WBC and lung tissue {37}, particularly in conjunction with GSTM1 null.

CYP1B1 present in lung, bioactivates many exogenous procarcinogens including PAH and also estrogens. There is polymorphic inducibility in lymphocytes {2004}. Five SNPs result in amino acid substitutions, of which 2 are located in the heme binding domain {1998}. Ser119 has been shown to be associated with SCC in Japanese {2111}. Ethnic variation in allelic frequency has been demonstrated.

CYP2D6 metabolizes clinically important drugs and also the tobacco specific nitrosamine, NNK (poor substrate). Among at least 40 SNPs and different allelic variants, many lead to altered CYP2D6 activity. The much-studied association between lung cancer and polymorphic expression of CYP2D6 has remained inconsistent: A meta-analysis reported a small decrease in lung cancer risk for the poor metaboliser phenotype, which the genotype analysis could not confirm {1696}.

CYP2A13, a highly polymorphic gene, is expressed in the human lung and efficiently bioactivates NNK. Among several variant alleles, only one SNP is located in the coding region, leading to an A257C amino acid change; the 257C variant was less active than the wild-type protein. Inter-ethnic differences in allelic variant frequencies have been found {2239A}. CYP2A6 is also important for the bioactivation of NNK. There are several polymorphisms for this gene, with some positive studies in Japanese {73} and Chinese {1968}, but overall the data are conflicting {1208,1642}.

The microsomal epoxide hydrolase (MEH3) may affect lung cancer risk based on pooled analysis of 8 studies (His/His OR = 0.70, CI = 0.51-0.96), which was not observed in a meta-analysis of the same studies {1154}. There are some positive studies for MEH4 {1303, 2175,2240}.

Phase II

Glutathione-S-transferases (GST) detoxify tobacco carcinogens such as PAH by conjugation. Individuals lacking GSTM1 (null polymorphism e.g. in 50% of Caucasians) appear to have a slightly elevated risk of lung cancer: A meta-analysis of 43 studies found an OR of 1.17 (CI 1.07 - 1.27) for the null genotype. When the original data from 21 case-control studies (9500 subjects) were analysed no evidence of increased lung cancer risk among null carriers, nor an interaction between GSTM1 genotype and smoking was found {144}. A base-substitution polymorphism in GSTM1 seems to affect squamous cell cancer risk in non-smokers {1228}. GSTM1 genotype affects internal carcinogen dose levels: DNA adduct levels were higher in lung tissue and white blood cells from GSTM1 null individuals exposed to PAH {37}. Because adduct levels are affected by a range of genetic polymorphisms {697} results from all GSTM1 studies were not consistent.

Among two GST-Pi polymorphisms studied, one in exon 6 has been associated with lung cancer risk {1891,2106}, although other studies did not {944, 1447}. Studies of environmental tobacco smoke further support a role of this polymorphism in lung cancer {1312}. Studies on a deletion polymorphism in GST-T1 are mostly negative {944,1447,1891} or contradictory for the "at-risk" allele {869}. A role for younger persons with lung cancer has been suggested {1943}.

N-Acetyltransferases (NAT) 1 and 2 with distinct but overlapping substrate specificities activate and/or detoxify aromatic amines. From 11 studies on lung cancer ORs, fast acetylation vs. slow NAT2 ranged from 0.5 – 3.0; most studies found no significant association, but in some, fast NAT2 acetylators were at increased risk {2243}. The NAT1*10 allele, (a putative fast allele) has inconsistently been associated with an increased risk for lung cancer.

Myeloperoxidase (MPO): 11 Lung cancer case-control studies have reported ORs from 0.54 - 1.39 for the G/A genotype, 0.20 - 1.34 for the A/A genotype and 0.58 - 1.27 for the (G/A + A/A) genotypes. A large study did not find the A-allele to be protective for lung cancer, while a meta-analysis (excluding this study) showed marginally significant inverse correlations of the A/A and/or G/A genotype prevalence and lung cancer risk {576}. Carriers of the A-allele had a significantly reduced capacity to bioactivate B(a)P into its epoxide in coal tar treated skin {1678}.

DNA repair genes

DNA repair genes are increasingly studied, for example PADPRP (193bp deletion), XPD (Codons 751, 312), AGT (Codons 143, 160), XRCC3 (Codon 241), and XRCC1 (codons 194, 280 or 399). As most study sizes were small, only a few were statistically significant, including an OR of 1.86 (CI 1.02 - 3.4) for XPD codon 312 (genotype AA) {260}, an OR of 1.8 (1.0 - 3.4) for XRCC1 codon 280 (AA+AG) {1641}, and an OR of 2.5 (1.1 - 5.8) for XRCC1 Codon 399 (AA) {500A}. In the latter study there was inconsistency among ethnic groups (Caucasians OR 3.3, 1.2 - 10.7; Hispanics OR 1.4, 0.3 - 5.9). In one study {744} a strong effect of PADPRP (193bp deletion) was observed only in African-Americans (OR 30.3, 1.7 - 547) and in Hispanics (OR 2.3, 1.22 - 4.4), but not in Caucasians (OR 0.5, 0.1 - 1.9); the biological plausibility is hard to assess {160, 161}.

hOGG1, which repairs oxidative DNA damage (8-oxo-dG) {1045} has been studied. Functional effects of the variants and a few positive lung cancer associations have been reported {914,1145, 1899}.

In the p53 gene there is a genetic polymorphism in codon 72, and several haplotypes are known. A functional effect by these variants has not been described, but an association with lung cancer risk was found {169,554,978,1193}. The risk was more elevated in persons, when combined with GSTM1 null {1193,2003} and GST Pi {1313} variants. Also, an interaction with CYP1A1 has been reported {978}.

Phenotypic DNA repair studies found consistently an increased risk of lung cancer associated with putative impaired repair functions {160,161}.

Smoking behaviour and addiction
Evidence for a genetic component for nicotine addiction (an obvious risk factor for lung cancer) comes from twin studies {291,805,806}. Most polymorphism studies have focused on dopamine neuronal pathways in the brain, including genes coding for dopamine receptors, dopamine transporter reuptake (SL6A3) and dopamine synthesis. Many of these polymorphic genes result in altered protein function, but the data for any specific candidate polymorphism are not consistent {396,1163-1166,1482,1715,1800, 1864}.

Combinations
The risk modifying effect of any one SNP may be more pronounced when it occurs in combination with other 'at risk' genotypes of biotransformation and repair enzymes implicated in pathways of a given carcinogen. The combined genotypes for CYPs and GSTs have shown an enhanced effect on lung cancer risk and an impact on intermediate end-points (e.g. DNA adduct level and mutations) {117,260}. Gene-gene interactions for a combination of GST polymorphisms {944,1006,1024,1891} are known and prospective studies confirmed the increased risk {1570}. An interaction for

p53 and GST genotypes {978,1193, 2003}, might be more important in younger persons {1313}.

Conclusions
Studies on genetic polymorphisms and lung cancer risk have identified a number of candidate genes involved in xenobiotic metabolism, DNA repair and possibly nicotine addiction. Certain variants of these genes and combinations thereof were shown to modify the risk of tobacco related lung cancer. Their influence varied by ethnicity, by histological lung tumour types, by exposure and by other host-/life-style factors. Due to this complexity, to date lung cancer risk cannot be predicted at an individual level.

Squamous cell carcinoma

S.P. Hammar
C. Brambilla
B. Pugatch
K. Geisinger
E.A. Fernandez
P. Vogt

N. Petrovitchev
Y. Matsuno
S. Aisner
R. Rami-Porta
V.L. Capelozzi
R. Schmidt

L. Carvalho
I. Petersen
A. Gazdar
M. Meyerson
S.M. Hanash
J. Jen
C.C. Harris

Definition

Squamous cell carcinoma (SCC) is a malignant epithelial tumour showing keratinization and/or intercellular bridges that arises from bronchial epithelium.

ICD-O code

Squamous cell carcinoma 8070/3
Papillary carcinoma   8052/3
Clear cell carcinoma   8084/3
Small cell carcinoma   8073/3
Basaloid carcinoma   8083/3

Synonym

Epidermoid carcinoma

Epidemiology - Etiology

Over 90% of squamous cell lung carcinomas occur in cigarette smokers {1860}. Arsenic is also strongly associated with squamous cell carcinoma and other causes are summarized in Table 1.

Sites of involvement

The majority of squamous cell lung carcinomas arise centrally in the mainstem, lobar or segmental bronchi {2007}.

Imaging

Radiography. In central SCC, lobar or entire lung collapse may occur, with shift of the mediastinum to the ipsilateral side {263,264,614,1676}. Central, segmental or subsegmental tumours can extend into regional lymph nodes and appear as hilar, perihilar or mediastinal masses with or without lobar collapse {264}. Peripheral tumours present as solitary pulmonary nodules (< 3 cm) or masses (> 3 cm). Squamous cell carcinoma is the most frequent cell type to cavitate giving rise to thick walled, irregular cavities with areas of central lucency on the chest film. When located in the superior sulcus of the lung, they are called Pancoast tumours and are frequently associated with destruction of posterior ribs and can cause Horner's syndrome. The chest radiograph may be normal in small tracheal or endobronchial tumours {1820}. Hilar opacities, atelectasis or peripheral masses may be associated with pleural effusions, mediastinal enlargement or hemidiaphragmatic elevation.

CT and spiral CT. The primary tumour and its central extent of disease is usually best demonstrated by CT scan {614}. Spiral CT may assess better the thoracic extension of the lesion, reveal small primary or secondary nodules invisible on chest radiograph, and exhibit lymphatic spread.

PET scan. This is now the method of choice to identify metastases (excluding brain metastases which may require MRI) {195,614,2061}. Bone metastases are typically osteolytic.

Cytology

The cytologic manifestations of squamous cell carcinoma depend on the degree of histologic differentiation and the type of sampling {673,936}. In a background of necrosis and cellular debris, large tumour cells display central, irregular hyperchromatic nuclei exhibiting one or more small nucleoli with an abundant cytoplasm. Tumour cells are usually isolated and may show bizarre shapes such as spindle-shaped and tadpole-shaped cells. They may appear in cohesive aggregates, usually in flat sheets with elongated or spindle nuclei. In well-differentiated squamous cell carcinoma keratinized cytoplasm appears robin's egg blue with the Romanowsky stains, whereas with the Papanicolaou stain, it is orange or yellow. In exfoliative samples, surface tumour cells predominate and present as individually dispersed cell with prominent cytoplasmic keratinization and dark pyknotic nuclei. In contrast, in brushings, cells from deeper layers are sampled, showing a much greater proportion of cohesive aggregates.

Macroscopy and localization

The tumours are usually white or grey and, depending on the severity of fibrosis, firm with focal carbon pigment deposits in the centre and star-like retractions on the periphery. The tumour may grow to a large size and may cavitate. Central tumours form intraluminal polypoid masses and / or infiltrate through the bronchial wall into the surrounding tis-

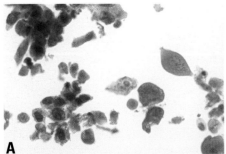
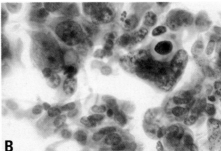
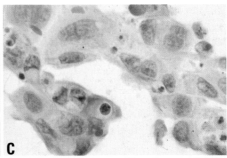

Fig. 1.08 Squamous cell carcinoma (SCC) cytology. **A** SCC with keratinization. Sheets of dysplastic and malignant cells. Isolated pleomorphic malignant cells with several squamous ghosts. Bronchial brushing. Papanicolaou stain. **B** SCC without keratinization. Clusters of malignant cells with variation in nuclear shape, distinct nuclear chromatin and high nuclear:cytoplasmic ratio. Bronchial brushing. Papanicolaou stain. **C** SCC without keratinization, fine needle aspiration cytology. Gaps between cells and distinct cell borders in this sheet of tumor cells identify the tumor as a squamous cell carcinoma. Papanicolaou stain.

sues and may occlude the bronchial lumen resulting in stasis of bronchial secretions, atelectasis, bronchial dilatation, obstructive lipoid pneumonia and infective bronchopneumonia. A minority of cases may arise in small peripheral airways. This may be changing since a recent study reported 53% of squamous cell carcinomas were found in the peripheral lung {640}.

Tumour spread and staging

Central squamous cell carcinoma is characterized by two major patterns of spread: intraepithelial (in situ) spread with or without subepithelial invasion, and endobronchial polypoid growth {391,1220}. Extensive intraepithelial spreading is common in major bronchi, and the epithelia of bronchial glands or ducts may often be involved. Two patterns of early invasive squamous cell carcinoma have been described: One grows laterally along the bronchial mucosa replacing surface epithelium, with submucosal microinvasion and involvement of the glandular ducts ("creeping type"); the other appears as small polypoid mucosal lesions with downward invasion ("penetrating type") {1424}. Direct involvement of hilar mediastinal tissue including lymph nodes may be encountered in advanced cases.

Peripheral squamous cell carcinoma characteristically forms a solid nodule, commonly with intrabronchiolar nodular growth, intraepithelial extension, or both {640}. In advanced cases, peripheral squamous cell carcinoma may involve the chest wall or diaphragm directly through the pleura.

Staging is usually performed according to the TNM system {738,2045}. In general, squamous cell carcinoma tends to be locally aggressive involving adjacent structures by direct contiguity. Metastases to distant organs is much less frequent than in adenocarcinoma or other histologic types of primary lung cancer {1629}. For peripheral tumours less than 2 cm in diameter, regional lymph node metastases are exceptional {77}. Tumours with poorly differentiated histology may metastasize early in their clinical course to organs such as the brain, liver, adrenals, lower gastrointestinal tract, and lymph nodes. Locoregional recurrence after surgical resection is more common in squamous cell carcinoma than in other cell types {276}.

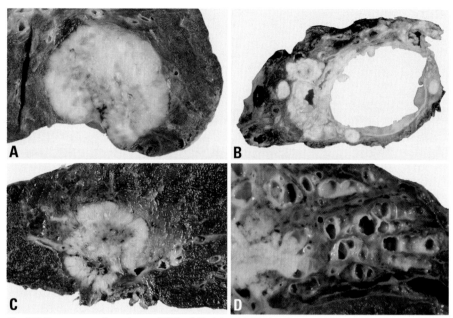

Fig. 1.09 Squamous cell carcinoma (SCC). **A** Peripheral SCC showing expansile growth, central necrosis and pleural puckering. **B** Marked cavitation of an SCC arising in an 18 year-old male with HPV11 infection and papillomatosis. **C** Central SCC arising in a lobar bronchus with bronchial and parenchymal invasion and central necrosis. **D** Central bronchogenic squamous carcinoma with extensive distal obstructive changes, including bronchiectasis.

Histopathology

Squamous cell carcinoma shows keratinization, pearl formation and/or intercellular bridges. These features vary with degree of differentiation, being prominent in well-differentiated tumours and focal in poorly differentiated tumours.

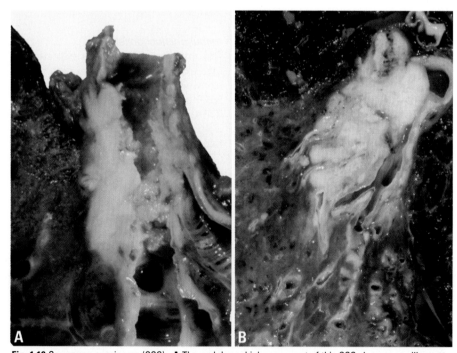

Fig. 1.10 Squamous carcinoma (SCC). **A** The endobronchial component of this SCC shows a papillary surface while the tumour has invaded through the bronchial wall superficially into the surrounding lung. Note the postobstructive bronchiectasis. **B** Central bronchogenic SCC arising in the proximal left lower lobe bronchus. Contiguous intralobar lymph node invasion, obstructive lipoid pneumonia and mucopurulent bronchiectasis in the basal segments.

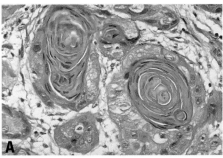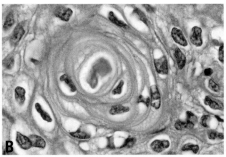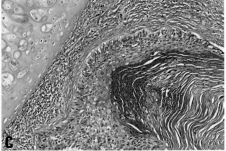

Fig. 1.11 Squamous cell carcinoma (SCC). **A** Invasion of fibrous stroma. Squamous cell differentiation is evident by the keratin pearls and prominent keratinization. Cytologic atypia with hyperchromatic nuclei indicates cytologic malignancy. **B** Squamous differentiation in these cytologically malignant cells, is manifest by the squamous pearl and distinct intercellular bridges. **C** The squamous differentiation reflected by layers of keratin. From Travis et al. {2024}.

Papillary variant of SCC. This may show exophytic and endobronchial growth in some proximal tumors. Sometimes there may be a very limited amount of intraepithelial spread without invasion; but invasion is seen in most cases {218,519}.

Clear cell variant of SCC is composed predominantly or almost entirely of cells with clear cytoplasm {634,971}. This variant requires separation from large cell carcinoma, adenocarcinoma of the lung with extensive clear cell change and metastatic clear cell carcinoma from kidney.

Small cell variant is a poorly differentiated squamous cell carcinoma with small tumour cells that retain morphologic characteristics of a non-small cell carcinoma and show focal squamous differentiation. This variant must be distinguished from combined small cell carcinoma in which there is a mixture of squamous cell carcinoma and true small cell carcinoma. The small cell variant lacks the characteristic nuclear features of small cell carcinoma having coarse or vesicular chromatin, more prominent nucleoli, more cytoplasm and more distinct cell borders. Focal intercellular bridges or keratinization may be seen {214,372,767,2024}.

Basaloid variant shows prominent peripheral palisading of nuclei. Poorly differentiated lung carcinomas with an extensive basaloid pattern but lacking squamous differentiation are regarded as the basaloid variant of large cell carcinoma {604,1892,2024}.

Alveolar space-filling type of peripheral SCC was recently described in which the tumor cells fill alveolar spaces without causing destruction of the alveolar framework; this contrasts with an expanding type which causes destruction of the alveolar framework and the lung architecture {640}. This type appears to comprised only approximately 5% of peripheral SCCs {640}. Rare non-keratinizing squamous cell carcinomas resemble a transitional cell carcinoma.

Electron microscopy
Squamous cell carcinomas show cytoplasmic intermediate keratin filaments, which frequently aggregate to form tonofilaments. The less well-differentiated carcinomas show few desmosomes and lesser amounts of cytoplasmic filaments.

Immunohistochemistry
The majority of squamous cell carcinomas express predominantly high molecular weight keratin (34ßE12), cytokeratins 5/6, and carcinoembryonic antigen (CEA). Many express low molecular weight keratin (35ßH11) and very few express thyroid transcription factor-1 (TTF-1) or cytokeratin 7 (CK7) {352,367, 634,1757}.

Differential diagnosis
Separation from large cell carcinoma is based on the presence of squamous differentiation. Focal intracellular mucin can be present. Even though invasive growth is not identified, papillary SCC can be diagnosed if there is sufficient cytologic atypia. Small biopsy specimens that show very well differentiated papillary squamous epithelium should be interpreted with caution since separation of a papillary squamous carcinoma from a papilloma can be difficult. The pattern of verrucous carcinoma is very rare in the lung and is included under papillary squamous carcinoma.

Massive involvement of the anterior mediastinal tissue can make differential diagnosis from thymic squamous cell carcinoma difficult and requires careful correlation with operative and radiologic findings. In the lung parenchyma, squamous cell carcinoma may entrap alveolar pneumocytes, which sometimes results in histological misinterpretation as adenosquamous carcinoma {391}. Squamous metaplasia with cytologic atypia in diffuse alveolar damage (DAD) may also raise concern for squamous carcinoma. The presence of overall features of DAD such as hyaline membranes, diffuse alveolar septal connective tissue proliferation with pneumocyte hyperplasia and bronchiolocentricity of the squamous changes would favor a metaplastic process.

Somatic genetics
Cytogenetics and CGH
Several differences have been found between lung squamous cell carcinomas and adenocarcinomas. Squamous cell carcinoma of the lung is either a near diploid or hyperdiploid-aneuploid neoplasm with mean chromosome numbers in the triploid range {104,1582}. Detection of aneuploidy by DNA measurement has been shown to be predictive for bad prognosis {1581}. Cytogenetics and CGH indicated a multitude of alterations with amplifications of the telomeric 3q region being most characteristic for the squamous carcinoma phenotype {1582}. Gain of 3q24-qter is present in the majority of squamopus cell carcinomas and in a minority of adenocarcinomas {104,176}. While the gene in the amplicon has not been identified with certainty, one candidate is the PIK3CA gene, which encodes the catalytic sub-

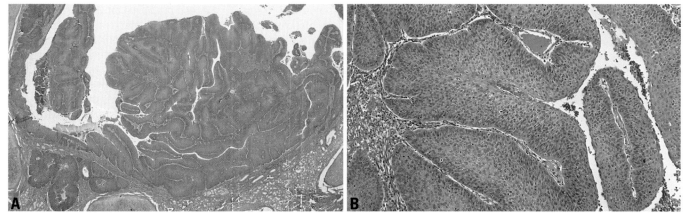

Fig. 1.12 A Exophytic, endobronchial SCC with papillary growth pattern. **B** Squamous cell carcinoma, papillary variant. The well-differentiated squamous carcinoma is growing in a papillary pattern. From Travis et al. {2024}.

unit of phosphatidylinositol-3 kinase, an essential component of many cell signaling pathways {104}. Deletions on the short arm of chromosome 3 are also frequent. Additional recurrent alterations are deletions on chromosomes 4q, 5q, 8p, 9p, 10q, 11p, 13q, 17p, 18q and 21q along with overrepresentations of chromosomes 5p, 8q, 11q13 and 12p {104, 125,898,1301,1330,1582}. The number of chromosomal imbalances accumulates during progression {370,1584}. Small interstitial deletions have a tendency to increase in size resulting into a deletion pattern similar to small cell carcinoma. In contrast, overrepresentations of entire chromosome arms may condense into smaller amplicons. Specific alterations, in particular deletions of 3p12-p14, 4p15-p16, 8p22-p23, 10q, 21q and overrepresentation of 1q21-q25, 8q11-q25 have been associated with the metastatic phenotype {1584}.

Molecular genetics

Squamous cell carcinoma commonly shows distinct molecular genetic characteristics. ErbB (EGFR, HER2/neu, KRAS) pathway abnormalities are common in non-small cell carcinoma but absent in SCLC. An average of 84% of squamous cell carcinomas are EGFR positive {608}. Lung cancers with detectable levels of epidermal growth factor receptor protein are significantly more frequent among squamous cell carcinomas than among other types of lung tumour {152}. HER2/neu expression, while relatively frequent in adenocarcinoma, is relatively rare in squamous cell carcinoma {845}. While activating mutations of the KRAS gene are frequent (~30%) in adenocarcinoma, they are rare in squamous cell carcinoma.

Disruption of normal p53 gene function, usually by point mutations, is frequent in all types of lung cancers. Mutations, while more frequent in SCLC, occur in the majority of NSCLC tumours including squamous cell carcinomas.

Disruption of the RB gene pathway is universal in lung cancers {981}. While mutations of the RB gene are the usual method of disruption in SCLC, they are rare in NSCLC. In NSCLC the mechanism of disruption is via the upstream pathway. In particular, inactivation of p16Ink4 as demonstrated by immunohistochemistry, occurs via epigenetic or genetic mechanisms (homozygous deletions, mutations, methylation), while cyclin D1 and E are overexpressed {215}.

Most squamous cell carcinomas demonstrate large 3p segments of allelic loss, whereas most adenocarcinomas and pre-neoplastic/preinvasive lesions have smaller chromosome areas of 3p allele loss {2158} One well studied gene is FHIT (fragile histidine triad) at chromosome 3p14.2, by deletions or by a combination

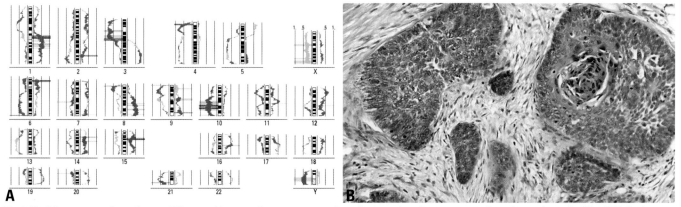

Fig. 1.13 A Squamous cell carcinoma. Difference histogram between metastatic and non-metastatic squamous cell carcinoma determined by CGH. Each tumor group consist of 25 cases. The chromosomal imbalances determined by CGH are shown as incidence curves along each ideogram. Left side loss, right side gains {1584}. **B** Squamous cell carcinoma, basaloid variant. The nests of tumour cells have prominent peripheral palisading of cells with less cytoplasm and more hyperchromatic nuclei than the tumour cells situated more centrally that have more abundant cytoplasm and prominent keratinization. From Travis et al. {2024}.

of deletion and promoter region methylation {1855}. The status of another gene located at 3p21.3, the RASSF1A gene, while more frequently inactivated in SCLC, does not demonstrate differences in the methylation frequencies between NSCLC types {238}.

Epigenetic gene silencing

The major mechanism is methylation, although histone deacetylation plays an important co-operative role. Most silenced genes are known or suspected tumour suppressor genes. The methylation profile varies with the tumour type and the methylation rates of APC, CDH13 and RAR-beta are significantly higher in adenocarcinomas than in squamous cell carcinomas {2017}.

Gene expression profiles

Squamous cell lung carcinoma is characterized by high-level expression of keratin genes and histologic evidence of keratinization. Markers of squamous cell lung carcinoma have been analyzed using oligonucleotide and cDNA microarray hybridisation {163,661} and serial analysis of gene expression or SAGE {623,1420}. When results are compared across experimental platforms, significant overlap can be seen. Genes for keratin 5, 6, 13, 14, 16, 17, and 19 are prominent among the gene expression markers for squamous cell lung carcinoma. Other genes found as squamous cell lung carcinoma markers in more than one data set include collagen VII alpha 1, galectin 7, the ataxia-telangiectasia group D-associated protein, the s100 calcium binding protein A2, and bullous pemphigoid antigen 1. In addition, squamous cell lung carcinomas are characterized by over-expression of the p53-related gene p63. Using gene expression profile generated by SAGE, a transcriptome map integrating the gene expression profile along each arm of the human chromosomes has been generated {623}. This transcriptome map revealed known chromosome regions and a novel locus with significantly altered gene expression patterns in squamous cell carcinoma. The identification of these molecular changes may provide potential markers for lung cancer.

Prognosis and predictive factors

Stage for stage, survival rate for squamous cell carcinoma is significantly better than for adenocarcinoma. Approximately 80% of patients with resected stage 1 (T1 N0 M0) squamous cell carcinoma are alive at five years after diagnosis compared to approximately 70% of similarly staged adenocarcinomas. Similar differences are seen in the rate of survival between stage 2 squamous cell carcinoma and stage 2 adenocarcinoma. Histologic factors important in prognosis are difficult to determine, although neoplasms that exhibit a great deal of necrosis are thought to be associated with a worse prognosis than those neoplasm that do not show necrosis.

Clinical criteria

Although clinical staging generally underestimates the extent of the lesions, the cTNM classification represents the main prognostic factor with clear-cut survival difference between the surgical cases and the rest (70% of the patients). In non-surgical cases weight loss, poor performance status and metastasis-related symptoms convey an adverse prognosis. In resectable tumours, advanced age is a cause of increased post operative morbidity. The female gender is a favourable factor in overall lung cancer survival, but it is mainly clinically significant in adenocarcinoma and less in squamous cancer. Race is not a prognosis factor when it can be separated from socio-economic factors which affect the outcome. Many biological tests have been published, such as elevation of Lactate Dehydrogenase (LDH) or serum tumour markers, but they are not independent prognostic factors of cTNM and/or weight loss in most cases.

Histopathological criteria

Currently, the stage of disease and the performance status at diagnosis remain the most powerful prognostic indicators for survival for primary squamous cell carcinoma. Nevertheless, histologic subtyping carries independent prognostic information. For example, well-differentiated squamous cell carcinoma tends to spread locally within the chest directly involving adjacent mediastinal structures. Poorly differentiated squamous cell carcinoma tends to metastasize early and to distant sites. The alveolar space-filling pattern of peripheral squamous cell carcinoma appears to carry a more favourable prognosis {641}

Genetic predictive factors

Prognostic biomarkers of nonsmall cell lung carcinoma (NSCLC) have been identified, but not ultimately confirmed, including the diminished expression of cyclin-dependent kinase inhibitors, e.g., p16INK4A, p21WAF1, and p27KIP1, the overexpression of cyclins, e.g., cyclin E, members of growth factor signal transduction pathways, e.g., HER2 and insulin-like growth factor-binding protein-3, and the inactivation of tumour suppressor genes, e.g., Rb, and FHIT, and p53 {146,251,279,332,348,836,875,1007, 1327,1406,1432,1817,1856,2012}. P53 inactivation is not of prognostic significance in squamous cell carcinoma {1331}. Epigenetic mechanisms such as DNA methylation transcriptional silencing of p16INK4A and genetic mutations of p53 are examples of the different molecular mechanisms responsible for their inactivation. p53 and FHIT mutations and epigenetic transcriptional silencing of p16INK4A are more frequent in squamous cell carcinomas compared to adenocarcinomas and in smokers compared to never smokers {1007,1856,2012}. Because most studies have examined a relatively small number of NSCLC, they have limited statistical power to compare squamous cell carcinoma with the other histological types. One strategy has been to perform a meta-analysis of multiple reports. For example, a meta-analysis of 43 articles revealed that p53 mutations and/or accumulation predicted poor prognosis of patients with adenocarcinoma, but not squamous cell carcinoma {1331}. Loss of Rb predicts poor survival of patients with squamous cell carcinoma or adenocarcinoma {279}, whereas the nuclear localization of the transcription factor YB-1 is a prognostic factor only for squamous cell carcinoma {1799}.

Small cell carcinoma

W. Travis
S. Nicholson
F.R. Hirsch
B. Pugatch
K. Geisinger
E. Brambilla
A. Gazdar

I. Petersen
M. Meyerson
S.M. Hanash
J. Jen
T. Takahashi
E.A. Fernandez
F. Capron

Definitions

Small cell carcinoma of the lung (SCLC)
A malignant epithelial tumour consisting of small cells with scant cytoplasm, ill-defined cell borders, finely granular nuclear chromatin, and absent or inconspicuous nucleoli. The cells are round, oval and spindle-shaped. Nuclear molding is prominent. Necrosis is typically extensive and the mitotic count is high.

Combined small cell carcinoma
Small cell carcinoma combined with an additional component that consists of any of the histologic types of non-small cell carcinoma, usually adenocarcinoma, squamous cell carcinoma or large cell carcinoma but less commonly spindle cell or giant cell carcinoma.

ICD-O code

Small cell carcinoma   8041/3
Combined small cell
carcinoma   8045/3

Synonyms

Previous classifications used terms such as oat cell carcinoma, small cell anaplastic carcinoma, undifferentiated small cell carcinoma, intermediate cell type, and mixed small cell/large cell carcinoma but these are no longer recognised.

Clinical features

Signs and symptoms
Symptoms reflect central location and locoregional spread, although stridor and haemoptysis are comparatively rare while hoarsness and vocal cord paralysis are more common, when compared to locoregional spread of squamous cell carcinoma. However, clinical symptoms more often reflect disseminated disease (e.g bone marrow and liver metastases). At the time of primary diagnosis, brain metastases are diagnosed in a minority of patients, but tend to develop during the course of disease {568,933,1797}. Paraneoplastic syndromes are also common in association with small cell carcinoma.

Imaging
Small cell carcinomas appear as hilar or perihilar masses often with mediastinal lymphadenopathy and lobar collapse {263,614}. Often, the primary tumour is

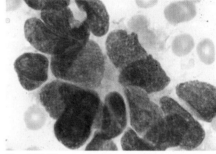

Fig. 1.15 Cluster of cells with scant cytoplasm, nuclear molding and finely granular chromatin. Absence of nucleoli. Incipient rosette formation.

not detected on radiographic studies. CT depicts mediastinal nodal involvement and superior vena caval obstruction with greater detail than the chest radiograph. Peripheral small cell carcinomas are radiographically indistinguishable from other pulmonary neoplasms.

Cytology
Cytologic specimens show loose and irregular or syncytial clusters, as well as individual tumour cells frequently arranged in a linear pattern {673, 936,2231}. Within cohesive aggregates, nuclear moulding is well developed. Mitoses are easily seen. Each neoplastic cell has a high nuclear/cytoplasmic ratio with an ovoid to irregular nuclear contour. Well-preserved cells feature finely granular and uniformly distributed chromatin, yielding the classic "salt and pepper" quality, while poorly preserved cells have a very dark blue structureless chromatin. Conspicuous nucleoli are absent or rare {1410,2099,2231}. Due to the fragility of the malignant nuclei, chromatin streaks are commonly seen in smears of all types, but especially in aspiration biopsies and brushings. In addition, the smear background often contains apoptotic bodies and granular necrotic debris.

Macroscopy and localization
Tumours are typically white-tan, soft, friable perihilar masses that show extensive necrosis and frequent nodal involve-

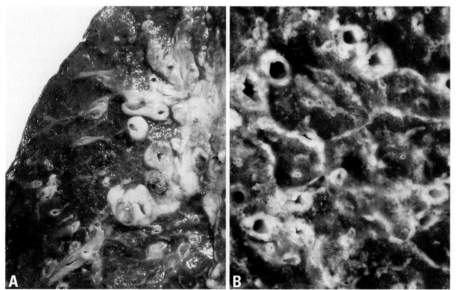

Fig. 1.14 Small cell carcinoma. **A** Central tumor extending toward the lung periphery in a sheath-like fashion around bronchovascular bundles. **B** Small cell carcinoma spreading along peribronchial lymphatics and interlobular septa.

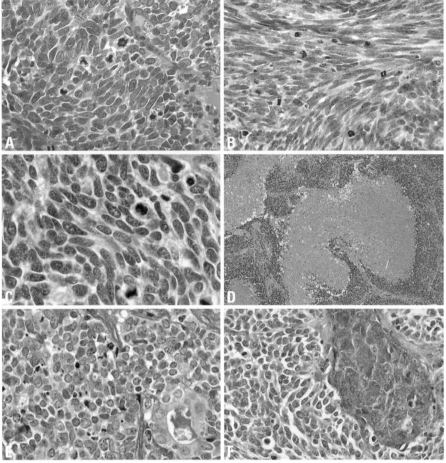

Fig. 1.16 Small cell carcinoma. **A** Tumour cells are densely packed, small, with scant cytoplasm, finely granular nuclear chromatin and absence of nucleoli. Mitoses are frequent. **B** The fusiform (spindle cell) shape is a prominent feature. The nuclear chromatin is finely granular and nucleoli are absent. **C** In this example, cells are somewhat larger and show some cytoplasm as well as a few inconspicuous nucleoli. **D** Small cell carcinoma with extensive necrosis. **E** Combined small cell carcinoma and adenocarcinoma. A malignant gland is present within the small cell carcinoma. **F** Combined small cell and large cell carcinoma. The large cell component has more cytoplasm and prominent nucleoli.

ment. Within the lung the tumour typically spreads along bronchi in a submucosal and circumferential fashion, often involving lymphatics. Approximately 5% of SCLC present as peripheral coin lesions {427}.

Tumour spread and staging
The tendency for widespread dissemination at presentation has led to small cell carcinoma being staged as limited versus extensive disease rather than using the TNM system {1871}.

Histopathology (including variants)
Architectural patterns include nesting, trabeculae, peripheral palisading, and rosette formation as shared by other neuroendocrine tumours. Sheet-like growth without these neuroendocrine morphologic patterns is common. Tumour cells are usually less than the size of three small resting lymphocytes and have round, ovoid or spindled nuclei and scant cytoplasm. Nuclear chromatin is finely granular and nucleoli are absent or inconspicuous. Cell borders are rarely seen and nuclear moulding is common. There is a high mitotic rate, averaging over 60 mitoses per 2mm². The tumour is by definition high grade, thus grading is inappropriate. No in-situ phase is recognized. In larger specimens, the cell size may be larger and scattered pleomorphic, giant tumour cells, dispersement of nuclear chromatin prominent nucleoli, extensive necrosis, brisk apoptotic activity, and crush artifact with encrustation of basophilic nuclear DNA around blood vessels (Azzopardi effect) may all be seen {1470,2024}.
The combined small cell carcinoma variant refers to the admixture of non-small cell carcinoma elements including squamous cell, adeno- and large cell carcinoma and less commonly spindle cell or giant cell carcinoma. For combined small cell and large cell carcinoma there should be at least 10% large cells present {1470}.

Immunohistochemistry
While small cell carcinoma is a light microscopic diagnosis, electron microscopy shows neuroendocrine granules approximately 100 nm in diameter in at least two-thirds of cases and immunohistochemistry is positive for CD56, chromogranin and synaptophysin in most cases {1470}. Less than 10% of SCLC are negative for all neuroendocrime markers {750}. Small cell carcinoma is also positive for TTF-1 in up to 90% of cases {600,975}.

Differential diagnosis 10314
The differential diagnosis includes lymphoid infiltrates, other neuroendocrine tumours, other "small round blue cell tumours" (SRBCT), and primary or metastatic non-small cell carcinomas. Crush artifact can occur not only with small cell carcinomas, but also carcinoids, lymphocytes of inflammation or

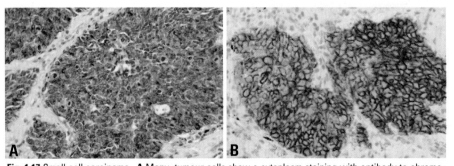

Fig. 1.17 Small cell carcinoma. **A** Many tumour cells show a cytoplasm staining with antibody to chromogranin. **B** CD56 immunoreactivity with a membranous staining pattern.

lymphomas and poorly differentiated non-small cell carcinomas. In crushed specimens some preserved tumour cells must be seen for a SCLC diagnosis. Immunohistochemical staining for cytokeratin vs leukocyte common antigen as well as neuroendocrine markers and TTF-1 may be helpful. Carcinoid tumours, typical and atypical, do not show the degree of necrosis, mitotic and apoptotic activity of small cell carcinomas {1470,2024}. Other SRBCTs including primitive neuroectodermal tumours (PNET) are less mitotically active than SCLC but also mark for MIC-2 (CD99) and not for cytokeratin or TTF-1 {765, 1214}. Positive staining for Cytokeratin 20, but not for Cytokeratin 7 or TTF-1 distinguishes Merkel cell carcinoma from SCLC {326,351}.

Morphologic separation of SCLC from NSCLC can be difficult {846,1240,1470, 2024,2089}. Examination of a good quality H&E stained section of well-fixed tissue is essential. The distinction does not rest on a single feature but incorporates cell size, nuclear: cytoplasmic ratio, nuclear chromatin, nucleoli, and nuclear molding. Corresponding cytology specimens may show much better-preserved tumour cell morphology.

Histogenesis

While the precise cell of origin is not known for SCLC, there is likely to be a pluripotent bronchial precursor cell that can differentiate into each of the major histologic types of lung cancer. However, within the spectrum of neuroendocrine tumours, there is closer morphologic and genetic similarity between large cell neuroendocrine carcinoma and small cell carcinoma than either typical or atypical carcinoid.

Somatic genetics

Cytogenetics and CGH

SCLCs are invariably aneuploid neoplasms although DNA cytometry frequently suggests a near diploid chromosome content. Cytogenetics and CGH revealed a characteristic pattern of chromosomal imbalances with a high incidence of deletions on chromosomes 3p, 4, 5q, 10q, 13q and 17p along with DNA gains on 3q, 5p, 6p, 8q, 17q, 19 and 20q {104}. Chromosome 3p deletions are present in nearly 100% of cases and are often associated with a 3q isochromosome formation. Amplification of chromo-

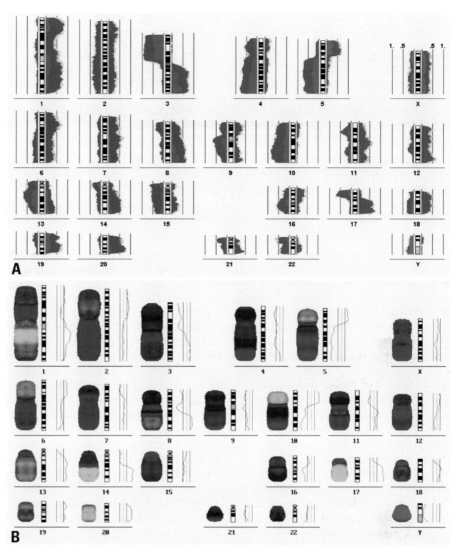

Fig. 1.18 Small cell carcinoma. Comparative genomic hybridization (CGH). **A** Chromosomal imbalances are shown as incidence curves along each chromosome. Areas on the left side of the chromosome ideogram correspond to loss of genetic material, those on the right side to DNA gains. **B** CGH analysis of the primary tumour (C) and the metastasis (D) reveals a clonal relationship as evidenced by the high number of common changes. Red, DNA losses. Green, DNA gains.

somal subregions occurs particularly during tumour progression and in pretreated patients. DNA gain of chromosome 17q24-q25 is a potential marker for brain metastasis formation {1583}.

Molecular genetic alterations

SCLC and pulmonary carcinoids are classic neuroendocrine (NE) tumours and they reflect all of the characteristic features of NE cells. However while SCLC is highly associated with smoking, carcinoids are not. While these two NE tumours share certain molecular abnormalities {269,727,1516}, there are also differences. SCLC tumours have a higher rate of p53 mutations {1516} while car-

cinoids are characterized by mutations in the menin gene {463}. There are similarities and differences in the genetic profiles of SCLC and NSCLC {269,727, 2244}. Most of these differences are relative. The absolute differences between these two major divisions of lung cancer are relatively few and include the presence of Ras gene mutations {1668} and Cox-2 {827,1248} over expression in NSCLC, while amplification of MYC {931} and methylation of caspase-8 {1814}, a key antiapoptotic gene, are characteristic of SCLC. While loss of cell cycle controls is a hallmark of cancers, the mechanism by which the two major types of lung cancer achieve this aim are very dif-

Table 1.10
Limited versus extensive staging system for small cell lung cancer (SCLC) {1796}.

Limited stage SCLC
> Patients with disease restricted to one hemithorax with regional lymph node metastases, including hilar, ipsi-, and contralateral mediastinal, or supraclavicular nodes. > Patients with contralateral mediastinal lymph nodes and supraclavicular lymph nodes since the prognosis is somewhat better than that of distant metastatic sites. > Patients with ipsilateral pleural effusion (benign or malignant)
Extensive stage disease
> All patients with disease who cannot be included in the limited stage.

ferent. Inactivation of the retinoblastoma (RB) gene and overexpression of E2F1 are almost universal in SCLC {549,981}. SCLC but rarely NSCLC, show more frequent inactivation of the 14-3-3 sigma and p14arf, two important G2 checkpoint genes {551,1471,1520}.

Most small cell lung carcinomas and squamous cell carcinomas demonstrate large 3p segments of allele loss, whereas most of the adenocarcinomas and preneoplastic/preinvasive lesions have smaller chromosome areas of 3p allele loss {2158}. Because these regions are gene rich, and the genes seldom demonstrate mutations, identification of the TSGs took nearly two decades. Putative TSGs have been identified at four widely separated regions, 3p12-13 (ROBO1/DUTT1), 3p14.2 (FHIT), 3p21.3 (multiple genes including RASSF1A, FUS1, HYAL2, BAP1, Sema3B, Sema3F, and beta-catenin at 3p21.3), and 3p24-6 (VHL and RAR-beta) {2228}. Of these, the FHIT, RASSF1A and RAR-beta genes are the best studied.

Mutations of the p53 gene are the most frequent genetic abnormality identified in human cancers, and are more common in SCLC than in NSCLC. Mutations are the most common mechanism of deregulation of gene activity. The frequency, type, and pattern of mutations in lung cancer are strongly related to cigarette smoking, with G to T transversions being more common in smokers (especially women) than in never smokers {1666}.

Multiple other changes occur frequently in SCLC, including upregulation of the proapoptotic molecule Bcl-2, activation of autocrine loops (bombesin like peptides, c-kit/stem cell factor), upregulation of telomerase, loss of laminin 5 chains and inhibitors of matrix matalloproteinases, and expression of vascular growth factors. In contrast to inactivation of TSGs (most often by epigenetic phenomena, especially methylation), the genes involved at sites of chromosomal gains have seldom been identified (with the exception of the MYC family). SCLC specific preneoplastic changes have not been identified and little is known about the molecular changes preceeding this tumour, although frequent allelic losses have been identified in histologically nor-

mal or hyperplastic bronchial epithelium adjacent to invasive tumours {2160}.

Gene expression profiles
Gene expression analysis can readily identify markers for small cell lung carcinoma. Given the histological and immunohistochemical features of neuroendocrine differentiation, it is not surprising that many of the gene expression markers are neuroendocrine genes including chromogranin B, chromogranin C, and l-aromatic amino acid decarboxylase. Experimental studies of gene expression in SCLC include analysis of primary tumours by oligonucleotide arrays {163}, analysis of primary tumours with cDNA arrays {661}, and analysis of cell lines with oligonucleotide arrays {1901}. Strikingly, the three studies identify sets of overlapping genes. All three studies identified insulinoma-associated gene 1 (IA-1) and the human achaete-scute homolog 1 (hASH1) as SCLC markers. Two of the three studies identified forkhead box g1b (FOXG1B), the Isl1 transcription factor, thymosin beta, and tripartite motif-containing 9.

Prognosis and predictive factors
Adverse clinical prognostic factors include 'extensive' stage of disease, poor performance status, elevated serum LDH or alkaline phosphatase, low plasma albumin and low plasma sodium levels {1523,1849}. No histologic or genetic factors are predictive of prognosis {1470}. A small percentage of low stage tumours may be successfully resected.

Adenocarcinoma

T.V. Colby
M. Noguchi
C. Henschke
M.F. Vazquez
K. Geisinger
T. Yokose

P. Ohori
R. Rami-Porta
T. Franks
Y. Shimosato
Y. Matsuno
A. Khoor
W.H. Westra

N.A. Jambhekar
I. Petersen
T. Takahashi
T. Kawai
M. Meyerson
S.M. Hanash
J. Jen

Definition

A malignant epithelial tumour with glandular differentiation or mucin production, showing acinar, papillary, bronchioloalveolar or solid with mucin growth patterns or a mixture of these patterns.

ICD-O codes

Adenocarcinoma	8140/3
Adenocarcinoma mixed subtype	8255/3
Acinar adenocarcinoma	8550/3
Papillary adenocarcinoma	8260/3
Bronchioloalveolar carcinoma	8250/3
Nonmucinous	8252/3
Mucinous	8253/3
Mixed nonmucinous and mucinous or indeterminate	8254/3
Solid adenocarcinoma with mucin production	8230/3

Variants

Fetal adenocarcinoma	8333/3
Mucinous ("colloid") carcinoma	8480/3
Mucinous cystadenocarcinoma	8470/3
Signet ring adenocarcinoma	8490/3
Clear cell adenocarcinoma	8310/3

Epidemiology

Adenocarcinoma has surpassed squamous carcinoma as the most common histologic subtype of lung cancer in many countries {391}. Although most cases are seen in smokers, it develops more frequently than any other histologic type of lung cancer in individuals (particularly women) who have never smoked {391,1002}.

Imaging

Compared to other lung cancers, adenocarcinomas are most frequently peripheral nodules under 4.0 cm in size {391, 614}. They infrequently present in a central location as a hilar or perihilar mass and only rarely show cavitation. Pleura and chest wall involvement is seen in approximately 15% of cases and this is more frequent than with other forms of lung cancer. Hilar adenopathy is less frequent with adenocarcinoma than with other forms of lung cancer.

Adenocarcinomas account for the majority of small peripheral cancers identified radiologically. By CT screening, adenocarcinoma is often distinct from the other histologic subtypes of lung cancer. Solid nodules (solid-density), ground glass opacities (non-solid, air-containing) and mixed solid/ground glass (part solid, subsolid) opacities are all recognized patterns of adenocarcinoma {817,1050, 1425,1952}.

Increased use of CT has lead to increased identification of small peripheral nodules, many of which prove to be adenocarcinomas. The larger the proportion of solid compared to ground glass component in a lung adenocarcinoma, the greater the likelihood of invasive growth and a less favorable outcome.

Cytology

Diagnosis of adenocarcinoma by cytology is based on a combination of individual cell cytomorphology and architectural features of cell clusters {673, 936,1826}. Adenocarcinoma cells may be single or arranged in three-dimensional morulae, acini, pseudopapillae, true papillae with fibrovascular cores and/or sheets of cells. Borders of cell clusters are typically sharply delineated. Cytoplasm varies in volume but is usually relatively abundant. It is typically cyanophilic and more translucent in comparison with squamous cell carcinoma. In most cells the cytoplasm is distinctly homogeneous or granular and in others is foamy due to abundant small indistinct vacuoles. A single large mucin-filled vacuole may be prominent and, in some cases, distends the cytoplasm and compresses the nucleus to one margin, forming a so-called signet-ring cell.

Nuclei are usually single, eccentric and round to oval with relatively smooth contours and minimal nuclear irregularity. Chromatin tends to be finely granular and evenly dispersed in better-differentiated tumours and coarse and irregularly distributed or hyperchromatic in poorly differentiated tumours. In most tumours,

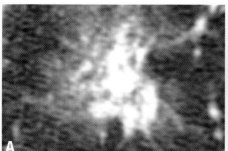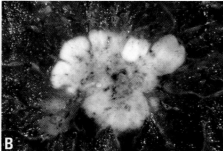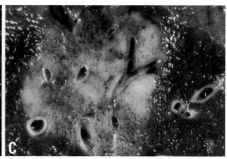

Fig. 1.19 A. Bronchioloalveolar carcinoma. High-resolution CT of a part-solid nodule in the right upper lobe in a 71 year-old women. Solid components are centrally located, surrounded by non-solid component. **B** Adenocarcinoma. This peripheral tumor consists of a lobulated white mass with central anthracosis and scarring. At the periphery there is a yellow area of bronchioloalveolar carcinoma with preservation of airspaces. **C** Adenocarcinoma. A predominantly bronchioloalveolar pattern prevailed histologically (alveolar spaces can just be seen on the tumour cut surface); the white and solid foci showed invasive disease.

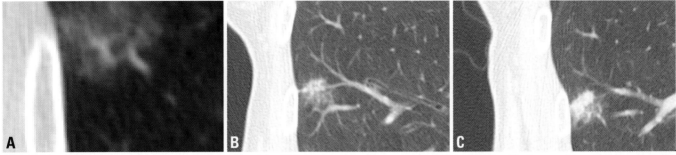

Fig. 1.20 Adenocarcinoma of mixed subtypes in a nonsolid nodule which developed a solid component. **A** High-resolution CT of a nonsolid nodule in the right middle lobe in a 76 year-old woman. **B** High resolution CT four years later shows the development of a solid component without any increase in the overall size of the nodule. **C** One year later the solid component has increased.

nucleoli are prominent and characteristically they are single, macronucleoli, varying from smooth and round to irregular.

Cytologic pleomorphism reflects histologic grade and has recently been reported to be related, in part, to tumour size. Morishita et al {1388} concluded that cells from BAC less than 2 cm in diameter are relatively small and round to ovoid when compared with other small-sized adenocarcinomas (invasive adenocarcinoma).

Although certain cytologic features have been proposed to favor a diagnosis of BAC over other adenocarcinoma patterns {1218,1607}, the diagnosis of BAC requires thorough histologic evaluation to exclude the presence of invasive growth. Mucinous BAC may be suggested based on the cytologic features in the appropriate radiologic setting. BAC cells in washings and bronchoalveolar lavage tend to be homogeneous with uniform, round, smooth, pale nuclei and inconspicuous nucleoli. BAC often shows clusters of uniform cells that display a three-dimensional "depth of focus", especially with the

mucinous type, presumably due to their abundant cytoplasm. Tissue fragments in aspiration specimens may show histologic features such as growth along intact alveolar septal surfaces {1218}, but this does not exclude an unsampled invasive component. On occasion, individual BAC cells resembling alveolar macrophages are dispersed in a smear but can be recognized because nuclei are rounder and larger than macrophage nuclei and a few cohesive clusters are usually present.

Currently, there are no established criteria for diagnosing AAH on cytology and to distinguish it from nonmucinous BAC. Anecdotally there is apparent overlap of the cytologic features. The Early Lung Cancer Action Project (ELCAP) has a cytology protocol, which includes a category of lesions designated "atypical bronchioloalveolar cell proliferation" when the findings are suspicious for, but not diagnostic of BAC {817,818}. The designation applies to lesions, which, when resected, may prove to be either atypical adenomatous hyperplasia (AAH) or BAC.

Macroscopy and localization

Pulmonary adenocarcinomas may be single or multiple and have a wide range in size. The vast majority of pulmonary adenocarcinomas present with one of six macroscopic patterns and these all have corresponding radiologic correlates. Combinations of these patterns may also occur.

The most common pattern is a peripheral tumour {1809}. Gray-white central fibrosis with pleural puckering may be apparent. The central area underlying pleural puckering is often a V-shaped area of desmoplastic fibrosis associated with anthracotic pigmentation. Invasion, when present histologically, is identified in areas of fibrosis and may be accompanied by necrosis, cavitation, and hemorrhage. The edges of the tumour may be lobulated or ill defined with stellate borders. In small tumours with a contiguous nonmucinous BAC pattern some alveolar structure may be grossly apparent at the edge of the solid portion of the nodule corresponding to the ground glass opacity noted radiologically in these lesions. Some peripheral adeno-

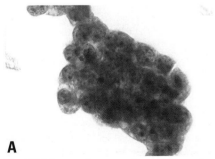
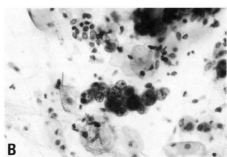
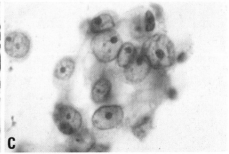

Fig. 1.21 Adenocarcinoma cytology. **A** Three-dimensional, large cluster of uniform malignant cells with distinct nuclear structure, nucleoli and finely vacuolated cytoplasm. Bronchial brushing. Liquid Based Cytology. Papanicolaou stain. **B** Cohesive three-dimensional cluster with papillary pattern. Fine needle aspiration, conventional cytology. Papanicolaou stain. **C** This cluster of malignant cells lacks definite cytoplasmic borders but shows vacuolization. Pale nuclei have small but distinct nucleoli. Fine needle aspiration, conventional cytology. Papanicolaou stain.

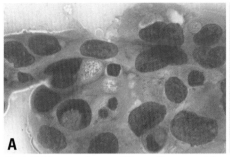 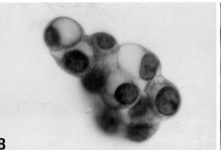 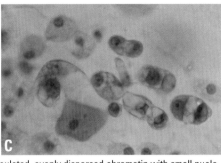

Fig. 1.22 Adenocarcinoma. **A** The malignant nuclei are ovoid with delicate smooth membranes and finely reticulated, evenly dispersed chromatin with small nucleoli and a single large nuclear pseudoinclusion. Cytoplasm is delicate and contains secretory vacuoles some of which contain mucin. Diff-Quik. **B** A cluster of tumor cells is present in this sputum sample from a patient with a bronchioloalveolar carcinoma cells, mucinous type. The cells have relatively small bland nuclei with smooth outlines, fine even chromatin, and inconspicuous nucleoli. The nuclear-to-cytoplasmic ratios are low as cytoplasmic mucin vacuoles occupy most of the cellular volume. Papanicolaou stain. **C** This bronchial washing demonstrates the alveolar macrophage pattern of bronchiolalveolar carcinoma. Neoplastic cells are individually dispersed. They have relatively low nuclear-to-cytoplasmic ratios and delicate, vacuolated cytoplasm. However, compared to the adjacent macrophages, the nuclei are larger and hyperchromatic. Papanicolaou stain.

carcinomas may have a gelatinous quality due to abundant mucin production.

A second pattern of adenocarcinoma is a central or endobronchial tumour {1042}. The neoplasm may grow as a plaque or in polypoid fashion with preservation of the overlying mucosa. With increasing degrees of bronchial luminal obstruction, the distal parenchyma may show obstructive "golden" (lipoid) pneumonia. The third pattern is a diffuse pneumonia-like, lobar consolidation with preservation of underlying architecture, typical of mucinous BAC.

A fourth pattern consists of diffuse bilateral lung disease. In some cases this manifests as widespread nodules (varying from tiny to large) involving all lobes; in other cases the appearance suggests an interstitial pneumonia due to widespread lymphangitic spread of carcinoma.

In the fifth pattern, the tumour preferentially invades and extensively disseminates along the visceral pleura, resulting in a rind-like thickening mimicking malignant mesothelioma (pseudomesotheliomatous carcinoma) {1060}.

Finally adenocarcinoma may develop in the background of underlying fibrosis, either a localized scar or diffuse interstitial fibrosis {391} Adenocarcinoma arising in association with a focal scar is quite rare, in contrast to the relatively common central secondary scarring that develops in localized peripheral adenocarcinomas.

Tumour spread and staging

Adenocarcinoma spreads primarily by lymphatic and hematogenous routes.

Aerogenous dissemination commonly occurs in bronchioloalveolar carcinoma and is characterized by spread of tumour cells through the airways forming lesions separate from the main mass. Aerogenous dissemination can include involvement of the same lobe or different lobes in the ipsilateral and/or contralateral lung resulting in the multicentricity seen in bronchioloalveolar cell carcinoma. Peripheral adenocarcinomas occasionally spread over the pleural surfaces mimicking mesothelioma.

Approximately one fifth of newly diagnosed adenocarcinomas present with distant metastases. Brain, bone, adrenal glands and liver are the most common metastatic sites {1629}. Isolated local recurrence after resection is less common in adenocarcinoma than in other non-small cell types {276}.

Adenocarcinomas are staged according to the international TNM system {738, 2045}.

Histopathology

Adenocarcinomas mixed subtype. These are the most frequent subtype, representing approximately 80% of resected adenocarcinomas {1993}. In addition to the mixture of histologic subtypes, different degrees of differentiation (well, moderate, poor) and cytologic atypia (mild, moderate, marked) are typically encountered, varying from field to field and block to block. Any of the histologic subtypes may have a component with a loss of cellular cohesion with individual tumour cells filling alveolar spaces.

The major individual histologic patterns/subtypes are *acinar, papillary,*

bronchioloalveolar, and solid adenocarcinoma with mucin production {2024}. Adenocarcinomas consisting purely of one of these histologic subtypes are uncommon compared to the mixed histologic subtype, especially in larger tumours. Well, moderate, and poorly differentiated histologies are recognized among the acinar and papillary tumours. The *bronchioloalveolar pattern* is virtually always moderately or well differentiated. The *acinar pattern* is characterized by acini and tubules composed of cuboidal or columnar cells which may be mucin

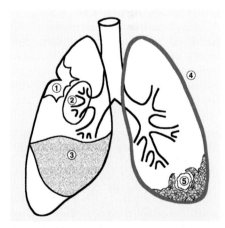

Fig. 1.23 Adenocarcinoma, summary of macroscopic growth patterns. Pattern 1 is the most common type: peripheral adenocarcinoma with desmoplastic fibrosis retracting the overlying pleura. Pattern 2 is the central or endobronchial adenocarcinoma. Pattern 3 is the diffuse pneumonia-like consolidation often associated with bronchioloalveolar or papillary growth. Pattern 4 represents the diffuse pleural thickening seen in 'pseudomesotheliomatous carcinoma' (see red line). Pattern 5 is the adenocarcinoma arising in the background of underlying fibrosis.

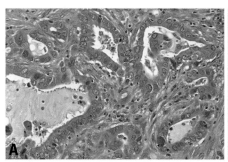
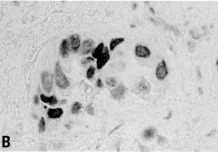

Fig. 1.24 Acinar adenocarcinoma. **A** This tumour forms irregular-shaped glands with cytologically malignant cells exhibiting hyperchromatic nuclei in a fibroblastic stroma. **B** Positive immunohistochemical staining for TTF-1 in an acinar adenocarcinoma. The nuclear staining varies.

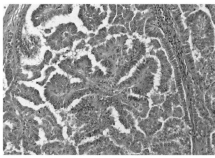

Fig. 1.25 Papillary adenocarcinoma. Tumour cells show a complex papillary glandular proliferation along fibrovascular cores. From Travis et al. {2024}.

producing and resemble bronchial gland or bronchial lining epithelial cells, including Clara cells {2024}.

The *papillary pattern* is characterized by papillae with secondary and tertiary papillary structures that replace the underlying lung architecture {2024}. Necrosis and lung invasion may be present. Bronchioloalveolar carcinomas that have simple papillary structures within intact alveolar spaces are excluded from this definition. The lining cells in papillary adenocarcinoma may be cuboidal to columnar, mucinous or non-mucinous and some cases may mimic papillary carcinoma of the thyroid. Some evidence suggests a micropapillary pattern of adenocarcinoma, in which papillary tufts lack a central fibrovascular core, may be prognostically unfavourable {1335}.

A *bronchioloalveolar carcinoma (BAC)* pattern shows growth of neoplastic cells along pre-existing alveolar structures (lepidic growth) without evidence of stromal, vascular, or pleural invasion {2024}. Septal widening with sclerosis is common in bronchioloalveolar carcinomas, particularly the non-mucinous variant. When there is marked alveolar collapse with increase in elastic tissue in the thickened alveolar septa, distinction between sclerosing BAC and early invasive adenocarcinoma may be difficult. Invasion is generally characterized by significant increase in cytologic atypia, a fibroblastic stromal reaction, and usually an acinar pattern of growth.

The non-mucinous variant of BAC typically shows Clara cell and/or type II cell differentiation {2024}. Clara cells are recognized as columnar with cytoplasmic snouts and pale eosinophilic cytoplasm. Nuclei may be apical in location. Type II cells are cuboidal or dome-shaped with fine cytoplasmic vacuoles or clear to foamy cytoplasm. Intranuclear eosinophilic inclusions may be present. In non-mucinous BAC there is no known clinical significance in distinguishing Clara from type II cells.

Mucinous BAC is by definition low grade, composed of tall columnar cells with basal nuclei and pale cytoplasm, sometimes resembling goblet cells, with varying amounts of cytoplasmic mucin and typically showing mucin production with mucus pooling in the surrounding alveolar spaces {2024}. Cytologic atypia is generally minimal. Aerogenous spread is characteristic and satellite tumours surrounding the main mass are typical. Extensive consolidation is common, sometimes with a lobar and/or pneumonic pattern. By convention small lesions, even those a few millimeters in size, showing this histology are considered mucinous BAC.

Rarely BACs are composed of a mixture of mucinous and non-mucinous cells.Mucinous and nonmucinous BAC may be solitary lesions, multifocal or consolidative (eg lobar) and the latter two are interpreted as aerogenous spread. Most solitary BACs encountered are of the nonmucinous subtype.

Solid adenocarcinoma with mucin is composed of sheets polygonal cells lacking acini, tubules, and papillae but

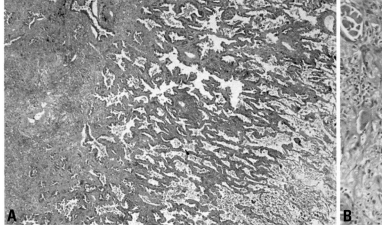
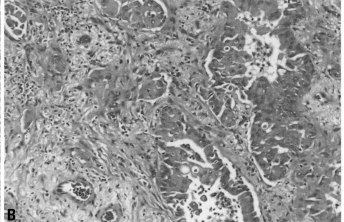

Fig. 1.26 **A,B** Invasive adenocarcinoma. Central area of invasion in an adenocarcinoma that at the periphery consisted of a non-mucinous bronchioloalveolar carcinoma. Invasion is associated with a significant increase in cytologic atypia and myofibroblastic stroma.

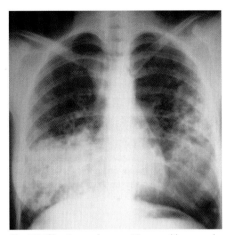

Fig. 1.27 Chest x-ray from an 18-year-old nonsmoking woman who presented with bilateral non-mucinous bronchioloalveolar carcinoma.

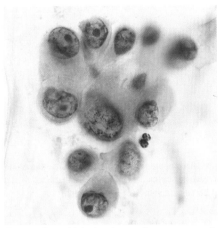

Fig. 1.28 Bronchioloalveolar carcinoma, non-mucinous subtype. Fine needle aspiration cytology shows a cohesive cell group with variable nuclear size, prominent nucleoli and perinucleolar clearing.

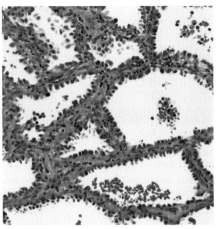

Fig. 1.29 Bronchioloalveolar carcinoma, non-mucinous. Cuboidal to columnar shaped cells grow along alveolar walls in a lepidic fashion.

with mucin present in at least 5 tumour cells in each of two high power fields confirmed with histochemical stains for mucin {2024}. Squamous carcinomas and large cell carcinomas of the lung may show rare cells with intracellular mucin production, but this does not indicate classification as adenocarcinoma.

Adenocarcinoma with mixed histologic patterns is an invasive tumour in which there is a mixture of histologic subtypes. The pathologic diagnosis of adenocarcinoma with mixed histologic patterns should include the histologic subtype with a comment about the pattern(s) identified: for example "adenocarcinoma with acinar, papillary and brochioloalveolar patterns". The extent of the stromal inflammation and fibrosis varies {391}. Small tumours (<2 cm.) with a BAC component should be histologically sectioned entirely to search for foci of invasion and to measure the size of fibrotic scars. Complete sampling is required for a diagnosis of localized nonmucinous BAC. In tumours that exhibit a component of nonmucinous BAC, the size and extent of invasion and scarring should be noted, as these may have prognostic importance. Tumours with localized fibrosis less than 5 mm. in diameter (regardless of the presence or absence of invasion) appear to have a 100% 5-year survival similar to localized BAC {1484, 1929,1993,2208} This localized fibrosis differs from the mild alveolar septal sclerosis and elastosis that is common in nonmucinous BAC. Central scars typically present as alveolar collapse with dense elastosis or active fibroblastic proliferation; when invasive carcinoma is present it is usually identified in regions of active fibroblastic proliferation and associated with increased atypia of the neoplastic cells. In some cases the distinction between elastotic sclerosis with trapping of airspaces lined by atypical cells from foci of fibroblastic proliferation with invasion may be difficult. In the setting of underlying diffuse interstitial fibrosis (from a variety of causes) there is significant fibrosis with honeycomb changes. However, all histologic types of lung cancer, not just adenocarcinoma, may arise in this setting {91}.

Multifocal invasive adenocarcinomas may be encountered. If a component of nonmucinous BAC can be confirmed contiguous with the invasive carcinoma, a presumptive diagnosis of a primary carcinoma can be made. Separate primary adenocarcinomas should be distinguished from satellite lesions that may be

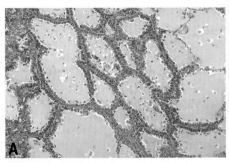

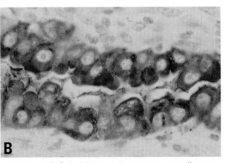

Fig. 1.30 Bronchioloalveolar carcinoma, non-mucinous, subtype. **A** Cuboidal to columnar tumor cells grow along alveolar walls. The monotony and crowding of the cells exclude a metaplastic process. From Travis et al. {2024}. **B** Immunohistochemistry for surfactant apoprotein A.

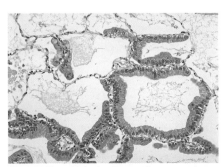

Fig. 1.31 Bronchioloalveolar carcinoma, mucinous subtype. There is a monotonous proliferation of well-differentiated mucinous epithelium growing along alveolar walls in a lepidic fashion with an abrupt transition from tumor to normal alveolar walls.

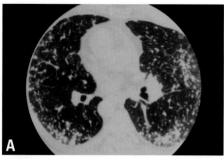 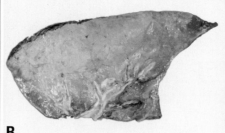 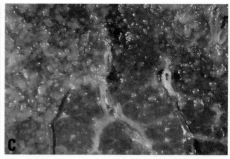

Fig. 1.32 Bronchioloalveolar carcinoma, mucinous subtype. **A** Computed tomography of a mucinous bronchioloalveolar carcinoma that presented as diffuse bilateral lung disease. **B** Macroscopy of mucinous bronchioloalveolar carcinoma, producing consolidation of a lobe without discrete mass formation. **C** Closer view of the macroscopy of another mucinous bronchioloalveolar carcinoma shows multiple tiny nodules.

encountered adjacent to the main tumour. Histologic disimilarity between the tumours also favors separate primaries. A definitive diagnosis of multifocality requires proof of molecular/genetic differences between the tumours, but such studies are often not feasible. Whether a tumour is classified as a separate primary or an intrapulmonary metastasis has implications regarding staging.

Fetal adenocarcinoma
Synonyms: well differentiated fetal adenocarcinoma, pulmonary adenocarcinoma of fetal type, pulmonary endodermal tumour resembling fetal lung.
This is a distinctive adenocarcinoma variant consisting of glandular elements composed of tubules of glycogen-rich, non-ciliated cells that resemble fetal lung tubules. Subnuclear and supranuclear glycogen vacuoles give the tumour an endometrioid appearance. Rounded morules of polygonal cells with abundant eosinophilic and finely granular cytoplasm are common {2024} (and resemble squamous morules in endometrioid adenocarcinomas). Some cases show a

clear cell pattern. Rarely, fetal adenocarcinomas are associated with other histologic types of lung cancer including other subtypes of adenocarcinoma. Most fetal adenocarcinomas are well differentiated; Nakatani, et al {1436} has recently described a variant designated poorly differentiated fetal adenocarcinoma. When fetal adenocarcinoma is associated with a sarcomatous primitive blastemal stroma the tumour is classified as pulmonary blastoma.

Mucinous ("colloid") adenocarcinoma
A lesion identical to their counterparts in the gastrointestinal tract, with dissecting pools of mucin containing islands of neoplastic epithelium {2024}. The epithelium in such cases may be extremely well differentiated and sometimes tumour cells float within the pools of mucin.

Mucinous cystadenocarcinomas
A circumscribed tumour that may have a partial fibrous tissue capsule. Centrally there is cystic change with mucin pooling and the neoplastic mucinous epithelium grows along alveolar walls.

Signet ring adenocarcinoma
Signet ring adenocarcinoma in the lung is usuallly a focal pattern associated with other histologic subtypes of adenocarcinoma. Exclusion of a metastasis, particularly from the gastrointestinal tract is important.

Clear cell adenocarcinoma.
This morphological feature is most often focal, but rarely it may be the major component of the tumour (clear cell adenocarcinoma) and it may occur in any of the major patterns of adenocarcinoma {391, 2024}. Metastatic renal cell carcinoma is an important consideration in such cases.

Immunohistochemistry
The immunohistochemical features of adenocarcinomas vary somewhat with the subtype and the degree of differentiation. Expression of epithelial markers (AE1/AE3, CAM 5.2, epithelial membrane antigen, and carcinoembryonic antigen) is typical {391}. CK7 is more frequently expressed than CK20 {1702}. TTF-1 staining is usually present, especially in better-differentiated tumours {1137, 2201}. In TTF-1 positive cases, a negative thyroglobulin helps to exclude metastatic thyroid carcinoma. Staining for surfactant apoprotein is seen less frequently than TTF-1 but is more problematic due to potential absorption of surfactant by metastatic tumour cells from the surrounding lung {14}. Mucinous tumours, especially mucinous BAC may represent exceptions, being TTF-1 negative and positive for CK7 and frequently CK20 {1136,1790}.

Differential diagnosis
The differential diagnosis includes metastatic adenocarcinoma, mesothe-

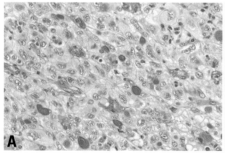 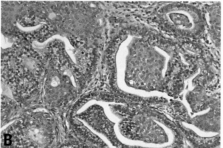

Fig. 1.33 A Solid adenocarcinoma with mucin formation. This poorly differentiated subtype of adenocarcinoma shows a substantial number of intracytoplasmic mucin droplets as seen on this periodic acid Schiff stain after diastase digestion. **B** Well-differentiated fetal adenocarcinoma, growing in glands with endometrioid morphology, including squamoid morules. Tumour cells are columnar, with clear cytoplasm that often has subnuclear vacuoles similar to endometrial glands. From Travis et al. {2024}.

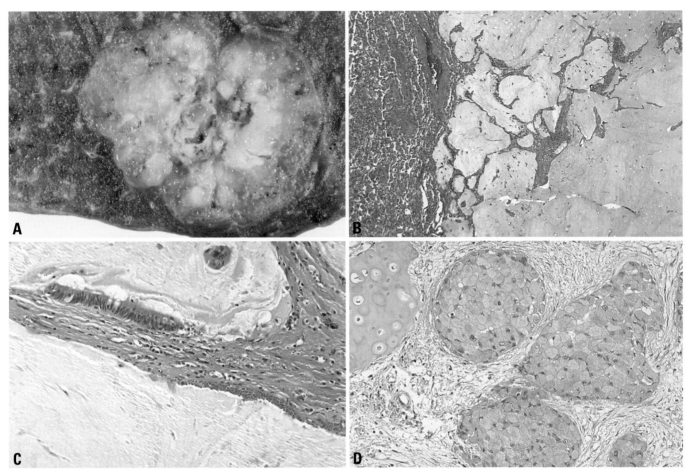

Fig. 1.34 **A** Mucinous ("colloid") adenocarcinoma. This subpleural tumor has a lobulated gelatinous tan-white surface. **B** Mucinous ("colloid") adenocarcinoma. The tumour consists of pools of mucin flooding airspaces and spreading in a permeative fashion into adjacent alveolar tissue. At low power microscopy the neoplastic cells are difficult to discern. **C** Mucinous ("colloid") adenocarcinoma. There is abundant mucin within alveolar spaces. Scattered clusters of tumour cells are present within the pools of mucin. Columnar mucinous epithelial cells line fibrotically thickened alveolar walls. **D** Signet ring adenocarcinoma. Tumour cells contain abundant cytoplasmic mucin that pushes the nucleus to the periphery. Stromal invasion adjacent to bronchial cartilage (left). From Travis et al. {2024}.

lioma, AAH, and reactive pneumocyte atypia associated with scars or organizing alveolar injury.

Patients with metastatic adenocarcinoma usually have a history of primary carcinoma and present with multiple lesions in the lung. Obtaining the histologic slides from the primary carcinoma for comparison with the histology of the lung lesion can be very informative. If the lesion in the lung is solitary, differentiation between primary and metastatic carcinoma may be more difficult. The presence of heterogeneity of histologic subtypes is characteristic of lung adenocarcinoma and this feature may be helpful in separating pulmonary primary from metastatic adenocarcinomas, since the latter tend to be more homogeneous. The presence of a bronchioloalveolar carcinoma (BAC) component favours primary adenocarcinoma of the lung over a

metastasis. However, some metastatic adenocarcinomas may rarely spread along the alveolar septa and mimic bronchioalveolar carcinoma.

Adenocarcinomas of the lung often show differentiation toward Type II cells or Clara cells and express markers found normally in these cell types. Up to 60% of pulmonary adenocarcinomas express surfactant proteins (SP-A, pro-SP-B, pro-SP-C) {138}. Thyroid transcription factor 1 (TTF-1), a transcription factor that plays an important role in the lung specific expression of surfactant proteins, is expressed in up to 75% of pulmonary adenocarcinomas {2232}. Metastatic adenocarcinomas with the exception of carcinomas of thyroid origin are negative for TTF-1. Negative mucin stains and positive staining for thyroglobulin help separate metastatic thyroid carcinoma from an adenocarcinoma of the lung.

This topic is discussed in more detail below in the section on metastases.

Cytokeratin (CK) 7 and CK20 may also be useful in differentiating primary versus metastatic adenocarcinoma {1702}. Most pulmonary adenocarcinomas have a CK7 positive, CK20 negative immunophenotype. One exception is mucinous BAC, which is usually positive for CK20 and negative with TTF-1. The differentiation of mucinous BAC from metastatic colonic adenocarcinoma, which is also typically CK20 positive, is aided with positive staining for the CDX2 homeobox gene {110,2124}. Prostate specific antigen, prostatic acid phosphatase and gross cystic disease fluid protein 15 may identify metastatic adenocarcinomas of prostate and breast origin, respectively {403,1780}.

Differentiation between pulmonary adenocarcinoma and epithelioid malignant mesothelioma should include clinical, macroscopic and microscopic, as well as immunohistochemical and/or electron microscopic analysis. This is addressed in detail in the pleural chapter. A typical workup should include a mucin stain, pan cytokeratin, and at least 2 general adenocarcinoma markers (e.g. CEA, CD15, or MOC 31), a marker specific for pulmonary adenocarcinoma (TTF-1) and 2 mesothelioma markers (e.g. calretinin, cytokeratin 5/6) {286,395}. When examined under the electron microscope, microvilli of malignant mesothelioma are more slender than those of pulmonary adenocarcinoma. In malignant mesothelioma, the ratio of length to diameter often exceeds 10 {2107}.

The separation of a small peripheral non-mucinous BAC from AAH may be difficult. No single criterion suffices and this distinction must be based on a constellation of features. Nonmucinous bronchioalveolar carcinoma is typically >5 mm. size with marked cellular stratification, high cell density and marked overlapping of nuclei, coarse nuclear chromatin and the presence of nucleoli, columnar cell change with cellular crowding, and micropapillary tufting.

AAH usually shows no more than one of these features. Marked pneumocyte atypia may be encountered adjacent to lung scars and associated with organizing alveolar injury. In the latter situation a history of pneumonia or prior chemotherapy or radiation is very helpful. In both situations the presence of a heterogeneous population of metaplastic cells, including ciliated cells, and a relative lack of cellular crowding and cytologic monotony (which favor adenocarcinoma) are important.

Prominent bronchiolar metaplasia in fibrotic lesions such as usual interstitial pneumonia may be confused with adenocarcinoma. The presence of papillary or invasive growth and abundant intracytoplasmic mucin favors adenocarcinoma.

Grading

Histological grading is a qualitative assessment of tumour differentiation and is an important component of the pathology report. Grading of pulmonary adenocarcinomas is based on conventional histological criteria, including the extent to which the architectural pattern of the tumour resembles normal lung tissue,

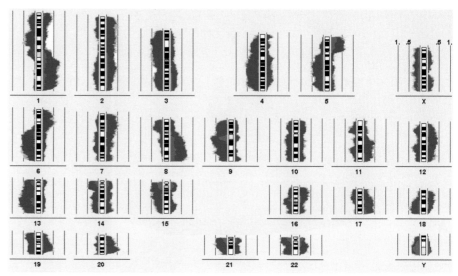

Fig. 1.35 Adenocarcinoma. Chromosomal imbalances of 30 primary lung adenocarcinomas. The chromosomal imbalances are shown as incidence curves along each chromosome. Areas on the left side of the chromosome ideogram correspond to loss of genetic material, those on the right side to DNA gains. The frequency of the alterations can be determined from the 50% and 100% incidence lines depicted parallel to the chromosome ideograms. DNA changes with 99% significance are coloured in blue, additional changes with 95% significance are depicted in green. The proportion of pronounced DNA imbalances are visualised in red. They are most likely to represent high copy amplifications or multi copy deletions.

and cytologic atypia. The amount of each component should be considered.

Typically, three grades are used. Well (grade 1), moderate (grade 2), and poorly differentiated (grade 3) tumours are recognized among acinar and papillary adenocarcinomas. The bronchioloalveolar pattern is virtually always well or moderately differentiated, whereas solid adenocarcinomas are poorly differentiated. If there is evidence of more than one grade of differentiation in a tumour, the least differentiated component should be recorded as the histological grade.

Histogenesis

Attempts to identify the cell of origin for lung adenocarcinomas has been frustrated by the diversity of epithelial cell types lining the airways, the propensity of lung adenocarcinomas to undergo phenotypic shifts during tumour progression, and the consequent morphologic heterogeneity among different lung adenocarcinomas and even within individual tumours. The phenotypic expression is influenced by anatomic location. Centrally located tumours arising from the large bronchi typically consist of a combination of columnar cells and mucinous cells. These central adenocarcinomas likely arise from the bronchial epithelium or bronchial glands. The

absence of a recognized preinvasive lesion for these central adenocarcinomas has handicapped efforts to trace their origin to a specific progenitor cell.

Most adenocarcinomas develop in the lung periphery. By light microscopy, electron microscopy, immunohistochemistry and gene expression analysis, these peripheral adenocarcinomas are composed of cells that closely resemble type II pneumocytes and Clara cells {163,481, 661,800} and these cells are identified as the likely cells of origin {1021,1377, 1521}. AAH is recognized as a preinvasive lesion for peripheral lung adenocarcinomas (particularly non-mucinous bronchioloalveolar carcinomas) {2125}. In AAH, the epithelial cells consist mostly of type II pneumocytes; Clara cells are more likely to be seen in bronchioloalveolar carcinomas than in AAH {481,800, 1022}.

Somatic genetics
Cytogenetics and CGH

Lung adenocarcinoma may be near diploid with only simple numerical chromosome changes, in particular loss of the Y chromosome and gains of autosomes 1 and 7. Alternatively, they may be hyperdiploid but also, even less commonly, hypodiploid, particularly the latter state being associated with extensive numerical and structural aberrations. The mean chromosome number is near the triploid range {104,1330}. The most frequent chromosomal imbalance is 1q overrepresentation {1582}. It is probably responsible for the inherent higher capacity of adenocarcinoma for hematogenous dissemination compared to squamous cell cancer because gain of the centromeric 1q region is also associated with metastasis formation {698}. Other frequently observed imbalances are deletions on chromosomes 3p, 4q, 5q, 6q, 8p, 9, 13q and gains on 5p, 8q, 20q {104,125,698,898,1301,1330,1582}. The CGH pattern can be helpful in the differentiation from squamous cell carcinoma {1582} and in particular mesothelioma {178,1075}.

Molecular genetics
The genetic alterations in adenocarcinoma include point mutations of dominant oncogenes, such as the K-ras gene, and tumour suppressor genes such as p53 and p16Ink4. K-ras mutations occur in approximately 30% of adenocarcinomas {1837} but are rare in other lung cancers. Most mutations are in codon 12, with smaller numbers in codon 13 and rarely in codon 61. They are more common in cancers arising in smokers. Mutations result in constant downstream signaling resulting in proliferative stimuli. Mutations have also been described in the putative precursor lesion, atypical adenomatous hyperplasia. p53 mutations are also a negative prognostic factor for limited stage adenocarcinoma {432,1331}. Increased expression of p27, one of the cell cycle regulators, correlates with better tumour differentiation and more favourable prognosis {2200}. p16Ink4 inactivation by multiple mechanisms occurs frequently in adenocarcinomas and may be smoking related {1300}. LKB1/STK11, the gene responsible for Peutz-Jeghers syndrome, is reported to be frequently inactivated in adenocarcinoma of the lung {1733}. Other important changes frequent in adenocarcinomas, but also present in smaller numbers of other non-small cell carcinomas, are over-expression of the HER2/Neu and COX-2 genes

Expression profiles
Recently, using the microarray technique, several genome-wide analyses have been reported. For example, using gene expression profiling, lung carcinomas have been subdivided into several groups and it has been possible to discriminate primary cancers from metastases of extrapulmonary origin {163,661, 1332,1638,2147}. The abnormal expression of genes involved in maintaining the mitotic spindle checkpoint and genomic stability contributes to the molecular pathogenesis and tumour progression of tobacco smoke-induced adenocarcinoma of the lung {1332}. Alterations in cell cycle genes have also been identified in lung adenocarcinoma using gene expression profiling {1830}.

Gene expression profiles revealed by microarray analyses have been found to be of prognostic significance in adenocarcinomas. Two studies have focused on classifying lung adenocarcinomas {163,661} using hierarchical clustering {535} to identify sub-classes in an unbiased fashion. Two of these subclasses are highlighted below. One adenocarcinoma subgroup is comprised of tumours that express neuroendocrine markers, such as l-aromatic amino acid decarboxylase, the human achaete-scute homolog 1 (hASH1), and insulinoma-associated 1. This expression pattern was associated with a significant decrease in patient survival when compared to other adenocarcinomas {163}.

Adenocarcinoma group 1 of the cDNA microarray expression study {661} shared significant patterns of relatively high-level gene expression with adenocarcinoma group C4 in the oligonucleotide array study {163}. These studies identified a subset of adenocarcinoma that appeared to express markers of alveolar type II pneumocytes {661}. High relative expression levels of surfactant protein genes and several other shared genes, including BENE, cytochrome b5, and selenium-binding protein 1, characterize these two groups. These samples were often diagnosed as bronchioloalveolar carcinomas {163} and appear to form a clear and distinct branch within the adenocarcinomas. More recently, a risk index compiling the relative expression of 50 genes was developed to identify high or low risk groups of Stage I adenocarcinomas that correlated inversely with patient survival {133} Using an independent, non-selective gene expression analysis method, serial analysis of gene expression or SAGE {623,1420} demonstrated that lung adenocarcinoma

exhibits distinct molecular characteristics as observed by the oligonucleotide microarray {163}. Furthermore, SAGE analyses also identified the down regulation of several p53 regulated genes and the over expression of immuno-related genes in lung adenocarcinoma {1420}.

Matrix-assisted laser desorption/ionisation mass spectrometry has been utilized to classify lung tumors based on their proteomic profile. In one study, proteomic spectra were obtained for 79 lung tumors and 14 normal lung tissues {2194}. More than 1600 protein peaks were detected from histologically selected 1 mm diameter regions of single frozen sections from each tissue. Class-prediction models based on differentially expressed peaks enabled the classification of lung cancer histologies, distinction between primary tumors and metastases to the lung from other sites, and classification of nodal involvement with 85% accuracy {2194}.

Prognostic and predictive factors
Radiologic features
Lesions with a component of ground glass opacity found in the context of CT screening, when resected, were found to be 1) atypical adenomatous hyperplasia, if very small, and when larger either 2) bronchioloalveolar carcinoma or 3) mixed adenocarcinoma with BAC and other patterns {819,1324,1425}. Kodama et al. {1039} showed that the ground-glass component correlates with the bronchioloalveolar carcinoma component in the histologic specimen.

CT screening which started in 1993 in Japan, showed long-term survival of patients with nodules to be associated with ground glass opacity {1038,1039, 2112,2192}. All of these studies show a more favourable prognosis for patients with tumours having a larger ground-glass component than a solid component, with long-term survival rates of up to 100%. Suzuki {1926} showed that none of the 69 cases of lung cancer found in sub-solid nodules had lymph node metastases and all were alive with a median follow-up time of 35 months. Takashima et al found that the presence of air bronchograms was an independent predictor of prognosis {1951}.

Histopathological criteria
Histological grading has prognostic implications. In general, patients with

poorly differentiated adenocarcinomas have more local recurrences and lymph node metastases than patients with well or moderately differentiated tumours {371}. However, histological grade may not be of prognostic importance in peripheral T1 adenocarcinoma {408}. The papillary pattern, including cases with a micropapillary pattern, appears to represent an unfavorable prognostic finding {1335,1484,1825}.

Histologic parameters that correlate with unfavourable prognosis include high histologic grade and vascular invasion {391}. Also considered promising, as unfavourable prognostic indicators are increased mitotic activity, relatively few tumour infiltrating lymphoid cells, and extensive tumour necrosis {391,1934}.

Histologic assessment that relates to stage (pleural invasion, evaluation of resection margins, assessment of sampled lymph nodes, search for intrapulmonary metastases) are all important and should be carefully evaluated in each case.

The diagnosis of bronchioloalveolar adenocarcinoma (BAC) is restricted to cases showing no pleural, vascular, or stromal invasion. In some series this applies to up to 20% of resected adenocarcinomas {1993}. The 5-year survival for localized resected BAC is 100% {1484,1929,1993, 2208} Recent studies {1929,1993,2208} suggest that adenocarcinomas with a predominant BAC pattern and central scarring less than 0.5 cm in tumours of 3 cm or less in diameter or p-T1 tumors, (regardless of the issue of invasion) have a similar, very favourable prognosis. Up to 30% of resected adenocarcinomas may be in this category {1993}.

In a study by Maeshima et al small adenocarcinomas (less than 2.0 cm) showing a bronchioloalveolar pattern without a central desmoplastic reaction showed 100% survival at ten years. The prognostic effect of the stromal reaction in small adenocarcinomas is important. Cases with central scars less than 0.5 cm in diameter (even if stromal invasion is

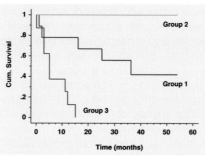

Fig. 1.36 Kaplan-Meier curves of lung adenocarcinoma subgroups based on cDNA microarray gene expression profiling. Group 3 carcinomas with the worst prognosis shared with large cell carcinomas the expression of genes involved in tissue remodeling. Reproduced from Garber et al. 2001 {661}.

present in this focus) have a very favourable prognosis {1222,1929,1993, 2208}.

These data, the radiologic studies above {1038,1039,1952,2112,2192}, and other recent studies {912} suggest that limited resection (eg. wedge resection) may be reasonable for small (< 2 cm., with good CT correlation, and entirely sectioned histologically) noninvasive peripheral tumours lacking active central fibrosis. Additional prospective confirmatory studies are necessary. This approach would render the distinction between AAH and BAC less critical for small lesions that have been entirely removed. Ishiwa et al. {912} showed that 13 of 54 patients (24%) with adenocarcinomas <2 cm. lacking fibroblastic proliferation and invasion (BAC) had no lymph node metastases on routine sectioning and with cytokeratin staining looking for micrometastases.

Bronchioloalveolar differentiation and never-smoking history predicts sensitivity to IRESSA in advanced non-small cell lung carcinoma {1321}.

Genetic predictive factors

There are no universally accepted genetic factors predictive of prognosis that have become part of routine clinical practice at the present time. Some prom-

ising preliminary studies have appeared. K-ras oncogene activation by point mutation correlates with poor survival and is also associated with the effect of chemotherapy at advanced stage {1670}. Another important prognostic factor is p53 gene mutation. The negative prognostic effect of p53 alteration is highly significant especially in adenocarcinoma both at the protein and DNA level {1331}. Also predictive of poor survival is the overexpression of p185neu (c-erbB2 oncogene-encoded protein) {1451}. Mutations in the EGFR gene have been found in patients who respond to the inhibor of the EGFR signaling pathway IRESSA (gefinitib) {1217,1530}.

Testing 3 molecular markers — c-Ki-ras, p53, and c-erbB2 – appears to improve the estimation of prognosis {1767}. In addition to these gene alterations, prognostic significance has been reported in many genes, although this is still controversial. For example, while expression of p21WAF1 is associated with favourable prognosis, expressions of cyclin D and bcl-2, and inactivation of retinoblastoma and p16 genes are associated with poor prognosis {589,1012,1479,2092}

Several studies using gene expression profiling have begun to identify prognostically significant subsets of lung adenocarcinoma {163,661,715}.

Loss of heterozygosity at chromosomes 2q, 9p, 18q, and 22q occurs frequently in advanced non-small cell lung carcinoma (NSCLC) plays an important role in the progression of NSCLC and predicts poor survival {1813}. Although reports of functional losses of the repair genes in adenocarcinoma have been infrequent, there have been reports that allelic imbalances at 9p and 22q with p53 alteration corre lates with shortened survival {2011}.

Large cell carcinoma

E. Brambilla
B. Pugatch
K. Geisinger
A. Gal
M.N. Sheppard
D.G. Guinee
S.X. Jiang

S. Lantuejoul
Y.L. Chang
I. Petersen
M. Meyerson
S.M. Hanash
M. Noguchi

Definition
Large cell carcinoma is an undifferentiated non-small cell carcinoma that lacks the cytologic and architectural features of small cell carcinoma and glandular or squamous differentiation.

ICD-O codes
Large cell carcinoma 8012/3

Large cell neuroendocrine
carcinoma 8013/3
Combined large cell neuroen
docrine carcinoma 8013/3
Basaloid carcinoma 8123/3
Lymphoepithelioma-like
carcinoma 8082/3
Clear cell carcinoma 8310/3
Large cell carcinoma with
rhabdoid phenotype 8014/3

Synonyms
Large cell carcinoma has previously been called large cell anaplastic carcinoma and large cell undifferentiated carcinoma. Before the description of large cell neuroendocrine carcinoma terms such as large cell neuroendocrine tumour {769}, neuroendocrine carcinoma with intermediate differentiation {2109}, atypical endocrine tumour of the lung {1283}, and large cell carcinoma of the lung with neuroendocrine differentiation {2135} were used for tumours that we now call large cell carcinoma with neuroendocrine differentiation. LCNEC was described in 1991 {2026}; basaloid car-

cinoma was described in 1992 {216} and both tumours were recognized as distinct clinicopathological entities by the WHO in the 1999 classification {2024}.

Epidemiology
Large cell carcinoma accounts for approximately 9% of all lung cancers {2029} in most studies {916,1957}. Large cell neuroendocrine carcinoma accounts for about 3% of lung cancer {916}. All types predominate in smokers, except lymphoepithelioma-like carcinoma. Average age at diagnosis is about 60 and most patients are male {216,916, 1390,2026}. Lymphoepithelioma-like carcinoma (LELC) is a very rare tumour, but represents 1% of lung tumours in China, affects younger, mostly female patients (mean age 57) and only 40% are smokers {324,331,340,770,771,2168}.

Clinical features
Signs and symptoms
Symptoms are common with those of other NSCLC. Most tumours are peripheral except basaloid carcinoma. Ectopic hormone production is uncommon in LCNEC {475}.

Relevant diagnostic procedures
Large cell carcinomas have no particular distinguishing radiological features. The appearance depends on the site of the tumour {614}. Large cell carcinomas, except basaloid carcinoma, occur pref-

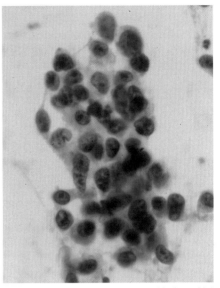

Fig. 1.38 Large cell carcinoma. In this bronchial brushing specimen, a loose syncytial aggregate of obviously malignant cells is present. The nuclei have thick very irregular membranes, coarsely granular and dark chromatin, and prominent and irregular nucleoli. No evidence of specific differentiation is apparent. Papanicolaou stain.

erentially in the lung periphery, so that tumours may be accessible by transthoracic fine needle aspiration biopsy as well at bronchoscopy. Specific diagnosis of LCC and variants can only be reliably achieved on surgical material.

Cytology
Most cases of LCC do not have specific discriminating cytologic features. Most cytologic samples show cellular aggregates; less often cells are dispersed. Cellular borders are indistinct so syncytia form haphazardly {673,936,1826}. Nuclei vary from round to extremely irregular {255} with irregular chromatin distribution. Nucleoli are generally very prominent. Cytoplasm is basophilic, usually scant with a high nuclear-to-cytoplasmic (N/C) ratio.
LCNEC shows neuroendocrine features (nuclear palisading and molding), but are distinguished from SCLC by the presence of prominent nucleoli and

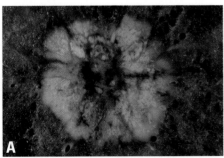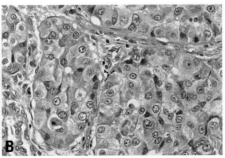

Fig. 1.37 A Peripheral LCC with cream-white foci of necrosis, central scar and anthracotic pigmentation. The periphery shows a homogeneous grey cut surface. **B** Large tumour cells have abundant cytoplasm with large nuclei, vesicular nuclear chromatin and prominent nucleoli. No glandular or squamous differenciation. From Travis et al. {2024}.

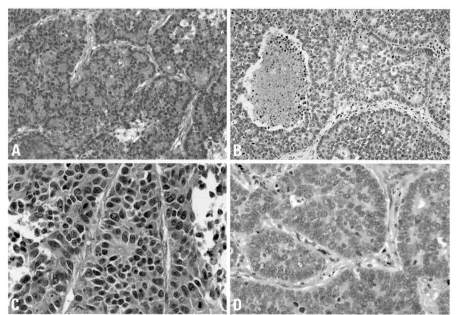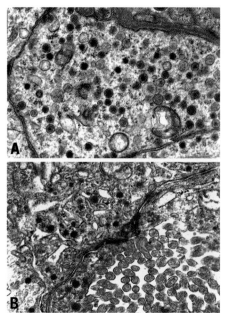

Fig. 1.39 Large cell neuroendocrine carcinoma. **A** Note numerous rosettes. **B** Palisading at the periphery of the nests of tumour cells and rosettes can been seen. Necrosis is present and mitoses are numerous From Travis et al. {2024}. **C** High magnification shows details of rosettes and nuclei with vesicular chromatin. **D** Palisading and rosette-like formations. Numerous mitoses. The nuclear chromatin is vesicular and many cells have prominent nucleoli. From Travis et al. {2024}.

Fig. 1.40 A Ultrastructural aspect of neuroendocrine cells in a large cell neuroendocrine carcinoma. Numerous dense core neurosecretory granules are present in the cytoplasm. **B** Ultrastructural features in a combined large neuroendocrine carcinoma showing within the same cell acinus formation with apical microvilli and typical neurosecretory granules.

nuclei larger than 3 times the diameter of a small resting lymphocyte. {2132,2197}. Basaloid carcinoma in smears consists of both individual tumour cells and cohesive aggregates. Well developed nuclear palisading can be discerned at the periphery of some cellular aggregates. Lymphoepithelioma-like carcinomas show cohesive flat syncytia {364}. Spindle-shaped tumour cells have solitary large nuclei with huge nucleoli, intimately admixed with numerous small lymphocytes.

Macroscopy and localization
Large cell carcinomas typically present as large, peripheral masses, frequently identified on chest radiographs, but which may also involve subsegmental or large bronchi. The tumour often invades visceral pleura, chest wall, or adjacent structures. Sectioning reveals a soft, pink-tan tumour with frequent necrosis, occasional hemorrhage and rarely, cavitation.
Large cell neuroendocrine carcinomas are often peripheral. In contrast basaloid carcinomas characteristically show exophytic bronchial growth {216}.

Tumour spread and staging
The pattern of spread of large cell carcinoma is similar to other non-small cell lung carcinomas. Metastases occur most frequently to hilar or mediastinal nodes followed by metastases to the pleura, liver, bone, brain, abdominal lymph nodes and pericardium {1875}. Micrometastases detected in hilar nodes have no significant impact on prognosis in otherwise stage I tumours {703}. Specific subtypes of large cell carcinoma differ in their pattern of spread, response to therapy and ultimate prognosis. Large cell neuroendocrine carcinoma {916,1272,1957,2028} combined large cell neuroendocrine carcinoma {1709}, large cell carcinoma with rhabdoid phenotype {304,350,1803} and basaloid carcinoma {216,1390} have a worse prognosis than classic large cell carcinoma. Recent studies have report-

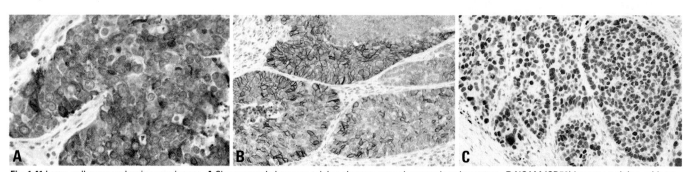

Fig. 1.41 Large cell neuroendocrine carcinoma. **A** Chromogranin immunostaining shows a granular cytoplasmic pattern. **B** NCAM (CD56) immunostaining with typical membrane pattern. **C** TTF1 (thyroid transcription factor one) immunoreactivity with a typical nuclear pattern.

ed both a better prognosis and better response by lymphoepithelial like carcinoma to both chemotherapy and radiation therapy {302,324,331,340,770}. The clinical behavior of clear cell carcinoma is similar to typical large cell carcinomas {971}.

Stage distribution for LCC at diagnosis is as seen in other NSCLC. Large cell neuroendocrine carcinomas are often stage III-IV at diagnosis. Basaloid carcinoma is frequently operable at presentation but prognosis is worse than that of other NSCLC and brain metastases are more frequent {1390}.

Histopathology

Large cell carcinomas

These are, by definition, poorly differentiated tumours. It is a diagnosis of exclusion made after ruling out the presence of a component of squamous cell carcinoma, adenocarcinoma or small cell carcinoma. They consist of sheets or nests of large polygonal cells with vesicular nuclei with prominent nucleoli, and a moderate amount of cytoplasm. Ultrastructurally minimal squamous or glandular differentiation is common.

Large cell neuroendocrine carcinoma

Large cell neuroendocrine carcinoma (LCNEC) shows histological features such as organoid nesting, trabecular growth, rosettes and perilobular palisading patterns, suggesting neuroendocrine differentiation {2024,2026} The tumour cells are generally large, with moderate

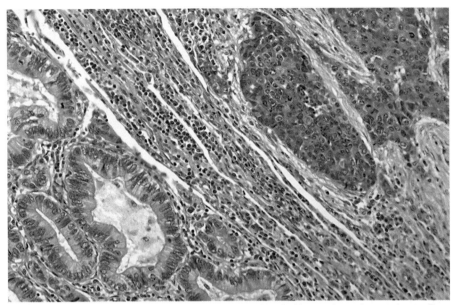

Fig. 1.42 This large cell neuroendocrine carcinoma is combined with an acinar adenocarcinoma. From Travis et al. {2024}.

to abundant cytoplasm. Nucleoli are frequent, prominent and their presence facilitates separation from small cell carcinoma. Mitotic counts are typically 11 or more (average 75) per 2 mm^2 of viable tumour. Large zones of necrosis are common. Confirmation of neuroendocrine differentiation is required using immunohistochemical markers such as chromogranin, synaptophysin and NCAM (CD56) {1128}. One positive marker is enough if the staining is clearcut. Around 50% of LCNEC express TTF-1 {1216,1892,1894}, but expression of CK 1, 5, 10, 14, 20 (34ßE12) is uncommon {1892,1893}.

Combined large cell neuroendocrine carcinoma:

A large cell neuroendocrine carcinoma with components of adenocarcinoma, squamous cell carcinoma, giant carcinoma and/or spindle cell carcinoma. Like small cell carcinoma, a small percentage of large cell neuroendocrine carcinomas are histologically heterogeneous. In view of the many shared clinical, epidemiologic, survival, and neuroendocrine properties between large cell neuroendocrine carcinoma and small cell carcinoma, we have arbitrarily chosen to classify these tumours as combined large cell neuroendocrine car-

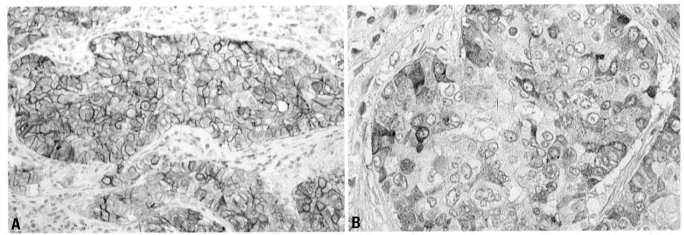

Fig. 1.43 Combined large neuroendocrine carcinoma. **A** NCAM (CD56) immunostaining in the large cell neuroendocrine component. Note the typical cell membrane pattern. **B** Combined large neuroendocrine carcinoma associated with an adenocarcinoma. The large neuroendocrine carcinoma is immunostained with chromogranin antibody.

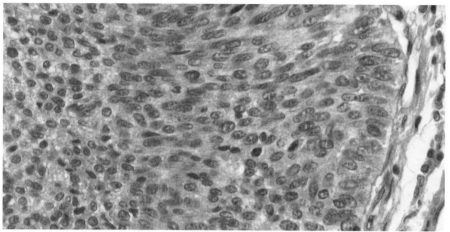

Fig. 1.44 Basaloid carcinoma at high magnification showing peripheral palisading and monomorphic cells with dense chromatin and unconspicuous nucleoli.

cinoma until future studies better define their biologic behavior. Combinations with small cell carcinoma also occur, but such tumours are classified as combined variants of small cell carcinoma.

Basaloid carcinoma
This tumour shows a solid nodular or anastomotic trabecular invasive growth pattern, with peripheral palisading. Tumour cells are relatively small, monomorphic, cuboidal fusiform, with moderately hyperchromatic nuclei, finely granular chromatin and absent or focal nucleoli. Cytoplasm is scant but nuclear molding is absent. Mitotic rate is high (15-50 per 2 mm²). Squamous differentiation is absent. Most basaloid carcinoma have hyalin or mucoid degeneration in the stroma. Frequent small cystic spaces are seen. Comedo type necrosis is common. Rosettes are seen in one third of cases. Immunohistochemical stains for neuroendocrine markers are geneally negative. In 10% of cases, one neuroendocrine marker may be positive in less than 20% of tumour cells. Cytokeratin

expression is as seen in NSCLC, and includes CK 1, 5, 10, and 14 (34ßE12), markers. Basaloid carcinoma does not express TTF-1 {1892}.

Lymphoepithelioma-like carcinoma
Pulmonary lymphoepithelial-like carcinoma is characterized by a syncytial growth pattern, large vesicular nuclei, prominent eosinophilic nucleoli, and heavy lymphocytic infiltration {302,324, 331,340,770} It has predominantly pushing border, infiltrating in the form of diffuse sheets. The prominent lymphoid reaction consists of mature lymphocytes often admixed with plasma cells and histiocytes with occasional neutrophils or eosinophils. The lymphoid component is seen even in metastatic sites. In rare cases, there is intratumoural amyloid deposition. EBER-1 RNA is present in the nuclei of the large undifferentiated neoplastic cells.

Clear cell carcinoma
Clear cell carcinomas have large polygonal tumours cells with water-clear or

foamy cytoplasm. Tumour cells may or may not contain glycogen.

Large cell carcinoma with rhabdoid phenotype
In large cell carcinoma with rhabdoid phenotype, at least 10% of the tumour cell population must consist of rhabdoid cells, characterized by eosinophilic cytoplasmic globules {304}, consisting of intermediate filaments, which may be positive for vimentin and cytokeratin {304,1803}. Pure large cell carcinomas with a rhabdoid phenotype are very rare. Small foci of adenocarcinoma {1803}, and positive neuroendocrine markers may be seen. Ultrastruscturally the eosinophilic inclusions are composed of aggregates of large intra cytoplasmic paranuclear intermediate filaments. Cells with rhabdoid features may be seen focally in other poorly differentiated NSCLC.

Differential diagnosis
The differential diagnosis of large cell carcinoma (NOS) includes poorly differentiated squamous cell carcinoma in which foci of keratinization and/or intercellular bridges are present and solid type adenocarcinoma, where a minimum of 5 mucinous droplets are present in at least 2 high power fields. The major differential diagnosis for LCNEC is atypical carcinoids (AC) and basaloid carcinoma. LCNEC is distinguished from atypical carcinoid primarily by a higher mitotic index (11 or more per 2mm²) and usually more extensive necrosis. Differential diagnosis between LCNEC and basaloid carcinoma is more difficult on H&E morphology alone and is usually achieved using neuroendocrine markers, since both tumours disclose palisading and one third of basaloid carcinoma show rosettes. Cytokeratins 1, 5, 10, 14 are

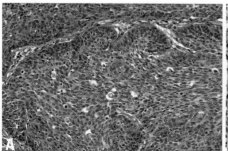
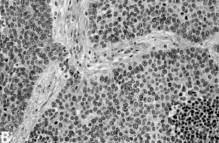
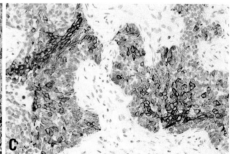

Fig. 1.45 Basaloid carcinoma. **A** Palisading is conspicuous at the periphery of the nests of tumour cells which are hyperchromatic, with relatively scant cytoplasm {2024}. **B** Lobular pattern with peripheral palisading, comedo type necrosis and some rosettes. **C** 34ßE12 immunostaining for cytokeratins 1, 5, 10, 14.

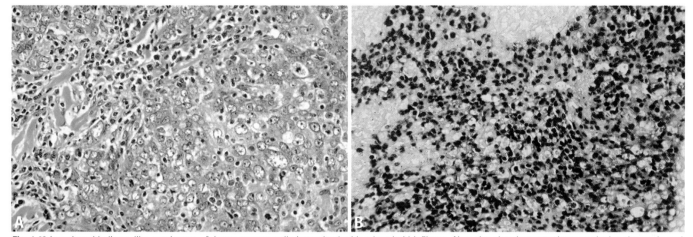

Fig. 1.46 Lymphoepithelioma-like carcinoma. **A** Large tumour cells intermixed with a lymphoid infiltrate. Note the abundant cytoplasm, vesicular chromatin and prominent nucleoli. From Travis et al. {2024}. **B** Epstein-Barr virus-encoded small RNA (EBER RNA) expression in the nuclei of large undifferentiated neoplastic cells but not in the surrounding lymphocytic infiltrate. *In situ* hybridization.

expressed (34ßE12) in other NSCLC but are typically negative in LCNEC {1892,1893}. Basaloid carcinoma must be distinguished from poorly differentiated squamous carcinoma. Although initially described with 2 forms, one pure and one mixed, the latter is now considered as the basaloid variant of squamous cell carcinoma. Occurrence of even focal squamous differentiation favors the diagnosis of basaloid variant of squamous carcinoma. Small cell carcinoma enters the differential diagnosis of basaloid carcinoma due to their small cell size and high mitotic rate, but nuclear to cytoplasmic ratio is higher in SCLC and nuclear chromatin is vesicular rather than finely granular.

The prominent inflammatory cell infiltrate, which characterises lymphoepithelioma-like carcinoma, may lead to considera-

tion of inflammatory pseudotumour, malignant lymphoma {1262}, or primary lymphoid hyperplasia of the lung. A panel of immunohistochemical stains allows recognition of the malignant epithelial cells, characteristically patchy in distribution, as well as CD8+ expression by the lymphocytic infiltrate.

Clear cell carcinoma of the lung resembles metastatic clear cell carcinomas arising in organs such as the kidney, thyroid and salivary gland. If squamous or glandular differentiation is seen, the tumour is classified as a clear cell variant of squamous cell or adenocarcinoma, respectively.

Precursor lesions

There is no precursor lesion identified for large cell carcinoma except for basaloid carcinoma. Adjacent squamous dyspla-

sia in one third of basaloid carcinoma, their pattern of infiltration, and both their immunophenotype and ultrastructure characteristic of bronchial reserve cells {216,222,1281}, supports an origin from bronchial preneoplastic lesions. Lympho-epithelioma-like carcinoma is characterised by the presence of EBV viral sequences, reflecting viral (EBER1) dependent transformation of lung epithelial cells.

Histogenesis

These tumours originate from a common pluripotent progenitor cell capable of multidirectional differentiation {1282, 2024}. Neuroendocrine differentiation in LCNEC does not imply origin from a specific neuroendocrine cell. In contrast to carcinoid tumours, LCNEC is not associated with diffuse neuroendocrine hyper-

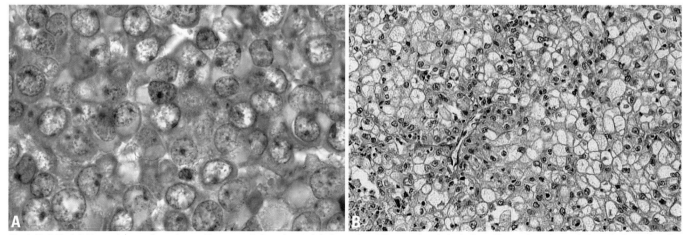

Fig. 1.47 A Rhabdoid type large cell carcinoma. Tumour cells have large globular eosinophilic cytoplasmic inclusions. The nuclear chromatin is vesicular and nucleoli are prominent. From Travis et al. {2024}. **B** Clear cell carcinoma with numerous tumour cells showing clear cytoplasm.

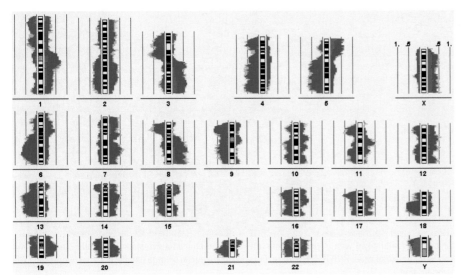

Fig. 1.48 DNA copy number changes in 18 classical (non-neuroendocrine) large cell carcinomas detected by CGH. Areas on the left side of the chromosome ideogram reflect loss of genetic material, those on the right side to DNA gains. DNA changes with 99% significance are coloured in blue, additional changes with 95% significance are depicted in green. The proportion of pronounced DNA imbalances are visualised in red; they typically represent high copy amplifications or multiple copy deletions.

plasia, tumourlets or MEN1 mutations {464} Cells of basaloid carcinoma display the immunohistochemical and ultrastructural phenotype of reserve suprabasal bronchial cells. {216,222, 1281} Clear cell and rhabdoid variants of LCC probably reflectf the pluripotent capacity of the LC progenitor cell.

Somatic genetics
Cytogenetics and CGH
Large cell carcinoma of the lung is mostly an aneuploid neoplasm with the highest mean chromosome number and DNA content of all lung cancer types being in the near triploid range or above {1581}. Accordingly, the karyotypes are complex and indicate a high chromosomal instability {1330} of which the major biological effect is probably the generation of DNA copy number changes. The CGH pattern of classical, non-neuroendocrine large cell carcinoma shows similarities to lung adenocarcinoma and squamous cell carcinoma like overrepresentations on 1q and 3q {178,898}. In particular, the tumours harbour imbalances that have been associated with progression and metastasis formation, e.g. amplifications of 1q21-q22, 8q and deletion of 3p12-p14, 4p, 8p22-p23, 21q. Large cell neuroendocrine carcinoma may carry very similar chromosomal imbalances as small cell lung carcinoma {898,2051, 2052}.

Molecular genetics
Large cell carcinomas share the molecular and genetic alterations commonly seen in NSCLC, since it is a poorly differentiated tumour issued from the same stem cells, exposed to the same carcinogens. K-ras mutations, P53 mutations and Rb pathway alteration (loss of P16INK4, hyperexpression of cyclin D1 or E) occurs with the same frequency as in other NSCLC. Large cell neuroendocrine carcinomas have P53 and Rb mutational patterns in addition to inactivation pathways similar to SCLC {212, 215,217,1516,1622}: a high frequency of P53 mutation, of bcl2 overexpression, lack of bax expression {217}, high telomerase activity, but lower frequency of Rb / P14ARF loss of protein, and of E2F1 overexpression than SCLC {549,550}. They display a low frequency of P16 loss, cyclin D1 and cyclin E overexpression, and lack MEN1 mutation and allelic deletion. Fas is downregulated but its ligand FasL is strongly upregulated {2083}.

Prognosis and predictive factors
Clinical criteria
Clinical prognostic criteria are not different from other NSCLC. The major criterion is performance status at diagnosis and the disease extension reflected by the TNM and stage. Although most basaloid carcinomas present as stage I-II tumours, they bear a dismal prognosis in

contrast with lymphoepithelioma-like carcinoma, which present at extended stage but have better prognosis than NSCLC. A direct correlation between larger tumour size and high stage and titre of EBV serology has been demonstrated in lymphoepithelioma-like carcinoma {331}. There is no significant difference in the prognosis between LCNEC and SCLC after stratification by stage. There is a significantly shorter survival for stage I LCNEC as compared with stage I NSCLC {1957} and stage I large cell carcinoma {916}. The outcome of carefully staged LCNEC may be better than prrevious studies have indicated {2229}.

Histopathological criteria
It is controversial whether the presence of neuroendocrine differentiation demonstrated by immunohistochemistry has any prognostic signficance in NSCLC (NSCLC-NED). Some studies indicate a worse prognosis {841,916,1566}, others a better prognosis {289,1759} and others show no difference in survival {651,1833, 1905}. In addition studies have suggested NSCLC-NED have a better prognosis {735} or no difference in response to chemotherapy {1448}.

Genetic predictive factors
The genetic predictive factors of large cell carcinoma should correspond to those of general primary lung carcinoma. However, one variant of large cell carcinoma – large cell neuroendocrine carcinoma (LCNEC) – has specific genetic characters similar to SCLC: allelic losses of 3p21, FHIT, 3p22-24, 5q21, 9p21, and the RB gene. All of these markers correlate with poor prognosis in neuroendocrine carcinoma including LCNEC. Both p53 gene loss and point mutation also correlate with poor survival {1516}.

Adenosquamous carcinoma

E. Brambilla
W.D. Travis

Definition

A carcinoma showing components of both squamous cell carcinoma and adenocarcinoma with each comprising at least 10% of the tumour.

ICD-O Code   8560/3

Clinical features

Signs and symptoms

The frequency of adenosquamous carcinoma is between 0,4-4% of lung carcinomas {586,909,1445,1867,1950,2203}. Their incidence might be rising parallel to the increase of adenocarcinoma {1868}. The majority of patients are smokers. Clinical presentation and behavior is similar to adenocarcinoma.

Imaging and relevant diagnostic procedures

Since most tumours are peripheral their diagnosis can be assessed by bronchoscopy in segmental or subsegmental bronchi, or by transthoracic needle biopsy. However their recognition is sampling dependent, the likelihood of identifying both components in small samples is small, and diagnosis is more definitive on surgical samples. Radiographic features are not different from those of non-small cell carcinoma; peripheral tumours may show central scarring and indentation or puckering of the overlying pleura. Some may display a rim of ground glass opacity.

Macroscopy and localization

Adenosquamous carcinomas are usually located in the periphery of the lung and may contain a central scar. They are grossly similar to other non-small cell carcinomas.

Tumour spread and staging

Metastases usually show the same combination of squamous and glandular differentiation as the primary. The spread of adenosquamous carcinoma is similar to other non-small cell carcinomas. They show early metastases and a poor prognosis {84}.

Histopathology

As there is a continuum of histological heterogeneity with both squamous cell and adenocarcinoma, the criterion of 10% for each component is arbitrary. Since some squamous cell carcinomas show focal mucin on histochemical stains the adenocarcinoma component is more easily defined if it shows an acinar, papillary or bronchioloalveolar pattern. Well-defined squamous cell carcinoma and adenocarcinoma are evident on light microscopy, the squamous cell carcinoma showing unequivocal keratin or intracellular bridges and the adenocarcinoma showing acini, tubules or papillary structures. The diagnosis of an adenocarcinoma component is difficult if it is confined to a solid pattern with mucin formation. More than 5 mucin droplets per high power field are then required for a diagnosis of adenocarcinoma. The two components may be separate or may merge and mingle. The squamous or the glandular component may be predominant or may be seen in equal proportion. The degree of differentiation of each component is not interdependent and is variable. A component of large cell carcinoma may be present in addition to the 2 other components but does not change the diagnosis. The same stromal features with or without inflammation occur as in other non-small cell lung carcinomas. Cases with amyloid-like stroma have been described {2217}, as seen in salivary gland type neoplasms. Ultrastructural features are those of squamous carcinoma and adenocarcinoma. By electron microscopy features of both cell types are common but tumour classification is based on light microscopy. Immunohistochemical findings also recapitulate both squamous and adenocarcinoma characteristics. They express cytokeratins with a wide molecular weight range including AE1/AE3, CAM 5.2, KL1, and CK7 but usually not CK20. EMA is positive and TTF-1 positivity is confined to the adenocarcinoma component.

Differential diagnosis

The differential diagnosis includes entrapment of alveolar or bronchiolar acinar structures within a squamous cell

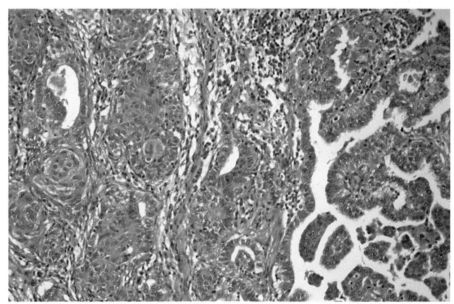

Fig. 1.49 Adenosquamous carcinoma. The tumour consists of squamous cell carcinoma (left) and papillary adenocarcinoma (right). From Travis et al. {2024}.

carcinoma. This should not be mistaken for glandular differentiation of the cancer. Similarly, adenocarcinoma may be associated with squamous metaplasia of entrapped bronchiolar structures.

Mucoepidermoid carcinoma enters the differential diagnosis. Arising from bronchial glands, low-grade mucoepidermoid carcinoma are centrally located and show histologic features identical to their salivary gland counterpart, with mixture of mucinous glands, intermediate or squamoid cells, with no or mild atypia. High grade mucoepidermoid carcinoma is more difficult to differentiate from adenosquamous carcinoma. In favour of mucoepidermoid carcinoma is the characteristic admixture of mucinous and squamoid cells, a proximal exophytic endobronchial location, areas of classic low grade mucoepidermoid carcinoma, absence of keratinisation or squamous pearl formation without overlying in situ squamous cell carcinoma {2217,2221}, or tubular, acinar, and papillary growth pattern. These two lung tumours cannot be distinguished reliably in all cases {1348}.

Histogenesis

The cell of origin is believed to be a pluripotential bronchial reserve cell. It has been proposed that adenocarcinomas according to their central (bronchial) or peripheral (alveolar parenchyma) location arise from two distant stem cells, bronchial epithelial and Clara cell type respectively {402} with different mutational patterns. Since most adenocarcinomas have mixed patterns combining both central (acinar, solid) and peripheral (bronchioloalveolar, papillary) adenocarcinoma patterns, it is likely they originate, like adenosquamous carcinoma, from a common intermediate bronchial-Clara type II cell type.

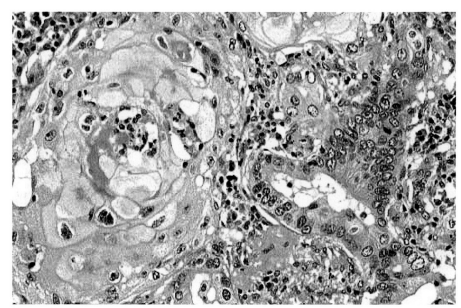

Fig. 1.50 Adenosquamous carcinoma showing a squamous cell lobule on the left, adjacent to an acinar adenocarcinoma on the right.

Somatic genetics

There is no information specifically available on adenosquamous carcinoma with regard to cytogenics and CGH, expression profile and proteomics. The molecular genetic alterations of each component are those characteristic of squamous and adenocarcinoma respectively. They may display Ras mutations similar to peripheral adenocarcinoma.

Prognosis and predictive factors

The histologic criteria for the diagnosis in these studies vary, and should be kept in mind when comparing results. They have a poor prognosis with a 5-year survival rate after resection of 62.5% for localized disease and 35% for resectable cases {909}. The prognosis is poorer than that of stage I-II squamous carcinoma or adenocarcinoma, and this histological type was shown to be an independent prognostic determinant at limited stage. The SEER results report an overall 21% 5-year survival.

Genetic predictive factors

There are no specific studies reported for adenosquamous carcinoma, although they have been included in non-small cell lung carcinomas. Ras and P53 mutations might be an unfavorable prognostic factor in stage I tumours.

Sarcomatoid carcinoma

B. Corrin
Y.L. Chang
G. Rossi
M.N. Koss
K. Geisinger

M.R. Wick
O. Nappi
S.D. Finkelstein
Y. Nakatani

Definition
Sarcomatoid carcinomas are a group of poorly differentiated non-small cell lung carcinomas that contain a component of sarcoma or sarcoma-like (spindle and/or giant cell) differentiation. Five subgroups representing a morphologic continuum are currently recognized: Pleomorphic carcinoma:, spindle cell carcinoma, giant cell carcinoma, carcinosarcoma and pulmonary blastoma.

ICD-O codes
Pleomorphic carcinoma	8022/3
Spindle cell carcinoma	8032/3
Giant cell carcinoma	8031/3
Carcinosarcoma	8980/3
Pulmonary blastoma	8972/3

Synonyms
An alternative classification recognizing monophasic and biphasic varieties with the latter further classified as homologous or heterologous {2138} is not currently recommended.

Epidemiology
These tumours are rare, accounting for approximately only 0.3-1.3% of all lung malignancies {584,1430,1695,2023,2029}. The average age at diagnosis is 60 years, and the male to female ratio is almost 4 to 1 {218,330,337,443,1440, 1857}. Biphasic blastomas are exceptional in that they afflict men and women equally with an average age in the fourth decade {1064,1665}.

Etiology
The factors implicated in the etiology of sarcomatoid carcinomas are similar to those involved in conventional histotypes. Tobacco smoking is the major factor; more than 90% of patients with pleomorphic carcinoma are heavy cigarette smokers {443,584,1430,1440,2029}. Some cases may be related to asbestos exposure {557,584}.

Localization
Sarcomatoid carcinomas can arise in the central or peripheral lung. A predilection for the upper lobes has been reported {443,584,1430,1695}. Pleomorphic carcinomas are often large peripheral tumours with a tendency to invade the chest wall {584}.

Clinical features
Signs and symptoms
Signs and symptoms are related to tumour localization {443,584,1430,1440, 1695,1857}. Since central endobronchial tumours tend to protrude into the lumina of large airways, patients often present with cough, haemoptysis, and progressive dyspnoea or fever due to recurrent pneumonia. Peripheral tumours, especially pleomorphic carcinoma, grow to large sizes and often present with chest pain due to pleural or chest wall invasion.

Relevant diagnostic procedures
Due to sampling issues and histologic heterogeneity the diagnosis of virtually all sarcomatoid carcinomas requires a surgical specimen. Based on cytology or a small biopsy specimens one might rarely suspect a diagnosis of pleomorphic, spindle cell or giant cell carcinoma, however it would be impossible to make a definitive diagnosis.

Cytology
Pleomorphic carcinoma consists of malignant giant and/or spindle cells and epithelial components such as squamous or adenocarcinoma in smears {582,878}. The spindle and/or giant cells occur as cohesive aggregates of tumour cell, generally lacking any glandular or squamous differentiation. The neoplastic spindle cells are pleomorphic and elongated, singly or in loose clusters, bundles or tissue fragments. Nuclei are solitary, large and spindled, with prominent nucleoli. Nuclear-to-cytoplasmic ratios are high. Fragments of myxoid matrix

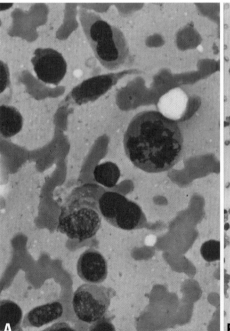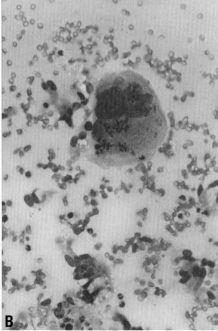

Fig. 1.51 Pleomorphic and sarcomatous carcinoma. **A** Huge individual neoplastic cells some of which have ovoid nuclei and one or two tails of basophilic cytoplasm. Several cells are multinucleated. Note the abnormal mitotic figure. Cohesion is distinctly lacking (Diff-Quik stain). **B** Solitary, huge multinucleated tumour giant cell in an aspiration biopsy of a giant cell carcinoma. The cell has multiple fused nuclei with coarse chromatin and distinct nucleoli (Diff-Quik stain).

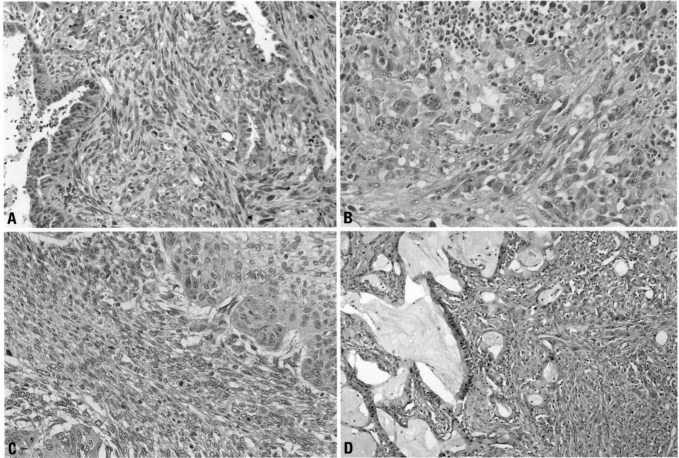

Fig. 1.52 A Pleomorphic carcinoma. Biphasic tumour with a clear-cut non-small cell carcinomatous component closely intermingled with a spindle cell carcinomatous component. **B** Mixed spindle cell carcinoma (SCC) and giant cell carcinoma (GCC). **C** Pleomorphic carcinoma consisting of a squamous cell carcinoma with a spindle cell component. **D** Pleomorphic carcinoma consisting of a mucinous adenocarcinoma (left) and spindle cell carcinoma (right). From Travis et al {2024}.

material may also be identified, as may malignant tumour giant cells. Both cell types are usually positive for cytokeratins in cell blocks.

Spindle cell carcinoma features malignant spindle cells with nuclear hyperchromasia and irregular, distinct nucleoli. Cohesion is generally better preserved than with true sarcomas, but isolated spindled epithelial cells may also be seen.

Giant cell carcinoma is cellular in cytological preparations and is characterized by a marked lack of intercellular cohesion {420,1489}. Accordingly, numerous individual multinucleated neoplastic giant cells are present. The nuclei vary from round and smooth to highly irregular with large nucleoli, which are often multiple, and coarse darkly stained chromatin granules. Cytoplasm may be abundant in these cells. Another characteristic feature is the smear background, which includes granular necrotic material and neutrophil leukocytes. Neutrophil emperipolesis is also characteristic.

When the malignant epithelial component is not evident within the smears, it could be difficult or impossible to distinguish a spindle cell or a giant cell carcinoma from a primary or metastatic spindle cell or pleomorphic sarcoma, respectively, based solely on cytomorphology {626,2182}. Here, immunocytochemistry performed on the smears or cell blocks, or obtaining an additional sample may be helpful.

In carcinosarcoma, and blastoma the cytologic smears contain heterologous sarcomatous elements, such as malignant cartilage, bone, or skeletal muscle, in addition to obvious carcinoma.

Macroscopy
Peripheral tumours are usually greater than 5 cm, well circumscribed and feature grey, yellow or tan creamy, gritty, mucoid and/or hemorrhagic cut surfaces

with significant necrosis. Sessile or pedunculated endobronchial tumours are smaller and often infiltrate underlying lung parenchyma {265,584,1213,1430, 1440,1442,1695}. Peripheral pulmonary blastomas are significantly larger than most NSCLC with a mean diameter of 10 cm.

Tumour spread and staging
These very aggressive tumours metastasize widely to the same sites as NSCLC, including unusual sites such as the esophagus, jejunum, rectum and kidney {154,265,330,584,1430}. Peripheral tumours usually present at a more advanced stage than central lesions. In general, stage at diagnosis is similar to that reported for the other non-small cell lung cancers {443,584,1213,1430,1440, 1695}.

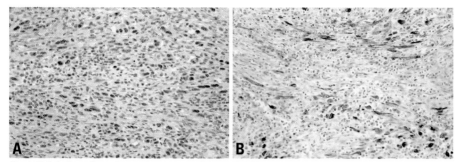
Fig. 1.53 Spindle cell carcinoma. Immunoreactivity for **A** TTF-1 and **B** cytokeratin 7.

Histopathology

Pleomorphic carcinoma:

A poorly differentiated non-small cell carcinoma, namely squamous cell carcinoma, adenocarcinoma or large cell carcinoma containing spindle cells and/or giant cells or, a carcinoma consisting only of spindle and giant cells. The spindle or giant cell component should comprise at least 10% of the tumour and while the presence of adenocarcinoma or squamous cell carcinoma should be documented, foci of large cell carcinoma need not be mentioned.

Histologic sections demonstrate conventional non-small cell carcinoma, namely adeno-, squamous cell or large cell subtypes, intimately associated with at least 10% malignant spindle cells and/or giant cells. Mitotically active spindle cells arranged haphazardly in a fascicular or storiform growth pattern have varying morphologic appearances ranging from epithelioid to mesenchymal sometimes with occasional smooth muscle features.

The stroma may be fibrous or myxoid. Dyscohesive malignant giant cells are polygonal, uni- or multinucleated, and have dense eosinophilic cytoplasm and pleomorphic nuclei. Emperipolesis is often present and large vessel invasion along with extensive necrosis are commonly seen. Rarely squamous cell carcinomas have an angiosarcomatoid component that has been called pseudoangiosarcomatous carcinoma. This is characterized by anastomosing channels lined by anaplastic, epithelioid cells focally aggregated in pseudopapillae and forming spaces filled with erythrocytes {1441,1442,1662}.

Spindle cell carcinoma

This variant is defined as a non-small cell carcinoma consisting of only spindle-shaped tumour cells. Identical to the spindle cell component of pleomorphic carcinoma, cohesive nests and irregular fascicles of overtly malignant cells feature nuclear hyperchromasia and distinct

nucleoli. Specific patterns of adenocarcinoma, squamous cell, giant cell or large cell carcinoma are not seen. Scattered and focally dense lymphoplasmacytic infiltrates surround and percolate through the tumoural mass. Rare cases with prominent inflammatory infiltrates may resemble inflammatory myofibroblastic tumour.

Giant cell carcinoma:

A non-small cell carcinoma composed of highly pleomorphic multi- and/or mononucleated tumour giant cells. Identical to the giant cell component of pleomorphic carcinoma, this tumour is composed entirely of giant cells and does not have specific patterns of either adenocarcinoma, squamous cell or large cell carcinoma. This tumour consists of very large, multinucleated and bizarre cells. Nuclei are pleomorphic, and often multilobed. The tumour cells are discohesive and tend to dissociate from each other {19,20,88,218,584,686,1695,2023, 2024}. There is generally a rich inflammatory infiltrate, usually of neutrophils, which frequently invade the tumour cells. This phenomenon was initially thought to represent phagocytosis by the tumour cells, but more probably reflects emperipolesis (active penetration of the leukocytes into the tumour cells) {934}. By electron microscopy, aggregates of paranuclear filaments and tonofibrils may be observed both in spindle cell and giant cell carcinomas {19,20,124,337, 584,1440,1664,1909,2023}. In giant cell

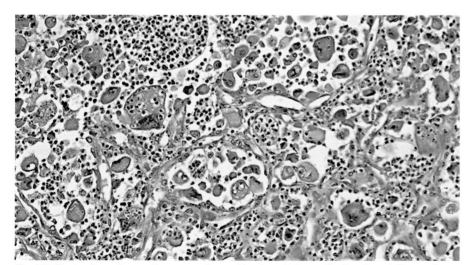
Fig. 1.54 Giant cell carcinoma. Numerous, often multinucleated giant cells. Prominent infiltrate of neutrophils, some of which permeate the tumour cell cytoplasm (emperipolesis). From Travis et al. {2024}.

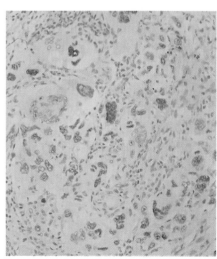
Fig. 1.55 TTF-1 expression in giant cell carcinoma (GCC).

carcinoma, only very occasional desmosomes are seen.

Carcinosarcoma:

This variant is defined as a malignant tumour with a mixture of carcinoma and sarcoma containing differentiated sarcomatous elements, such as malignant cartilage, bone or skeletal muscle.

The tumour is histologically biphasic, with a mixture of a conventional non-small cell lung carcinoma and true sarcoma containing differentiated elements. The carcinomatous component is most often squamous cell carcinoma (45-70%), followed by adenocarcinoma (20-31%), and large cell carcinoma (10%) {1061}. An epithelial component resembling so-called high grade fetal adenocarcinoma can occur in nearly 20% of cases, but the blastematous stroma of pulmonary blastoma is lacking {1061, 1436}. The malignant stroma often forms the bulk of carcinosarcomas, and only small foci of carcinoma may be seen. A significant component of these sarcomas is often poorly differentiated "spindle cell" sarcoma, but a careful search always shows areas of more specific sarcomatous differentiation, most often rhabdomyosarcoma, followed by osteosarcoma or chondrosarcoma or combinations of osteosarcoma and chondrosarcoma {1061}. More than one differentiated stromal component can be present. While metastatic foci usually feature both epithelial and mesenchymal com-

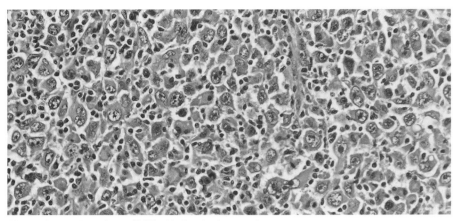

Fig. 1.56 Giant cell carcinoma (GCC) with discohesive growth pattern.

ponents, lesions may contain only one pattern.

Pulmonary blastoma:

This is a biphasic tumour containing a primitive epithelial component that may resemble well-differentiated fetal adenocarcinoma and a primitive mesenchymal stroma, which occasionally has foci of osteosarcoma, chondrosarcoma or rhabdomyosarcoma {2024}.

Pulmonary blastoma shows histologically a biphasic pattern with malignant gland growing in tubules that resemble fetal bronchioles, embedded in a sarcomatous embryonic-appearing mesenchyme {1857}. The glycogen-rich, non-ciliated tubules and primitive stroma resemble that seen in fetal lung between 10-16 weeks gestation (the pseudoglandular

stage of lung development) {2225}. The tubules can be well differentiated, resembling those reported in well-differentiated fetal adenocarcinomas, but they are usually less abundant. The tubules may also resemble a high-grade fetal adenocarcinoma. These tubules are lined by pseudostratified, non-ciliated columnar cells that have clear or lightly eosinophilic cytoplasm. The nuclei of the epithelial cells are oval or round and fairly uniform, but there can be cytologic atypia in the form of large multinucleated cells {2225}. The glands often have subnuclear or supranuclear vacuoles, producing an endometrioid appearance. The cytoplasmic vacuoles are due to abundant glycogen, readily demonstrated in periodic acid-Schiff stains. There may be small amounts of mucin within the glandular

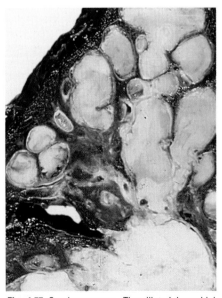

Fig. 1.57 Carcinosarcoma. The dilated bronchial tree is filled with a fleshy, cream-coloured masses.

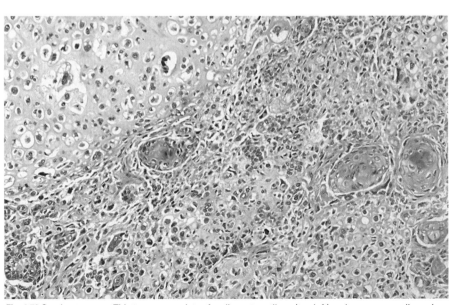

Fig. 1.58 Carcinosarcoma. This tumour consists of malignant cartilage (top left) and squamous cell carcinoma (bottom right). From Travis et al. {2024}.

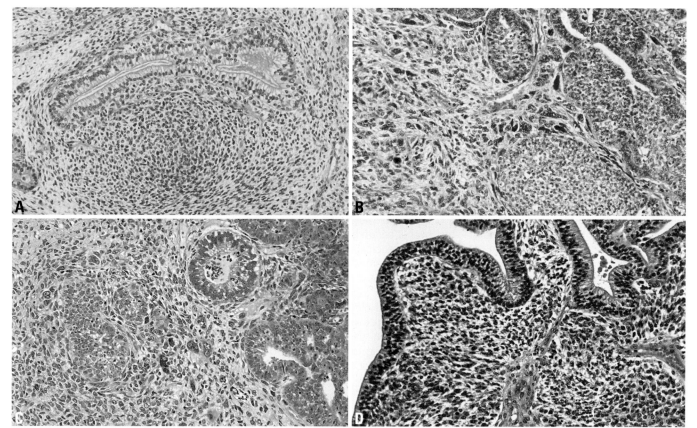

Fig. 1.59 Pulmonary blastoma. **A** Biphasic appearance, with a fetal-type gland and embryonic stroma. **B** Solid nests of epithelial cells and glands adjacent to an area of poorly differentiated spindle cell sarcoma. **C** The tumour consists of a spindle cell (left) and malignant glandular component (right). The glandular component resembles a well-differentiated fetal adenocarcinoma with endometrioid morphology. **D** Glandular pattern of a well-differentiated fetal adenocarcinoma with palisading of nuclei and abundant clear cytoplasm. The spindle cell component has a primitive malignant mesenchymal pattern. From Travis et al. {2024}.

lumens, but intracellular mucin is unusual. Similar to fetal adenocarcinomas, morular structures consisting of squamoid nests may be seen {605,917, 1064,1435,2225}.

Stromal cells generally have a blastema-like configuration. There is condensation of small oval and spindle cells in a myxoid stroma around neoplastic glands, similar to the appearance of Wilm's tumour of the kidney. Small foci of adult-type spindle cell sarcoma (most commonly showing a fascicular or storiform pattern) can be present. Foci of differentiated sarcomatous elements such as rhabdomyosarcoma, chondrosarcoma or osteosarcoma may be found {605,1064}.

Immunohistochemistry

Pleomorphic, spindle and or giant cell carcinoma:
Expression of epithelial markers in the spindle and/or giant cell component of a pleomorphic carcinoma is not required for the diagnosis so long as there is a component of squamous cell carcinoma,

adenocarcinoma, or large cell carcinoma {218,584,1430,1695,2023,2024}. Since these are poorly differentiated tumours, in some cases, multiple keratin antibodies and EMA are necessary to demonstrate epithelial differentiation in the sarcomatoid component. When pure spindle cell carcinomas fail to stain with any epithelial marker, separation from sarcoma may be difficult. The tumour cells often co-express cytokeratin, vimentin, carcinoembryonic antigen, and smooth muscle markers {20,88,337,584,1695}. TTF-1 may be positive in giant cell carcinomas.

Carcinosarcoma
The epithelial component of carcinosarcomas may stain with keratin antibodies. Chondrosarcoma will stain with S-100 protein and rhabdomyosarcoma with muscle markers.

Pulmonary blastoma
The fetal adenocarcinoma component of pulmonary blastomas will stain for

epithelial markers (keratin, EMA and CEA) and it may be positive for neuroendocrine markers such as chromogranin A as well in both morular and glandular cells {1064,1435}. The tumour cells can also express specific hormones, such as calcitonin, gastrin-releasing peptide, bombesin, leucine and methionine enkephalin, somatostatin and serotonin. This type of staining mimics that seen in developing fetal lung tubules {2225}. The epithelial component of blastomas diffusely stains with antibodies to epithelial markers, such as cytokeratin, carcinoembryonic antigen, and epithelial membrane antigen. Pulmonary blastomas rarely stain with alpha-fetoprotein {1824}. Both Clara cell antigen and surfactant apoprotein are expressed in epithelial cells and particularly in morules {1435, 2225}. Of interest, these antigens can also be seen in developing fetal lung tubules, which show differentiation towards Clara cells beginning at 13 weeks of gestation and towards Type II pneumocytes at 22 weeks {2225}.

Stromal cells of blastomas contain vimentin and muscle-specific actin. Desmin and myoglobin or S-100 protein can be seen when there is striated muscle or cartilage respectively. There is generally restriction of vimentin and cytokeratin to mesenchymal and epithelial tissues respectively {1064}, but vimentin can occur in glands and stromal cells can occasionally express cytokeratin {2225}.

Differential diagnosis

The differential diagnosis for pleomorphic carcinoma includes other tumours in this section as well as both primary and metastatic sarcomas. Identification of areas of non-small cell carcinoma and immunohistochemical confirmation of epithelial differentiation aid in the distinction.

Pleomorphic carcinoma may be difficult to distinguish from reactive processes and sarcomas {390,391,1440,2139}. A generous sampling (at least one section per centimeter of tumour diameter) to disclose a clear-cut carcinomatous component may be helpful in pleomorphic carcinomas, together with the use of ancillary techniques. It should be kept in mind that, although spindle cell carcinomas are rare, they are more common than primary sarcomas of the lung {1440, 2138}. Separation of spindle cell carcinoma from cytokeratin-positive sarcomas, particularly synovial sarcoma may be difficult {546,957,2236}. However, synovial sarcoma has a characteristic morphology, it tends to be only weakly or focally positive for keratin and demonstration of the X:18 translocation can be helpful. Spindle cell carcinomas may show a marked inflammatory infiltrate and therefore may be confused with an inflammatory myofibroblastic tumour or a localized area of organizing pneumonia; such a tumour with particularly bland neoplastic cells has been referred to as an inflammatory sarcomatoid carcinoma {390,391, 1440,2139}. Features favouring carcinoma include nuclear atypia coupled with brisk mitotic activity, vascular invasion, and positive immunostaining for cytokeratins, epithelial membrane antigen and thyroid transcription factor-1.

The differential diagnosis of giant cell carcinoma includes not only other types of lung carcinomas, but also primary and metastatic sarcomas including pleomorphic rhabdomyosarcoma, metastatic adrenocortical carcinoma, metastatic choriocarcinoma and other pleomorphic malignant tumours, most of which can be distinguished by their own distinctive markers. Beta-HCG staining can be seen in up to 20-93% of non-small cell carcinomas {207} and thus does not indicate a diagnosis of metastatic choriocarcinoma, even if serum beta-HCG is elevated. Benign osteoclast-like giant cells can populate non-small cell carcinomas, but these rare tumours should not be mistaken for giant cell carcinoma {187}.

The differential diagnosis of carcinosarcoma includes other tumours considered in this section as well as metastatic lesions including teratomas arising from the female gynaecologic tract and male genital tract.

Biphasic blastoma should be distinguished from a fetal adenocarcinoma, pleuropulmonary blastoma as well as primary and metastatic sarcomas including synovial sarcoma. Immunohistochemical and molecular studies in addition to morphologic features should differentiate these tumours.

Histogenesis

Sarcomatoid carcinomas represent malignant epithelial neoplasms that have undergone divergent connective tissue differentiation ("tumour metaplasia" or "divergence hypothesis") and not "collision" tumours (multiclonal hypothesis) {431,866,1078,1440,1738,2002}. The light microscopic finding of transition between epithelial and spindle cell components of most tumours, the finding of carcinoma in-situ in some, and the immunohistochemical and ultrastructural identification of epithelial differentiation in the spindle cell components support this theory {745}. P53 mutational genotyping of a small number of pleomorphic carcinomas, carcinosarcomas and blastomas demonstrated identical mutations in spindle cells and epithelium, supporting the contention that both epithelial and mesenchymal components originate from a single clone {189,866}.

Somatic genetics

Molecular studies have established that the epithelial and sarcomatoid components of pleomorphic carcinoma have identical molecular profiles, including equivalent patterns of acquired allelic loss {431}, p53 mutation profile {866} and X chromosome inactivation {2002}. A high percentage of pleomorphic carcinomas were reported to have variant CYP1A12 {1624}. The molecular profiles of these tumours are not unlike those of other non-small cell tumours. Mutations in beta-catenin were recently shown in blastomas {1779,1801}.

Prognosis and predictive factors
Clinical criteria

Clinical outcome is stage dependent but these tumours have a worse prognosis than conventional non-small cell carcinomas {330,584,1261,1430,1695,1976}. Despite the fact that one half of patients present with stage I disease, the 5-year survival is only 20% {218,584,1430,1695, 2023,2029}. Adjuvant chemotherapy and radiotherapy do not appear helpful {330, 443,584,1430,1440,1664,1695,1741, 1870}.

Carcinoid tumour

M.B. Beasley
F.B. Thunnissen
Ph.S. Hasleton
M. Barbareschi
B. Pugatch

K. Geisinger
E. Brambilla
A. Gazdar
W.D. Travis

Definitions

Carcinoid tumours are characterized by growth patterns (organoid, trabecular, insular, palisading, ribbon, rosette-like arrangements) that suggest neuroendocrine differentiation. Tumour cells have uniform cytologic features with moderate eosinophilic, finely granular cytoplasm, and nuclei with a finely granular chromatin pattern.
Typical carcinoid (TC): A carcinoid tumour with fewer than 2 mitoses per 2 mm^2 and lacking necrosis.
Atypical carcinoid (AC): A carcinoid tumour with 2-10 mitoses per 2 mm^2 and/or foci of necrosis.

ICD-O codes

Carcinoid	8240/3
Typical carcinoid	8240/3
Atypical carcinoid	8249/3

Synonyms

The following synonyms have been used, but are no longer recommended.
Typical carcinoid: Well differentiated neuroendocrine carcinoma, Kultchitsky cell carcinoma – grade 1, mature carcinoid.
Atypical carcinoid: malignant carcinoid, moderately differentiated neuroendocrine carcinoma, grade 2 neuroendocrine carcinoma.

Localization

TC is uniformly distributed throughout the lungs {391,2026} whereas AC is more commonly peripheral {128}.

Clinical features

Signs and symptoms

Up to half of all bronchopulmonary carcinoids indentified as an incidental radiographic finding {580}. The most common symptoms cough and haemoptysis typically relate to bronchial obstruction. Cushing's syndrome due to ectopic ACTH production is uncommon {2026}. The carcinoid syndrome is rare and only occurs when there are widespread metastases {580}. MEN1 syndrome is another rare association {1439}.

Imaging

Carcinoid tumours are seen as well defined pulmonary nodules {613}. Calcification is often seen. Cavitation and irregular margins are rare and pleural effusions are uncommon. Endobronchial tumours can sometimes be directly demonstrated on CT and obstructive atelectasis or consolidation and mucoid impaction may be evident distal to the mass. Because of their vascularity, carcinoid tumours often show intense contrast enhancement. PET scaning may be negative. TC and AC tumours are indistinguishable radiographically.

Diagnostic procedures

Carcinoid tumours can be diagnosed reliably by cytology of fine needle aspiration or bronchoscopic specimens, but sputum samples are often hypocellular {53,673,936,1329,1457,1940}. In most cases the diagnosis can be made by bronchoscopic biopsy. However, separation of TC from AC usually requires examination of a resected specimen unless mitoses and/or necrosis are seen on a bronchoscopic biopsy.

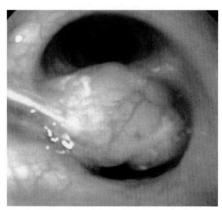

Fig. 1.60 Bronchoscopic image of a typical carcinoid, presenting as a polypoid endobronchial mass.

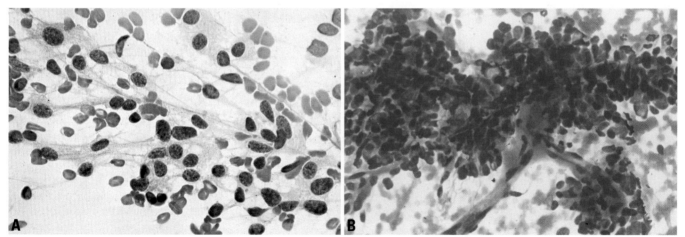

Fig. 1.61 Carcinoid. **A** Loose aggregates of slightly irregular small sized tumor cells. Delicate, capillaries with loosely attached radiating tumor cells. Round or oval nuclei with a irregular 'salt and pepper' chromatin pattern. **B** Aspiration biopsy showing the classic association of carcinoid tumor cells with arborizing delicate capillaries. Note the striking uniformity of the neoplastic elements. Diff-Quik stain.

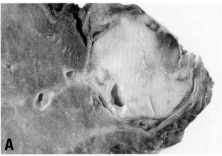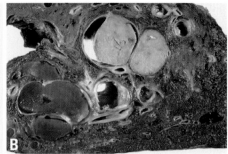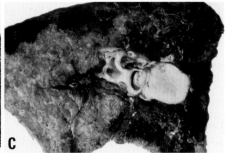

Fig. 1.62 A Central bronchial carcinoid tumour in a 26 year old woman. **B** More peripherally located carcinoid tumour with bronchiectasis. **C** Typical carcinoid presenting as round, partially endobronchial mass. Note the post-stenotic pneumonia.

Cytology

Carcinoid tumours are generally identifiable in cytological specimens although haemorrhage may dilute brush samples {53,673,936,1329,1457,1940}. The neoplastic cells are generally present both individually and in cohesive aggregates. The latter include acini, flat sheets, trabeculae, and vascularized connective tissue fragments; the latter typically present solely in aspiration smears {1329}.

There is a striking uniformity of the neoplastic cells. These are small and may be difficult to distinguish from plasma cells, especially in aspiration specimens. Usually, they are oval with moderate amounts of cytoplasm. The latter is basophilic and occasionally granular. The nuclei are uniformly round or ovoid.

Finely stippled chromatin granules give the nucleus a characteristic "salt and pepper" pattern. Nucleoli are small and inconspicuous. Isolated tumour cells have more peripheral nuclei. Infrequently, carcinoids are composed of spindle cells {421,566}.

In most cytologic specimens, the smear background is clean but in aspiration biopsies it often contains abundant basophilic granular material.

In AC, the neoplastic cells may be more pleomorphic and larger {619,942,1940} and the nuclei show slightly greater chromatin staining.

Macroscopy

TC and AC both form firm, well demarcated, tan to yellow tumours. TC in particular is typically associated with bronchi and are frequently endobronchial. The overlying mucosa may be intact or ulcerated. Squamous metaplasia may be seen. Other bronchial carcinoids push down into the adjacent lung parenchyma. Association with an airway may not be readily evident in peripheral tumours {391,1844}.

Tumour spread and staging

At presentation approximately 10-15% of TC have metastasized to regional lymph nodes and 5-10% of cases eventually metastasize to distant sites such as liver or bone. At presentation, 40-50% of AC have metastasized to regional lymph nodes and beyond with approximately 20% Stage II, 15% Stage III and 10% Stage IV {128}. Although the TNM classification applies to carcinomas of the lung, it has been used to stage carcinoids of the lung.

Histopathology

Carcinoid tumours are classically composed of uniform polygonal cells with finely granular chromatin, inconspicuous nucleoli and scant to moderate amounts of eosinophilic cytoplasm {1844}. Oncocytic tumours have abundant eosinophilic cytoplasm {391,2026}. Rarely the tumour cell cytoplasm is clear or it may contain melanin {647,653}. Intracytoplasmic mucus is very unusual. Nuclear atypia and pleomorphism may be quite marked, even in TC, but these features are unreliable criteria for distinguishing TC from AC {2028}. Prominent nucleoli may be observed {1844,2026}. A variety of growth patterns are encountered frequently within one tumour. The most common patterns are the organoid and trabecular, in which the tumour cells are respectively arranged in nests or cords. Other patterns include spindle

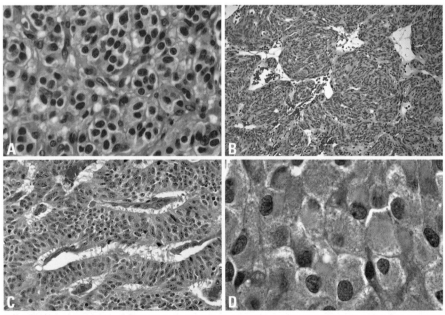

Fig. 1.63 Typical carcinoid. **A** Tumour cells grow in an organoid nesting arrangement, with a fine vascular stroma. The moderate amount of cytoplasm is eosinophilic and the nuclear chromatin finely granular. **B** Prominent spindle cell pattern. **C** Trabecular pattern. **D** Oncocytic features with abundant eosinophilic cytoplasm. From W. Travis et al. {2024}.

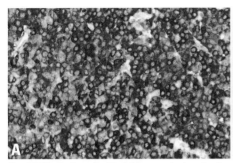 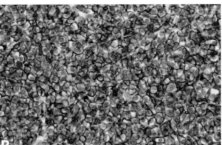 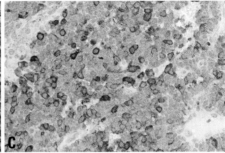

Fig. 1.64 Typical carcinoid. **A** Strong cytoplasmic chromogranin staining. **B** The tumour cells show strong membranous staining for CD56. **C** Scattered tumour cells show strong cytoplasmic ACTH staining in patient presenting with Cushing syndrome due to ectopic ACTH production.

cell, papillary, pseudoglandular, rosette formation and follicular {391,1246,2026}. True gland formation is rare.

There is generally a highly vascularized fibrovascular stroma, but in some tumours the stroma is hyalinized, or it shows cartilage or bone formation {391}. Stromal amyloid is rare {35,537}. The adjacent airway epithelium may show neuroendocrine cell hyperplasia, sometimes associated with airway fibrosis, as described in diffuse idiopathic neuroendocrine cell hyperplasia {29,1317}. This is seen most often in association with peripheral carcinoids. In rare cases there are also multiple tumourlets or multiple carcinoid tumours {1314}.

AC shows either focal necrosis or mitoses numbering between 2-10/2mm^2 {2026,2028}. AC may exhibit all of the growth patterns and cytologic features listed above for TC.

Immunohistochemistry

Most carcinoid tumours stain for cytokeratin but up to 20% may be keratin negative {128,272,2026}. Neuroendocrine markers such as chromogranin, synaptophysin, Leu-7 (CD57) and N-CAM (CD56) are typically strongly positive, particularly in TC {600,2026,2028}. However, in AC, staining for these markers may be patchy or focal. S-100 protein may highlight the presence of sustentacular cells {108,718}. Varying results are published for TTF-1 with some indicating TC and AC are usually negative {1894} but others finding approximately a third of TC and most AC are positive {600, 1513,2134}. The explanation for this discrepancy is not known. CD99, is also positive in many carcinoids {1565,2134}. Ki 67 is more often positive in AC than TC and is related to survival {416}. EM demonstrates desmosomes and dense core neurosecretory granules {2110}.

Differential diagnosis

The differential diagnosis of carcinoid tumours includes separation from other neuroendocrine tumours, and a wide variety of other tumours depending on the cytology or pattern of the carcinoid. It may be difficult to address the differential diagnosis based on small specimens obtained by bronchoscopy or fine needle aspiration. Carcinoid tumourlets resemble TC and are only distinguished by size, being less than 5 mm in diameter {373}. TC and AC are distinguished by the criteria outlined above and this distinction usually requires a surgical specimen. The high-grade neuroendocrine tumours, large cell neuroendocrine carcinoma (LCNEC) and small cell lung carcinoma (SCLC) are distinguished by having a mitotic rate greater than 10 / 2mm^2. Ordinarily the rate is much higher than this, making these two tumours easily distinguishable from AC. The presence of large areas of necrosis is also against the diagnosis of AC {128, 2026,2028}.

Pseudoglandular or gland-like patterns in carcinoid tumours can be mistaken with adenocarcinoma, mucoepidermoid carcinoma, and adenoid cystic carcinoma. Adenocarcinomas usually show more cytologic atypia, mucin production and less staining for neuroendocrine markers than carcinoids. Mucoepidermoid carcinomas are negative for neuroendocrine markers and they produce mucin. The solid component of adenoid cystic carcinomas may be mistaken for carcinoid, but these cells are negative for neuroendocrine markers {1368}.

The organoid nesting pattern of carcinoid tumours can be confused with paragangliomas, which are very rare in the lung. The presence of S-100 positive sustentacular cells in some carcinoids may also cause confusion {108,718}. A key discriminating feature is the lack of cytokeratin staining in paraganglioma, which is frequently positive in carcinoids {391}. Glomus tumour may also resemble carcinoid but it is positive for smooth muscle actin and negative for neuroendocrine markers {645}.

Spindle cell carcinoids may be confused with various mesenchymal tumours, particularly smooth muscle tumours; recognition of the finely granular nuclear chromatin and organoid nesting pattern this can generally be resolved morphologically and with appropriate immunohistochemical stains.

Carcinoids with a prominent papillary pattern may be confused with sclerosing hemangioma but this tumour is negative with neuroendocrine stains {488}.

The epithelial pattern of a carcinoid can be mimicked by metastatic breast or prostate carcinoma. Although the architecture may be the same, the nuclei in the latter have a more vesicular chromatin pattern. In addition, immunohistochemistry is helpful for the distinction since PSA is positive in prostate carcinoma, while neuroendocrine markers and TTF1 are negative {61,391}.

Grading

Carcinoid tumours are divided into the low grade TC and intermediate grade AC based on the criteria outlined above.

Histogenesis

Pulmonary carcinoid tumours are derived from neuroendocrine cells known to exist in normal airways. In fetal lung, neuroendocrine cells are numerous and are known to play an important role in lung development {539,761,1141}. They are less common in the lungs of adults, but various stimuli result in neuroendocrine cell hyperplasia {28,719,720}. However, none of these stimuli is recognized to be

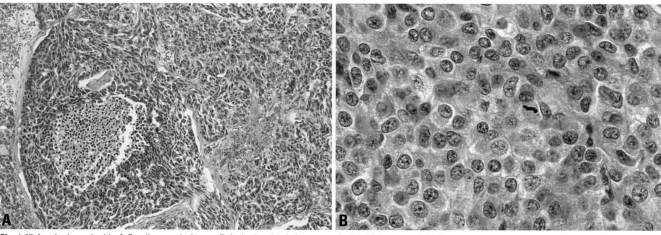

Fig. 1.65 Atypical carcinoid. **A** Small necrotic focus. **B** A single mitosis is present in this high power field. The tumour cells show carcinoid morphology with moderate eosinophilic cytoplasm and finely granular nuclear chromatin. From Travis et al. {2024}.

of importance of carcinoid tumours. The very rare condition of diffuse idiopathic pulmonary neuroendocrine cell hyperplasia (DIPNECH) is recognized to be a preinvasive lesion for carcinoids {29, 2024}.

Somatic genetics
Cytogenetics and CGH
Unbalanced chromosomal aberrations as observed by comparative genomic hybridization (CGH) are rare in carcinoids except underrepresentation of 11q material including MEN1 gene in 0-50% of typical carcinoids and 50-70% of atypical carcinoids {2052,2097}. Atypical carcinoids but not typical carcinoids may show 10q and 13q underrepresentation {2097}.

Molecular genetics
Carcinoids have features of neuroendocrine cells, in common with small cell lung cancer and also share some genetic alterations. In general, atypical carcinoids (AC) have more extensive changes than typical carcinoids. A distinctive feature of carcinoids not found in other lung cancers is the frequent presence of mutations of the MEN1 gene and absence of its protein product, menin {463,1516}, even though virtually all bronchial carcinoids are sporadic and not familial tumours. The mutations are accompanied by allelic loss at the MEN1 locus at 11p13. These features are also found in gastrointestinal carcinoids.
Loss of heterozygosity (LOH) at 3p, 13q, 9p21 and 17p is rare in TC but present in AC but at frequencies lower than in SCLC {1516}.

LOH at 3p (3p14.3-21.3) at has been found in 40% of AC, which is significantly lower than other NSCLC including the high-grade neuroendocrine tumours LCNEC and SCLC (p<0,001). LOH at Rb locus (13p14) and retinoblastoma gene pathway inhibitor (Rb) is rare in typical carcinoids {127,269,726,727} but present in 20% of AC {127}. Similarly, Rb expression is normal in typical carcinoids but lost in 21% of atypical carcinoids. Cyclin D1 is overexpressed in 6% of TC {127} LOH is at 9p21 (P16) is observed in a few (20%) AC and TC {1516}. In contrast to smoking associated lung cancers that often show G:T transversions, AC show P53 point mutation of an unusual type (G:C to A:T transitions or nonsense mutations) {1516}. The p53 pathway is infrequently affected and inactivated in carcinoids, and is extremely rare in TC. Accordingly P53 aberrant stabilization is not seen in TC and seen in rare cases of AC {217,1622}. Other proteins of Rb/P53 pathways such as E2F1 are rarely affected in TC but more often in AC. P14ARF protein loss occurs in 6% of TC and 43% of AC {549,669}. Methylation of tumour suppressor genes is infrequently seen in TC and AC {1814,2019}. Methylation index was lower in carcinoids than in SCLC There was no difference in methylation frequencies and index between TC and AC except for RASSF1A methylation (a gene with functions similar to Ras), which is observed in 71% of AC (as frequently as in SCLC) and in 45% of TC {2019}. Caspase 8 promoter methylation occurs in 18% of carcinoids {1814}. Except for this important proapoptotic molecule, methylation and silencing of

tumour suppressor genes is relatively rare in carcinoids compared to other lung cancers {1814,2017,2019}.

Expression profiles
Limited expression data are available for carcinoid tumours. Those data, which are available, indicate that carcinoid tumours are more similar to neuronal tumours than to normal bronchial epithelial cells or small cell carcinoma {52}.

Prognosis and predictive factors
Clinical and histopathological criteria
The overall 5- and 10-year survival rates are worse for AC (61-73% and 35-59%) than TC (90-98% and 82-95%, p<0.001) {128,1844,2028}. After separation of TC from AC, stage is the most important prognostic factor {128,2028}. However, even with lymph node metastasis, TC carries an excellent prognosis {1999}. With AC size over 3.5 cm also conveys a worse prognosis {128}. Further histopathological prognostic criteria (beyond necrosis and mitoses) include vascular invasion and nuclear pleomorphism {2028}. Negative predictors of prognosis in AC include mitotic rate, pleomorphism, and aerogenous spread, whereas palisading, papillary formation, and pseudoglandular patterns are favourable prognostic features {128}.

Mucoepidermoid carcinoma

S.A. Yousem
A.G. Nicholson

Definition
A malignant epithelial tumour characterized by the presence of squamoid cells, mucin-secreting cells and cells of intermediate type. It is histologically identical to the salivary gland tumour of the same name.

ICD-O code
Mucoepidermoid carcinoma 8430/3

Synonyms
Mucoepidermoid tumour.

Epidemiology
Mucoepidermoid tumours comprise less than 1% of all lung tumours {732,2040, 2221}. They have an equal sex distribution with a slight predilection for men and have an age range of 3-78 years with 50% of tumours occurring in individuals less than 30 years, and most patients presenting in the third and fourth decade {811,2221}. There is a suggestion of predilection for Caucasians over Blacks. They form a significant proportion of pediatric endobronchial tumours.

Etiology
There appears to be no association with cigarette smoking or other risk factors.

Localization
The majority arise from bronchial glands in the central airways. Tumours with this histology that are encountered in the peripheral lung should raise the question

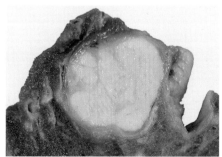

Fig. 1.66 Mucoepidermoid carcinoma. The well circumscribed, light tan mass does not grossly infiltrate the underlying lung parenchyma.

of metastatic tumour or adenosquamous carcinoma.

Clinical features
Signs and symptoms
Signs and symptoms are related to the polypoid endobronchial growth of this tumour and tracheal and large airway irritation {398,1011,1646}. Wheeze, haemoptysis, and recurrent pneumonia with post-obstructive changes are most often noted, although up to 25% of patients may be asymptomatic.

Imaging
Chest radiographs and CT scans demonstrate a well-circumscribed oval or lobulated mass arising within the bronchus {612}. Calcification is occasionally seen. Post-obstructive pneumonic infiltrates are often noted, occasionally with cavitation.

Macroscopy
Grossly, these tumours usually occur in the main, lobar or segmental bronchi, ranging in size from 0.5-6 cm with an average size of approximately 2.2 cm {811,2221}. They are soft, polypoid, and pink-tan in colour often with cystic change and a glistening mucoid appearance. Extension between bronchial cartilaginous plates is occasionally noted. Distal obstructive / cholesterol pneumonia may be seen. High-grade lesions are usually more infiltrative.

Tumour spread and staging
Low-grade mucoepidermoid tumours spread to regional lymph nodes by local growth in less than 5% of cases, although distant spread rarely occurs. High-grade tumours involve not only regional nodes but may metastasize to liver, bones, adrenal gland, and brain.

Histopathology
On the basis of morphological and cytological features, tumours are divided into low and high-grade types. In low-grade tumours, cystic changes often dominate and solid areas typically comprise mucin

secreting and columnar epithelium forming small glands, tubules, and cysts. Necrosis is inconspicuous. These cysts often contain inspissated mucus, which has a colloid-like appearance and frequently is calcified. The lining cells are cytologically bland with round to oval nuclei, abundant eosinophilic, mucin-rich cytoplasm, and infrequent mitotic figures. Often, intimately admixed with this mucinous epithelium are non-keratinizing squamoid cells that grow in a sheet-like pattern with intercellular bridges. The third cellular component is an intermediate or transitional cell that is oval in shape, has a round nucleus and faint eosinophilic cytoplasm. The accompanying stroma is often oedematous with foci of dense stromal hyalinization, particularly around the glandular elements, that may have an amyloid-like appearance. Stromal calcification and ossification, with a granulomatous reaction is seen around areas of mucus extravasation.

High-grade mucoepidermoid carcinomas are rare and have histologic features that overlap with adenosquamous carcinoma {811,1445,2221}. They consist largely of intermediate and squamoid cells with a minor component of mucin secreting elements. They demonstrate nuclear atypia with hyperchromatism, pleomorphism, brisk mitotic activity and a high nuclear to cytoplasmic ratio. These lesions often invade the pulmonary parenchyma and may be associated with positive regional lymph nodes. Controversy exists in their separation from adenosquamous carcinoma. Criteria more typical of high grade mucoepidermoid tumours include: (1) exophytic endobronchial growth, (2) surface epithelium lacking changes of in-situ carcinoma, (3) absence of individual cell keratinization and squamous pearl formation, (4) transitional areas to low grade mucoepidermoid carcinoma.

Histogenesis
Mucoepidermoid carcinomas are histologically similar to their counterparts in the salivary glands and it has been pre-

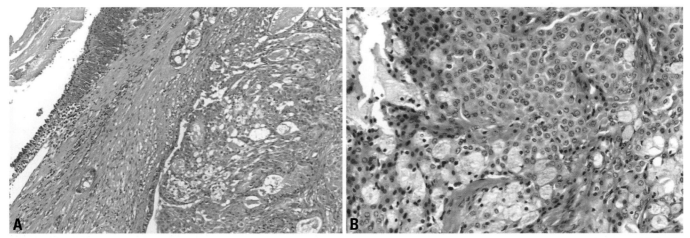

Fig. 1.67 Mucoepidermoid carcinoma. **A** Mucoepidermoid carcinomas arise in the submucosa of the airways, in association with the tracheobronchial glands. Variably solid and cystic appearance. **B** Goblet cells containing abundant mucin and form glandular arrays with centrally located extracellular mucosubstance. Squamoid cells with a polygonal appearance, round nuclei, irregularly distributed chromatin, inconspicuous nucleoli and abundant cytoplasm. Intercellular bridges and keratinization are absent. Transitional cells occupy an intermediate cytomorphology between squamoid and mucin producing elements.

sumed that they are derived from primitive cells differentiating within the tracheobronchial mucous glands.

Somatic genetics

No consistent cytogenetic abnormalities have been noted with mucoepidermoid carcinomas of the tracheobronchial tree.

Genetic susceptibility

No genetic susceptibilities are noted with mucoepidermoid tumours. It should be noted, however, that the pediatric population comprises a significant percentage of patients with this lesion.

Prognosis and predictive factors

Low-grade mucoepidermoid tumours have a much better prognosis than high-grade tumours, the latter being similar to non-small cell carcinomas {732,811, 2221}. Low-grade tumours rarely metastasize with less than 5% of reported cases metastasizing to regional lymph nodes. Children have a particularly benign clinical course. Low-grade tumours are often treated with bronchoplastic procedures such as sleeve resection.

High-grade mucoepidermoid carcinomas are generally treated similar to non-small cell carcinomas. Their prognosis is much more guarded as they tend to behave as non-small cell carcinomas.

Diagnostic features, which indicate a high likelihood of recurrence, metastasis, or death include constitutional signs and symptoms including pain, weight loss, malaise. Positive margins of resection; positive hilar lymph nodes and local aggressive behaviour, such as chest wall invasion are also adverse factors {398, 732,2221}.

Adenoid cystic carcinoma

S.A. Yousem
A.G. Nicholson

Definition

Adenoid cystic carcinoma is a malignant epithelial neoplasm, recapitulating its counterpart in the salivary glands, with a distinctive histologic pattern of growth of the epithelial cells in cribriform, tubular and glandular arrays orientated around and associated with a variably mucinous and hyalinized basement membrane-rich extracellular matrix, with the cells showing differentiation characteristics of duct lining and myoepithelial cells.

ICD-O code   8200/3

Synonyms

Cylindroma and adenocystic carcinoma.

Epidemiology

Adenoid cystic carcinoma of the lung and bronchus comprises less than 1% of all lung tumours {809,2029}. It has an equal sex distribution and tends to occur in the fourth and fifth decades of life {1368}. In the majority of cases adenoid cystic carcinoma behaves in an insidious and indolent fashion with multiple local recurrences preceding metastases.

Etiology

There appears to be no association with cigarette smoking or other risk factor(s).

Localization

90% of cases originate intraluminally within trachea, main stem or lobar bronchi {1621}.

Clinical features

Presentation reflects proximal airway obstruction with shortness of breath, cough, wheeze, chest pain and haemoptysis described {833,1271,1487,1560, 2014}. Radiographs show a centrally located mass that may have an endobronchial component or may form plaques or annular lesions in the wall of bronchi {1271}. Extension into the pulmonary parenchyma is often present and occasionally into mediastinal fat.

Macroscopy

Adenoid cystic carcinoma typically forms gray-white or tan polypoid lesions thickening the submucosa of the bronchus, sometimes with no alteration of the surface mucosa. It also may form diffuse infiltrative plaques that extend in a longitudinal and/or circumferential fashion beneath the submucosa. Size ranges from 1–4 cm with an average of 2 cm {1368}. A distinctive feature is that it has deceptively infiltrative margins, which extend far beyond the localized nodule noted grossly and therefore sampling of peribronchial soft tissue is worthwhile.

Tumour spread and staging

Staging of adenoid cystic carcinomas is performed according to the AJCC and UICC TNM staging system. Adenoid cystic carcinoma is predisposed to recur within the lung parenchyma, the pleura, chest wall, and mediastinum before metastasizing late to liver, brain, bone, spleen, kidney, and adrenal glands. Regional lymph node metastases are seen in approximately 20% of cases and systemic metastases in approximately 40%.

Histopathology

Architecturally, adenoid cystic carcinoma often breaches the cartilaginous plate extending into the pulmonary parenchyma, hilar and mediastinal soft tissues. Its growth pattern is typically heterogeneous, with neoplastic cells arranged in cribriform arrays, tubules or solid nests. The most characteristic cribriform pattern shows cells surrounding cylinders in a sclerotic acid mucopolysaccharide-rich basement membrane-like material. The neoplastic cells are small with scant cytoplasm and dark hyperchromatic

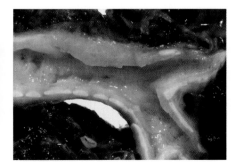

Fig. 1.68 Adenoid cystic carcinoma arising within the bronchus.

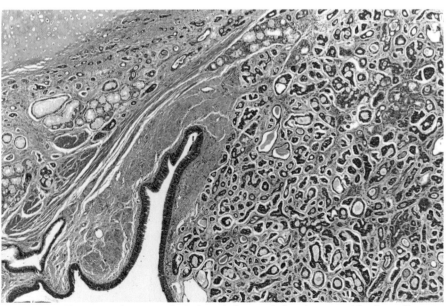

Fig. 1.69 Adenoid cystic carcinoma growing in the typical pattern in the submucosa of the airway. Note preserved, intact respiratory mucosa.

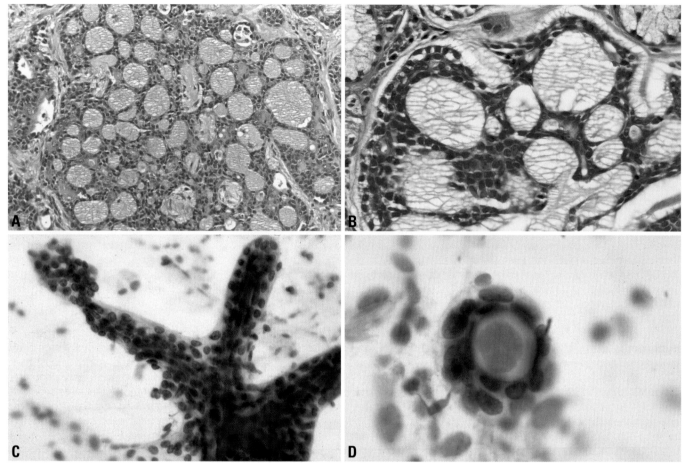

Fig. 1.70 Adenoid cystic carcinoma. **A** Adenoid cystic carcinoma was historically termed cylindroma: neoplastic cells typically form cylinders of basophilic mucoid and basement membrane-like material surrounded by hyperchromatic angulated epithelial cells. **B** Cylinders are surrounded by small hyperchromatic cells with dense oval nuclei having scant eosinophilic cytoplasm. Occasional tubular differentiation is noted. **C** Finger-like stromal structure. Cohesive cells with oval nuclei and little cytoplasm. Bronchial brushing. Papanicolaou stain. **D** Translucent hyaline globule surrounded by small uniform epithelial cells. Bronchial brushing. Papanicolaou stain.

nuclei that are oval to angulated, and show infrequent mitotic figures. Occasionally, these cells form tubules lined by two to three cells, with the luminal cells having a low cuboidal appearance and the peripheral cells forming a myoepithelial layer. Perineural invasion is seen in 40% of cases and extension along vascular structures, bronchi and bronchioles, and lymphatics is characteristic.

Immunoperoxidase stains show that the neoplastic cells have a variable ductal and myoepithelial phenotype, the cells expressing cytokeratin but also vimentin, smooth muscle actin, calponin, S-100 protein, p63, and GFAP. The surrounding matrix recapitulates a basement membrane like material in that it stains positive with antibodies directed at Type IV collagen, laminin, and heparin sulfate.

Histogenesis

Adenoid cystic carcinoma is derived from a primitive cell, presumably of tracheobronchial gland origin, which shows differentiation characteristics of ductal and myoepithelial cells.

Prognosis and predictive factors

The behavior of adenoid cystic carcinoma is one of multiple recurrences with late metastases and survival needs to be analyzed over a prolonged period (10-15 years) {398,1271,1560,1621}. Patients are prone to develop local recurrence because of difficulty obtaining clear margins and it is recommended that margins of resection be analyzed by frozen section at the time of primary surgery. Primary treatment is surgery with supplemental radiation, especially by linear accelerator. Poor prognosis is related to stage of the tumour at the time of diagnosis, the presence of positive margins, and a solid cellular growth pattern.

Epithelial-myoepithelial carcinoma

S.A. Yousem
A.G. Nicholson

The tracheobronchial tree may be the site of origin for a wide variety of salivary gland tumours {1187,1364,1563,1883, 1883}. These include epithelial-myoepithelial carcinoma, acinic cell carcinoma, carcinoma ex pleomorphic adenoma and malignant endobronchial myxoid tumour. Of these only epithelial-myoepithelial carcinomas have been analysed in significant numbers.

Definition
Epithelial-myoepithelial carcinomas consist of myoepithelial cells with spindle cell, clear cell or plasmacytoid morphology and varying amounts of duct-forming epithelium.

ICD-O code   8562/3

Synonyms
Adenomyoepithelioma, myoepithelioma, epithelial-myoepithelial carcinoma, epithelial-myoepithelial tumour, epimyoepithelial carcinoma, epithelial-myoepithelial tumour of unproven malignant potential and malignant mixed tumour comprising epithelial and myoepithelial cells.

Epidemiology
Age ranges from 33 to 71 years with no sex predominance.

Etiology
There appears to be no association with cigarette smoking or other risk factor(s).

Localization
The tumors are nearly all endobronchial in location.

Clinical features
Presenting symptoms and imaging reflect airway obstruction {639,1480, 2037}.

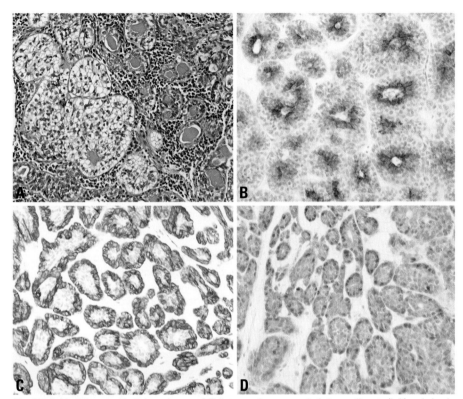

Fig. 1.71 Epithelial-myoepithelial carcinoma. **A** This tumour is composed of clear cell nests (left) and glands (right) some of which have a double layer of cells with an inner layer of eosinophilic cells and an outer layer of clear cells. **B** The inner layer of ductal cells is immunostained by cytokeratin 7. **C** The outer layer of myoepithelial cells is immunostained by smooth muscle actin. **D** The outer layer of myoepithelial cells is immunostained by S100 protein.

Macroscopy
The cut surface ranges from solid to gelatinous in texture and white to gray in colour {639,1480,2037}.

Histopathology
Tumours comprise myoepithelial cells that are spindled or rounded and contain eosinophilic or clear cell cytoplasm, plus a variable proportion of duct-forming epithelium {639,1480,2037}.
Occasional purely myoepitheliomatous tumours are described. Ducts are typically lined by a dual layer of cells, comprising an inner layer of cuboidal cells with eosinophilic cytoplasm and an outer layer of cells with predominantly clear cytoplasm. Mitotic activity is generally low. Generally, the inner layer of ducts stains for MNF116 and EMA and the outer layer plus solid components stain for SMA and S-100, although there may be some overlap.

Prognosis and predictive factors
Surgical resection is the treatment of choice and usually curative, although late recurrence may occur {639,1480, 2037}.

Squamous dysplasia and carcinoma in situ

W.A. Franklin
I.I. Wistuba
K. Geisinger
S. Lam
F.R. Hirsch

K.M. Muller
G. Sozzi
E. Brambilla
A. Gazdar

Definition

A precursor lesion of squamous cell carcinoma arising in the bronchial epithelium. Squamous dysplasia and carcinoma in situ are a continuum of recognizable histologic changes in the large airways. They can occur as single or multifocal lesions throughout the tracheobronchial tree. Dysplasia or carcinoma in situ may exist as an isolated finding or as a bronchial surface lesion accompanying invasive carcinoma

ICD-O code

Squamous cell carcinoma
in situ   8070/2

Synonyms and historical annotation

Squamous atypia, angiogenic squamous dysplasia, bronchial premalignancy, preinvasive squamous lesion, high-grade intraepithelial neoplasia, early non-invasive cancer.

The existence of central airway squamous lesions regarded as progenitors of squamous carcinoma has been recognized for decades {93}. They were initially graded according to complicated descriptive criteria including the loss of cilia, thickness (number of cell layers) of the epithelium, the degree of atypia and the percentage of atypical cells {94,95}, but a manageable and reproducible classification was recently published {1465,2024}.

Clinical features

Squamous dysplasia is nearly always asymptomatic but occurs in individuals with heavy tobacco exposure (more than 30 pack years of cigarette smoking) and with obstructive airway disease {849, 1389}. Pre-invasive squamous bronchial lesions are found more frequently in men than in women {1118}.

Relevant diagnostic procedures

Sputum cytology examination

Currently, the only non-invasive test that can detect pre-invasive lesions is sputum cytology examination {620,993}.

20% of patients with greater than a 30 pack year history of smoking, airway obstruction with forced expiratory volume 1 (FEV1) <70% of expected have moderate dysplasia or worse by fluorescence bronchoscopy {1533}. Of those with moderate atypia on sputum cytology, at least 55% have dysplasia detectable by fluorescence bronchoscopy. Sputum atypia as an independent variable in predicting dysplasia at fluorescence bronchocoscopy has not yet been tested in a controlled trial evaluating high-risk smokers with airway obstruction.

White-light bronchoscopy

Approximately 40% of cases of carcinoma in situ can be detected by white-light reflectance bronchoscopy. About 75% of detected carcinoma in situ lesions

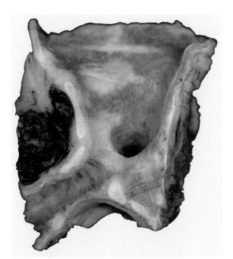

Fig. 1.72 Carcinoma in situ at the bronchus bifurcation. Note the plaque-like greyish lesions resembling leukoplakia.

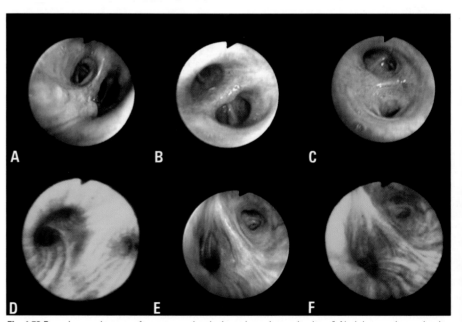

Fig. 1.73 Bronchscopy images of squamous dysplasia and carcinoma in situ. **A** Nodular carcinoma in-situ of the left lower lobe. White-light image. **B** Carcinoma in situ right upper lobe with focal thickening of the bronchial bifurcation and slight irregularity of the bronchial mucosa. **C** Carcinoma in situ upper divisional bronchus, left upper lobe. Focal increase in vascularity was observed under white-light bronchoscopy. **D** Carcinoma in situ left upper lobe. The lesion is visible as an area of reddish-brown fluorescence under autofluorescence bronchoscopy {1117,1120}, using the LIFE-Lung Device. **E** Severe dysplasia left upper lobe. No abnormality under white-light bronchoscopy. **F** Same case as E. The dysplastic lesion is visible as an area of reddish fluorescence under autofluorescence bronchoscopy {1117,1120}, using the Onco-LIFE Device (Xillix Technologies Inc. Vancouver, Canada).

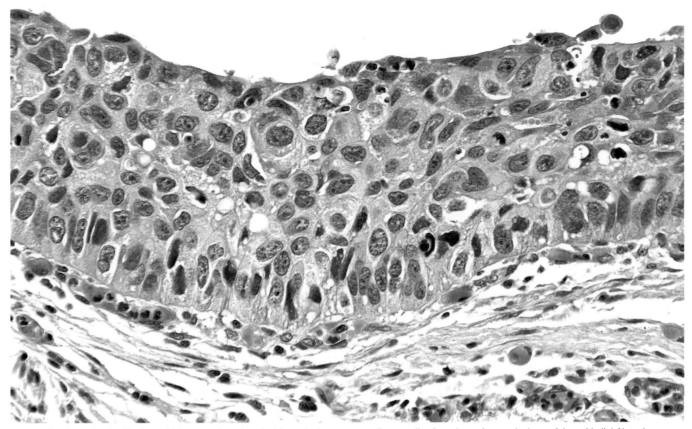

Fig. 1.74 Carcinoma in situ. The bronchial mucosa is replaced with atypical squamous cells extending from the surface to the base of the epithelial. Note the severe nuclear polymorphism, hyperchromasia and enlarged nuclei.

appear as superficial or flat lesions; the remaining 25% have a nodular or polypoid appearance {967,1423}. Because nodular/polypoid lesions are elevated from the adjacent normal mucosa, lesions as small as 1-2 mm in diameter can be seen. Flat or superficially spreading lesions greater than 1-2 cm in surface diameter are generally visible as areas of focal thickening, increase in vascularity or marked irregularity of the mucosa. Flat lesions 5-10 mm in diameter usually produce non-specific thickening, redness, fine roughening, loss of luster or a slight increase in granularity which are difficult to distinguish from inflammation or squamous metaplasia {2057}. Lesions <5 mm are usually invisible on white light bronchoscopy. Bronchial dysplasia usually presents as non-specific mucosal swelling or thickening at a bronchial bifurcation.

Autofluorescence bronchoscopy
Pre-invasive lesions that have subtle or no visible findings on white-light bronchoscopy can be localized by autofluo-

rescence imaging using a violet or blue light for illumination instead of white-light and special imaging sensors attached to a fiberoptic bronchoscope for detection of the abnormal autofluorescence {1117, 1120}. Dysplastic and malignant tissues have a significant decrease in the green autofluorescence intensity relative to the red autofluorescence. These pre-invasive lesions are identified by their brown or brownish-red autofluorescence. Lesions as small as 0.5 mm can be localized by this method.

Cytology
Sputum cytological classification schemes for preneoplastic lesions have been published by Saccomanno {1717} and Frost {621} and consist of gradations of microscopic abnormality similar to those observed in histological sections from lower airways of smokers. Squamous metaplasia presents in sputum smears as individual cells, but mostly as flat loosely cohesive clusters. The cytologic manifestations of dysplasia occur as increasingly severe cellular

changes, ranging from mild, moderate, and severe atypia to carcinoma in situ (CIS) {1717}. There are progressive alterations including increasing variability in cellular and nuclear sizes, increasingly variable nuclear-to-cytoplasmic ratios, increasing proportions of cells with cytoplasmic eosinophilia (orangeophilia), increasing coarseness of chromatin granularity until a pyknotic-like pattern is reached in CIS, increasing irregularity in the distribution of chromatin granules, and increasing irregularities in the outlines of nuclear membranes {844,1717, 1718}. This last feature first appears in moderate atypia {1717}. According to Koprowska et al {1055}, it is this deviation from smooth nuclear outlines that is most strongly associated with the presence of carcinoma.

Localization and macroscopy
Foci of carcinoma in situ usually arise near bifurcations in the segmental bronchi, subsequently extending proximally into the adjacent lobar bronchus and distally into subsegmental branches.

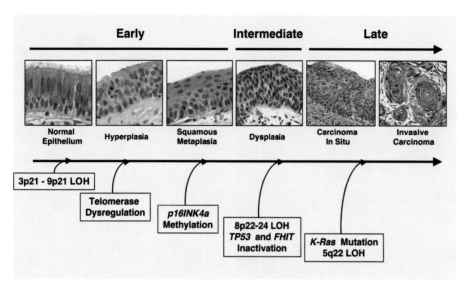

Fig. 1.75 Preinvasive lesions. Sequential molecular changes during the multistage pathogenesis of squamous cell lung carcinoma. Molecular changes occurring during lung pathogenesis may commence early (normal or slightly abnormal epithelium), at an intermediate (dysplasia) stage, or relatively late (carcinoma in situ, invasive carcinoma).

The lesions are less frequent in the trachea. Bronchoscopically and grossly there is often no macroscopical alteration. When gross abnormalities are present, focal or multi-focal plaque-like greyish lesions resembling leukoplakia, nonspecific erythema and even nodular or polypoid lesions may be seen.

Histopathology

A variety of bronchial epithelial hyperplasias and metaplasias may occur that are not regarded as preneoplastic including goblet cell hyperplasia, basal cell (reserve cell) hyperplasia, immature squamous metaplasia, and squamous metaplasia. The term preinvasive does not imply that progression to invasion will necessarily occur. These lesions represent a continuum of cytologic and histologic changes that may show some overlap between defined categories. Squamous dysplasia does not invade the stroma. The basement membrane remains intact and is variably thickened. There may be vascular budding into the epithelium, termed angiogenic squamous dysplasia {986}. The latter lesion has also been previously reported as micropapillomatosis {724, 1407}.

Immunohistochemistry

A series of immunohistochemical changes accompany squamous dysplasia. These include increased expression of EGFR {607,1101,1710}, HER2/neu {608}, p53 {145,211,1251}, MCM2 {1966}, Ki-67 {607,1149,1966}, cytokeratin 5/6 {54}, bcl-2 {211}, VEGF {602,1126}, maldistribution of MUC1, and loss of several proteins including FHIT {1855}, folate binding protein {609,676}, and p16 {213,1122}. A linear progression of proliferative activity, assessed with immunohistochemical staining for the proliferation marker Ki-67 (MIB-1), correlates with the extent and grade of the preneoplasia {1966}. Loss of RAR-beta expression is very frequent in the bronchial epithelium of smokers {1252,2017}. Type IV collagen staining highlights discontinuities in basement membranes that increase from basal cell hyperplasia to dysplasia, progressing to destruction in carcinoma in situ and invasive carcinoma {657}. Changes also occur in matrix metalloproteinase (MMP) and tissue inhibitor of metalloproteinase (TIMP) expression corresponding to progression in severity of dysplasia, in situ carcinoma and invasive carcinoma {657}.

Electron microscopy

There is an increase in atypical basal cells with loss of polarity. The nuclei show considerable hyperchromasia, and variations in shape with numerous invaginations. The number of nucleoli is increased, and so-called pseudoinclusion bodies may be seen within the nuclei. Some cells exhibit atypical development via an atypical array of organelles {711,712,1407}. A special feature is seen in the basement membrane in CIS. It is subdivided by multiple tentacle-like cytoplasmic protrusions, which vary considerably in shape and size but are always directed towards and between the fibrous structures of the basement membrane {711,712,1407}.

Histogenesis

The stem cell for the squamous epithelium of the proximal airway is not certain, but it is presumed that the basal cells represent a relatively quiescent zone that is the precursor for preneoplastic epithelium. It is of interest that these cells express a different cytokeratin profile with high levels of cytokeratin 5/6 and are the only cells in the normal respiratory mucosa and express significant levels of epidermal growth factor receptor. In the earliest preinvasive lesions, this basal zone is expanded with phenotypic changes that mirror the quiescent basal zone in normal epithelium including the overexpression of EGFR, transformation from cytokeratin 5/6 negative to positive, and increased proliferative activity with high expression of Ki-67 and MCM2. It is widely supposed that low grade changes such as basal cell hyperplasia and squamous metaplasia may (with or without micropapillomatosis) progress through mild, moderate and severe dysplasia up to carcinoma in situ {392,994,2022} to invasive carcinoma. However, such a progression is rarely observed in individual subjects and the predictive power of specific grades of premalignant change for the future development of invasive carcinoma is still under investigation.

Somatic genetics
Cytogenetics and CGH

Relatively few cytogenetic studies have been performed on preneoplastic lesions because of their small size and because of the difficulty of identifying them {1449, 1854}. Classic cytogenetic studies are further limited by the necessity for short-term cultures and the inability to identify the cell of origin of metaphase spreads. For these reasons most analyses have utilized fluorescence in situ hybridization (FISH) for detection of chromosomal or numerical changes in bronchial epithelial cells. As part of the field effect resulting from widespread smoking damage to the entire upper aerodigestive tract, cytoge-

Table 1.11
Microscopic features of the squamous dysplasia and carcinoma *in situ*.

Abnormality	Thickness	Cell size	Maturation/orientation	Nuclei
Mild Dysplasia	Mildly increased	Mildly increased Mild anisocytosis, Pleomorphism	Continuous progression of maturation from base to luminal surface Basilar zone expanded with cellular crowding in lower third Distinct intermediate (prickle cell) zone present Superficial flattening of epithelial cells	Mild variation of N/C ratio Finely granular chromatin Minimal angulation Nucleoli inconspicuous or absent Nuclei vertically oriented in lower third Mitoses absent or very rare
Moderate Dysplasia	Moderately increased	Mild increase in cell size; cells often small May have moderate anisocytosis, pleomorphism	Partial progression of maturation from base to luminal surface Basilar zone expanded with cellular crowding in lower two thirds of epithelium Intermediate zone confined to upper third of epithelium Superficial flattening of epithelial cells	Moderate variation of N/C ratio Finely granular chromatin Angulations, grooves and lobulations present Nucleoli inconspicuous or absent Nuclei vertically oriented in lower two thirds Mitotic figures present in lower third
Severe Dysplasia	Markedly increased	Markedly increased May have marked anisocytosis, pleomorphism	Little progression of maturation from base to luminal surface Basilar zone expanded with cellular crowding well into upper third Intermediate zone greatly attenuated Superficial flattening of epithelial cells	N/C ratio often high and variable Chromatin coarse and uneven Nuclear angulations and folding prominent Nucleoli frequently present and conspicuous Nuclei vertically oriented in lower two thirds Mitotic figures present in lower two thirds
Carcinoma in situ	May or may not be increased	May be markedly increased May have marked anisocytosis, pleomorphism	No progression of maturation from base to luminal surface; epithelium could be inverted with little change in appearance Basilar zone expanded with cellular crowding throughout epithelium Intermediate zone absent Surface flattening confined to the most superficial cells	N/C ratio often high and variable Chromatin coarse and uneven Nuclear angulations and folding prominent Nucleoli may be present or inconspicuous No consistent orientation of nuclei in relation to epithelial surface Mitotic figures present through full thickness

netic changes may be detected both in preneoplastic lesions as well as histologically normal appearing cells. Numerical changes of chromosme 7 are frequent and may predict risk for cancer development {1147,2245}. Only one study to date has performed comparative genomic hybridization on preneoplastic lesions and found that numerical alterations of chromosome 3 were the most frequent change {813}.

Molecular genetics
Precise microdissection of epithelial cells followed by molecular genetic analysis of such lesions has provided a sequence of molecular changes similar to that observed in other epithelial cancers {844,2161}. These studies have also indicated similarities and differences between the sequential changes leading to central and peripheral tumours. The histological changes preceding squamous cell carcinomas are well documented because of accessibility of these lesions, and the developmental sequence of molecular changes is nonrandom. DNA aneuploidy is frequent in dysplastic lesions particularly in high-grade lesions. Small foci of allelic loss are common at multiple sites in the bronchial epithelium and persist long after smoking cessation {1549}.
LOH occurs at one or more chromosome 3p regions and 9p21 early in neoplastic development, commencing in histologically normal epithelium. Later changes include 8p21-23, 13q14 (RB) and 17p13 (P53) being detected frequently in histologically normal epithelium {1236,2157, 2158,2162}. In contrast, allele loss at 5q21 (APC-MCC region) mutations has been detected at the carcinoma in situ stage, and P53 mutations appear at variable times {1900,2157,2162}. Chromosome 3p losses in normal epithelium, basal cell hyperplasia and squamous metaplasia are small and multifocal, commencing at the central (3p21) region of the chromosomal arm, while in later lesions such as carcinoma in situ, allelic loss is present along nearly all of the short arm of chromosome 3p {2157, 2158}. The clonal patches of bronchial epithelium having molecular changes (allelic loss and genetic instability) are usually small, and have been estimated to be approximately 40,000 to 360,000 cells {1549}. p16INK4a methylation has also been detected at early stages of squamous preinvasive lesions with frequency increasing during histopathologic progression from basal cell hyperpla-

sia to squamous metaplasia to carcinoma in situ {140}. Detection of such changes in sputum samples may be of predictive value in identifying smokers at increased risk of developing lung cancer {141}. Similar changes have been detected in telomerase activation {2199}. While weak telomerase RNA expression is detected in basal layers of normal and hyperplastic epithelium, dysregulation of telomerase expression increases with tumour progression with moderate to strong expression throughout the multilayers of the epithelium in squamous metaplasia, dysplasia and carcinoma in situ.

While specific premalignant changes associated with SCLC have not been identified, extensive genetic damage occurs in the accompanying normal and hyperplastic bronchial epithelium and is characteristic of SCLC tumours {2160}. These changes are much more extensive than changes accompanying similar epithelia from lung resections of patients with squamous cell carcinoma or adenocarcinoma. These findings suggest major differences in the pathogenesis of the three major lung cancer types.

Our knowledge of the changes preceding peripheral tumours is much more limited, mainly because of the inability to identify and have access to such lesions. However, careful examination of lung cancer resections indicates that peripheral tumours, especially adenocarcinoma, may be accompanied by specific morphologic changes known as atypical adenomatous hyperplasia (AAH). The advent of CT scans for the detection of early lung cancers has greatly increased the identification of such lesions, both in smokers with and without lung cancer {844,2078}. Inflation of the lungs prior to fixation greatly enhances the ability to detect these lesions. Multiple molecular changes have been described in these lesions {1021} including aneuploidy, ras gene mutations, COX-2 over expression, active proliferation, 3p and 9p deletions, K-ras codon 12 mutations, and disruption of the cell cycle control, but p53 gene aberrations are rare and telomerase activation is absent.

Prognostic factors
Carcinoma in situ, being a preneoplastic lesion, is classified as "Stage 0 disease." Resection of specific lesions at this stage means 100% curability, although frequent multifocality means that other foci are liable to present elsewhere in the airways. In general, higher grades of dysplasia are more closely associated with synchronous invasive carcinomas, although the prognostic significance of identifying dysplasia in isolation is uncertain. Currently, there are no recommendations to screen asymptomatic individuals with a history of dysplasia for development of invasive lesions {1119,1408, 1860}. There are no data to allow prediction of progression to invasive disease, depending on grade of dysplasia. It is likely that severe dysplasia/CIS carries a high risk. Progression of disease, from the early stages, probably takes many years.

Genetic predictive factors
There is a general consensus that numerous genetic and molecular abnormalities occur in very early stages of lung carcinogenesis including hyperplasia and metaplasia and even in normal appearing bronchial epithelium in smokers {1236,2162}. None of these isolated molecular abnormalities have been shown to predict progression to cancer, but their cumulative rate may be associated with the risk of cancer in the bronchial tree {926}.

Atypical adenomatous hyperplasia

K. M. Kerr
A.E. Fraire
B. Pugatch
M.F. Vazquez
H. Kitamura
S. Niho

Definition
Atypical adenomatous hyperplasia (AAH) is a localised proliferation of mild to moderately atypical cells lining involved alveoli and, sometimes, respiratory bronchioles, resulting in focal lesions in peripheral alveolated lung, usually less than 5mm in diameter and generally in the absence of underlying interstitial inflammation and fibrosis.

Synonyms
Atypical alveolar cuboidal cell hyperplasia {1807}, alveolar epithelial hyperplasia {1434}, atypical alveolar hyperplasia {288}, atypical bronchioloalveolar cell hyperplasia {2123}, bronchioloalveolar cell adenoma {1316}.

Background
AAH is a putative precursor of peripheral pulmonary adenocarcinoma, including bronchioloalveolar carcinoma (BAC) {1807}; the 'adenoma' in an adenoma-carcinoma sequence in the peripheral lung {1318}. Epidemiological, morphological, morphometric, cytofluorometric and genetic evidence support this hypothesis {392,994,1021,1378,2022}.
AAH is most frequently found as an incidental histologic finding in lungs already bearing primary cancer, especially adenocarcinoma. Lungs with very high num-

bers of AAH (>40) have been reported in conjunction with multiple synchronous peripheral primary adenocarcinomas or BAC {51,333,1316,1434,1928,2123}. Autopsy studies have reported AAH in 2-4% of non-cancer bearing patients {1879,2206,2207}.
AAH has been reported in up to 19% of women and 9.3% of men with lung cancer and up to 30.2% and 18.8%, respectively, in women and men with pulmonary adenocarcinoma {333}. In Japan, this gender relationship is inconsistent {1429, 2123}. Almost all Caucasians reported with AAH have been smokers, while in Japan, an association is not clear. Data on the association of AAH with either a personal or family history of malignancy are conflicting {334,1429,1960}.

Clinical features
Signs and symptoms
There are no clinical signs or symptoms directly referable to AAH. The lesions are usually encountered as incidental findings at gross or, more often, microscopic examination of lung.

Imaging
Radiological experience of AAH is largely confined to screening studies using High Resolution CT scanning (HRCT) {979,1108}, though some have been

Table 1.12
AAH in lung cancer resection specimens.
From references: {33,1041,1316,1387,1434,2123}

Cancer type	Prevalence
All primary lung cancer	9 - 21%
Adenocarcinoma	16 - 35%
Squamous cell carcinoma	3 - 11%
Large cell carcinoma	10 - 25%
Metastatic disease	4 - 10%

described during follow-up of patients with lung cancer {1038,1198}. In this context, small non-solid nodules, also described as localised areas of pure ground glass opacity (GGO), may be identified as areas of increased opacification with distinct borders, not completely obscuring the underlying lung parenchyma on CT scan, measuring 2-24mm in diameter, and typically not visualized on chest radiographs. Resection of GGOs has shown a range of pathology including benign disease in up to 30%, AAH in 10-77%, BAC in up to 50% and invasive adenocarcinoma in 10-25% of cases {979,1038,1108,1431}.

Relevant diagnostic procedures
AAH may rarely be visualised radiologically and a presumptive diagnosis made. Most likely as part of an HRCT screening

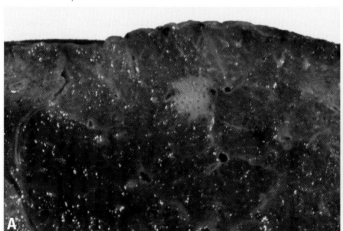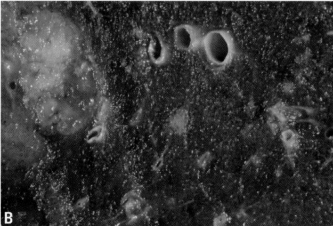

Fig. 1.76 Atypical adenomatous hyperplasia. **A** Unusually prominent AAH lesion. Alveolar spaces are visible within the lesion. **B** AAH (center) detected incidentally in a lung resected for mucinous adenocarcinoma, present on the left.

programme for lung cancer, any detected lesion, which necessitates further investigation, can be sampled by fine needle aspiration or local resection.

Cytology
A diagnosis of AAH cannot be made on a cytology specimen. This issue is discussed further in the chapter on adenocarcinoma.

Macroscopy and localization
Most lesions are only incidentally found at microscopy but AAH may be visible on the cut surface of lung as discrete, grey to yellow foci ranging from less than 1mm to, rarely, over 10mm {408,994}. Most are less than 3mm. AAH is easier to see by flooding the lung surface with water, or after tissue fixation with Bouin's fluid {1316}. Occasionally the alveolar spaces within the lesion create a stippled pattern of depressions. AAH lesions are more often found close to the pleura {1434} and in the upper lobes {1429}. It is likely that most occur as multiple lesions.

Histopathology
AAH is a discrete parenchymal lesion arising often in the centriacinar region, close to respiratory bronchioles. The alveoli are lined by rounded, cuboidal, low columnar or 'peg' cells, which have round or oval nuclei. Up to 25% of the cells show intranuclear inclusions {1434} and many have light microscopic {1434} and ultrastructural {1022} features of Clara cells and type II pneumocytes. Ciliated and mucous cells are never seen. Double nuclei are common; mitoses are extremely rare. There is some blending with normal alveolar lining cells peripherally, but most lesions are well defined. The alveolar walls may be thickened by collagen, occasional fibroblasts and lymphocytes. Lesions with these components in abundance are unusual. These interstitial changes do not extend beyond the limits of the lesion, as defined by the epithelial cell population.
Cellularity and cytological atypia vary. Many lesions show a discontinuous lining of cells with small nuclei and minimal nuclear atypia. Fewer show a more continuous single cell layer with moderate atypia. Pseudopapillae and tufts may be present. Some authors separate lesions into low and high grades: LGAAH and HGAAH {1023,1040}. This practice is not

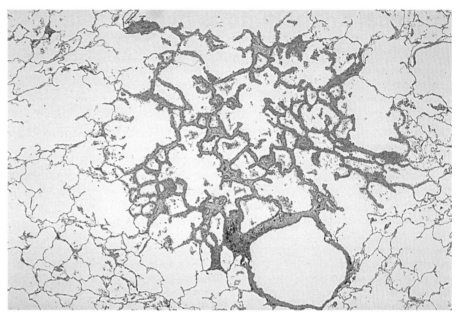

Fig. 1.77 Atypical adenomatous hyperplasia showing localised centriacinar alveolar wall thickening and increased numbers of alveolar lining cells. From Travis et al. {2024}.

universally accepted, has no known clinical significance, its reproducibility is untested, and this panel does not recommend it. The features of AAH fall short of those accepted as BAC. This issue is addressed in the discussion on BAC.
The postulated progression of disease, apparent from the increasingly atypical morphology, is supported by numerous morphometric and cytofluorometric studies {1375,1379,1438}. AAH and nonmucinous BAC probably represent a continuum of progression of pulmonary alveolar intraepithelial neoplasia.
AAH must be distinguished from reactive hyperplasia, secondary to parenchymal inflammation or fibrosis, where the alveolar lining cells are not the dominant feature and are more diffusely distributed. Generally, AAH cannot be identified in the presence of inflammatory or fibrosing disease. Distinction between more cellular and atypical AAH and BAC is difficult. BAC is generally >10mm in size, has a more pleomorphic, homogeneous columnar cell population, which is densely packed with greater cell-cell contact, overlap, mild stratification, and, usually, a less graded, more abrupt transition to adjacent alveolar lining cells. True papillae suggest papillary adenocarcinoma.

Immunohistochemistry
AAH expresses SPA, CEA {1640}, MMPs {1084}, E-cadherin, ß-catenin, CD44v6

and TTF-1. The expression of oncogene and tumour supressor gene products (TP53, C-ERB2, RB, MST1(p16), WAF1/CIP1 (p21) and FHIT) essentially reflects neoplastic progression from AAH to BAC and invasive adenocarcinomas {802,995,1021,1100}. In contrast to the data on TP53 mutations, TP53 protein accumulation seems to occur early in the proposed sequence of events {995}.

Histogenesis
The origin of AAH cells is still unknown but the differentiation phenotype derived from immunohistochemical and ultrastructural features suggests an alveolar origin. Surfactant apoprotein {1041}, and Clara cell specific 10kDd protein {1021, 1379} are expressed in almost all AAH lesions. Ultrastructurally, cytoplasmic lamellar bodies and nuclear branching microtubles, both typical of type II pneumocytes {768,1021,1316,1521}, and electron-dense Clara cell-type granules {1021,1434,1521} are found. AAH cells are likely derived from a progenitor cell with the potential for both type II pneumocyte and Clara cell differentiation.

Somatic genetics
KRAS. Mutations of the K-ras gene, particularly at codon 12, are specific for peripheral lung adenocarcinomas, as opposed to bronchogenic carcinoma, suggesting an alternative pathway of peripheral lung tumourigenesis {287,

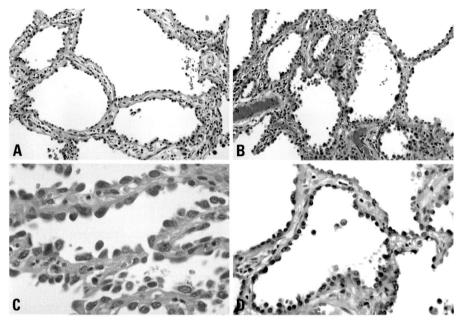

Fig. 1.78 Atypical adenomatous hyperplasia. **A,B** Slightly thickened alveolar walls are lined by an intermittent single layer of cuboidal cells. Occasional large cells are present. **C** Cuboidal pneumocytes line the alveolar walls with gaps between the adjacent cells. **D** Slightly thickened alveolar walls lined by an intermittent single layer of cuboidal cells, some with apical cytoplasmic snouts.

402}. K-ras codon 12 mutations are reported in 15-39% of AAH lesions, and up to 42% of concurrent adenocarcinomas. Most of the time, the K-ras mutations are different. One study found K-ras codon 12 mutations in 15% of AAH, 33% of 'early' BAC and 24% of 'advanced' BAC. {1021}, suggesting that K-ras codon 12 mutation is a very early event in the development of peripheral adenocarcinoma {1021,2126}.

TP53. Abnormalities of the P53 gene (17p), with impaired protein function, promote neoplastic transformation in affected cells. Many lung adenocarcinomas show missense mutations of the P53 gene with abnormal nuclear protein accumulation. LOH and mutations of the P53 gene are very rare in AAH compared with adenocarcinoma; however p53 protein overexpression is frequent in AAH {1021}. P53 mutation has been demonstrated with increasing frequency in the progression from AAH, through BAC to early invasive adenocarcinoma {1836}.

LOH Allelic-specific losses at 3p and 9p loci have been detected in AAH {1044, 2187}. Some AAH lesions have shown LOH in 9q {51} and both 17q {2187} and 17p {51} LOH in the 3p and 9p loci probably occurs at a very early stage and may represent the earliest and crucial event in neoplastic transformation, with 17p events occurring later.

FHIT. The fragile histidine triad (FHIT) gene (3p) is deleted in many lung carcinomas {1856}.

p16INK4. Loss and inactivation plays an important role in the pathogenesis of lung carcinoma. However, loss of expression of p16INK4 is relatively rare in both AAH and adenocarcinoma {1021}.

TSC. A recent study on lung adenocarcinoma with concurrent multiple AAH lesions showed frequent LOH of tuberous sclerosis complex (TSC)-associated regions (TSC1 at 9q and TSC2 in 16p), suggesting that these are candidate loci for tumour suppressor genes in peripheral lung adenocarcinoma {1949}.

Aneuploidy. FISH studies of AAH have shown frequent aneuploidy of chromosome 7. The percentages of aneuploid cells and mean chromosome copy number increased from AAH to invasive adenocarcinomas, suggesting increasing polyploidy during malignant change {2245}. Some cases of AAH have been shown to be monoclonal, suggesting that it is a true preneoplastic lesion {1475}.

Prognosis and predictive factors

Assuming that AAH is always multifocal, several studies have compared postoperative survival in groups of patients with, and without AAH {333,1198,1927, 1960}. None showed any difference in outcome.

There is no indication for surgical or medical therapy in patients without cancer who are incidentally found to have AAH. In such a clinical setting, careful followup is warranted.

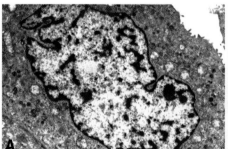
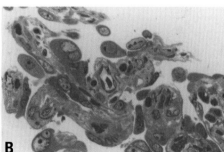
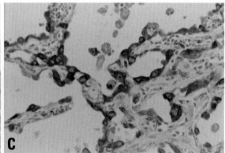

Fig. 1.79 Atypical adenomatous hyperplasia. **A** Transmission electron photomicrograph of a formalin-fixed AAH lesion showing a cuboid AAH cell having many intracytoplasmic small inclusion bodies and granules. Note scattered short microvilli on the free surface of the cell, the irregular contour of the nucleus and basal membrane. **B** Light photomicrograph of a thin section of a formalin-fixed, epoxy-resin-embedded AAH lesion showing a cell with an intranuclear inclusion body at the middle upper portion as well as several binucleated cells. Toluidine blue stain. **C** Immunostaining with a mouse monoclonal antibody against surfactant apoprotein A (PE10), showing uniformly strong positive staining of the cytoplasm of almost all the AAH cells as well as many nuclear inclusion bodies.

Diffuse idiopathic pulmonary neuroendocrine cell hyperplasia

J.R. Gosney
W.D. Travis

Definition

Diffuse idiopathic pulmonary neuroendocrine cell hyperplasia (DIPNECH) is a generalised proliferation of scattered single cells, small nodules (neuroendocrine bodies), or linear proliferations of pulmonary neuroendocrine cells (PNCs) that may be confined to the bronchial and bronchiolar epithelium, include local extraluminal proliferation in the form of tumourlets, or extend to the development of carcinoid tumours. It is sometimes accompanied by intra- and extraluminal fibrosis of involved airways, but other pathology that might induce reactive PNC proliferation is absent.

Synonyms

The entity of DIPNECH was not fully recognised and named until 1992 {29}, but cases with its clinical and pathological features appear in the literature from the early 1950s {570}.

Clinical features

Signs and symptoms

DIPNECH may occur at any age, but presents typically in the fifth or sixth decades, and is perhaps commoner in women {29,74,1150,1317}. The history is one of a very slowly worsening dry cough and breathlessness, often over many years, sometimes misdiagnosed as mild bronchial asthma. Physical examination usually reveals no signs, but pulmonary function tests show an obstructive or mixed obstructive/restrictive pattern of impairment with reduced diffusing capacity.

Imaging

Plain thoracic radiography is often normal, but tomographic scanning reveals a mosaic pattern of air trapping, sometimes with nodules and thickened bronchial and bronchiolar walls {1150}. Multiple nodules corresponding to tumourlets or carcinoid tumours may be present.

Macroscopy and localization

The early lesions of DIPNECH are invisible to the naked eye, but tumourlets and microcarcinoids, when present, can be just discerned as small, gray-white nodules, the latter often well-demarcated and resembling 'miliary bodies'. Larger carcinoid tumours are firm, homogeneous, well-defined, grey or yellow-white masses. The lesions of DIPNECH usually affect one or both lungs uniformly.

Histopathology

Histopathological examination reveals widespread proliferation of PNCs {29,74, 1317}. The earliest lesions comprise increased numbers of individual cells, small groups, or larger, nodular aggregates, confined to the bronchial or bronchiolar epithelium, the larger lesions bulging into the lumen, but not breaching the subepithelial basement membrane. The bronchiolar wall sometimes is fibrotically thickened. Bronchiolar occlusion may occur due to fibrosis and/or PNC proliferation. These are sufficient for the diagnosis of DIPNECH providing other defining criteria are met. In particular inflammatory or fibrous lesions that might cause secondary PNC hyperplasia are not seen. However, more advanced lesions are often present. These develop when the proliferating PNCs break through the basement membrane to invade locally, developing a conspicuous fibrous stroma to form small (2-5 mm) aggregates traditionally known as 'tumourlets'. This proliferation of PNCs is sometimes accompanied by intra- and extramural fibrosis of the involved airways that often obliterates them, but the surrounding lung is otherwise unremarkable. Once PNCs reach a size of 5mm or greater, they are classified as carcinoids.

Differential diagnosis

Clinically and on imaging, DIPNECH may be indistinguishable from other diffuse lung diseases characterised by cough,

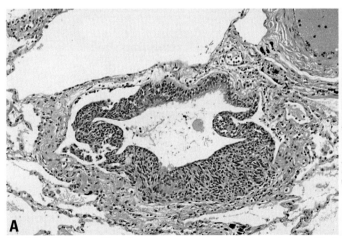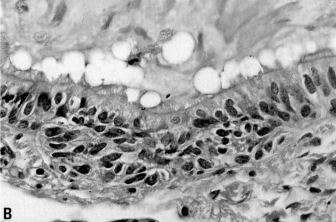

Fig. 1.80 Diffuse idiopathic pulmonary neuroendocrine cell hyperplasia. **A** The bronchiolar epithelium is almost entirely replaced by proliferating neuroendocrine cells. **B** Hyperplastic neuroendocrine cells form a nest at the base of the bronchiolar epithelium. From Travis et al {2024}.

breathlessness, mixed obstructive/restrictive pulmonary impairment and a nodular pattern of pulmonary infiltration, so that the diagnosis is usually impossible to make without recourse to biopsy. Histopathologically, DIPNECH must be distinguished from the PNC proliferation that may accompany a variety of pulmonary conditions, particularly chronic inflammatory diseases such as bronchiectasis and chronic lung abscess {717}; in the latter situation, progression of the proliferation to carcinoid tumours does not occur. DIPNECH must also be distinguished from the proliferation of PNCs not uncommonly seen adjacent to peripheral carcinoids {29,1317}.

Histogenesis

As with neuroendocrine neoplasms arising in the lungs, the origin of the proliferating PNCs that characterize DIPNECH is likely to be a yet-to-be-defined uncommitted precursor cell that is stimulated by unknown influences to differentiate along a neuroendocrine line. However, the PNCs that proliferate in DIPNECH are found in normal lungs of adults {719, 1141}.

Somatic genetics

There are no genetic markers of DIPNECH such that it might be possible to distinguish it genetically from the limited, reactive, reversible proliferative response of PNCs that occurs after pulmonary injury. It is of interest, however, that allelic imbalance at the 11q13 region that closely approximates to the MEN1 tumour suppressor gene appears to be rare in tumourlets, but is present in the majority of carcinoid tumours {581}.

Prognosis and predictive factors

DIPNECH is a slowly progressive condition with a benign course spanning many years. Associated carcinoid tumours are indolent and atypical features have not been described. There are no predictive histologic or genetic data for DIPNECH.

Squamous cell papilloma

D.B. Flieder
F. Thivolet-Bejui
H. Popper

Definition

A papillary tumour consisting of delicate connective tissue fronds with a squamous epithelial surface. Squamous papillomas can be solitary or multiple and can be exophytic or inverted.

ICD-O codes

Squamous cell papilloma	8052/0
Exophytic	8052/0
Inverted	8053/0

Epidemiology

Solitary squamous papillomas are very rare representing less than 0.50% of lung tumours at one large institution {1612}. Exophytic lesions far outnumber the inverted growth pattern {592}. Solitary squamous papillomas are seen predominantly in men, with a median age of 54 years {592}. Juvenile and adult laryngotracheal papillomatosis rarely involve the lower respiratory tract are always related to laryngotracheal papillomatosis {1223}.

Etiology

An association with human papilloma virus (HPV) subtypes 6 and 11 suggests a possible pathogenetic role for the virus {592}. Human papilloma virus subtypes 16,18 and 31/33/35 in squamous papillomas associated with carcinomas and in squamous cell carcinomas have been reported, suggesting that HPV infection might be related to tumoural progression {139,1611,1612}. More than half of patients are tobacco smokers, but an etiologic role has not been established {592,1937}.

Localization

Papillomas are endobronchial.

Clinical features

While up to one-third of lesions are incidental radiographic findings, patients most often present with obstructive symptoms. Computed tomography scans demonstrate a small endobronchial protuberance or nodular airway thickening. Involvement of distal airways may lead to nodular opacities and/or thin-walled cavity nodules {2213}. An endobronchial biopsy may be diagnostic, but distinction from well-differentiated squamous cell carcinoma can be difficult, especially with superficial tissue fragments. Bronchoscopic cytologic specimens will only demonstrate the squamous nature of the lesion. Parakeratotic cells, cytologic atypia and viral cytopathic effect should not be misinterpreted as invasive carcinoma {1677}.

Macroscopy

Solitary squamous papillomas arise from the wall of either mainstem bronchi or major subdivisions and appear as cauliflower-like tan-white soft to semi-firm excrescences protruding into bronchial lumens. Tumours range from 0.7-9.0 cm with a median of 1.5 cm. Distal airways may be bronchiectatic with secondary atelectasis and consolidation {965}.

Tumour spread and staging

Squamous papillomas may recur at their original site and laryngotracheal papillomatosis can spread into the lower respiratory tract. It has been suggested that electrical or laser fulguration is responsible for alveolar parenchymal seeding.

Histopathology

Squamous papillomas are composed of a loose fibrovascular core covered by stratified squamous epithelium. Exophytic lesions feature orderly squamous maturation from the basal layer to the superficial flattened and oftentimes keratinized cells. Acanthosis may be prominent. While non-keratinized epithelium may resemble transitional epithelium, the squamous nature of these cells has been demonstrated ultrastructurally and use of this term is discouraged. Over 20% of solitary squamous papillomas feature wrinkled nuclei, binucleate forms and perinuclear halos, i.e., koilocytosis related to HPV infection {592}. Scattered

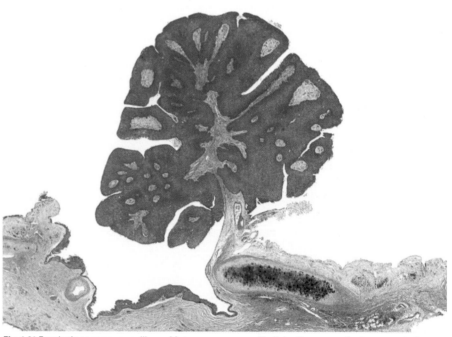

Fig. 1.81 Exophytic squamous papilloma. Mature squamous epithelial cells are growing in an exophytic papillary pattern on the surface of thin fibrovascular cores. The papilloma is attached to the underlying bronchial wall by a stalk. .

dyskeratotic cells, large atypical cells and occasional mitotic figures above the basal layer can be seen. Dysplasia should be graded according to the World Health Organization classification {2024}. Squamous cell carcinoma infrequently arises in solitary squamous papillomas {1611,1612}.

Inverted lesions feature both exophytic and random invaginations of squamous epithelium. The basal lamina investing the endophytic nests is continuous with the basal lamina underlying the surface epithelium. Basal cells are perpendicular to the basement membrane while central cells are parallel and whorling. Tumour can involve adjacent seromucinous glands.

Alveolar parenchymal involvement manifests as either well circumscribed solid intraalveolar nests of cytologically bland non-keratinizing squamous cells surrounded by hyperplastic type II pneumocytes or large cysts lined by similar benign epithelium. Lower respiratory tract involvement with laryngotracheal papillomatosis is morphologically similar with the exception that virtually all lesions feature viral cytopathic effect. Neither immunohistochemical nor in situ hybridization studies are helpful in diagnosis.

Differential diagnosis

Inflammatory endobronchial polyps may show focal squamous metaplasia but generally have voluminous granulation tissue-like stroma and subepithelial dense lymphoplasmacytic infiltrates with a lack of continuous proliferative epithelial surface. Well-differentiated squamous cell carcinoma can be entirely papillary and endobronchial, but usually demonstrates malignant cytologic features if not also stromal invasion and/or angiolymphatic invasion. Entrapped glands within the papillary stalk of a benign papilloma should not be mistaken for invasion. Inverted papillomas with

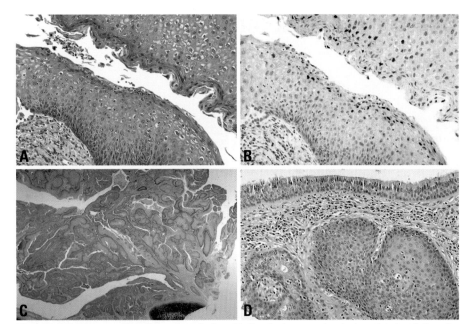

Fig. 1.82 A Squamous cell papilloma. Acanthotic epithelium features parakeratosis and dyskeratotic cells. **B** Squamous cell papilloma. In situ hybridization staining for human papillomavirus subtypes 6/11. **C** Inverted squamous cell papilloma. Mature squamous epithelial cells are growing in an inverted papillary pattern within the lumen of this bronchus. From Flieder et al {592} and Travis et al. {2024}. **D** Inverted squamous cell papilloma. Mature squamous cells are growing in an papillary configuration with an inverted pattern of growth. From Flieder et al. {592} and Travis et al. {2024}

even minimal cytologic atypia may be indistinguishable from invasive squamous cell carcinoma. Parenchymal destruction, cellular pleomorphism, loss of maturation, prominent dyskeratosis and hyperkeratosis favour a diagnosis of carcinoma.

Precursor lesions-Histogenesis
Squamous papillomas most likely arise from metaplastic respiratory epithelium.

Prognosis and predictive factors
While solitary squamous papillomas are considered benign lesions, the presence of focal cytologic atypia, a recurrence rate approaching 20% and reports of squamous cell carcinomas arising at papilloma excision sites indicate a low malignant potential. Thus, lesions should

be completely excised when feasible. Human papilloma virus subtyping may be prognostically significant as condylomatous papillomas have malignant potential {1611,1612,1937,2030}. Solitary papillomas may progress to papillomatosis, but lower respiratory tract involvement usually represents spread of juvenile or rarely adult laryngotracheal papillomatosis. Papillomatosis may be lethal even in the absence of malignant transformation owing to obstructive complications. Increased topoisomerase alpha II and p53 expression along with reduced RB gene protein product and p21 expression may serve as markers of transformation to so-called invasive papillomatosis and squamous cell carcinoma {753}.

Glandular papilloma

D.B. Flieder
F. Thivolet-Bejui
H. Popper

Definition
A papillary tumour lined by ciliated or non-ciliated columnar cells, with varying numbers of cuboidal cells and goblet cells.

ICD-O code
8260/0

Synonym
Columnar cell papilloma

Epidemiology
Glandular papillomas are exceedingly rare. An equal sex distribution and median age of 68 years are established based on the few reported cases {85,118,592,1858}.

Etiology
No specific etiologies have been implicated in the evolution of glandular papillomas.

Localization
Endobronchial

Clinical features and diagnostic procedures
Individuals present with obstructive symptoms including wheezing or haemoptysis {592}; a minority are asymptomatic and radiographic studies demonstrate either a small endobronchial protuberance or nodular airway thickening. While bronchoscopic biopsy can identify a central lesion, complete excision is necessary for definitive diagnosis.

Macroscopy
Glandular papillomas are white to tan endobronchial polyps that measure from 0.7-1.5 cm. Bronchiolar lesions can appear solid without obvious papillary fronds.

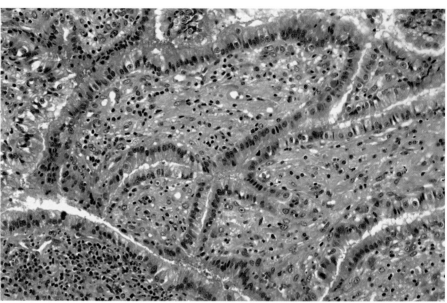

Fig. 1.83 Glandular papilloma. Columnar epithelial cells proliferate in a papillary fashion along the surface of fibrovascular cores. From Flieder et al. {592} and Travis et al. {2024}.

Histopathology
Central lesions have relatively non-inflamed thick arborizing stromal stalks with prominent thin-walled blood vessels or hyalinization covered by glandular epithelium. Necrosis is absent. Pseudostratified or columnar epithelium lacks micropapillary tufts and cellular desquamation. Epithelium can be non-ciliated or ciliated, cuboidal or columnar or a mixture and interspersed mucin-rich cells can be seen. The cytoplasm can be clear and the nuclei lack atypia and mitoses. Peripheral lesions demonstrate attachment to bronchiolar mucosa and contain scattered ciliated cells.

Differential diagnosis
Primary and metastatic papillary adenocarcinomas feature epithelial crowding, malignant cytologic features and often show bronchial wall invasion. Inflammatory polyps and the papillary variant of mucus gland adenoma lack true fibrovascular stromal cores and inflammatory polyps lack a proliferative epithelial component. Papillary adenomas are parenchymal lesions without attachment to airways and usually demonstrate type II pneumocyte differentiation.

Prognosis and predictive factors
Glandular papillomas are benign tumours that may recur following incomplete resection, but neither extension into alveolar parenchyma nor malignant transformation has been reported {85, 118,592,1858}.

Mixed squamous cell and glandular papilloma

D.B. Flieder
F. Thivolet-Bejui
H. Popper

Definition
Mixed squamous and glandular papilloma is an endobronchial papillary tumour showing a mixture of squamous and glandular epithelium. One-third of the epithelium should be composed of the second epithelial type.

ICD-O code　　　　　8560/0

Synonyms
These tumours were formely called transitional papillomas {1072}.

Epidemiology
Mixed papillomas are exceedingly rare with seven cases reported in the world literature. An equal sex distribution and median age of 64 years are compiled from the few reported cases {592,1858}.

Etiology
No specific etiologies have been implicated in the evolution of mixed papillomas. Human papilloma virus has not been detected in the few cases studied. 60% of patients are tobacco smokers, but an etiologic role has not been established {592}.

Clinical features and diagnostic procedures
Individuals present with obstructive symptoms {592,1858}. While endobronchial biopsy can demonstrate the neoplastic nature of a central lesion, complete excision is necessary for definitive diagnosis.

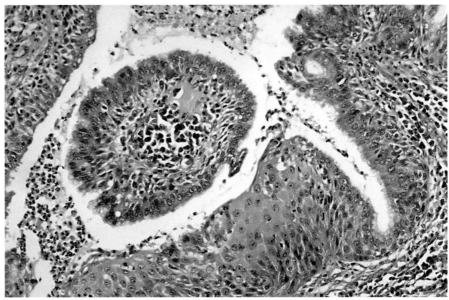

Fig. 1.84 Mixed squamous cell and glandular papilloma. Flieder et al. {592} and Travis et al. {2024}.

Macroscopy
Endobronchial lesions are tan to red, polypoid and measure from 0.2-2.5 cm. A lobar preference is not seen.

Histopathology
Endobronchial lesions are composed of fibrovascular cores with scattered lymphoplasmacytic infiltrates lined by squamous and glandular epithelium. Pseudostratified ciliated and nonciliated cuboidal to columnar cells with occasional mucin-filled cells are distinct from acanthotic and focally keratinizing squamous epithelium. Squamous atypia ranging from mild to severe dysplasia can be seen but viral cytopathic change has not been reported. Glandular atypia and necrosis are not seen.

Differential diagnosis
This is the same as for pure squamous and glandular papillomas.

Prognosis and predictive factors
Complete resection appears to be curative {592}.

Alveolar adenoma

L.M. Burke
D.B. Flieder

Definition
A solitary well-circumscribed peripheral lung tumour consisting of a network of spaces lined by a simple low cuboidal epithelium associated with a variably thin and inconspicuous to thick spindle cell-rich stroma, sometimes with a myxoid matrix.

ICD-O code   8251/0

Synonyms
This tumour has been mistakenly reported under the term lymphangioma.

Epidemiology
This tumour is very rare. The age range is 39-74 years (mean, 53 years), with a slight female predominance {194,252, 624,792,1054,1297,1464,1514,1782, 1811,1822,2219}.

Localization
Alveolar adenoma has been reported in all five lobes with a predilection for the left lower lobe {1116}. Most tumours are intraparenchymal peripheral or subpleural although a hilar location has been noted.

Clinical features
Patients are usually asymptomatic and the tumour is an incidental radiographic finding. {1116}. Chest X-ray and CT appearances are those of a well circumscribed, homogenous, non-calcified, solitary mass, although one report, unconfirmed histologically, raises the possibility of multifocality {624}. Contrast enhancement on CT and MRI displays cystic spaces with central fluid and rim enhancement {624}.

Macroscopy
Tumours measure from 0.7-6.0 cm and feature well demarcated smooth, lobulated, multicystic, soft to firm and pale yellow to tan cut surfaces {252}.

Histopathology
Alveolar adenomas are well-circumscribed unencapsulated multicystic masses with ectatic spaces filled with eosinophilic granular material. Spaces are lined by cytologically bland flattened, cuboidal and hobnail cells. Cystic spaces are usually larger in the centre of the lesion and squamous metaplasia can be seen. The myxoid and collagenous interstitium varies in thickness and contains scattered to dense groups of cytologically bland spindle cells.

Immunohistochemistry
Epithelial lining cells are type 2 pneumocytes that stain for broad-spectrum keratin, CEA, surfactant protein and TTF-1 while stromal cells show focal positivity for smooth-muscle actin and muscle-specific actin and negativity for desmin , TTF-1, proSPB, proSPC and CC10 {252}. Low proliferation indices in both the epithelial and mesenchymal cells have been reported {194,1297}.

Electron microscopy
By electron microscopy, lining cells contain lamellar bodies, blunt surface microvilli and cell junctions of the zonula adherens type.

Differential diagnosis
Lymphangioma, sclerosing hemangioma, and adenocarcinoma including bronchioloalveolar carcinoma comprise the differential diagnosis. Cytokeratin positivity of cells lining the cystic spaces differentiates this lesion from a lymphangioma {252}. The single architectural growth pattern, large ectatic spaces lacking blood and stromal cell negativity for TTF-1 discern the tumour from a sclerosing haemangioma {252,1464}. The well-circumscribed growth pattern, lack of lepidic growth and cytologic atypia discern alveolar adenoma from bronchioloalveolar carcinoma {252}. Primary and metastatic spindle cells tumours may

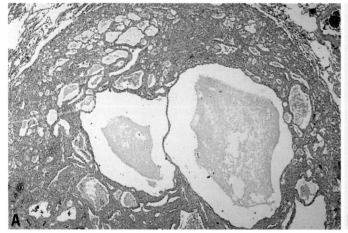
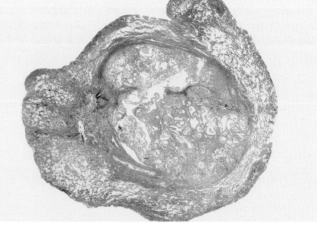

Fig. 1.85 Alveolar adenoma. **A** This tumour nodule is circumscribed, but not encapsulated. There are large cysts and smaller spaces resembling alveoli. From Burke et al. {252} and Travis et al {2024}. **B** This whole-mount section demonstrates the well circumscribed nature of the multicystic neoplasm.

also become cystic, with foci resembling alveolar adenoma.

Histogenesis
This lesion appears to represent a combined proliferation of alveolar pneumocytes and septal mesenchyme {252, 1514}.

Somatic genetics
The neoplastic nature of alveolar adenoma was demonstrated in a cytogenetic study of one tumour. A pseudodiploid karyotype, 46,XX, add (16) (q24), was described and fluorescence in situ hybridization studies revealed the add (16) (q24) to be a der(16)t(10;16) (q23;q24) {1682}.

Prognosis and predictive factors
Alveolar adenomas are benign tumours and surgical excision is curative.

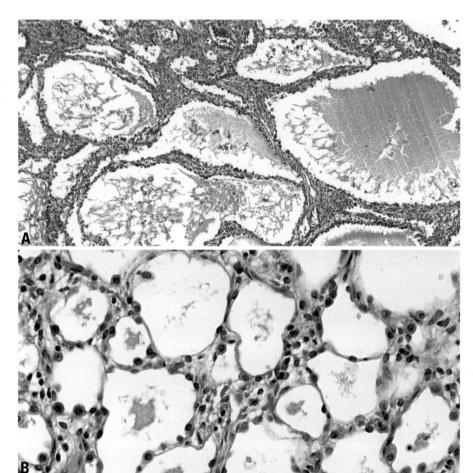

Fig. 1.86 Alveolar adenoma. **A** Cystic spaces of varying sizes are filled with eosinophilic fluid and PAS-positive granular material. Intervening stroma is focally prominent. **B** Alveolus-like spaces are lined by flat or cuboidal pneumocytes on the surface of a thin layer of vascular connective tissue resembling an alveolar wall. A few macrophages are present within the alveolar-like spaces. From Burke et al. {252} and Travis et al. {2024}.

Papillary adenoma

D.B. Flieder

Definition
Papillary adenoma is a circumscribed papillary neoplasm consisting of cytologically bland cuboidal to columnar cells lining the surface of a fibrovascular stroma.

ICD-O code   8260/0

Synonyms
Bronchiolar adenoma, papillary adenoma of type II pneumocytes, type II pneumocyte adenoma, adenoma of type II pneumocytes, peripheral papillary tumour of type II pneumocytes.

Epidemiology
The papillary adenoma is a rare tumour with less than 20 cases reported. Individuals range in age from 7-60 years (mean 32 years) and males predominate {484,555,579,635,808,1103,1376,1483, 1858,2185}.

Etiology
The etiology in humans is unknown but a similar lesion can be chemically induced in mice {974}.

Localization
The tumour has no lobar predilection and involves alveolar parenchyma but not airways {484,555,579,635,808,1103,1376, 1483,1858,2185}.

Clinical features
Individuals are usually asymptomatic and the tumour is incidentally noted on chest radiographs as a well-defined pulmonary nodule {484,555,579,635,808, 1376,1483,1858,2185}.

Macroscopy
Grossly, the tumour is a well defined, sometimes encapsulated, soft, spongy to firm mass with a granular gray white/brown cut surface measuring from 1.0-4.0 cm {484,555,579,635,808,1376, 1483,1858,2185}. Although generally separate from the airways, protrusion into the lumen of a small bronchiole can occur {1483}.

Histopathology
Papillary adenomas are generally well circumscribed but infiltrative growth has been described. The tumour has a papillary growth pattern sometimes mixed with more solid areas. Focally inflamed fibrovascular cores are lined with cuboidal to columnar epithelial cells with round to oval nuclei. Cilitated {635,1376} and oxyphilic cells {555,579} can be seen. Occasional eosinophilic intranuclear inclusions are noted but nuclear atypia and mitosis are rare to absent. Intracellular mucin is not present.

Immunohistochemistry and electron microscopy
Both type II and Clara cells can be found in papillary adenomas resulting in positive staining for broad-spectrum cytokeratin, Clara cell protein, TTF-1 and surfactant apoprotein as well as CEA. Neuroendocrine markers are negative {484,555,579,635,808,1376,1483,1858, 2185}. Ultrastructurally lamellar bodies, surface microvilli, with membrane bound electron dense deposits have been observed {635,2185}.

Differential diagnosis
Sclerosing haemangioma demonstrates varied architectural growth patterns including hemorrhagic, sclerotic and solid tumour cell growth {488}. Alveolar adenoma does not display a papillary growth pattern, Clara cells or ciliated cells {252}. Papillary adenocarcinomas including metastatic thyroid carcinoma and bronchioloalveolar carcinoma have a greater degree of cellular proliferation with micropapillary tufts and nuclear pleomorphism. Papillary carcinoid tumour has granular cytoplasm and a finely granular chromatin pattern.

Histogenesis
Pulmonary papillary adenoma is thought to arise from a multipotential stem cell/immature bronchioloalveolar cell that differentiates towards type II pneumocytes, Clara cells or ciliated respiratory epithelial cells {555,635,1483,1858}.

Prognosis and predictive factors
Papillary adenoma is benign and surgical excision is curative. {484,555, 635,808,1103,1376,1483,2185}.

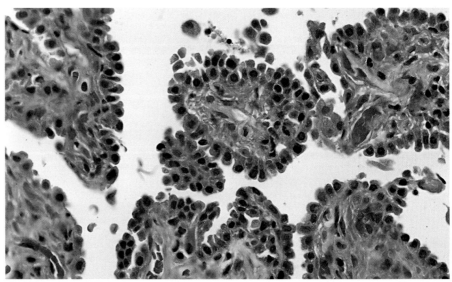

Fig. 1.87 Papillary adenoma. Cuboidal epithelial cells line the surface of the fibrovascular cores. From Travis et al. {2024}.

Mucous gland adenoma

D.B. Flieder
F. Thivolet-Bejui
H. Popper

Definition
A benign predominantly exophytic tumour of the tracheobronchial seromucinous glands and ducts featuring mucus-filled cysts, tubules, glands and papillary formations lined by a spectrum of epithelium including tall columnar cells, flattened cuboidal cells, goblet cells, oncocytic cells and clear cells.

ICD-O code   8480/0

Synonyms
Bronchial cystadenoma, mucous cell adenoma, polyadenoma, bronchial adenoma arising in mucous glands

Epidemiology
The tumour is extremely rare {1561}. There is no sex predilection and tumours have been reported in both children and the elderly with a mean age of 52 years {543,1077}.

Localization
Most tumours are central but peripheral lesions have been described {543,2117}.

Clinical features
Individuals present with signs and symptoms of obstruction. Radiographic studies demonstrate a coin lesion. CT scans may show a well-defined intraluminal mass with air-meniscus sign {1109}. Excision is usually required for definitive diagnosis {472}.

Macroscopy
Grossly, white-pink to tan, smooth and shiny tumours with gelatinous mucoid solid and cystic cut surfaces measure from 0.7-7.5 cm (mean 2.3 cm) {543}.

Histopathology
Mucous gland adenomas are well-circumscribed, predominantly exophytic nodules above the cartilaginous plates of the bronchial wall. Tumours comprise numerous mucin-filled cystic spaces and non-dilated microacini, glands, tubules and papillae may also be seen. Neutral and acid-mucin filled cysts are lined by

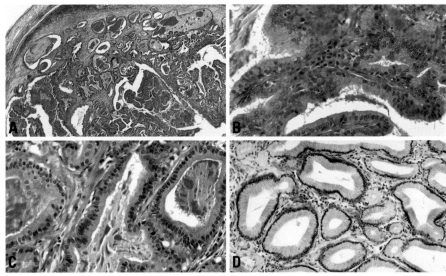

Fig. 1.88 Mucous gland adenoma. **A** Endobronchial mass is comprised of numerous mucin-filled cystic spaces, microacini, glands, tubules and papillae. **B** Papillary fronds are a minor architectural pattern. **C** Neutral and acid-mucin filled cysts are lined by cytologically bland columnar, cuboidal or flattened mucus secreting cells. **D** Glands lined by columnar epithelium with small basally oriented nuclei and abundant apical mucinous cytoplasm. From Travis et al. {2024}.

cytologically bland columnar, cuboidal or flattened mucus secreting cells. Oncocytic and clear cell change can also be seen as well as focal ciliated epithelium. Hyperchromasia, pleomorphism and mitoses are rare while squamous metaplasia only involves overlying surface respiratory epithelium. Bands of spindle cell-rich stroma may be hyalinized or with prominent lymphocytes and/or plasma cells.

Immunohistochemistry and EM
Immunohistochemistry demonstrates similar staining to non-neoplastic bronchial glands with epithelial cells positive for EMA, broad-spectrum cytokeratins and CEA. Focal stromal cell positivity for broad-spectrum keratins, smooth-muscle actin and S-100 protein indicate a myoepithelial component. Proliferating cell nuclear antigen and Ki-67 staining performed in several cases demonstrate rare tumour cell positivity {543}. Mucinous and myoepithelial cell types have been identified by electron microscopy {543,804}.

Differential diagnosis
Low-grade mucoepidermoid carcinoma including the papillary and cystic variants may closely mimic mucus gland adenoma. Despite architectural similarities, the presence of squamous and intermediate cells confirms mucoepidermoid carcinoma. Mucinous cystadenomas are located in the lung periphery and consist of a cystic lesion filled with mucus and lined by uniform, bland mucus cells. Adenocarcinomas are usually infiltrative and feature cytologic atypia, mitoses and necrosis.

Histogenesis
The tumour is postulated to arise from the mucus glands of the bronchus.

Prognosis and predictive factors
Mucus gland adenomas are benign and conservative lung-sparing bronchoscopic or sleeve resection is recommended {543}.

Pleomorphic adenoma

D.B Flieder
F. Thivolet-Bejui
H. Popper
C. Moran

Definition
A tumour with both epithelial and connective tissue differentiation consisting of glands intermingled with myoepithelial cells in a myxoid and chondroid stroma.

ICD-O code
8940/0

Synonym
Benign mixed tumour

Epidemiology
Although rare, pulmonary pleomorphic adenoma has been reported in individuals ranging from 11-74 years, but most often affects those in their sixth and seventh decades of life. A gender predilection is not seen {803,1364,1727,1958}.

Etiology
No specific etiologies have been implicated in the evolution of the tumour.

Localization
Most tumours are centrally located endobronchial polypoid masses but peripheral lesions occur {803,1364,1727,1958}.

Clinical features
Tumours most often present with obstructive symptoms {1364}. A minority of lesions are incidental X-ray findings demonstrating either discrete endobronchial mass with minimal bronchial wall thickening or well-circumscribed peripheral nodules. Cytologic and bronchoscopic biopsy material can suggest the diagnosis but complete excision is required for a definitive diagnosis.

Macroscopy
Tumours range in size from 1.5-16 cm {803,1364,1727,1958}. Typically, endobronchial lesions are usually associated with a major or secondary bronchus and are polypoid, with some degree of luminal occlusion. Peripheral lesions are not intimately associated with airways. Tumours are circumscribed, unencapsulated with a gray-white, rubbery or myxoid cut surface.

Histopathology
Pulmonary pleomorphic adenomas are biphasic like their salivary gland counterpart, but do not often feature either a prominent glandular component or chondroid stroma. Rather, tumours exhibit features of the so-called "cellular mixed tumour" manifesting sheets, trabeculae or islands of epithelial and/or myoepithelial cells and a myxoid matrix. When present, ducts composed of an outer layer of myoepithelial cells and an inner layer of epithelial cells containing small amounts of periodic acid-Schiff (PAS)-positive luminal secretion. Mitotic activity, pleomorphism and necrosis are unusual.

Immunohistochemistry
Ductal and myoepithelial cells stain for both low-molecular weight and broad spectrum keratin while myoepithelial and stromal cells are positive for vimentin, smooth-muscle actin and glial fibrillary acidic protein. S-100 protein immunoreactivity can also be seen in both epithelial and myoepithelial cells {1364,1727}.

Differential diagnosis
Pulmonary pleomorphic adenoma must be discerned from head and neck or even breast metastasis by thorough clinical history and examination. A solitary tumour associated with a cartilage-bearing airway suggests a pulmonary origin. The morphologic differential diagnosis includes hamartoma, pulmonary blastoma and carcinosarcoma. Hamartomas usually show cartilage and other mesenchymal elements while the latter tumours feature obviously malignant stroma and epithelium.

Histogenesis
This neoplasm with epithelial and connective tissue differentiation is regarded as arising from the submucosal bronchial gland epithelium. However, peripheral and subpleural locations unrelated to bronchi raise the possibility that the tumour may originate from a primitive stem cell.

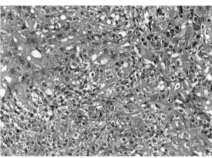

Fig. 1.89 Pleomorphic adenoma. Sheets of epithelial and/or myoepithelial cells are embedded in a myxoid matrix.

Prognosis and predictive factors
Pleomorphic adenomas of the lung exhibit a spectrum of clinical behavior ranging from benign to malignant. On the basis of several studies, small well-circumscribed lesions are cured with lobectomy while larger, infiltrative or poorly circumscribed lesions tend to recur and metastasize. Tumours with greater than 5 mitoses per 10 high-power fields may be associated with aggressive behavior {1364}, but in the absence of malignant cytology, necrosis and angiolymphatic invasion such lesions should be diagnosed as benign pleomorphic adenoma rather than carcinoma ex pleomorphic adenoma.

Other benign salivary gland-like tumours

Well-defined salivary gland tumours including monomorphic adenoma, oncocytoma, and myoepithelioma are extremely rare primary lung tumours {429,1812,1883,1977,2037}. Adenomyoepithelioma {2037} is discussed under epimyoepithelial carcinoma in the section on malignant salivary gland tumours. In the absence of known salivary gland primaries and exclusion of mimics such as metastatic and primary malignancies including typical carcinoid tumour, these solitary lesions in the lung can be diagnosed as primary lung neoplasms.

Mucinous cystadenoma

D.B. Flieder
F. Thivolet-Bejui
H. Popper
B. Pugatch

Definition
A localized cystic mass filled with mucin and surrounded by a fibrous wall lined by well-differentiated columnar mucinous epithelium.

ICD-O code   8470/0

Epidemiology
This exceedingly rare tumour is most often seen in both men and women in their sixth and seventh decades of life {730,1067,1068,1699}. Most reported cases occur in tobacco-smokers but no specific etiologies have been implicated in the evolution of the tumour {730,1067, 1068,1699}.

Localization
These tumours are usually located in the peripheral lung.

Clinical features and diagnostic procedures
Mucinous cystadenoma are asymptomatic lesions that present as incidental rounded well demarcated masses on X-ray and CT scans {1067,1068}. Fine needle aspirates and transbronchial biopsies may sample mucin or goblet cells, but a definitive diagnosis requires surgical excision and complete histologic sampling.

Macroscopy
Grossly, unilocular mucous-filled cysts measure from less than 1.0-5.0 cm and are not associated with airways. Cyst walls are thin (0.1 cm) and lack mural nodules {1067,1068}.

Tumour spread and staging
One instance of tumour seeding the parietal pleura (so-called pleural pseudomyxoma) has been reported {730}.

Histopathology
Microscopically, the cystic lesion is filled with mucus and the fibrous connective tissue wall is lined by a discontinuous layer of low cuboidal to tall columnar, mucin-secreting epithelium. Lining cells feature basally located hyperchromatic nuclei and abundant cytoplasmic mucin. Focal cellular stratification, papillary infoldings and rare mitoses may be seen, but micropapillary fronds, necrosis and overt cytologic atypia are by definition absent. Foreign body giant cell reaction associated with extravasated mucus and stromal chronic inflammation are prominent adjacent to areas of denuded epithelium.

Immunohistochemistry
Lesional epithelium is broad-spectrum keratin positive, rarely CEA positive and surfactant-associated protein A negative {1067,1699}. Proliferating cell nuclear antigen and Ki-67 antibodies stain less than 10% and 5% of lesional cell nuclei, respectively {1699}.

Differential diagnosis
Mucinous cystadenoma should not be confused with mucinous cystadenocarcinoma or the colloid mucinous variant of adenocarcinoma. Mucus extravasation, lepidic spread of epithelium beyond the fibrous capsule or into adjacent lung invasion or cytologic anaplasia indicates adenocarcinoma. Other considerations include mucinous bronchioloalveolar carcinoma, and non-neoplastic lesions, such as congenital cystic adenomatoid malformation as well as developmental and post-infectious bronchogenic cysts.

Prognosis and predictive factors
Mucinous cystadenomas are benign tumours. Complete excision is curative.

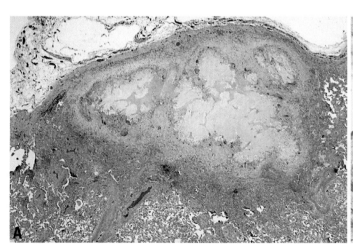 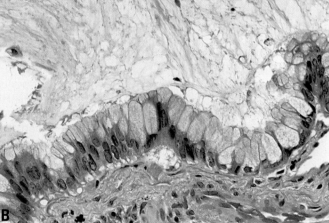

Fig. 1.90 Mucinous cystadenoma. **A** A subpleural cystic tumour is surrounded by a fibrous wall and contains abundant mucus. From Travis et al. {2024}. **B** Columnar epithelial cells line the wall of the cyst. Most of the nuclei are basally oriented but there is focal nuclear pseudostratification. The apical cytoplasm is filled with abundant mucin. From Travis et al. {2024}.

Marginal zone B-cell lymphoma of the mucosa-associated lymphoid tissue (MALT) type

A.G. Nicholson
N.L. Harris

Definition

Pulmonary marginal zone B-cell lymphoma of mucosa-associated lymphoid tissue (MALT) is an extranodal lymphoma comprising morphologically heterogeneous small B-cells, cells resembling monocytoid cells, and/or small lymphocytes, with scattered immunoblasts and centroblasts-like cells. There is plasma cell differentiation in a proportion of the cases. The infiltrate is in the marginal zone of reactive B-cell follicles and extends into the interfollicular region. The neoplastic cells typically infiltrate the bronchiolar mucosal epithelium, forming lymphoepithelial lesions.

ICD-O code   9699/3

Synonyms

The term pseudolymphoma is considered obsolete, and lymphocytic interstitial pneumonia is now limited to inflammatory lesions. Terms such as BALT (bronchial associated lymphoid tissue) lymphoma and BALTOMA should now also be avoided.

Historical annotation

Primary pulmonary non-Hodgkin's lymphoma was originally defined as a lymphoma that presented primarily in the lungs, with or without hilar node involvement but without clinical evidence of disease elsewhere {1731}. Those tumours

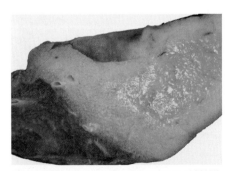

Fig. 1.91 Marginal zone B-cell lymphoma of MALT. Macroscopy. A diffuse consolidation of the middle lobe with a solid cream-coloured cut surface that is similar in texture to the cut surface of a lymph node involved by lymphoma.

not fulfilling these criteria were classified as pseudolymphomas, but this term is now obsolete as most of these cases are now believed to be neoplastic and the rare localized reactive lesions are classified as nodular lymphoid hyperplasia. Early series of pulmonary lymphoma were categorised according to lymph node classifications {1063,2041}, but it is now accepted that the majority of cases arise from bronchial mucosa-associated lymphoid tissue (MALT) {21,137,407,577, 1104,1176,1467}. The REAL classification currently recommends the term 'Marginal Zone B-Cell Lymphoma of the Mucosa-Associated Lymphoid Tissue (MALT) Type' for those with 'low-grade' features and 'diffuse large B-cell non-Hodgkin's lymphoma' for those with 'high-grade' features.

Epidemiology

Approximately 70-90% of primary pulmonary lymphomas are marginal zone lymphomas of MALT type but they account for less than 0.5% of all primary lung neoplasms and a similarly low proportion of all lymphomas {21,1063,1176}. Patients tend to be in their fifth, sixth or seventh decades, with a slight male preponderance. Presentation in younger patients is rare without underlying immunosuppression {21,137,407,577, 1176,1467}.

Etiology

Pulmonary marginal zone B-cell lymphomas of MALT type are thought to arise in acquired MALT secondary to inflammatory or autoimmune processes. Bronchial MALT is not thought to be a normal constituent of the human bronchus, and it likely develops as a response to various antigenic stimuli, for example smoking {1659} and autoimmune disease {1469}. However, a common association, as seen between gastric lymphomas of MALT origin and Helicobacter pylori infection {2171}, has not been found. The etiology of most cases of pulmonary MALT lymphoma is not known.

Localization

Tumours have no zonal or lobar predisposition, are typically peripheral in location, and range from solitary nodules to diffuse bilateral disease (the pattern that mimics lymphocytic interstitial pneumonia).

Clinical features

The most common presentation is a mass discovered on a chest radiograph in an asymptomatic patient, with symptomatic patients presenting with cough, dyspnoea, chest pain and haemoptysis. Previous or synchronous MALT lymphomas at other extranodal sites are not uncommon. A monoclonal gammopathy may be present, but if present may indicate pulmonary involvement by lymphoplasmacytic lymphoma in a patient with Waldenstrom macroglobulinemia. Rarely patients manifest systemic or 'B' symptoms.

Chest radiographs and high resolution computerized tomograph (HRCT) scanning show multiple, solitary masses or alveolar opacities with associated air bronchograms. HRCT scans may also show airway dilatation, positive angiogram signs and haloes of ground glass shadowing at lesion margins {1014}.

Diagnosis can be made by bronchoscopic or transbronchial biopsy, although not infrequently a surgical lung biopsy will be required. Broncholaveolar lavage and fine-needle aspiration biopsy specimens can be diagnostic of lymphoma if a clonal B-cell population can be demonstrated, but the specific type of lymphoma can rarely be diagnosed by these techniques.

Macroscopy

Nodular areas of pulmonary involvement by pulmonary marginal zone B-cell lymphomas of MALT type typically show a consolidative mass that is yellow to cream in colour, not dissimilar in texture to the cut surface of a lymph node involved by lymphoma. Rarely, tumours are focally cystic.

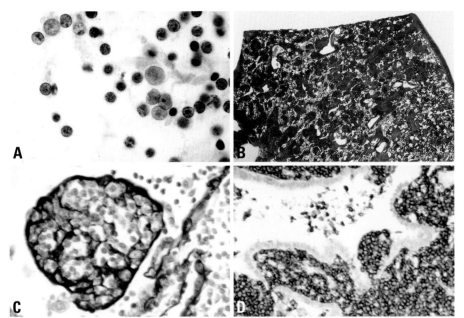

Fig. 1.92 Marginal zone B-cell lymphoma of MALT. **A** Cytology. Loosely cohesive and single cells with well preserved nuclei without nuclear molding. Occasional prominent nucleoli. Bronchial brushing. Papanicolaou stain. **B** A monotonous population of small lymphoid cells diffusely infiltrates the lung. From Travis et al., {2024}. **C** Lymphoepithelial lesions are highlighted by this cytokeratin stain. **D** Neoplastic lymphoid cells stain for CD20, indicating B-cell phenotype.

Histopathology

Pulmonary marginal zone B-cell lymphomas of MALT type generally appear as a diffuse infiltrate of small lymphoid cells, which surround reactive follicles that are typically smaller and less conspicuous than those arising in the stomach. Follicles, best seen when highlighted with a CD21 stain, may be overrun by tumour cells (follicular colonisation). Tumours are composed of lymphocyte-like, lymphoplasmacytic-like, centrocyte-like (marginal zone), or monocytoid B cells, which are all thought to be variations of the same neoplastic cell {904, 1104}. Infiltration of bronchial, bronchiolar and alveolar epithelium (lymphoepithelial lesions) is characteristic but not pathognomonic, since this phenomenon can be seen in non-neoplastic pulmonary lymphoid infiltrates. Plasma cells may be numerous and may accumulate along bronchovascular bundles or interlobular septa and may or may not show light chain restriction. Scattered transformed large cells (centroblasts and immunoblasts) are typically seen, but these are in the minority. The term, marginal zone B-cell lymphoma of MALT type refers only to tumours with a predominance of small cells ('low grade'). Areas with sheets of large cells should receive a separate diagnosis of diffuse large B-cell lymphoma. Lymphoid cells often track along bronchovascular bundles and interlobular septa at the periphery of masses but alveolar parenchyma is destroyed towards their centres. Airways are often left intact, correlating with the presence of air bronchograms on HRCT. Central sclerosis may also be a feature. Giant lamellar bodies are seen in about 20% of cases, most likely reflecting the indolent nature of the neoplasm {1576}. Vascular infiltration, pleural involvement and granuloma formation are not uncommon, but have no prognostic significance. Necrosis is very rare. Amyloid deposition forming nodules with a ring of lymphoma cells can be seen.

Immunophenotype

The neoplastic cells are monoclonal B cells, and may be identified by CD20 or CD79a staining, with a variable reactive T-cell population in the background. Light chain restriction is present in all cases if studied in fresh tissue; it can be demonstrated in paraffin sections in a variable proportion of the cases depending on the laboratory. Cytoplasmic secretory immunoglobulin indicating plasmacytic differentiation is observed in about 30% of cases. The majority of the cases express mu heavy chain, but some express gamma or alpha. They are CD5-, CD10-, CD23-, BCL6-, and CD43 is expressed in some cases. The tumour cells are usually BCL2+ in contrast to reactive monocytoid B cells. Stains for follicular dendritic cells (FDC) such as CD21, CD23, and CD35 highlight reactive follicles and often demonstrate expanded meshworks associated with disrupted follicles overrun by tumour cells. The proliferation fraction (Ki67) is usually very low (<10%); residual follicles show numerous Ki67+ cells. Stains for cytokeratin highlight lymphoepithelial lesions.

Differential diagnosis

From the clinical and imaging aspect, the differential diagnosis includes sarcoidosis, bronchioloalveolar cell carcinoma, organizing pneumonia, infections and rarer alveolar filling disorders and amyloidosis. The histologic differential diagnosis includes lymphocytic interstitial pneumonia, nodular lymphoid hyperplasia, extrinsic allergic alveolitis, inflammatory myofibroblastic tumour and plasma cell granuloma.

In relation to lymphocytic interstitial pneumonia, pulmonary marginal zone B-cell lymphomas of MALT type tend to infiltrate and destroy the alveolar architecture, with greater widening of alveolar septa by the lymphoid infiltrate. Lymphoepithelial lesions may be seen in reactive conditions, but are more prominent in the lymphomas. Using immunohistochemical stains, the presence of expanded infiltrates of B cells outside of follicles is characteristic of MALT lymphoma, while in reactive infiltrates. B cells are present as small aggregates or follicles with a peribronchial and/or septal distribution. Demonstration of immunoglobulin light chain restriction is important in this differential diagnosis, but is optimally done on fresh frozen tissue; anaylsis of immunoglobulin heavy gene rearrangement by PCR can also be very helpful.

Nodular lymphoid hyperplasia (NLH) refers to the rare occurrence of one or several pulmonary nodules consisting of reactive lymphoid cells {1066}. Patients have similar presentation and epidemiology to those with pulmonary marginal zone B-cell lymphomas of MALT type although associated lymphadenopathy and pleural effusions suggest the diagnosis of lymphoma {611}.

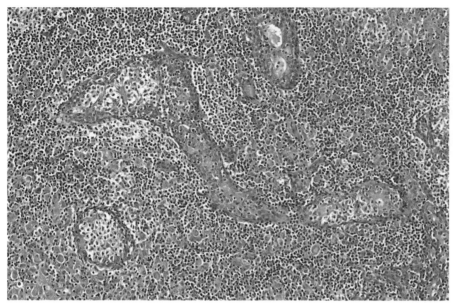

Fig. 1.93 Marginal zone B-cell lymphoma of MALT. The lymphoid cells infiltrate the bronchiolar epithelium forming lymphoepithelial lesions. From Travis et al. {2024}.

Histologically, NLH comprises numerous reactive germinal centres with well-preserved mantle zones and interfollicular sheets of mature plasma cells, with varying degrees of interfollicular fibrosis. Plasma cells may show Russell bodies, but not Dutcher bodies. Invasion of the visceral pleura or invasion of bronchial cartilage are not found. Immunohistochemical stains demonstrate a reactive pattern of B cells and T cells. In particular, the germinal centers stain for the B-cell marker CD20, while interfollicular lymphocytes are immunoreactive for CD3, CD43 and CD5 {10}. Antibodies to CD45RA stain the mantle zone lymphocytes, but stains for bcl-1 and bcl-2 do not decorate the follicles. The CD20-positive lymphocytes do not co-express either CD43 or CD5. Staining for immunoglobulin light chains shows a polyclonal pattern among the plasma cells. Molecular genetic analysis has shown no rearrangement of the immunoglobulin heavy chain gene {10}. Assays for the chromosomal rearrangement t(14;18) have been negative.

Pulmonary marginal zone B-cell lymphomas of MALT type may produce amyloid and must be distinguished from nodular amyloidomas {430}. The morphologic finding of a dense plasma cell infiltrate, light chain restriction in plasma cells, numerous B cells expressing CD20 and coexpression of CD43 by B cells have been shown to be useful in confirming the diagnosis of lymphoma.

The differential diagnosis, particularly on small biopsy specimens, also includes other small B-cell lymphomas, such as follicular lymphoma, mantle cell lymphoma, small lymphocytic lymphoma (CLL) and lymphoplasmacytic lymphoma. Lack of CD5 is helpful in excluding small lymphocytic and mantle cell lymphoma, lack of cyclin D1 in excluding mantle cell lymphoma, and lack of CD10 and BCL6 in excluding follicular lymphoma. Distinction from lymphoplasmacytic lymphoma requires finding the characteristic morphologic features of pulmonary marginal zone B-cell lymphomas of MALT type (follicles and marginal zone differentiation) or the characteristic clinical features of lymphoplasmacytic lymphoma (disseminated disease with bone marrow involvement and macroglobulinemia).

Histogenesis
Lymphocytes within bronchial MALT.

Somatic genetics
Immunoglobulin genes are clonally rearranged. Rearrangements can be detected by Southern blot in all cases if fresh or frozen tissue is used. Amplification of the immunoglobulin heavy chain gene from paraffin sections with the polymerase chain reaction can detect monoclonality in 60% of marginal zone lymphomas {137,1467}.

T(11;18)(q21;q21) translocation, is the most common genetic abnormality in pulmonary marginal zone B-cell lymphoma of MALT type (50-60% of cases). T(1;14) or trisomy 3 may also occur. The t(11;18) involves the API2 anti-apoptosis gene on chromosome 11 and a recently recognized gene called MLT on chromosome 18, and produces a fusion protein. Both the t(1;14) and the t(11;18) lead to nuclear Bcl-10 expression {1504}. One recent study has shown that t(11;18) and aneuploidy are primarily mutually exclusive events, especially in the lung, suggesting different pathogenetic pathways in the development of this type of lymphoma. Both abnormalities were associated with recurrent disease {1104}.

Tumour spread and staging
It has been recommended that cases with unilateral or bilateral pulmonary involvement be staged as IE, and cases with regional lymph node (hilar/mediastinal) involvement be staged as IIE {2053}. When distant spread occurs, there is preferential spread to other mucosal sites rather than to lymph nodes (just as other lymphomas of MALT origin may spread to the lung) {407,1467}.

Prognosis and predictive factors
In patients with resectable disease, surgery has resulted in prolonged remission {2053}, but for those with either bilateral or unresectable unilateral disease, treatment has been governed by the principles that apply to more advanced nodal lymphomas. Indeed, elderly patients with asymptomatic lesions may well be followed up without treatment. Five-year survival for marginal zone lymphomas of MALT origin is quoted at 84-94% {577,1176,1467}. A small percentage of MALT lymphomas progress to diffuse large B-cell lymphoma.

Primary pulmonary diffuse large B-cell lymphoma

A.G. Nicholson
N.L. Harris

Definition
Diffuse large B-cell non-Hodgkin's lymphoma (DLBCL) is a diffuse proliferation of large neoplastic B lymphoid cells with nuclear size equal to or exceeding normal macrophage nuclei or more than twice the size of a normal lymphocyte. Primary pulmonary DLBCL is used for tumours that are localized to the lungs at presentation.

ICD-O code   9680/3

Synonyms
High-grade MALT lymphoma has been used for these tumours, but this term should no longer be used.

Epidemiology
DLBCL comprise about 5-20% of primary pulmonary lymphomas {21,407,577, 1063,1176,1467}. Patients usually present between 50-70 years of age, similar to patients with pulmonary marginal zone B-cell lymphoma of MALT type. There is no sex predisposition. Primary pulmonary DLBCL may occur as a complication of immunosuppression for allografts.

Etiology
The etiology of most diffuse large B-cell lymphomas is not known. However, an association between diffuse large B-cell non-Hodgkin lymphomas arising in the lung and collagen vascular diseases, both with and without fibrosing alveolitis, has been reported {1469}. Other associations of B-cell lymphomas include AIDS and immunodeficiency conditions.

Localization
Tumours have no zonal or lobar predisposition, and are typically peripheral in location.

Clinical features
Patients are nearly always symptomatic and present with cough, haemoptysis and dyspnoea. Some patients complain of systemic ('B') symptoms. Imaging shows solid and often multiple masses.

Macroscopy
Nodules are typically solid and cream-coloured, and may also exhibit paler and softer areas that correlate with necrosis.

Tumour spread and staging
It has been recommended that cases with unilateral or bilateral pulmonary involvement be staged as IE, and cases with regional lymph node (hilar/mediastinal) involvement be staged as IIE {2053}.

Histopathology
DLBCL of the lung are morphologically similar to DLBCL in other sites. Tumours consist of diffuse sheets of large, blastic lymphoid cells, 2-4 times the size of normal lymphocytes, infiltrating and destroying the lung parenchyma. Vascular infiltration and pleural involvement are commonly seen, but lymphoepithelial lesions are rare. Necrosis is common.

Immunohistochemistry
The neoplastic cells are of B-cell phenotype, expressing pan-B antigens (CD20, CD79a) with a variable reactive T-cell population in the background. Monotypic immunoglobulin light chain expression may be detected if frozen tissue is available.

Differential diagnosis
The differential diagnosis includes other malignant tumours, including undifferentiated carcinoma of either large cell or small cell type, some variants of Hodgkin's lymphoma, anaplastic large cell lymphoma and rarely germ cell tumours. The diagnosis can usually be made using an immunohistochemical panel including cytokeratins, placental alkaline phosphatase, CD20, CD3, CD30, ALK1, CD15, CD45 and EMA Primary pulmonary DLBCL must be distinguished from mediastinal large B-cell lymphoma infiltrating the lung. Knowledge of the clinical features, including the age and sex of the patient and the presence of a mediastinal mass, is important in establishing the correct diagnosis. A lung biopsy in a young woman showing DLBCL should raise the suspicion of mediastinal large B-cell lymphoma. Distinction from pulmonary lymphomatoid granulomatosis may be difficult as both entities show a B-cell phenotype and angiocentricity and necrosis may not be apparent on a small biopsy specimen. In lymphomatoid granulomatosis, the T-cell infiltrate is usually much more prominent than in DLBCL. Identification of Epstein-Barr virus may be of value as atypical B-cells in lymphomatoid granulomatosis and immunodeficient patients are usually positive, whilst those in immunocompetent patients with diffuse large B-cell lymphoma are negative {1716}.

Histogenesis
DLBCL originates from proliferating peripheral B cells and or dedifferentaition of bronchial MALT lymphocytes.

Somatic genetics
Immunoglobulin genes are clonally rearranged. Evidence of monoclonality via amplification of the immunoglobulin heavy chain gene with the polymerase chain reaction can be demonstrated in about 25% of DLBCL {1467}. Little is known about genetic abnormalities in primary pulmonary DLBCL.

Prognosis and predictive factors
Patients may inadvertently undergo resection for localised disease , but are usually treated with combination chemotherapy as for DLBCL in other sites, often with high response rates to adriamycin-based regimens {1203, 1320}. Overall, five-year survival ranges from 0-60% {577,1176,1467}.

Lymphomatoid granulomatosis

M.N. Koss
N. L. Harris

Definition
Lymphomatoid granulomatosis (LYG) is an extranodal angiocentric and angiodestructive lymphoproliferative disorder, composed of a polymorphous infiltrate of atypical appearing Epstein Barr virus-infected B cells and numerically more abundant admixed reactive T cells {752}. Lymphomatoid granulomatosis shows a spectrum of histologic grade and clinical aggressiveness, which is related to the proportion of EBV positive large B cells. LYG may progress to an EBV positive diffuse large B-cell lymphoma.

ICD-O code   9766/1

Synonyms and historical annotation
These lesions were first described nearly 30 years ago by Averill Liebow, who could not decide whether they were a variant of Wegener's granulomatosis or a malignant lymphoma - hence, the unusual name "lymphomatoid granulomatosis" {1182}. More recently, the term "angiocentric immunoproliferative lesion" (AIL) was proposed, which included what we now know as nasal-type NK/T-cell lymphoma, and suggested that the disease is a lymphoproliferative disorder with the capability of evolving into lymphoma {919} Neoplasms of T or NK-cell origin with an angiocentric growth pattern should not be classified as LYG, but rather as extranodal peripheral T-cell lymphomas. The term LYG is currently preferred.

Epidemiology
LYG is rare. It typically presents in middle-aged adults (although both younger and older patients have been reported) {562,969,1062,1182,1603}. The disease can occur as an apparently idiopathic lesion, but it more often occurs in patients who have been immunosuppressed. Examples include patients who have AIDS or Wiskott-Aldrich syndrome, those who have had organ transplants or who have been treated for acute lymphoblastic lymphoma or follicular lymphoma and those who have agnogenic myeloid metaplasia {1468}. In patients without known prior immunodeficiency, anergy, impaired in vitro responsiveness to mitogens, diminished humoral and cell-mediated responsiveness to Epstein-Bar virus and decrease in total T cells, CD4 and CD8 lymphocytes, have all been reported {920,2154}.

Etiology
LYG is an EBV-driven B-cell lymphoproliferative disorder, probably arising in a background of immunodeficiency in most cases.

Localization
Masses or nodules can involve a variety of organs, most often lung and central nervous system, and kidney; skin may be involved (in the form of ulcerated or non-ulcerated subcutaneous nodules, erythematous dermal papules or plaques) {131}.

Clinical features
There is a complex array of symptoms, corresponding to the sites of involvement. Up to 70% of patients show bilateral, usually peripheral, lung nodules that measure up to 9 cm. in diameter {969, 1062,1603}. Cavitation may or may not be present. Other radiographic patterns include diffuse reticulonodular or alveolar infiltrates, localized infiltrates or a solitary mass. The upper respiratory tract can be involved by ulcero-destructive lesions but lymphadenopathy is infrequent.

Macroscopy
The lungs usually show yellow-white well-demarcated masses that can have a solid or granular, cheesy appearance. They often have a "cannon ball" appearance. They may be cavitated. Similar masses can be found in other organs, such as the kidney or brain.

Histopathology
The lymphoid infiltrate often surrounds muscular pulmonary arteries and veins early in the course of the disease, and typically invades the walls of these vessels. Necrosis is a frequent, although not universal, feature of the disease and it can range from extensive in larger masses or high-grade lesions to minimal in low-grade lesions.

LYG consists of small round lymphocytes, some of which may show slight cytologic atypia and variable numbers of atypical large mononuclear lymphoid cells in a background of histiocytes and occasional plasma cells {969,1062,

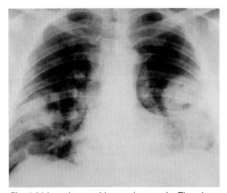

Fig. 1.94 Lymphomatoid granulomatosis. The chest radiograph shows multiple bilateral cavitary masses.

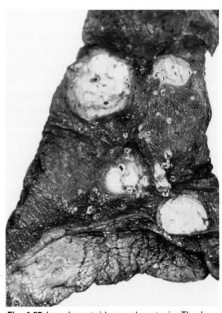

Fig. 1.95 Lymphomatoid granulomatosis. The lung shows multiple yellow-white necrotic masses.

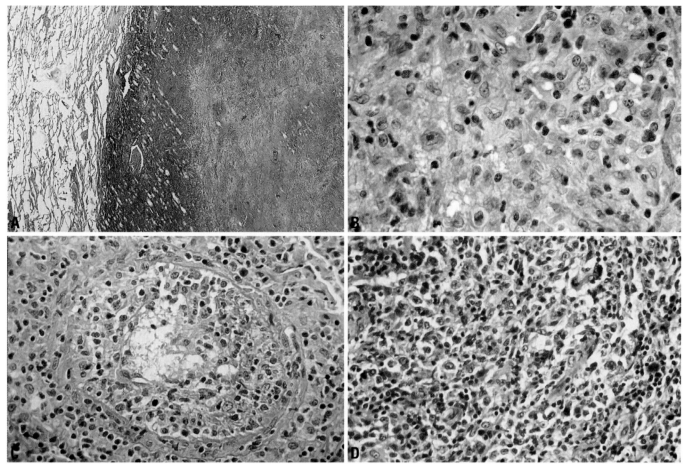

Fig. 1.96 Lymphomatoid granulomatosis. **A** The lesion is well demarcated, with a central area of bland necrosis and a rim of residual lymphoid tissue. **B** Lymphomatoid granulomatosis (grade 2). The lesion shows a mixed cell population of small lymphocytes, macrophages and a single immunoblast with a prominent nucleolus. **C** Vasculitis in lymphomatoid granulomatosis. The arterial wall is infiltrated by small lymphocytes. **D** Lymphomatoid granulomatosis (grade 3), containing sheets of markedly atypical cells, consistent with large cell lymphoma.

1182}. Eosinophils and neutrophils are usually not conspicuous. The large cells resemble immunoblasts; some of the atypical cells may have double nuclei, suggesting Reed-Sternberg cells, but classic Reed-Sternberg cells are not seen. Despite the term "granulomatosis" in the name, epithelioid granulomas and giant cells are almost always absent.

Sample size is important: Less than 30% of transbronchial biopsies are diagnostic, so a surgical lung biopsy will be necessary in most cases to achieve a diagnosis {1603}.

There is a histologic grading system for LYG that is based on the number of atypical large EBV-infected cells {1192}. Grade 1 lesions contain few or no EBV-infected cells (less than 5 per high-power field), usually lack necrosis, and are polymorphous. Grade 2 lesions have scattered EBV-infected cells (5-20 per high-power field) and foci of necrosis (extensive at times), but they remain polymorphous; this is the classic and most frequently encountered type of case. Grade 3 lesions show sheets of EBV-infected cells, necrosis, and cellular monomorphism, and are considered a subtype of diffuse large B-cell lymphoma {919}.

Immunophenotype
LYG is a T-cell-rich, B-cell lymphoproliferative process, as shown by a number of studies, both in lung and in other sites, such as skin {131,752,776,1382,1468, 1973}.

Histogenesis
EBV-infected peripheral B cell.

Genetics and pathogenesis
In grade 2 and 3 lesions, the B-cells are either clonal or oligoclonal by methods such as VJ-PCR and Southern blot and appear to be proliferating, at least by proliferation indices {751,919}. The EBV sequences also are typically clonal. Different monoclonal B-cell clones can occur in different sites in the same patient {131,2154}. In grade 1 lesions, monoclonality can be more difficult to demonstrate, possibly because of the paucity of neoplastic B cells, or alternatively because some of these lesions may not be truly neoplastic The T cells that are so abundant in LYG are polyclonal by molecular methods {751}.

These results suggest that in most cases LYG is a T-cell-rich B-cell lymphoma. However, some grade 1 cases may be EBV driven polyclonal lymphoproliferations, and grade 2 cases may be similar to polymorphous, monoclonal post-transplant lymphoproliferative disorders (PTLD), in which some degree of immunodeficiency allows proliferation of clonal EBV+ B cells. These cases may evolve

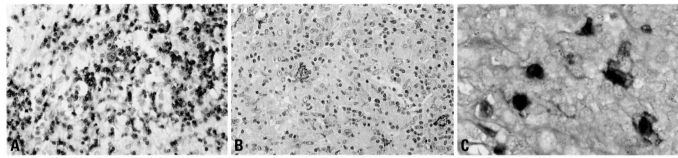

Fig. 1.97 Lymphomatoid granulomatosis (grade 2). **A** Immunohistochemical staining for CD3 shows the numerous background lymphocytes to be T cells. Scattered larger atypical lymphocytes (B-cells) are negative. **B** The same microscopic field stained for CD20. The scattered large immunoblastic cells are B cells. **C** Double labeling in situ hybridization for Epstein-Barr Virus with immunohistochemical staining for CD20. Immunohistochemical staining for CD20 (brown) decorates cells which are also positive for EBV by in situ hybridization (black). From Guinee et al. {752}.

into an autonomous, monomorphous diffuse large B-cell lymphoma, analogous to the situation in PTLD {751,919,920}. EBV in a partially immunocompetent host may explain the vascular damage that is a hallmark of the disease. Chemokines, such as IP-10 and Mig, elaborated as a result of the EBV infection may be responsible for vascular damage by promoting T-cell adhesion to endothelial cells {1994}.

Differential diagnosis

Some lesions that are histologically similar to LYG do not show atypical EBV-infected B cells, but rather contain atypical cells that are CD3+ T cells {1382, 1417}. These T-cell lesions are peripheral T-cell lymphomas, that, because they are angiocentric and polymorphous, are histologically similar to LYG {1382}. Cases of enteropathy-associated T-cell lymphoma and of acute T-cell lymphoblastic leukemia have been confused as cases of LYG in some series {1468}. T-cell lymphomas of other types, such as nasal-type CD56+ NK/T-cell lymphomas may also mimic LYG histologically. Immunophenotypic analysis to demonstrate the B or T/NK-cell nature of the large cells is important in distinguishing these entities. In many peripheral T cell lymphomas the proliferation fraction of the T cells (Ki67+) is higher than that of the T cells in LYG. The diagnosis of LYG should be made only in cases in which the proliferating large cells are B cells. Cases of grade 1 LYG may lack EBV-positive B cells. Skin lesions also often have very few EBV-infected B cells and are subject to sampling problems {131}. These cases give rise to a differential diagnosis of reactive inflammatory processes. Clinical correlation and biopsy of other sites may be necessary to establish the diagnosis.

Prognosis and predictive factors

Outcome is variable. Patients may show waxing and waning of their disease. When disease is confined to the lung, or skin, it may resolve without treatment (14-27% of patients) {919,920}. Still, the most common result is death, with median survival of 2 years {919}. The histologic grade of the lesion is correlated with outcome {969,1192}. Most patients have grades 1 or 2 disease. Only one-third of patients with grade 1 lesions progress to malignant lymphoma (grade 3), whereas two-thirds of patients with grade 2 lesions develop lymphoma (all patients with grade 3 lesions have lymphoma by definition) {1192}. It is less clear whether stage of disease correlates with outcome: one study reported a worse prognosis in patients with neurologic lesions, while another did not {969,1062}. Lesions in the central nervous system are often of high histological grade. Long-term survival may occur even in untreated patients with grade 1 and 2 lesions, particularly those whose disease is restricted to lung {969,1062}. Currently, grade 3 lesions are typically treated as diffuse large B cell lymphoma {1168} with aggressive chemotherapy; grade 1 and 2 lesions are often treated with interferon alpha 2b {920,2154}.

Table 1.13
Immunoprofile of lymphomatoid granulomatosis. From references {776,1382,2154}.

B cells (immunoblasts) CD20+, CD79a+, CD30+ (EBV-induced), CD43+/-, CD15- EBV+ (by in situ hybridization for EBER 1/2 RNA or by immunohistochemistry for LMP)
T cells CD3+, CD4+, CD8+ Cytotoxic markers: TIA-1, granzyme B

Pulmonary Langerhans cell histiocytosis

T.V. Colby
W.D. Travis

Definition

Pulmonary Langerhans cell histiocytosis (PLCH) is an interstitial lung disease caused by the proliferation of Langerhans cells and their associated changes in the lung. Most affected patients are adults and in most the lung is the sole site of involvement.

Many Langerhans cell proliferation syndromes are considered clonal and neoplastic {919} but clonality studies on PLCH in adults suggests that this may represent a reactive proliferation of Langerhans cells {2218}.

ICD-O code   9751/1

Synonyms

Pulmonary histiocytosis X, pulmonary eosinophilic granuloma, pulmonary Langerhans cell granulomatosis.

Epidemiology

PLCH is an uncommon form of interstitial lung disease {2025,2075,2076}. The sex predilection has varied in series; it is probably roughly equal. The mean age at diagnosis is approximately 40 years with a broad range (18-70 years) when children with disseminated LCH syndromes are excluded {2075,2076}.

Etiology

95% or more of patients are current or former cigarette smokers {2075,2076}.

Localization

Predominantly upper and mid zones with sparing of the costophrenic angles.

Clinical features

Signs and symptoms

Patients may be asymptomatic (15-25%), or may present with pulmonary symptoms (cough, dyspnoea, chest pain) or with systemic complaints (malaise, weight loss, fever) {2025,2075,2076}. Approximately 15% of adults with PLCH have extrapulmonary involvement {2075}. PLCH in adults may rarely be part of a systemic Langerhans cell histiocytosis or Langerhans cell sarcoma, which are best considered a neoplastic haematologic problem {919}.

Pulmonary function studies are abnormal in most (85% or more) patients and include (in order of frequency) restrictive deficits, obstructive deficits, isolated decreased diffusing capacity, and mixed restrictive/obstructive deficits {2076}.

Imaging

Chest radiographs show interstitial lung disease with predilection for the mid and upper lung zones {2025,2075,2076}. High-resolution CT scanning is distinctive, most typically showing nodules or nodules and cystic change with mid and upper lung zone predilection {2025, 2075,2076}.

Macroscopy

The gross findings depend on the extent of involvement and the amount of scarring. Small nodules, generally 2-5 mm in size (rarely up to 2 cm), may be palpated {2025}. In progressive disease there is extensive interstitial fibrosis with or without associated emphysematous changes.

Histopathology

Histologically most cases of PLCH show concomitant changes of smoking including emphysema and respiratory bronchiolitis {2025,2075,2076}. The lesions of PLCH begin as cellular proliferations of Langerhans cells along small airways, primarily bronchioles and alveolar ducts. As the lesions enlarge, rounded or stellate nodules develop and the bronchiolocentricity is less easy to discern. The nodules undergo a natural history from cellular lesions rich in Langerhans cells to fibrotic lesions which, in their end-stage, are entirely devoid of identifiable Langerhans cells. In healed PLCH cases the diagnosis is possible based on the presence of stellate centrilobular scarring in the setting of typical HRCT changes.

Langerhans cells are recognized by their distinctive morphology with pale eosinophilic cytoplasm and delicate nuclei with prominent folding of the nuclear membranes {919,2025,2075, 2076}. Their presence may be confirmed with S-100 protein and/or CD1a staining.

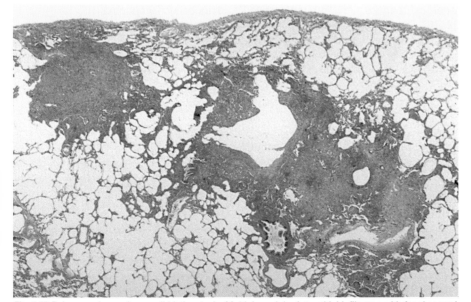

Fig. 1.98 Pulmonary Langerhans cell histiocytosis. Multiple nodular interstitial infiltrates with focal central cavitation. The edge of the nodular infiltrates shows a stellate shape. From Travis et al. {2024}.

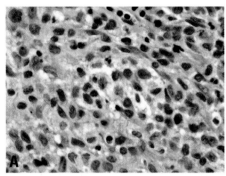 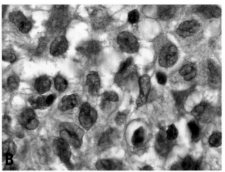 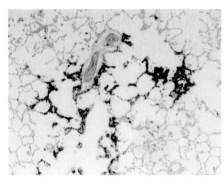

Fig. 1.99 Pulmonary Langerhans' cell histiocytosis. **A** Langerhans' cells are readily recognizable by their distinctive morphology with pale cytoplasm and delicate folded nuclei. Interspersed eosinophils and pigmented alveolar macrophages are also common. **B** The infiltratre consists of Langerhans cells with a moderate amount of eosinophilic cytoplasm and nuclei with prominent grooves. From {2024}.

Fig. 1.100 Pulmonary Langerhans cell histiocytosis. CD1a shows an infiltrate of strongly positive Langerhans cells in the interstitium along an alveolar duct.

The morphologic features are sufficiently characteristic that immunohistochemical staining is unnecessary for diagnosis in classic cases.

Precursor lesions
Langerhans cell hyperplasia in association with smoking {2075}.

Histogenesis
Proliferation of Langerhans cells {2075}.

Somatic genetics
Yousem et al used the X-linked polymorphic human androgen receptor assay (HUMARA) locus to assess clonality in female patients with pulmonary LCH and found that seven (29%) were clonal and 17 (71%) were nonclonal. A nonclonal population was found in three of six cases with multiple nodules. In one biopsy with five nodules, two nodules were clonal with one allele inactivated, one nodule was clonal with the other allele inactivated, and two nodules were nonclonal. These findings indicate that pul-

monary LCH appears to be primarily a reactive process with clonal proliferation of Langerhans cells developing in the setting of nonclonal Langerhans cell hyperplasia, probably in response to antigens in cigarette smoke {2218}.

Treatment
Steroids have been the mainstay therapy for PLCH {2075,2076}. With the recognition of the association of PLCH with cigarette smoking, smoking cessation is also important. Refractory cases may respond to immunosuppressive therapy. Some cases of PLCH clear spontaneously, making the effects of treatment difficult to determine.

Prognosis and predictive factors
Approximately 15% of patients have progressive respiratory disease that may be fatal or lead to lung transplantation {2076}. Progression may be slow, spanning decades and be dominated by clinical features of obstructive lung disease. Predictors of shorter survival include

older age, lower forced expiratory volume in one second (FEV1), higher residual volume, lower ratio of FEV1 to forced vital capacity, and reduced carbon monoxide diffusing capacity {2076}.

Pulmonary involvement by other haematolymphoid malignancies

The lung may rarely be the primary site of presentation of most types of lymphomas recognized in lymph nodes {391} including both non-Hodgkin lymphoma (follicle center cell lymphoma, mantle cell lymphoma, intravascular large B-cell lymphoma, anaplastic large-cell lymphoma, etc.) and Hodgkin lymphoma. Primary plasmacytomas are also recognized. The lung is also a very common site of relapse in patients who already carry a diagnosis of lymphoma.
Similarly, virtually any leukaemia may affect the lung, either primarily (and be the initial site of presentation) or in patients with known disease {391}.

Table 1.14
Table 1. Classification of Langerhans cell histiocytosis in adults.

Single-organ disease
Lung (occurs in isolation in > 85% of cases with lung involvement)
Bone
Skin
Pituitary
Lymph nodes
Other sites; thyroid, liver, spleen, brain
Multisystem involvement
Multiorgan disease with lung involvement (in 5-15% of cases with lung involvement)
Multiorgan disease without lung involvement
Multiorgan histiocytic disorder

Epithelioid haemangioendothelioma / Angiosarcoma

W.D. Travis
H.D. Tazelaar
M. Miettinen

Definition
Pulmonary epithelioid haemangioendothelioma (PEH) is a low-to-intermediate-grade vascular tumour composed of short cords and nests of epithelioid endothelial cells embedded in a myxohyaline matrix. The tumours are distinctive for their epithelioid character, sharply defined cytoplasmic vacuoles, intraalveolar and intravascular growth and central hyaline necrosis. High-grade epithelioid vascular tumours are called epithelioid angiosarcomas.

ICD-O code
Epithelioid haemangioendothelioma
                                          9133/1
Angiosarcoma   9120/3

Synonyms and historical annotation
Epithelioid haemangioendothelioma was previously called intravascular 'sclerosing' bronchioloalveolar tumour (IVBAT) in the lung.

Clinical features
Signs and symptoms
Most patients with PEH are Caucasian, 80% are women. The mean age is 36 with a range of 12-61 years {435,533, 2120}. The presentation is usually indolent and almost half of the patients are asymptomatic. Symptomatic patients may present with pleuritic chest pain, dyspnoea, mild nonproductive cough, haemoptysis, and clubbing. PEH may rarely present with alveolar hemorrhage {225,298} or as thromboembolic disease {2205}. Up to 15% of patients may have substantial liver involvement. PEH with histology similar to that seen in the lung occur in the liver, bone and soft tissue {510,536,1227,1453}.

Imaging
CT scans or chest x-rays characteristically demonstrate multiple, bilateral, small nodules 1-2 cm in size. However, PEH may present as a solitary lung mass {1399}. The radiographic pattern of the multiple smaller lesions may mimic that of pulmonary Langerhans' cell histiocytosis {1606}. Occasionally the lung nodules may appear calcified {1212}. The most common initial interpretation of the radiographic picture is that of metastatic tumour or old granulomatous disease.

Macroscopy and localization
The most common gross appearance of PEH is that of a 0.3-2.0 cm circumscribed mass of gray-white or gray-tan firm tissue with occasional yellow flecks {435,2081}. The center of the nodules may be calcified and the cut surface reveals a cartilaginous consistency. PEH may involve the pleura in a pattern resembling diffuse malignant mesothelioma {424,1184,2222,2239}.

Histopathology
Low power histologic examination reveals round to oval-shaped nodules, which typically have a central sclerotic, hypocellular zone and a cellular peripheral zone. The necrotic center of the nodules sometimes can be calcified and ossified. The tumour typically spreads into adjacent bronchioles and alveolar spaces in a micropolypoid manner and can be seen passing through pores of Kohn in alveolar walls. Extensive lymphangitic spread may mimic metastatic carcinoma. The intercellular stroma consists of an abundant matrix that may appear chondroid, hyaline, mucinous or myxomatous. Intracellular vacuoles are common, sometimes creating a signet-ring appearance, and suggest an attempt to form unicellular vascular channels. The nuclei of the tumour cells are usually round to oval. Intranuclear cytoplasmic inclusions are common.

Immunohistochemistry and electron microscopy
Commonly used endothelial markers include CD31, CD34 and factor VIII (von Willebrand factor), and most PEH express these markers {462}. Recently, Fli1 (a member of the ETS family of DNA binding transcription factors) and FKBP12 (a cytosolic FK506 binding protein interacting with calcineurin) have been shown to be reliable endothelial markers {599,828}. In epithelioid haemangioendotheliomas, CD31, CD34 and Fli1 protein are more sensitive and reliable markers than von Willebrand factor. Vimentin is strongly positive and present in abundance in these tumour cells in

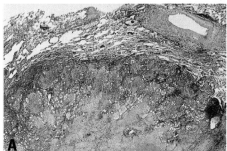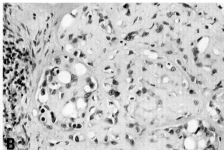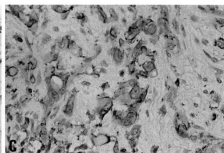

Fig. 1.101 Epithelioid haemangioendothelioma. **A** Tumour nodule showing increased cellularity at the periphery and abundant eosinophilic stroma with focal necrosis in the center. **B** Abundant eosinophilic stroma; cells have prominent cytoplasmic vacuoles or intracytoplasmic lumina. From Travis et al. {2024}. **C** CD31 stain. The tumour cells stain positively; several show prominent cytoplasmic vacuoles.

comparison with normal endothelial cells. Focal cytokeratin expression is reported in 20-30% of cases. Angiosarcomas are also known to express endothelial markers such as von Willebrand factor, CD31, CD34 and Fli1 in the majority of cases. Among them, von Willebrand factor is more specific, but least sensitive. It is often present in a minority of cases with focal weak staining. CD31 is relatively specific and extremely sensitive, being positive in about 90% of the cases. Cytokeratin is expressed in about 30% of the cases, emphasizing the importance of antibody panels to distinguish these vascular tumours from carcinoma {1184,1308}.

Electron microscopic studies reveal an external lamina or basement membrane surrounding the tumour cells and occasional tight junctions {409,1798,2122}. Pinocytotic vesicles may be seen. Conspicuous 100-150 µm thick cytofilaments are present. Weibel-Palade bodies have been described, but may not be detectable in every case. Intracytoplasmic lumens are characteristically present.

Differential diagnosis

The differential diagnosis of PEH includes a variety of benign non-neoplastic conditions such as old granulomatous disease, organizing infarcts, amyloid nodules; several benign neoplasms such as hamartomas, sclerosing haemangioma, and chemodectomas; and malignant neoplasms such as mesothelioma, adenocarcinoma (both primary and metastatic), angiosarcoma, chondrosarcoma, or leiomyosarcoma.

Most of these considerations can be excluded by recognition of the characteristic architecture of the nodular lesions of PEH with a cellular periphery and a central zone, which is often necrotic. The

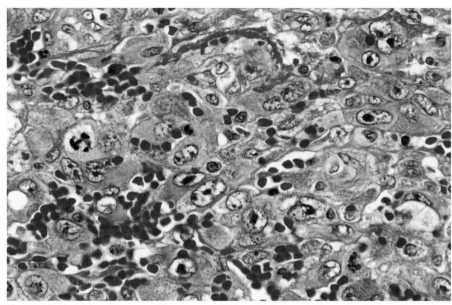

Fig. 1.102 Epithelioid angiosarcoma. The tumour cells show marked cytologic atypia with large hyperchromatic nuclei, vesicular chromatin, prominent nucleoli and mitotic activity.

possibility of lung metastases should be considered since EH can also arise in the liver, soft tissue, and bone. When these tumours metastasize to the lungs, they may present with histologic features identical to cases of PEH {510,536, 2081}. In the presence of a dominant mass in an extrapulmonary site, the lung involvement may represent metastatic disease. Some cases of multifocal bilateral pulmonary disease suggesting metastases, do not have extrathoracic tumours {435}.

Grading: PEH are low or intermediate grade tumours. High grade epithelioid vascular tumours are called epithelioid angiosarcoma, and show more nuclear atypia (mitoses, nucleoli, hyperchromatic chromatin) and less eosinophilic matrix and may have spindle cell foci. Epithelioid angiosarcomas also tend to present as large solitary masses.

Histogenesis

Epithelioid haemangioendotheliomas are derived from endothelial cells.

Somatic genetics

Little is known about the genetics of epithelioid haemangioendothelioma. In two cases an identical chromosomal translocation involving chromosomes 1 and 3 [t(1;3)(p36.3;q25)] was detected {1295}. In another case karyotyping revealed several clonal abnormalities: a complex unbalanced translocation [7;22] involving multiple breakpoints (confirmed by fluorescence in situ hybridization), a Robertsonian t(14;14), and loss of the Y chromosome {208}. Monosomy for chromosome 11 was noted in a subset of the tumour cells {208}.

Pleuropulmonary blastoma

L.P. Dehner
H.D. Tazelaar
T. Manabe

Definition

Pleuropulmonary blastoma is a malignant tumour of infancy and early childhood arising as a cystic and/ or solid sarcomatous neoplasm, in the lung or less often from the parietal pleura {99,1231}. The cystic component is lined by benign metaplastic epithelium that may be ciliated. This embryonic or dysontogenetic neoplasm of the lung and/or pleura is the nosologic counterpart to other like neoplasms of childhood including Wilms tumour, neuroblastoma, hepatoblastoma and retinoblastoma.

ICD-O code   8973/3

Synonyms

Rhabdomysarcoma arising in congenital cystic adenomatoid malformation, pulmonary blastoma of childhood, pulmonary sarcoma arising in mesenchymal cystic hamartoma, embryonal rhabdomysarcoma arising within congenital bronchogenic cyst, pulmonary blastoma associated with cystic lung disease, pleuropulmonary blastoma in congenital cystic adenomatoid malformation {565}.

Epidemiology

Owing to the fact that the pleuropulmonary blastoma came to be recognized as a clinicopathologic entity in 1989, systematic data are not available on its incidence. There are presently over 100 cases registered with The Pleuropulmonary Blastoma Registry (www.ppbregistry.org). It is certainly less common than Wilms tumour, neuroblastoma and even hepatoblastoma. Approximately 25% of cases are accompanied by an apparent constitutional and heritable predisposition to dysplastic or neoplastic disease in keeping with a familial cancer syndrome {1620}. Cystic nephroma, ovarian teratoma, multiple intestinal polyps, and a second pleuropulmonary blastoma have been observed in affected children {910, 1025,1115,1393,1593}.

Age and sex distribution

The age at diagnosis ranges from one month to 12 years, with a median age of 2 years. Most are diagnosed at or before 4 years of age {1619}. The male to female ratio is approximately equal.

Etiology

The origin of this tumour remains unknown, but it may represent the expression of the mesodermally derived thoracic splanchnopleural mesenchyme in the absence of any neoplastic epithelial elements, as in a classic pulmonary blastoma {1231 Since one type of pleuropulmonary blastoma is exclusively cystic, a controversial suggested origin is from congenital cystic adenomatoid malformation {1207}.

Localization

Pleura and/or lung.

Clinical features

The clinical manifestations are variable and depend on age and pathologic type. Respiratory distress with or without pneumothorax is the most common presentation of the cystic pleuropulmonary blastoma in the first 12-18 months of life {892, 1619}. Asymptomatic lesions may be incidental findings during investigation of seemingly unrelated clinical problems {1544,1545,1619}. Fever, chest pain and cough are the presenting complaints in the 2-4 year old child with a cystic and solid or exclusively solid neoplasm, which may be suspected initially to be pneumonia or empyema.

Imaging

Unilateral, rarely bilateral, localized air-filled cysts are a common finding on images that have been obtained subsequent to the onset of respiratory distress {468,1207,1545,1619,1650}. A pneumothorax is rarely present. Septal thickening or an intracystic mass(es) is another feature which should suggest the possibility of something other than a congenital adenomatoid malformation or congenital lobar emphysema. Other patterns of masses lesions and/ or cysts are described {99}.

Macroscopy

Three basic pathologic types are currently recognized with associated gross and microscopic features {468,2173}. The purely cystic pleuropulmonary blastoma is characterized as a filmy, thin-walled multicystic structure, which collapses after resection {321}. Another pattern is a solid, firm to gelatinous creamy white, sometimes hemorrhagic tumour, measuring over 15 cm in greatest dimension and weighing over 500 g. The solid tumours may occupy an entire lobe or lung and in a minority of cases, the mass has arisen from the visceral or parietal pleura, including the dome of the diaphragm.

Histopathology

The purely cystic or type I pleuropulmonary blastoma is characterized by the presence of a multicystic structure lined by respiratory type epithelium beneath which is a population of small primitive malignant cells with or without apparent rhabdomyoblastic differentiation The malignant cells may be identified as a continuous or discontinuous cambium layer-like zone, but may be difficult to find. Small nodules of fetal appearing cartilage or a hyalinzed septal stroma are features which should prompt careful search for malignant cells, if they are not initially apparent. Type II pleuropulmonary blastoma shows partial or complete overgrowth of the septal stroma by sheets of primitive small cells without apparent differentiation, embryonal rhab-

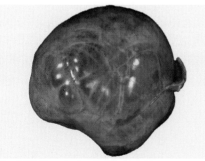

Fig. 1.103 Type I pleuropulmonary blastoma, presenting as round, sharply circumscribed multicystic lesion.

domysarcoma or fascicles of a spindle cell sarcoma with the formation of plaques or nodules. Other examples of type II tumours are those with a grossly visible solid component and microscopically identifiable type I foci. Type III tumours are solid. The solid areas of the types II and III neoplasms have mixed blastematous and sarcomatous features. Nodules of malignant appearing cartilage, small aggregates of anaplastic and pleomorphic appearing cells, fibrosarcoma-like areas, rhabdomyosarcomatous foci and condensed blastema-like islands separated by loosely arrayed short spindle cells may also be seen alone, or in combination. Foci of necrosis, haemorrhage and fibrosis are variably present. Though respiratory epithelium may be entrapped within a field of tumour, neoplastic epithelial elements have not been seen in this tumour type to date, in contrast to the classic pulmonary blastoma. The primitive small cell pattern with or without apparent rhabdomyoblastic differentiation is seen in the purely cystic lesion whereas a more complex mixed sarcomatous pattern is present in those neoplasms with a solid component.

Immunohistochemistry
Based upon the microscopic features, the immunophenotype is predictable in that most neoplastic cells are reactive for vimentin, and the only cytokeratin-positive cells are the respiratory-type cells lining the cysts and the entrapped small airspaces within solid areas of the tumour. Muscle specific actin and desmin are consistently expressed in cells identifiable histologically as rhabdomyoblastic and less consistently in the primitive small cells in the cambium layer-like subepithelial zones in the cystic areas {1619}. The nodules of cartilage express S-100 protein. Immunohistochemistry is useful in the differential diagnosis in those rare cases of a cystic synovial sarcoma of the lung and chest wall {546}. When the latter is a consideration, epithelial membrane antigen, cytokeratin and CD99 are useful since these three markers are not expressed in the pleuropulmonary blastoma.

Histogenesis
The cell of origin for pleuropulmonary blastoma is not known. However, it is

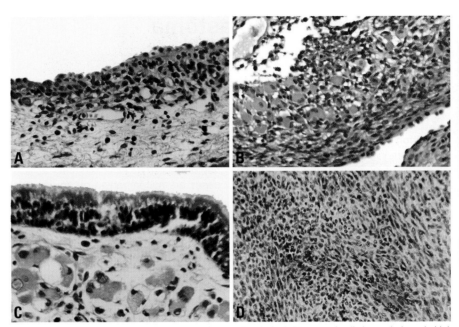

Fig. 1.104 A Type I pleuropulmonary blastoma. Narrow band of primitive round cells beneath the cuboidal epithelium. **B** Cystic tumour with a type 2 pneumocyte epithelial lining beneath which is a cellular cambium layer of spindle cell and epithelioid rhabdomyoblasts. **C** Type II pleuropulmonary blastoma. Differentiated rhabdomyoblasts with abundant eosinophilic cytoplasm are present beneath the epithelium. This tumour showed solid as well as cystic areas. **D** Type III pleuropulmonary blastoma. A portion of the tumor is composed of interlacing fibrosarcoma-like foci. This tumour was purely solid.

probably derived from primitive mesenchymal cells in the lung and or pleura.

Somatic genetics
Several reports have documented gains in chromosome 8 detected by karyotyping and fluorescence in situ hybridization {111,910,991,1035,1107,1492,1620, 1773,2073,2196}. Though this finding appears to be consistent in these tumours, gains in chromosome 8 have been observed in infantile fibrosarcoma, desmoid fibromatosis and mesoblastic nephroma. It is interesting that the latter tumour has been reported on occasion in children who also have a pleuropulmonary blastoma. An unbalanced translocation between chromosomes 1 and X has been described resulting in addition copies of 1q and Xq and loss of part of Xp. Mutations in p53 are also reported.

Prognosis and predictive factors
The pure cystic or type I pleuropulmonary blastoma has a generally favourable prognosis of 80-90% 5-year disease-free survival, whereas the types II and III have a poorer outcome of less than 50% {1569,1619}. The importance of recognizing this neoplasm in its cystic form has been emphasized in the recent

literature {1545,1941}. It would appear that the occult type II neoplasm with microscopic overgrowth of the septal areas, and without the formation of grossly visible masses or plaques, may have a similar favourable outcome as the type I pleuropulmonary blastoma. These tumours locally recur and have a predilection for metastasis to the brain-spinal cord and skeletal system {1619}. Ocular and pancreatic metastases have also been reported {494,1115,2100}.

Chondroma

J.A. Carney
H.D. Tazelaar
T. Manabe

Definition

A benign tumour composed of hyaline or myxohyaline cartilage. It is usually found in Carney triad (gastric stromal sarcoma, pulmonary chondroma and paraganglioma).

ICD-O code   9220/0

Synonyms

Osteochondroma, chondroma

Clinical features

Signs, symptoms and imaging

These are usually asymptomatic tumours. Radiologically, they appear as circumscribed lesions with "pop-corn" calcification, usually multiple, and predominantly in young women {292,689, 2006}.

Macroscopy and localization

These are peripheral solid lesions, which may be calcified and easily enucleated at surgery.

Histopathology

These lesions consist of encapsulated lobules of hypocellular neoplastic cartilaginous tissue. Features of malignancy are absent {292,689,2006}.

Differential diagnosis

Pulmonary hamartoma (mesenchymoma), in the majority of cases, shows cleft-like spaces between cartilaginous lobules lined by a component of respiratory epithelium, with, less often, other differentiated mesenchymal elements. Metastatic chondrosarcoma may also be considered. Clinical history and cytological evidence of malignancy will aid distinction.

Prognostic factors

These patients are cured upon removal of their pulmonary chondroma. Clinical problems in these patients are more likely to relate to their gastric leiomyosarcomas or paragangliomas {294,1772}.

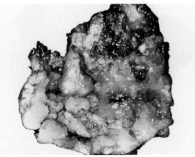

Fig. 1.105 Chondroma. Circumscribed, bosselated tumour composed of white glistening, irregularly-shaped lobules, some with a bluish tinge.

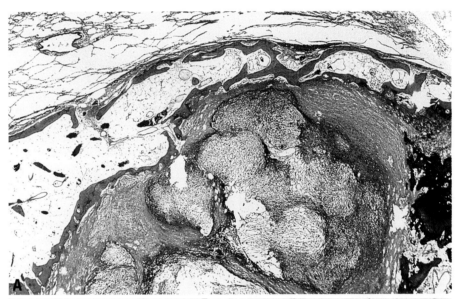

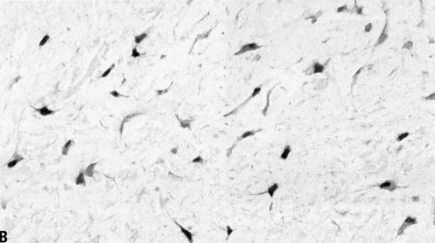

Fig. 1.106 Chondroma. **A** Encapsulated, hypocellular (left) to moderately cellular (right) tumour with dispersed cells set in a chondromyxoid stroma. A fibrous capsule with spicules of mature bone containing marrow fat separates the tumour from the surrounding compressed pulmonary parenchyma. **B** Paucicellular tumour featuring elongated fusiform and stellate cells with eosinophilic cytoplasm and hyperchromatic, polymorphic nuclei set in a loose chondromyxoid matrix.

Congenital peribronchial myofibroblastic tumour

W.D. Travis
L.P. Dehner
T. Manabe
H.D. Tazelaar

Definition
An interstitial and peribronchovascular proliferation of uniform, plump to more fusiform cells arranged in broad, interlacing fascicles; cellularity and mitotic activity may be marked. This spindle cell neoplasm is reminiscent of the congenital infantile fibrosarcoma.

ICD-O codes   8827/1

Synonyms
Congenital fibrosarcoma, congenital leiomyosarcoma, congenital bronchopulmonary leiomyosarcoma, congenital pulmonary myofibroblastic tumour, congenital mesenchymal malformation of lung, neonatal pulmonary hamartoma

Epidemiology
This rare neoplasm is documented in the literature as individual case studies with less than 15 cases to date {45,930,1001, 1082,1284}.

Etiology
This tumour occurs sporadically and has neither syndromic association nor relevant maternal history, at least to date.

Clinical features
As a congenital tumour, it is recognized shortly after birth although the pregnancy may be complicated by polydramnios and non-immune hydrops fetalis. However, its detection by prenatal ultrasonography should be anticipated {45, 930,1001,1082,1284}.

Macroscopy
The well-circumscribed, non-encapsulated mass has a smooth or multinodular surface with or without fine trabeculations. The cut surface has a tann-grey to yellow-tan fleshy appearance. Haemorrhage and necrosis are variable features. The maximum dimension varies from 5-10 cm and the tumour may weigh in excess of 100 gms. The bronchus is often distorted or totally obliterated.

Histopathology
The lung parenchyma is replaced by fascicles of uniform spindle cells {903}, arranged in intersecting fascicles with or without a herringbone pattern. The nuclei are elongated and have finely dispersed chromatin, an absence of pleomorphism or anaplasia and variable mitotic activity. Atypical mitotic figures are not present. Bronchial invasion is often seen, and the peribronchial distribution is implicit in the name. The growth may diffusely obliterate the parenchyma or form islands and nodules of spindle cells with interspersed foci of uninvolved parenchyma {930}. Tumour growth in septa or on the pleural surface may occur. In less cellular perivascular areas, the tumour cells appear less sarcomatous with a more fibromyxoid or myofibroblastic proliferation. Cystic foci of haemorrhage may be present.

Immunoprofile and electron microscopy
A myofibroblastic immunophenotype is not demonstrable in all cases.
The spindle cells are consistently positive for vimentin whereas staining for desmin and smooth muscle actin is absent or restricted to isolated cells {1082,1284}. Ultrastructural studies suggest myofibroblastic differentiation {1284}. Muscle specific actin immunoreactivity is present in less than 5% of the cells and desmin reactivity may be observed on rare occasion. This tumour is considered to be identical with, or at least related to, the lesions reported as congenital leiomyosarcoma, fibrosarcoma, and fibro-leiomyosarcoma. Immunoprofiles in the tumours diagnosed as such are non-specific and have been reported to express neuron-specific enolase, alpha-smooth muscle actin, HHF 35 actin and muscle-specific actin {382}. Desmin, S-100 protein, CD34, CD57, CD68, factor XIIIa, and CAM 5.2 are also occasionally expressed.

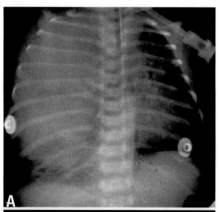
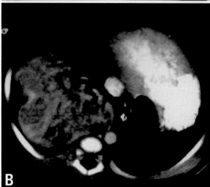

Fig. 1.107 Congenital peribronchial myofibroblastic tumour. **A** Plain view chest roentegenograph shows opacification of the right hemithorax of a 7-week-old female who presented with respiratory distress. **B** Computed tomogram reveals a well circumscribed mass lesion with a collage of high and low density foci, representing areas of tumour and compressed uninvolved parenchyma."

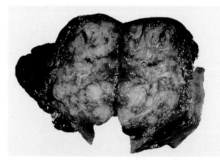

Fig. 1.108 Congenital peribronchial myofibroblastic tumour. The resected tumour required a pneumectomy in a 7-week-old female. The cross-section reveals a circumscribed, tan-grey, multinodular mass measuring 10 cm in greatest dimension.

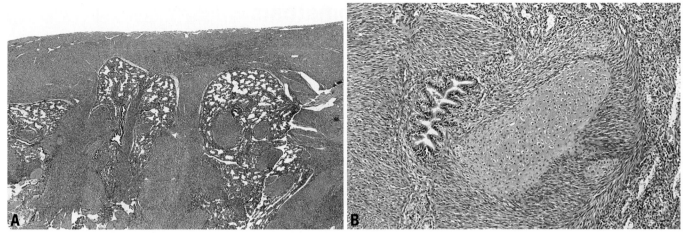

Fig. 1.109 Congenital peribronchial myofibroblastic tumour. **A** There is an extensive infiltrate of spindle cells along lymphatic routes: pleura, septa and broncho-vascular bundles. **B** The spindle cells resemble smooth muscle cells and inflitrate around bronchial cartilage, epithelium and vessels. From Travis et al. {2024}.

Imaging

A large mass lesion partially or totally opacifying the hemithorax is the usual appearance on a plain chest radiograph. Computed tomography reveals a well-circumscribed heterogeneous mass {45, 930,1001,1082,1284}.

Somatic genetics

One case has been reported with a complex karotype which included a t(8;10) (p11.2;p15) translocation {45}. Although these tumours resemble congenital-infantile fibrosarcoma and congenital mesoblastic nephroma in their gross and microscopic features, there are no reports to date of the detection of t(12;15) (p13;q25-26) translocation in a congenital peribronchial myofibroblastic tumour {1734}.

Prognosis and predictive factors

Surgical resection of the involved lobe or lung is the treatment of choice. However, the presence of fetal hydrops with its own associated morbidity and mortality may compliate the clinical outcome.

Diffuse pulmonary lymphangiomatosis

K.O. Leslie
H.D. Tazelaar

Definition
A diffuse proliferation of lymphatic vascular spaces and smooth muscle, distributed with the normal lymphatics of the lungs, pleura and mediastinum.

Synonyms
Lymphangiomatosis, lymphangiectasis, lymphatic dysplasia

Clinical features
The process affects children and young adults of both sexes who present with progressive symptoms of "asthma," dyspnoea or haemoptysis {230,563,832, 925,1319,1637,1933,1985,2039}.

Imaging
Chest radiographs show increased interstitial markings. Computed tomography shows smooth thickening of the interlobular septa, major fissures, central airways and pleura.

Macroscopy and localization
There is prominence of the bronchovascular bundles and other structures, including pleura, interlobular pulmonary septa, and mediastinum, reflecting the lymphatic distribution of the disease.

Histopathology
Anastomosing endothelial-lined spaces of varying size are diffusely distributed along lymphatic routes in pleura, intralobular septa, and bronchovascular sheaths and often contain acellular, sometimes eosinophilic, material {230, 563,832,925,1319,1637,1933,1985, 2039}. Variable numbers of spindle cells with bland oval to cigar shaped nuclei are present between channels. Mass lesions and cysts are not identified. Intra-alveolar siderophages are often present in surrounding lung parenchyma.

Immunophenotype and electron microscopy
The immunophenotypic profile of the lining cells is compatible with endothelium (FVIIIrAg positive, vimentin positive, UEA positive) {1985}. The spindle cells commonly express vimentin, desmin, actin, and progesteron receptor but are negative for estrogen receptor, keratin, and HMB-45. Ultrastrucurally, the spindle cells resemble smooth muscle cells.

Differential diagnosis
In lymphangiectasis the lymphatic vessels are not increased in number and do not anastamose {230,563,832,925,1319, 1637,1933,1985,2039}.
Lymphangioleiomyomatosis exhibits a more random distribution in association with cysts. Kaposi sarcoma does not exhibit the complex anastomosing lymphatic channels. In diffuse pulmonary haemangiomatosis vascular spaces are blood-filled and in interstitial emphysema spaces are airfilled and lack smooth muscle.

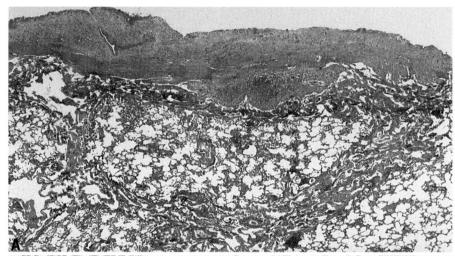

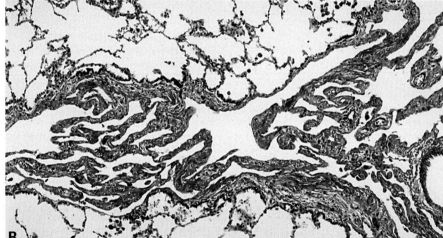

Fig. 1.110 Diffuse pulmonary lymphangiomatosis. **A** The pleura and septa are infiltrated by a proliferation of lymphatics. **B** The lymphatic proliferation infiltrating along the interlobular septa are highlighted with trichrome stain. From Travis et al. {2024}.

Inflammatory myofibroblastic tumour

S.A. Yousem
H.D. Tazelaar
T. Manabe
L.P. Dehner

Definition

Inflammatory myofibroblastic tumour is a subgroup of the broad category of "inflammatory pseudotumours" and is composed of a variable mixture of collagen, inflammatory cells, and usually cytologically bland spindle cells showing myofibroblastic differentiation.

ICD-O code   8825/1

Synonyms

Inflammatory myofibroblastic tumour has acquired a wide array of synonyms including the following {654,1259,1292}: inflammatory pseudotumour, plasma cell granuloma, fibroxanthoma, fibrous histiocytoma, pseudosarcomatous myofibroblastic tumour, and invasive fibrous tumour of the tracheobronchial tree.

Epidemiology

Inflammatory myofibroblastic tumour has an equal sex distribution and occurs in all ages, though most occur in individuals less than 40 years {654,1850}. Inflammatory myofibroblastic tumour is the most common endobronchial mesenchymal lesion in childhood.

Etiology

Some believe inflammatory myofibroblastic tumour is a reactive inflammatory condition, others that it represents a low-grade mesenchymal malignancy {1292}. Pulmonary lesions have been associated with previous viral infections, and some reports have indicated an association with HHV8 {707}.

Localization

Chest radiographs show a solitary mass with regular borders in 80% of the cases {309,384}. The mass may have a spiculated appearance and if endobronchial in location, may be accompanied by a post-obstructive pneumonia and atelectasis.

Clinical features

The clinical presentation of patients with inflammatory myofibroblastic tumour is protean, with signs and symptoms relating to the site of involvement {38,381, 384}. Endobronchial lesions present with complaints reflecting bronchial irritation, with cough, wheeze, haemoptysis, and chest pain. Constitutional symptoms are rare. Peripheral pulmonary parenchymal nodules are often asymptomatic although local invasion into the chest wall may elicit pleuritic or chest wall pain.

Macroscopy

These lesions are typically solitary round rubbery masses, which have a variable degree of a yellowish-gray discoloration reflecting the histiocytic component of the inflammatory infiltrate. The size range is wide (1-36 cm) with an average size of 3.0 cm {38,381,384}. The lesions do not appear encapsulated and local involvement of hilar soft tissues or chest wall is seen in 5-10% of cases. Gritty calcification is occasionally noted. Cavitation is rare.

Tumour spread and staging

Inflammatory myofibroblastic tumour is usually localised. Involvement of the chest wall, mediastinum, or pleura is rare, as are recurrences and metastases.

Histopathology

Inflammatory myofibroblastic tumour contains a mixture of spindle cells showing fibroblastic and myofibroblastic differentiation arrayed in fascicles, or with storiform architecture. The spindle cells have oval nuclei, fine chromatin, inconspicuous nucleoli, and abundant bipolar lightly eosinophilic cytoplasm. Mitoses are infrequent. Cytologic atypia is not obvious. Admixed with the spindle proliferation, and often obscuring it, is an inflammatory infiltrate containing lymphocytes, plasma cells, and histiocytes, including Touton type giant cells. Plasma cells may be prominent and are often associated with lymphoid follicles. The spindle cells, in rare instances, will infiltrate blood vessels or the pleura.

Immunohistochemistry

Pulmonary and extrapulmonary inflammatory myofibroblatic tumours (IMT) show similar immunoprofiles {384,1636, 2223}. Immunostains demonstrate that

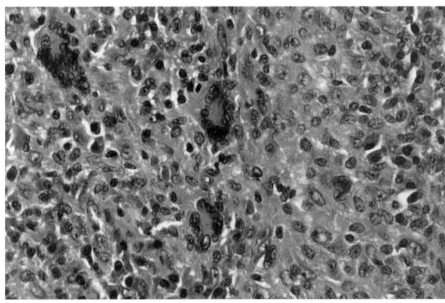

Fig. 1.111 Inflammatory myofibroblastic tumour, containing Touton-like giant cells, foamy histiocytes, and abundant inflammatory cells, all within the context of the background bland spindle cell proliferation.

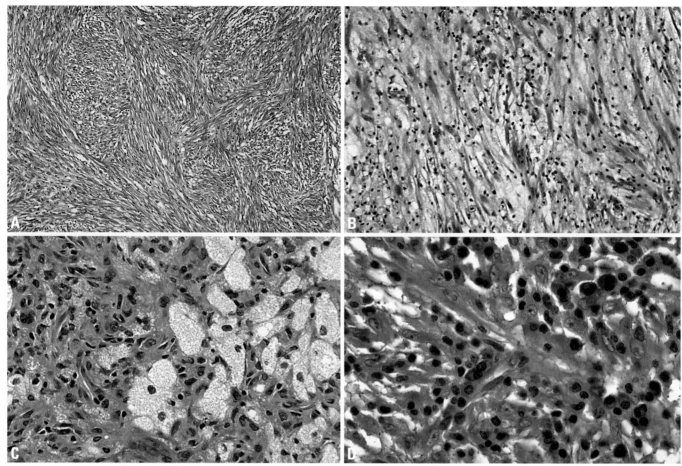

Fig. 1.112 Inflammatory myofibroblastic tumour. **A** Spindle cells growing in interlacing fascicles. **B** Spindle cells with myxoid stroma and mild chronic inflammatory infiltrate. **C** Numerous foamy histiocytes give this lesion a fibroxanthomatous appearance. **D** Prominent lymphocytes and plasma cells infiltrate among the myofibroblastic cells in this lesion. From Travis et al. {2024}.

the spindle cells express vimentin and smooth muscle actin, and rarely desmin {107,309,882}. They fail to express myogenin, myoglobin, CD117 (cKit) and S-100 protein. Focal cytokeratin reactivity is noted in about one third of the cases, perhaps due to alveolar entrapment. Expression of ALK1 and p80 is noted in IMT in about 40% of the cases. {312,322, 383,401,741}. P53 immunoreactivity is rare and reported in association with recurrence and malignant transformation {882}.

Histogenesis
Inflammatory myofibroblastic tumour is a proliferation of cells showing myofibroblastic differentiation.

Somatic genetics
Inflammatory myofibroblastic tumour is most often euploid, but may occasionally be aneuploid {170,882}. Similarly, some cases may show TP53 mutations. IMT

show clonal changes in 2/3 of cases involving chromosome 2 at the 2p23 location of the ALK gene {1771,1842, 1895,1896,2223}. Translocations involving the ALK gene to chromosome 5 create ALK fusion gene products, which are thought to play a role in the development of malignancy {1701}. Few inflammatory myofibroblastic tumours have complete cytogenetics reported, and they indicate the presence of ring chromosomes and translocations involving chromosome 1, 2, 4, and 5.

Prognosis and predictive factors
In most instances complete excision of pulmonary inflammatory myofibroblastic tumour leads to excellent survival {654}. A minority (5%) of inflammatory myofibroblastic tumours may show extrapulmonary invasion, recurrence or metastases, recurrence usually occurring in cases, which were incompletely excised. Histologic features that may be associat-

ed with a poor prognosis include focal invasion, vascular invasion, increased cellularity, nuclear pleomorphism with bizarre giant cells, a high mitotic rate (greater than 3/50 hpf), and necrosis {38,381,384}.

Lymphangioleiomyomatosis

H. Tazelaar
E.P. Henske
T. Manabe
W.D. Travis

Definition
Lymphangioleiomyomatosis (LAM) is a widespread interstitial infiltrate of immature short spindle cells resembling smooth muscle cells, usually associated with cystic change, most commonly occurring in women of reproductive age.

ICD-O code   9174/1

Synonyms
Lymphangiomyomatosis

Clinical features
LAM is very rare with an estimated incidence of 1 per 1,000,000 in the United States, France, and United Kingdom. It most often occurs as a sporadic disease, but also occurs in women with tuberous sclerosis complex (TSC). Among women with TSC, 26-39% show radiographic evidence of LAM {414,610,1391}. Renal angiomyolipomas occur in most TSC patients and in approximately 50% of sporadic LAM patients {97}. LAM is the third most frequent cause of TSC-related death, after renal disease and brain tumours {303}. LAM has been reported in both postmenopausal women and in at least one man {92}.

Signs and symptoms
These include progressive dyspnoea on exertion, pneumothorax (often recurrent), cough, haemoptysis and chylous pleural effusions.

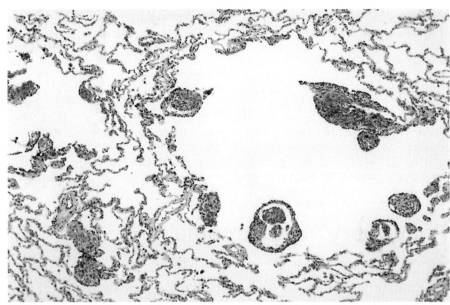

Fig. 1.114 Lymphangioleiomyomatosis. Cystic spaces are surrounded by abnormal smooth muscle bundles. From Travis et al. {2024}.

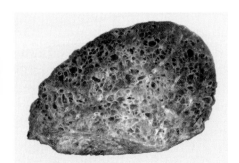

Fig. 1.113 Lymphangioleiomyomatosis. The lung shows diffuse cystic changes characteristic of lymphangioleiomyomatosis.

Imaging
Chest radiograph may be normal, but as the disease progresses, it typically shows diffuse reticular infiltrates with hyperinflation. Computed tomography shows cystic lesions between 2-20 mm, uniformly distributed in both lungs.

Macroscopy and localization
In advanced cases the lungs show diffuse cystic changes from apex to base. Early lesions may show only a few scattered cysts.

Histopathology
The two major lesions of lymphangioleiomyomatosis are cysts and immature smooth muscle proliferation. The variably sized cystic spaces are lined by plaque-like or nodular aggregates of smooth-muscle-like spindle cells. These may be admixed with more rounded epithelioid cells, perhaps representing perivascular epitheliod cells (PECs) or epithelioid smooth muscle cells. Micronodular pneumocyte hyperplasia may also be present in patients with tuberous sclerosis.

Immunohistochemistry
The cells of lymphangioleiomyomatosis show smooth muscle differentiation and express. alpha-smooth muscle actin and desmin, as well as vimentin. Unlike normal smooth muscle cells, however, they also show immunoreactivity with a melanocytic marker, HMB-45 {200, 1083}. Not all the cells stain, but when present, together with consistent histological changes, is highly specific and sensitive for LAM. Estrogen and progesteron receptors are present in some cases {153,393}.

Differential diagnosis
Benign metastasizing leiomyoma is not usually associated with cysts and the nodules of smooth muscle are generally larger than those seen in LAM. Emphysema lacks the spindle cells. Langerhans' cell histiocytosis shows the pathognomonic cells, eosinophils and has a characteristic gross and microanatomical distribution.

Histogenesis

The perivascular epithelioid cell (PEC) has been suggested.

Somatic genetics

Germline mutations in both TSC1 and TSC2 are associated with LAM, including missense mutations in the final exon of TSC2 (exon 41) {610,1885}. No genotype-phenotype correlation has been identified. Most women with sporadic LAM do not have germline TSC2 gene mutations {86,1747}, but TSC2 mutations have been found in angiomyolipomas, lymph nodes, and microdissected pulmonary LAM cells from sporadic LAM patients {297,961,1747,1839}. These mutations are not present in morphologically normal kidney or lung, or in the peripheral blood, indicating that they arise somatically, and leading to the hypothesis that LAM cells migrate or metastasize to the lung from angiomyolipomas or lymph nodes. LAM can recur after lung transplantation {174,1477, 1495}. In one case, a somatic TSC2 gene mutation was used to prove that recurrent LAM cells in the allograft lung arose from the patient's native LAM {961} consistent with hypothesis that LAM cells migrate in vivo.

Prognosis and predictive factors

The prognosis for women with pulmonary LAM is variable. Progression is common with a median survival of 8 to 10 years from diagnosis {1019,1260,1983}. An elevated TLC and a reduced FEV1/FVC ratio are associated with poor survival {1019}. Kitaichi showed that patients with a predominantly cystic type of LAM had a worse prognosis than those with a predominantly muscular type {1019}. Matusi et al recently showed that the 5- and 10-year survivals for LAM patients were 100% for LAM histology score (LHS)-1, 89.9% and 74.6% for LHS-2 and 59.1% and 47.3% for LHS-3, respectively {1260}. He also found that increasing degrees of hemosiderin deposition were associated with higher LHS scores (p=0.029) and a worse prognosis (p=0.0012) {1260}.

Pulmonary vein sarcoma

H.D. Tazelaar
D.B. Flieder

Definition

A sarcoma arising in a pulmonary vein which almost always shows features of leiomyosarcoma.

ICD-O code
8800/3

Epidemiology

Pulmonary vein sarcomas are rarer than pulmonary artery sarcomas and less than 20 cases have been reported {1512}.

Clinical features

The tumours tend to occur in women ranging from 23-67 years (mean 49 years). The most common presenting symptoms are dyspnoea, haemoptysis and chest pain. In most cases, the clinical impression is that of a left atrial or lung tumour.

Macroscopy and localization

The tumours are generally fleshy-tan and tend to occlude the lumen of the involved vessel. They range from 3.0-20.0 cm in greatest dimension. Invasion of either wall of the vein to involve hilar structures of pulmonary parenchyma is common.

Histopathology

The majorities of pulmonary vein sarcomas show smooth muscle differentiation and, therefore, represent leiomyosarcomas. They are moderate to highly cellular spindle cell neoplasms with varying degrees of mitotic activity and necrosis. Epithelioid morphology may be present. Immunohistochemically, the tumours are reactive with antibodies to vimentin, desmin and actin, confirming the presence of smooth muscle differentiation. Aberrant keratin reactivity may be observed in as many as 40% of cases.

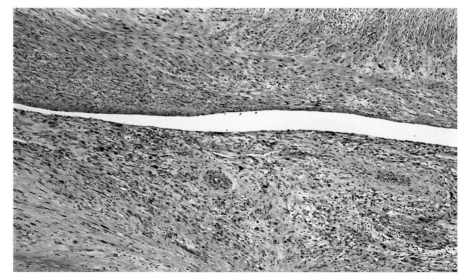

Fig. 1.115 Pulmonary vein sarcoma. The wall of the vein is infiltrated by spindle and pleomorphic sarcoma cells.

Pulmonary artery sarcoma

J. E. Yi
H.D. Tazelaar
A. Burke
T. Manabe

Definition

A sarcoma of the large pulmonary arteries with two types. Intimal sarcomas have an intraluminal polypoid growth pattern and usually show fibroblastic or myofibroblastic differentiation. Mural sarcomas are considered distinct from intimal sarcomas, and are classified separately according to the histologic subtype as in soft tissue sarcomas (leiomyosarcoma).

ICD-O code   8800/3

Synonyms

Intimal sarcoma of the pulmonary artery has been used interchangeably with pulmonary artery sarcoma, since intimal sarcomas comprise the vast majority of pulmonary artery sarcomas. Mural sarcomas are exceedingly rare.

Epidemiology

Pulmonary artery sarcomas are a rare tumour with only a few hundred cases reported. The incidence is unknown and probably underestimated, since many cases are still misdiagnosed as pulmonary embolism preoperatively and may remain unrecognized if not examined histologically. The average age at diagnosis is 49.3 years (range 13-81 years) with a roughly equal sex distribution {419,1079,1488}.

Localization

These tumours occur in the pulmonary trunk, most commonly, right pulmonary artery, left pulmonary artery, pulmonary valve, and, least often, the right ventricular outflow tract {419}.

Clinical features

The most common presenting symptom is dyspnoea, followed by, in decreasing order, chest / back pain, cough, haemoptysis, weight loss, malaise, syncope, fever, and rarly sudden death {419}. These clinical findings are often indistinguishable from those of chronic thromboembolic disease, but progressive weight loss, anemia and fever are unusual for benign pulmonary vascular diseases and should raise a suspicion for malignancy {1547}. Common physical signs include systolic ejection murmur, cyanosis, peripheral oedema, jugular venous distension, hepatomegaly, and clubbing {1547}.

Imaging

Radiologic findings overlap with those of chronic thromboembolic disease, but the rate of preoperative diagnosis has increased remarkably in the last decade with advances in imaging {419,959,973}. Solid appearing expansion of the proximal pulmonary artery branches is highly suggestive of a sarcoma, especially in the presence of pulmonary nodules, cardiac enlargement and decreased vascularity {419}. The features in computed tomography (CT) and magnetic resonance imaging (MRI) that favor a diagnosis of sarcoma over thrombi include: heterogeneous soft tissue density, smooth vascular tapering without abrupt narrowings and cut-offs {973}, and unilateral central pulmonary emboli {419,973}. Vascularization in sarcomas may be seen with bronchial arteriography {419}.

Macroscopy and localization

Intimal sarcomas resemble mucoid or gelatinous clots filling vascular lumens. Distal extension may show smooth tapering of the mass. The cut surface may show firm fibrotic areas and bony/gritty or chondromyxoid foci may be present in mural lesions. Haemorrhage and necrosis are common in high-grade tumours. Most cases have bilateral pulmonary artery involvement, although one side is usually dominant.

Tumour spread and staging

Pulmonary artery sarcomas metastasize primarily to the lung and mediastinum (50%). Distant metastases have been reported in 16% cases {419}. There is no recognized staging sytem.

Histopathology

Intimal sarcomas typically show a proliferation of spindle cells in a myxoid background, alternating with hypocellular collagenized stroma. Recanalized thrombi may be intimately admixed, especially as tumour extends distally. Some intimal and most mural tumours will show foci of more differentiated sarcomas: osteosarcoma, chondrosarcoma or rhabdomyosarcoma {101,182,246,1285,1488,1559, 1816}.

Immunohistochemistry / Electron microscopy

Most intimal sarcomas show immunohistochemical and ultrastructural evidence of myofibroblastic differentiation {101, 182,246,1285,1488,1559,1816}. The tumour cells, in general, exhibit strong and diffuse immunoreactivity for vimentin {728}. Osteopontin expression can also be expressed {667}. Reactivity for smooth muscle actin is variable. Tumor cells may express desmin or endothelial

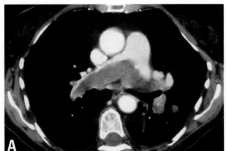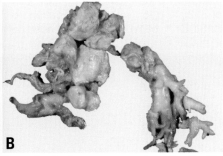

Fig. 1.116 Pulmonary artery sarcoma (PAS). **A** Axial CT scan showing large tumor mass (arrow) outlined by contrast material straddling the bifurcation of the pulmonary artery and extending into the left lower lobe branches. **B** Gross photograph of PAS resected by pulmonary thromboendarterectomy procedure.

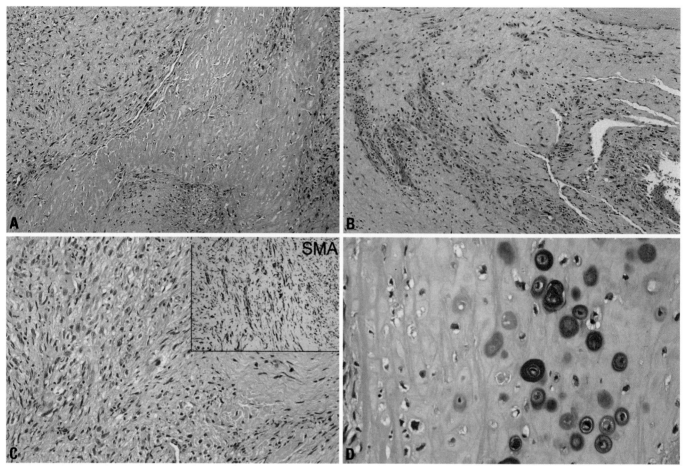

Fig. 1.117 Pulmonary artery sarcoma (PAS). **A** Spindle cell proliferation, alternating with hypocellular collagenous stroma. **B** PAS intimately incorporated with recanalizing thrombi. **C** PAS with myofibroblastic differentiation as shown by smooth muscle actin (SMA) immunostain in inset. **D** Chondrosarcomatous area within a pulmonary artery sarcoma.

markers, such as factor VIII, CD31, and CD34 when they show evidence of smooth muscle or vascular differentiation {728}.

Differential diagnosis and grading
The diagnosis is fairly straightforward in most cases, though some thrombi may have highly cellular foci. Metastases should always be excluded. There is no specific grading system; NCI and FNCLCC systems for soft tissue sarcoma can be used.

Histogenesis
Intimal sarcomas presumably arise from pluripotential mesenchymal cells of the intima {246,1488}, but primitive cells of the bulbus cordi in the trunk of pulmonary artery have been also proposed as the origin {1285}.

Somatic genetics
Comparative genomic hybridization revealed frequent gains or amplification of 12q13-q15 with amplification of SAS/CDK4, MDM2 and GLI. In addition,

there was amplification of PDGF receptor A on 4q12. Less consistent alterations have been identified including losses on 3p, 3q, 4q, 9p, 5p, 6p, and 11q.

Prognosis and predictive factors
Overall prognosis is very poor regardless of therapy with the mean survival ranging from 14-18 months {246,485,1488}. Surgical resection is the single most effective modality for short-term palliation and the role of adjuvant therapy is yet to be determined {55,485}.

Pulmonary synovial sarcoma

M.C. Aubry
S. Suster
H.D. Tazelaar
T. Manabe

Definition
Pulmonary synovial sarcoma (SS) is a mesenchymal spindle cell tumour, which variably displays areas of epithelial differentiation. While it can be seen as a metastasis from an extrapulmonary site, it also occurs in the lung in the absence of primary elsewhere.

ICD-O codes
Synovial sarcoma   9040/3
Synovial sarcoma, spindle cell
                                  9041/3
Synovial sarcoma, biphasic
                                  9043/3

Synonyms
Synovial cell sarcoma, malignant synovioma, synovioblastic sarcoma

Clinical features
Pulmonary SS usually presents in young to middle age adults and shows no gender predilection {68,546,694,850,957, 1777,1992,2234,2236}. Cough, often with haemoptysis is the most common clinical manifestation, followed by chest pain. Low-grade fever and weight loss are rare. These tumours can also present as incidental tumours on chest X-ray. Prognosis is in general poor with almost half of patients dying of disease (mean 23 months) {68,546,694,850,957,1777,

1992,2234,2236}. However, prolonged survival without disease, over 5 years, has occurred.

Macroscopy and localization
Pulmonary SS are usually peripheral, well-circumscribed but non-encapsulated, solid tumours. Size ranges between 0.6-17.0 cm (mean 5.6 cm) {546}. Rare cases involving the tracheobronchial tree with formation of an endobronchial mass have been described. Occasionally, the tumour diffusely infiltrates chest wall or mediastinal structures. The cut surface of the tumour can show cystic degenerative changes and necrosis.

Tumour spread and staging
Pulmonary SS mainly spreads and recurs regionally, involving chest wall, pericardium, diaphragm, paraspinal soft tissue. Direct extension to the abdominal cavity may also occur {68,546,694,850,957, 1777,1992,2234,2236}. Metastases to mediastinal lymph nodes are extremely uncommon (5%). Systemic metastases, mainly to liver, bone, brain, and lung, occur in almost a quarter of patients.

Histopathology
Histologic features of pulmonary SS are identical to its soft tissue counterpart {68,546,694,850,957,1777,1992,2234,

2236}. Both biphasic and monophasic subtypes have been described. Monophasic SS, the most common pulmonary subtype is comprised solely of the spindle cell component. The spindle-cell component consists of interweaving fascicles of densely packed elongated cells. This subtype often displays a prominent haemangiopericytomatous vascular pattern, and focal areas of dense hyaline fibrosis. Biphasic SS comprises both epithelial and spindle components. Epithelial areas contain cleft-like glandular spaces with scattered tubulo-papillary differentiation. The cells are cuboidal with moderate eosinophilic cytoplasm, round nuclei with granular chromatin and occasional nucleoli. Mucoid secretions are commonly seen. Care should be taken not to confuse the epithelial component with entrapped alveolar epithelium that will be TTF-1 positive and could be mistaken for biphasic synovial sarcoma {2234}. The cells contain scant cytoplasm with oval nuclei. Most pulmonary SS contain focal necrosis. Mitotic activity varies greatly (5-25/10HPF). Calcification and mast cell infiltrates may be seen.

Immunohistochemistry
Most synovial sarcomas show immunoreactivity for cytokeratins (CK) and/or

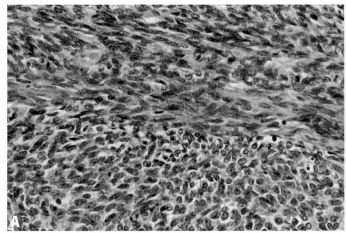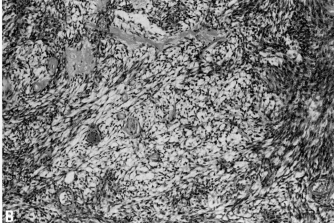

Fig. 1.118 Synovial sarcoma. **A** Round to oval and spindle shaped cells with minimal cytoplasm, hyperchromatic nuclei, inconspicuous mitoses and only slight fibrous stroma. **B** Alternating myxoid and cellular areas with some vessels showing hyalinization.

epithelial membrane antigen (EMA) {410}. The intensity of staining is more prominent in the epithelial rather than the spindle cell component. EMA tends to be expressed more often and more widely than CK. In monophasic lesions, reactivity may be scanty. Cytokeratins 7 and 19 are particularly useful because synovial sarcoma cells express these types of cytokeratins, and these are generally negative in other spindle cell sarcomas {1306,1838}. Vimentin is usually expressed in the spindle cells of synovial sarcoma. Intranuclear and intracytoplsmic immunoreactivity for S-100 protein can be identified in up to 30% of the tumours {585,749}. BCL-2 and CD99 are frequently positive {469,1652,1908} CD34 is virtually usually negative {2064}. Desmin is absent but focal reactivity for muscle specific actin or smooth muscle actin is noted on occasion in monophasic synovial sarcomas. Lastly, given the differential diagnosis with mesothelioma, it is relevant to note that synovial sarcomas commonly contain foci of calretinin-positive cells {1310}.

Differential diagnosis
The most important and common differential diagnosis is metastatic SS to the lung, which needs to be excluded with a thorough clinical and radiologic exam. Otherwise the differential diagnosis is wide and includes both more common epithelial and other rare mesenchymal tumours, such as spindle cell carcinoma, malignant mesothelioma, small cell carcinoma, thymoma, pleuropulmonary blastoma, localized fibrous tumour, fibrosarcoma, smooth muscle tumour, and malignant peripheral nerve sheath tumour and Ewing sarcoma. The distinction is usually made on the basis of histologic and immunohistochemical features. In difficult cases, detection of specific cytogenetic/molecular abnormality might be useful.

Histogenesis
This remains unknown, though is thought to be a totipotential mesenchymal cell.

Somatic genetics
The cytogenetic hallmark of synovial sarcoma is the t (X; 18)(p11; q11) {68,546, 850,957,1992}. This translocation results usually in the fusion of the SYT gene on chromosome 18 to either the SSX1 or SSX2 gene on chromosome X. The translocation has been found in >90% of SS, regardless of histologic type and the fusion transcript, identified either by FISH, RT-PCR, or real time PCR, is considered specific. The translocation or the fusion transcript was present in all evaluated pulmonary SS.

Hamartoma

A.G. Nicholson
J.F. Tomashefski Jr.
H. Popper

Definition
Pulmonary hamartomas are benign neoplasms composed of varying proportions of mesenchymal tissues, such as cartilage, fat, connective tissue and smooth muscle, typically combined with entrapped respiratory epithelium.

Synonyms
The popular term chondroid hamartoma denotes the usual predominance of cartilagenous matrix. Other terms include benign mesenchymoma, hamartochondroma, chondromatous hamartoma, adenochondroma and fibroadenoma of the lung.

Epidemiology
The population incidence is 0.25% {1065} with a two- to four-fold male predominance and peak incidence in the sixth decade {2066}. Hamartomas are rare in children.

Localization
Hamartomas are usually peripheral and less than 4 cm in diameter. About 10% arise endobronchially {2006,2066}.

Clinical features
Presentation is typically as an asymptomatic, solitary, well-circumscribed nodule on routine chest x-ray. Hamartomas represent approximately 7-14% of coin lesions. Multiple lesions are rare. Occasionally, the distinctive radiographic appearance of "popcorn calcification" is seen. Endobronchial lesions tend to cause symptoms due to bronchial obstruction {2006,2066}.

Macroscopy
Parenchymal tumours are multilobulated, white or gray, firm masses that "shell out" from the surrounding parenchyma. The consistency is cartilaginous, with occasional gritty specks of dystrophic calcification or bone. Endobronchial lesions, which tend to be more lipomatous, are situated within the larger airways as broad-based polyps.

Histopathology
Hamartomas are composed predominantly of lobulated masses of mature cartilage surrounded by other bland mesenchymal elements such as fat, smooth muscle, bone, and fibrovascular tissue. These latter elements rarely predominate. Clefts of respiratory-type epithelium frequently extend as slit-like spaces between the lobules of mesenchymal components. In endobronchial hamartomas, adipose tissue may predominate, and epithelial inclusions tend to be shallow or absent. Cytologic diagnosis of chondroid hamartoma is based on recognition of the mesenchymal components. Immunohistochemistry and ultrastructural studies rarely contribute to the diagnosis.

Differential diagnosis
Hamartomas are separated from monomorphic benign soft tissue tumours by the presence of at least two mesenchymal elements, and from chondrosarcoma by the lack of cytologic atypia. "Cystic mesenchymal hamartoma" refers mainly to neoplasms of children, is readily distinguishable from chondroid hamartoma, and is preferably classified as pleuropulmonary blastoma. Hamartomas must also be distinguished from bronchopulmonary chondromas that tend to be multiple in Carney's triad (pulmonary chondromas, epithelioid gastric smooth muscle tumours and extra-adrenal paraganglioma). These consist solely of cartilage without cleft-like spaces lined by respiratory epithelium.

Histogenesis
Histogenesis is unknown, although genetic studies indicate a neoplastic rather than hamartomatous origin {2006, 2066}.

Somatic genetics
Pulmonary hamartomas have a high frequency of genetic mutations, similar to those seen in other benign mesenchymal neoplasms such as lipomas. Most notable are mutations of high-mobility group (HMG) proteins, a family of non-histone, chromatin-associated proteins, which are important in regulating chromatin architecture and gene expression. Mutations in the regions 6p21 and 12q14-15 are most commonly found {591,824,982,983}.

Prognosis and predictive factors
Conservative surgery is appropriate, either by enucleation or wedge resection for parenchymal lesions or by bronchoplastic resection for endobronchial lesions. Recurrence or sarcomatous transformation is exceedingly rare {2066}.

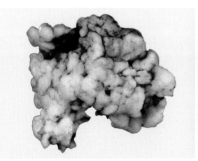 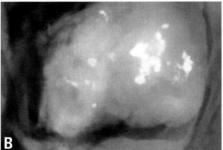

Fig. 1.119 A Hamartoma, 'shelled-out' of the lung parenchyma, with a lobulated cream-coloured external surface. **B** Hamartoma, specimen radiograph. The irregularly shaped white area represents "popcorn" calcification.

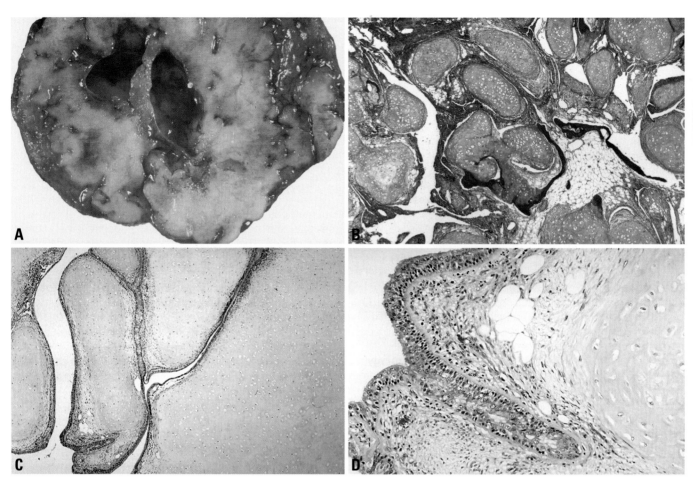

Fig. 1.120 Hamartoma. **A** A bisected, circumscribed hamartoma revealing lobules of firm cartilagenous tissue interspersed by fibrovascular and adipose tissue. Focal cystic change is also seen. **B** At low power, a hamartoma shows lobules of cytologically bland cartilagenous tissue interspersed by mature adipose tissue. Focal ossification. **C** Lobules of mature cartilage with deep clefts lined by bronchiolar type epithelium From Travis et al. {2024}. **D** Adjacent to the cartilage are fat vacuoles and a spindle cell mesenchymal stroma. The cleft-like space is lined by bronchiolar-type epithelium From Travis et al. {2024}.

Sclerosing haemangioma

M. Devouassoux-
Shisheboran
A.G. Nicholson
K. Leslie
S. Niho

Definition
A lung tumour with a distinctive constellation of histologic findings including: solid, papillary, sclerotic, and haemorrhagic patterns. Hyperplastic type II pneumocytes line the surface of the papillary structures. Cholesterol clefts, chronic inflammation, xanthoma cells, haemosiderin, calcification, laminated scroll-like whorls, necrosis, and mature fat may be seen.

ICD-O code   8832/0

Synonyms and historical notation
Pneumocytoma, papillary pneumocytoma {992}. It was named sclerosing haemangioma as it was originally believed to be vascular in origin due to prominent angiomatoid features. Current consensus favors a benign or very low-grade neoplasm arising from primitive respiratory epithelium.

Epidemiology
Sclerosing haemangioma predominantly affects middle-aged adults (median = 46, from 11–80 years-old) {1456,1859}, with a female predominance (80% of cases) {488}. It is rare in western countries. In East Asia (e.g Japan), its frequency is higher and is similar to that of carcinoid tumour.

Localization
Most tumours are solitary and peripheral; 4% of cases are multiple {1153}. The

Table 1.15
Immunoprofile of sclerosing haemangioma. From M. Devouassoux-Shisheboran et al. {488}.

Markers	Round cells (% of cases)	Surface cells (% of cases)
Pan-cytokeratin	-	+
EMA	+ membranous	+ membranous
Low molecular weight keratin (CAM 5.2)	+ focal (17%)	+
Cytokeratin 7	+ focal (31%)	+
Cytokeratin 20	-	-
High molecular weight keratin (CK 5/6; K903)	-	-
TTF-1	+ nuclear (92%)	+ nuclear (97%)
Pro-Sp A and pro-SpB	-	+
Clara cell antigen	-	+
Vimentin	+	+
S-100 protein	-	-
SMA	-	-
Factor VIII	-	-
Calretinin	-	-
Estrogen receptors	+ (7%)	-
Progesterone receptors	+ (61%)	-
Chromogranin	-	-
Synaptophysin	-	-
Leu-7	-	-

EMA (epithelial membrane antigen); CK 5/6 (cytokeratin 5/6), K903 (keratin 903), TTF-1 (thyroid transcription factor-1), pro-SpA and pro-SpB (surfactant apoproteins A and B), SMA (smooth muscle actin).

tumour may involve visceral pleura (4%), mediastinum (1%), and rarely occurs as endobronchial polyps (1%) {488}.

Clinical features
Most patients are asymptomatic (80%). Haemoptysis, cough, and thoracic pain may occur. Chest x-ray shows a solitary circumscribed mass, rarely calcified, and occasionally cystic. CT scans show a well-circumscribed mass with marked contrast enhancement, and foci of sharply marginated low attenuation and calcification {890}. By MRI, a haemorrhagic component may help differentiate SH from other coin lesions {627}.

Macroscopy
SH presents as a well-circumscribed mass without a preferential lobar distribution. Size ranges from 0.3-8 cm. Sections show a solid, grey to tan-yellow

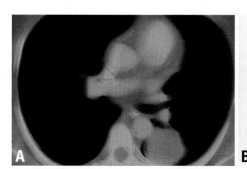
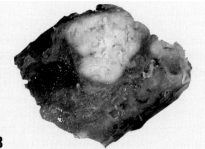
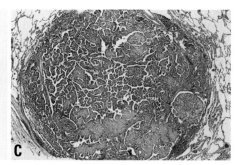

Fig. 1.121 Sclerosing haemangioma. **A** CT scan shows a circumscribed, solid yellow tan mass lying within the posterior segment of the left upper lobe. **B** Sclerosing haemangioma, presenting as a well-circumscribed solid white tumour at its periphery. **C** Well-circumscribed unencapsulated nodule with a mixture of papillary, solid and sclerotic patterns.

surface with foci of haemorrhage and occasionally cystic degeneration {1464} or calcification.

Tumour spread and staging
These tumours may spread to regional lymph nodes in approximately 1% of cases {488,1009,1334}. Rarely SH may present in the mediastinum without apparent connection to the lung {1728}.

Histopathology
Two cell types occur: round stromal cells and surface cells, both of which are thought to be neoplastic in origin {970}.
Round cells are small with well-defined borders and centrally located round to oval bland nuclei with fine dispersed chromatin, an absence of discernible nucleoli. Mitotic index is low (usually less than 1 per 10 high power fields). Their cytoplasm is eosinophilic but may be foamy or vacuolated with a signet ring appearance. Cuboidal surface cells display the morphology of bronchiolar epithelium and activated type II pneumocytes. They may be multinucleated, or demonstrate clear, vacuolated, foamy cytoplasm or intranuclear inclusions. Focal mild to marked nuclear atypia can be seen in either cell type.
1. Papillary pattern: complex papillae lined by cuboidal surface cells. The stalk of the papillary projections contains the round cells. It can be sclerotic or occasionally myxoid.
2. Sclerotic pattern: dense foci of hyaline collagen at the periphery of the haemorrhagic areas, within papillary stalks, or within the solid areas.
3. Solid pattern: sheets of round cells, with scattered cuboidal surface cells forming small tubules.
4. Haemorrhagic pattern: large blood-filled spaces lined by epithelial cells or foci of haemorrhage and debris containing haemosiderin deposits, foamy macrophages, and cholesterol clefts, rarely surrounded by granulomatous and chronic inflammation.
Calcifications sometimes display a psammoma-like configuration. Lamellar structures in the spaces between papillae are also encountered. Rarely, mature fat may be seen. Neuroendocrine cells, isolated or in solid nests (tumourlets) may rarely occur SH combined with typical carcinoid has been described {1153}.

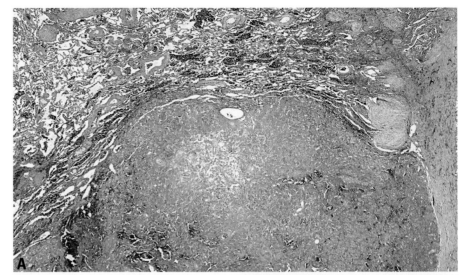
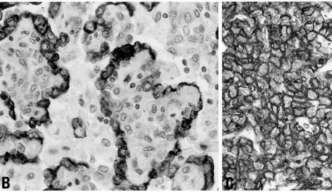
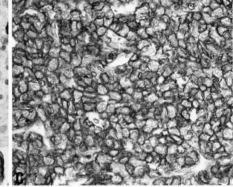

Fig. 1.122 Sclerosing haemangioma. **A** The tumour is circumscribed, but not encapsulated and shows a sclerotic and papillary pattern. From Travis et al. {2024}. **B** Cytokeratin (AE1/AE3) staining shows positive staining of the surface cells but negative staining of the round cells. **C** EMA shows membranous staining of round and surface cells.

Immunohistochemistry
Round cells express TTF-1 and EMA, but are pancytokeratin negative. Surface cells express TTF-1, epithelial membrane antigen (EMA), surfactant apoprotein A and pancytokeratin.

Cytopathology
Trans-thoracic fine needle aspiration cytology {655} typically shows a moderately cellular, dual cell population.
Round cells are small, round or spindle-shaped, with granular cytoplasm, uniform nuclei arranged in cohesive papillary clusters or in flat pavement-type orientation. The nuclei may be atypical, but the absence of nucleoli helps in distinguishing SH from adenocarcinoma. Hyalinized stromal tissue fragments may be seen. Foamy macrophages, haemosiderin, and red cells are seen in the background.

Differential diagnosis
The differential diagnosis includes clear cell tumours involving the lung (metastatic renal cell carcinoma, clear cell 'sugar' tumours, and clear cell carcinomas of the lung), carcinoids and papillary pulmonary epithelial neoplasms. SH can be usually be distinguished from these by bland cytology, heterogeneous architecture and a characteristic immunostaining pattern.

Histogenesis
Since the first description in 1956 {1183}, vascular {1183}, mesothelial {972}, mesenchymal {883}, epithelial {1751}, and neuroendocrine {2180} origins have been postulated. Immunohistochemical findings suggest that sclerosing haemangioma derives from primitive, undifferentiated respiratory epithelium. Molecular studies have demonstrated

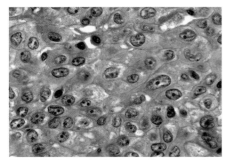

Fig. 1.123 These epithelioid cells of sclerosing haemangioma are growing in the solid pattern. From Travis et al. {2024}.

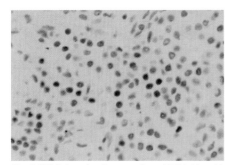

Fig. 1.124 Sclerosing haemangioma TTF-1 (thyroid transcription factor-1) is expressed in tumour cells.

the same monoclonal pattern in both the round and surface cells, consistent with a true neoplasm rather than a hamartoma {1474} There is no normal counterpart for the neoplastic stromal cell recognized in the human lung.

Prognosis and predictive factors

Sclerosing haemantioma behaves in a clinically benign fashion. No recurrence or disease-related deaths have been reported. Reported cases with hilar or mediastinal lymph node involvement do not have a worse prognosis {1464,2198}.

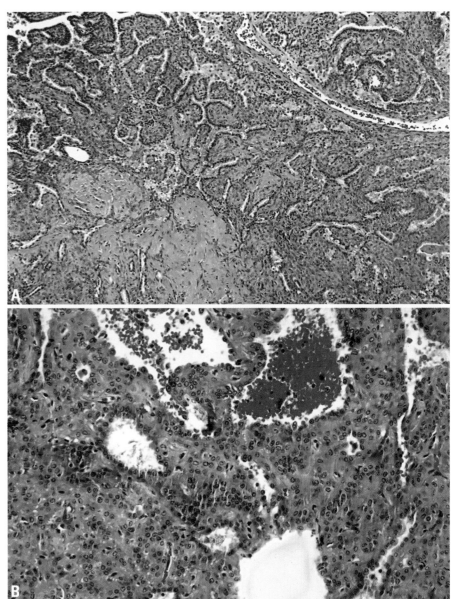

Fig. 1.125 Sclerosing haemangioma. **A** Sclerotic, solid and papillary patterns are present . **B** In this haemorrhagic pattern the tumour forms ectatic spaces filled with red blood cells that are surrounded by type II pneumocytes. From Travis et al. {2024}.

Clear cell tumour

A.G. Nicholson

Definition
Clear cell tumours are benign tumours probably arising from perivascular epithelioid cells (PEC). They comprise cells with abundant clear or eosinophilic cytoplasm that contain abundant glycogen.

ICD-O code   8005/0

Synonyms
Other terms include 'sugar tumour' in the lung and PEComa (perivascular epithelioid cell-oma), or myomelanocytomas at other sites.

Epidemiology
This tumour is extremely rare. There is a slight female predominance, with age range of 8-73 years.

Etiology
There is a very rare association with tuberous sclerosis and lymphangioleiomyomatosis {594}.

Localization
Most are solitary and peripheral in location.

Clinical features
Clear cell tumours are generally asymptomatic and discovered incidentally {646}.

Macroscopy
Tumours are usually about 2 cm in diameter (range 1 mm to 6.5 cm) {59,646}. They are well circumscribed and solitary, with red-tan cut surfaces.

Histopathology
Clear cell tumours comprise rounded or oval cells with distinct cell borders and abundant clear or eosinophilic cytoplasm. There is mild variation in nuclear size, nucleoli may be prominent, but mitoses are usually absent. The presence of necrosis is extremely rare and should lead to consideration of malignancy {646}, as should significant mitotic activity and an infiltrative growth pattern {1984}. Thin-walled sinusoidal vessels are characteristic. Due to the glycogen-rich cytoplasm, there is usually strong diastase-sensitive PAS positivity {1127}.

Immunohistochemistry and electron microscopy
Tumours stain most consistently for HMB-45 {59,646,648,652,1127}. Electron microscopy shows abundant free and membrane bound glycogen {646,648, 1127}. Melanosomes have also been identified {646,648,1127}.

Differential diagnosis
Clear cell tumours are distinguished from clear cell carcinomas, both primary and metastatic, on the basis of a lack of cytologic atypia, the presence of thin-walled sinusoidal vessels within the tumour, positive staining for S-100 and HMB-45 (melanocytic markers) and negative staining for cytokeratins. Metstatic renal cell carcinomas may contain intracytoplasmic glycogen but show necrosis and stain for epithelial markers. Granular cell tumours stain for S-100 but not for HMB-45 and do not contain abundant glycogen in their cytoplasm. Metastatic melanomas and clear cell sarcomas will have a similar immunophenotype and ultrastructure, but the tumour cells will not show significant atypia and there is usually a history of a previous neoplasm.

Histogenesis
Recent data suggest a pericytic origin and clear cell tumours have been proposed to represent one of the family of PEComas, neoplasms originating from the perivascular epithelioid cells (PEC) {201}.

Prognosis and predictive factors
Virtually all tumours have been cured by excision {646,652,1127}.

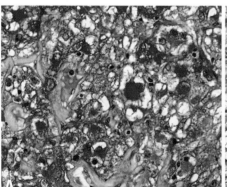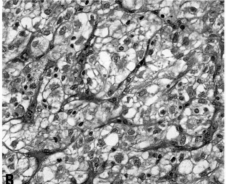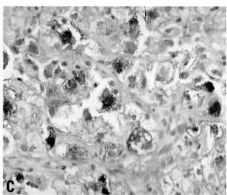

Fig. 1.126 Clear cell tumour. **A** The abundant cytoplasmic glycogen is stained with periodic acid-Schiff (PAS). **B** The glycogen is removed in this PAS stain with diastase digestion. **C** The tumour cells stain positively with immunohistochemistry for HMB-45. From Travis et al. {2024}.

Teratoma

A.G. Nicholson

Definition
Teratomas are tumours consisting of tissues derived from more than one germ cell line. They may be mature or immature. Criteria for pulmonary origin are exclusion of a gonadal or other extragonadal primary site and origin entirely within the lung.

ICD-O code
Teratoma mature   9080/0
Teratoma immature   9080/3

Epidemiology
The majority of cases occur in the second to fourth decades (range 10 months to 68 years) with a slight female preponderance.

Localization
Teratomas are more common in the upper lobes, principally on the left side {78,1373,1931}.

Clinical features
Patients present most often with chest pain, followed by haemoptysis, cough and pyothorax {78,1373,1969}. Expectoration of hair (trichoptysis) is the most specific symptom {1373,1971, 2056}. Radiologically, the lesions are typically cystic masses, often with focal calcification {1373}.

Macroscopy
Tumours range from 2.8-30 cm in diameter. They are generally cystic and multiloculated, but may rarely be predominantly solid, the latter tending to be immature. Cysts are often in continuity with the bronchi and may have an endobronchial component {1373}.

Tumour spread and staging
Pulmonary mature teratomas are benign. Rupture may result in spillage of cyst contents that may cause bronchopleural fistulas and a marked inflammatory and fibrotic reaction.

Histopathology
Mesodermal ectodermal and endodermal elements are seen in varying proportions {78}. Most pulmonary teratomas are composed of mature, often cystic somatic tissue, although malignant or immature elements may occur. Of 31 cases reviewed, 65% were benign and 35% were malignant {1373}. Mature teratomas of the lung generally take the form of squamous-lined cysts similar to those of the ovary, also known as dermoid cysts. Malignant elements consisted of sarcoma and carcinoma. Immature elements, such as neural tissue, infrequently occur. In mature teratomas, thymic and pancreatic elements are often seen.

Differential diagnosis
Metastatic teratoma requires exclusion via thorough clinical investigation. Of note, teratomas treated by chemotherapy often comprise wholly mature elements in their metastases {268}. Carcinosarcomas, pleuropulmonary blastomas and pulmonary blastomas do not recapitulate specific organ structures.

Histogenesis
Pulmonary teratomas are thought to arise from ectopic tissues derived from the third pharyngeal pouch.

Prognosis and predictive factors
Surgery is the treatment of choice with all mature teratomas being cured {1373}. Complete surgical resection may be complicated if the tumour has ruptured with bronchopleural fistula and a marked fibroinflammatory reaction. Resection of malignant teratomas has also led to prolonged disease remission, although most cases were unresectable and died within 6 months of diagnosis.

Other germ cell tumours

Germ cell malignancies other than immature teratomas are extremely rare and require exclusion of an extrapulmonary primary. They should also be distinguished from carcinomas of the lung (including pleomorphic and giant cell carcinomas), which may produce alphafoetoprotein, chorionic gonadotrophins, or placental lactogen.

Most cases reported as choriocarcinoma of the lung are pleomorphic carcinomas with ectopic beta-HCG production. Instead of a dual population of cytotrophoblasts and syncytiotrophoblasts typical of choriocarcinoma, there is a continuous spectrum of morphology from large to pleomorphic tumour cells.

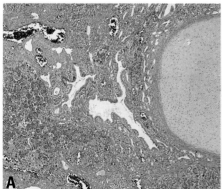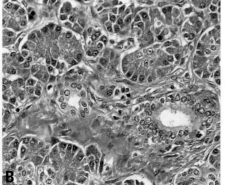

Fig. 1.127 Mature teratoma. A Mature cartilage, glands and pancreatic tissue. **B** Pancreatic tissue with acinar and ductal epithelium. From Colby et al. {391} and Travis et al. {2024}.

Intrapulmonary thymoma

A.G. Nicholson
C. Moran

Definition
Intrapulmonary thymomas are epithelial neoplasms histologically identical to mediastinal thymoma thought to arise from ectopic thymic rests within the lung {1238,1367}.

ICD-O code
8580/1

Epidemiology
Sex distribution differs between series, with one series showing a female preponderance {1367} whilst others show greater equality. Ages range from 17-77 years, with a median of about 50 years.

Localization
Tumours may be hilar or peripheral. Pleural tumours are addressed in the pleural chapter.

Clinical features
Symptoms include cough, weight loss, chest pain, fever and dyspnoea. Tumours may occasionally be asymptomatic. Myasthenia gravis has been rarely described {1367}.

Macroscopy
Sizes range from 0.5-12cm. Tumours are usually circumscribed encapsulated solitary masses although multiple cases are described. The cut surface is frequently lobulated and may be focally cystic, with variable coloration.

Histopathology
Intrapulmonary thymomas show the same features as those arising in the mediastinum (see thymus chapter).

Immunohistochemistry
Immunohistochemical stains for keratin and epithelial membrane antigen highlight the epithelial cells scattered against the variable lymphoid cell background. Staining CD5 may stain the epithelial elements and the lymphocytes stain for CD1a {632,1609}.

Differential diagnosis
Predominantly epithelial thymomas may be mistaken for carcinomas and spindle cell carcinoids, and lymphocyte-rich variants for lymphoma and small cell carcinoma {1367}. Conversely, radiographic studies and/or surgical inspection must exclude primary mediastinal thymomas infiltrating the lung. Thymomas usually lack cytologic atypia and have a more lobulated architecture than small and non-small cell carcinomas.

Histogenesis
Probable derivation from thymic epithelial rests.

Prognosis and predictive factors
Surgical resection appears the treatment of choice with disease-free survival in most patients when tumour is confined to the lung. However, invasive tumours will likely require additional treatment. Nodal involvement is also described and nodal dissection should therefore be considered.

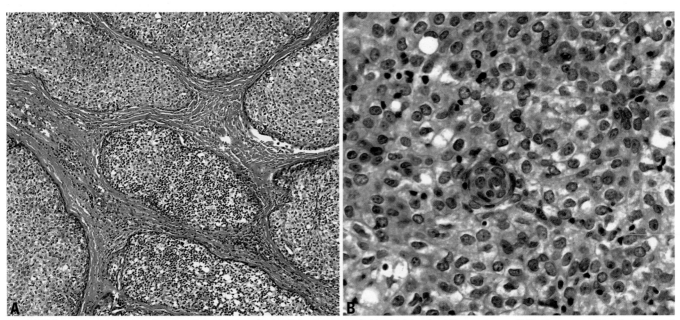

Fig. 1.128 Thymoma. **A** This pleural tumour shows lobules of epithelial cells surrounded by thick bands of fibrous stroma. **B** The tumour consists of a mixture of thymic epithelial cells with a few lymphocytes. From Travis et al. {2024}.

Melanoma

A.G. Nicholson

Definition
Melanomas are malignant tumours derived from melanocytes. Criteria for a primary pulmonary origin include an infiltrating tumour arising from junctional change in the bronchial epithelium, a concomitant naevus-like lesion, no history of previous melanoma and no tumour demonstrable at another site at the time of diagnosis.

ICD-O code   8720/3

Epidemiology
Metastatic melanoma to the lungs is common, but primary pulmonary melanoma is extremely rare.

Localization
Most cases are endobronchial but origin in the trachea is also described {515, 928}. Solitary melanomas in peripheral lung are usually metastatic.

Clinical features
There is an equal sex distribution, with a median age of 51 years (range 29-80 years) {928,1522}. Presentation is with obstructive symptoms.

Macroscopy
Most tumours are solitary and polypoid {928,2152}, although cases of 'flat' melanomas have been described in the trachea {1374}. Most show variable pigmentation.

Histopathology
The tumour is typically lobulated and ulcerative. Architecturally and cytologically, the tumour cells are similar to those of melanoma at other sites. Often, the tumour spreads in Pagetoid fashion within the adjacent bronchial mucosa and rarely, benign nevus-like lesions can also be seen {928,2152}. Immunohistochemistry shows positivity for S-100 protein and HMB-45. Ultrastructural analysis shows melanosomes within the cytoplasm {2152}.

Differential diagnosis
Metastatic disease is the most common differential diagnosis and it may be impossible to prove primary pulmonary origin with absolute certainty. Bronchial carcinoids may be pigmented, but will stain for neuroendocrine markers and are typically cytokeratin positive.

Precursor lesions
No precursor lesion is recognized. Nevus-like proliferation of melanocytic cells can be seen in the mucosa adjacent to some primary pulmonary melanomas, but benign naevi are not known to occur in the bronchus and these may be a cytologically bland form

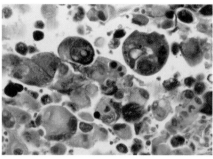

Fig. 1.130 Cytology of an aspirate of metastatic malignant melanoma. Highly pleomorphic and dissociated malignant cells. Note the presence of nuclear pleomorphism, massive nucleoli, and occasional nuclear pseudoinclusion.

of tumour spread, rather than a precursor lesion.

Histogenesis
It is uncertain whether they arise from melanocytic metaplasia or from cells that migrated during embryogenesis.

Prognosis and predictive factors
Once pulmonary origin has been confirmed, treatment is by surgical resection,. Prognosis varies between series, but is generally poor {2152}. However, some patients remain free of disease for up to 11 years {928}.

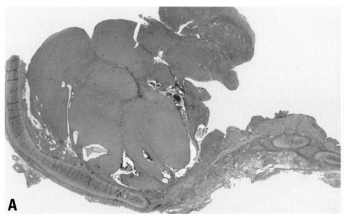
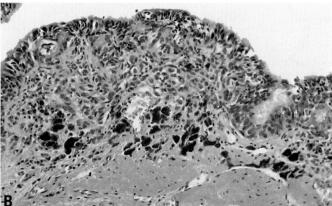

Fig. 1.129 Primary malignant melanoma. **A** Polypoid endobronchial mass with spread along the adjacent bronchial mucosa. **B** Tumour cells infiltrate the bronchial mucosa and involve the epithelium in a pagetoid fashion. From Colby et al. {391} and Travis et al. {2024}.

Metastases to the lung

D.H. Dail   B. Pugatch
P.T. Cagle   S.D. Finkelstein
A.M. Marchevsky   K. Kerr
A. Khoor   C. Brambilla
K. Geisinger

Definition
Tumours in the lung that originate from extra-pulmonary sites or that are discontinuous from a primary tumour elsewhere in the lung.

Synonyms
Secondary tumours in the lung.

Epidemiology
Most common sources of metastatic tumours to lung, in relative order of frequency: breast, colon, stomach, pancreas, kidney, melanoma, prostate, liver, thyroid, adrenal, male genital, female genital.

At autopsy, the lungs are involved with tumour spread from extra-pulmonary solid malignancies in 20-54% of cases {13,426,558,935,1692,2148} and in 15-25% of cases the lungs are the sole site of tumour spread {558}. In some 3-7% of cases of diagnosed primary lung tumours, there is another known primary cancer elsewhere {2202}.

Pathogenesis
Secondary tumours are the commonest form of lung neoplasm and the lungs receive the most secondary tumours of any organ. This is because the lungs are the only organ to receive the entire blood and lymph flow and they have the dens-est capillary network in the body, that network also being the first encountered by tumour cells entering the venous blood via the ductus lymphaticus {548, 578,2237}. Also there is probably favourable "seed and soil" deposition in the lungs as orignally proposed by Paget in 1889 {1531}.

Localization
Some generalizations apply to secondary tumours in the lungs. They are usually, peripheral, have more discrete borders, are harder to reach with fiberbronchoscopy forceps and less often shed cells for cytological examination than lung primaries.

Pulmonary metastases usually present as multiple, bilateral pulmonary nodules but can also appear as solitary masses {13,319,442,935,1784,1961,2129}. Metastatic tumour nodules to the lungs can be present in any intrathoracic location but are most common in the lower lobes {13,126,290,595,781,922,1605}.

Clinical features
Signs and symptoms
Most patients with lung metastases do not have pulmonary symptoms. The few with endobronchial spread simulate primary tumours by causing cough, haemoptysis, wheezing, and signs of obstruction such as obstructive pneumonia, atelectasis, dyspnoea and fever {2131}. Those with pleural infringment and/or effusion may have chest pain and/or dyspnoea. Those with vascular or lymphangitic spread may have signs of cor pulmonale.

The following considerations are important in estimating the likelihood of a lesion in the lung being metastatic in a patient with known extrapulmonary malignancy: the patient's age, smoking history, stage of the extrathoracic primary, cell type and the disease free interval {2131}.

Imaging
Typical metastatic disease to the lungs presents radiographically as multiple well-defined pulmonary nodules. Cavitation may be present and in rare instances, the margins of the nodules may be poorly defined. Calcification is uncommon but may be seen with metastatic osteogenic sarcoma, teratomas and certain adenocarcinomas. On CT, more nodules are routinely detected and their distribution and internal characteristics are better defined. Endobronchial metastases are uncommon but when present cause the same patterns of atelectasis as with primary lung neoplasms. When mediastinal or

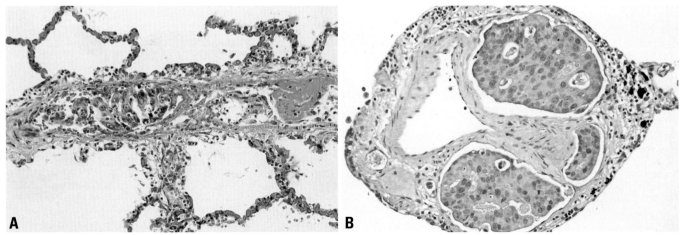

Fig. 1.131 A Metastatic carcinoma, intra-arterial spread. Small artery with endoluminal cancer cells and focal thrombus. **B** Metastatic adenocarcinoma, lymphatic spread. Lymphatic spaces are distended by metastatic adenocarcinoma.

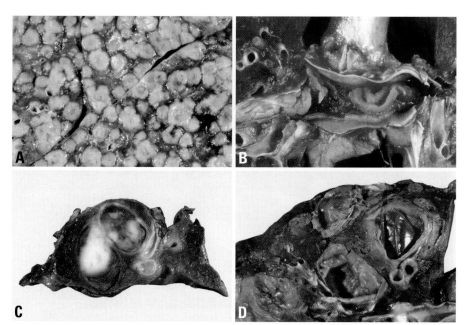

Fig. 1.132 Secondary tumours. **A** Multiple nodules of similar size, metastatic from cholangiocarcinoma. From Dail and Hammar {434}. **B** Large tumour thrombus to main pulmonary artery. From Colby et al. {391}. **C** Metastatic renal cell carcinoma, situated in major brochus. **D** Metastatic leiomyosarcoma. Higher gross power of cystic metastatic uterine leiomyosarcoma. From Dail and Hammar {434}.

hilar lymph nodes are involved, CT scanning detects enlargement much earlier than conventional radiographs. In lymphangitic carcinomatosis the interstitial markings of the lung become prominent and irregular.

Relevant diagnostic procedures

Routine chest radiography is the most effective means of detection. CT scans give higher resolution, sometimes showing additional lesions that are hard to detect on plain chest radiographs. At times, perfusion scans are useful for detecting tumour emboli. PET scans are very helpful, although inflammatory conditions can also be PET scan positive.

Pulmonary function tests are rarely helpful except when there is endobronchial obstruction or extensive endovasular spread.

Sputa, bronchial washes, brushes and lavages, and fine needle apirations, either transtracheal, transbronchial or transthoracic, are as helpful in detecting metastasis as they are with primary lung tumours. Transbronchial biopsy is valuable with proximal lesions but less so with small peripheral ones.

Cytology

Generally, there is little to allow distinction of primary neoplasms from metas-

tases on morphology alone {582}. However, immunocytochemical, cytogenetic, and molecular analyses, can be applied directly to cytological material just as readily as to histological specimens.

Metastatic colonic carcinoma classically presents in smears as cohesive flat sheets with peripheral nuclear palisading, elongated nuclei, and a background of necrotic debris. Similarly, signet ring cell carcinomas are more likely to be metastatic from sites such as the stomach. Lobular adenocarcinoma of the breast may also have a sufficiently distinct morphology: the tumour cells are relatively small and homogeneous with solitary nuclei without hyperchromatism or prominent nucleoli, and may possess cytoplasmic vacuoles. Linear arrays of tumour cells without well developed nuclear molding may be present.

Squamous cell carcinomas metastatic to the lungs generally do not have any distinguishing morphological attributes {582}.

Melanomas typically show little intercellular cohesion and melanin pigment is sometimes evident {618}.

In the paediatric population, most tumours fall into the small round cell category and the primary neoplasm is often known at the time of detection of metas-

tases {672}. A major distinguishing point is lymphoreticular versus nonlymphoreticular. For the former, diagnostic features in the smears include an almost total lack of intercellular cohesion, relatively finely granular chromatin, and lymphoglandular bodies in the background.

Macroscopy

Metastatic neoplasms presenting with multiple pulmonary nodules are variable in gross appearance according to their site of origin, histopathology and pattern of spread {1605,1961} They vary in size from small, miliary lesions (e.g. melanoma, ovarian carcinoma, germ cell neoplasms) to large, confluent, "cannonball" masses (e.g. sarcomas, renal cell carcinoma) {781,1605}. Metastatic adenocarcinomas are usually firm, grey-tan with areas of necrosis and haemorrhage {1633}. Mucin-secreting adenocarcinomas of gastrointestinal, pancreatic, breast, ovary and other site origin exhibit a wet, slimy, glistening yellow-tan surface {13,126,935}. Metastatic colonic adenocarcinomas usually exhibit extensive necrosis with/without cavitation {595}. Metastatic squamous cell carcinomas have a grey, dry surface with punctate areas of necrosis {13,126,442}. Renal cell carcinomas usually present as yellow nodule/s {1605}. Metastatic sarcomas and malignant lymphomas usually have a firm, grey, glistening, "fish-flesh" surface. Metastatic angiosarcomas tend to exhibit a dark red, haemorrhagic surface, while melanomas may be black.

Histopathology

Patterns of spread of metastatic neoplasms to the lung are well known {442,911,1590,1605} but are seldom helpful in identifying the site of origin of the metastatic neoplasm. Metastatic tumour emboli (e.g. sarcomas, others) may occlude the main pulmonary artery or present as multiple pulmonary emboli (breast, stomach, others) {90,876}. Metastatic neoplasms may also present as single or multiple endobronchial polypoid lesions (e.g. head and neck, breast, kidney, others), interstitial thickening due to lymphangitic spread (e.g. lung, breast, gastrointestinal, others), cavitary lesions (e.g. squamous cell carcinoma, sarcomas, teratoma, others) pleural nodules or diffuse areas of consolidation that simulate a pneumonia (e.g. pancreas, ovary, others).

Immunohistochemistry

This is a valuable tool for the distinction between primary and metastatic lung neoplasms. For example, approximately 80% of primary lung adenocarcinomas exhibit nuclear TTF-1 immunoreactivity, an epitope that can also be seen in thyroid neoplasms but is absent in other adenocarcinomas {138,352,704,773, 1564}. Thyroid neoplasms exhibit cytoplasmic thyroglobulin immunoreactivity with a high frequency; this is absent in primary lung tumours and it is useful to demonstrate thyroglobulin negativity in TTF-1 positive lung tumours to exclude a metastasis from the thyroid. Primary adenocarcinomas of the lung usually exhibit keratin 7 and variable keratin 20 cytoplasmic immunoreactivity unless the tumour expresses mucin {184,366,368}. In contrast, colonic adenocarcinomas exhibit a cytoplasmic keratin profile of CK 20 positive/ CK 7 negative as well as CDX-2. {184,352,366,368,704,766,773, 1307,2082}. Breast neoplasms can exhibit nuclear immunoreactivity for estrogen receptor, a finding that is absent in primary lung lesions {976, 1528,1657,1737}. Renal cell carcinomas usually stain weakly with keratin AE1/AE3, and keratin 7 and exhibit strong cytoplasmic vimentin immunoreactivity. Metastatic carcinomas of the ovary usually express immunoreactivity for CA125, N-cadherin, vimentin, oestrogen receptor, and inhibin and negative CEA immunoreactivity {976,1486,2189}.

Differential diagnosis

Some adenocarcinomas have characteristic histopathological features. For example, a cribriform pattern characterizes colonic adenocarcinoma {595}. Necrosis with nuclear debris is also common in metastatic colonic adenocarcinomas. Renal cell carcinomas typically have clear cells arranged in nests surrounded by a rich vascular network {1605}. In squamous cell carcinoma, severe dysplasia or in situ carcinoma favours a primary lung neoplasm {13,935}.

Somatic genetics

Cytogenetics and CGH

In poorly differentiated secondary neoplasms of unknown primary site in which conventional light microscopic, immunohistochemical, and electron microscopic techniques fail to yield a specific diagno-

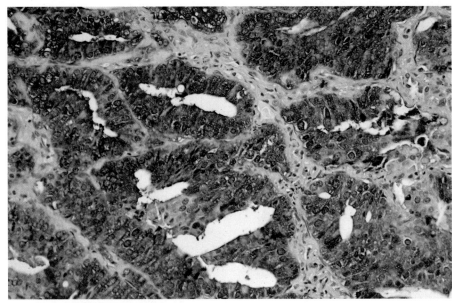

Fig. 1.133 Metastatic prostate carcinoma staining for prostate specific antigen. Typically, PSA is not expressed in primary lung tumours.

sis, cytogenetic analysis promises to increase diagnostic acuity. However, information on nonrandom (recurrent) chromosomal aberrations in solid tumours is currently limited.

When data from different cytogenetic studies are combined, a pattern of nonrandom genetic aberrations appears {1890}. As expected, some of these aberrations are common to different types of tumours {270}, whereas others are more tumour-specific. For example, recent studies suggest that CGH analysis may be helpful in separating benign mesothelial proliferation, malignant mesothelioma, and metastatic adenocarcinoma {1427}. Continued technical refinement of cytogenetic techniques will lead not only to improved understanding of tumour pathobiology, but also to greater clinical applicability.

Molecular genetic alterations

Many of the same molecular genetic alterations of tumour suppressor genes and oncogenes can be found in both primary pulmonary carcinomas and in metastatic carcinomas. Only those molecular genetic markers that are specific or relatively restricted to metastatic carcinomas are candidates for diagnosis of a metastasis with identification of the primary site. For diagnostic purposes, expression of putative primary site specific molecular markers can be most conveniently accomplished by reverse-

transcriptase-polymerase chain reaction amplification (RT-PCR) and immunohistochemistry. Adenocarcinomas metastatic to the lungs are a common problem in differential diagnosis due to their histopathologic resemblance to primary lung adenocarcinomas. Among the molecular markers that are specific or relatively restricted for site of origin of adenocarcinomas are prostate specific antigen for prostate, mammaglobin 1 for breast, TFF2 for pancreas, pepsinogen C for stomach, PSCA for pancreas, metallothionein IL for pancreas, uroplakin II for bladder, MUC II for colon, A33 for colon, lipophilin B for breast, ovary and prostate and glutathione peroxidase 2 for colon and pancreas. Diagnostic genes detectable by RT-PCR are recognized for a number of sarcomas that might metastasize to the lung. Examples include the SYT-SSX fusion genes in synovial sarcomas and EWS-ETS fusion genes in the Ewings family of sarcomas. There is promise that comparative molecular profiles may enable recognition of primary versus metastatic tumours in the lung {1681,1745,1750}.

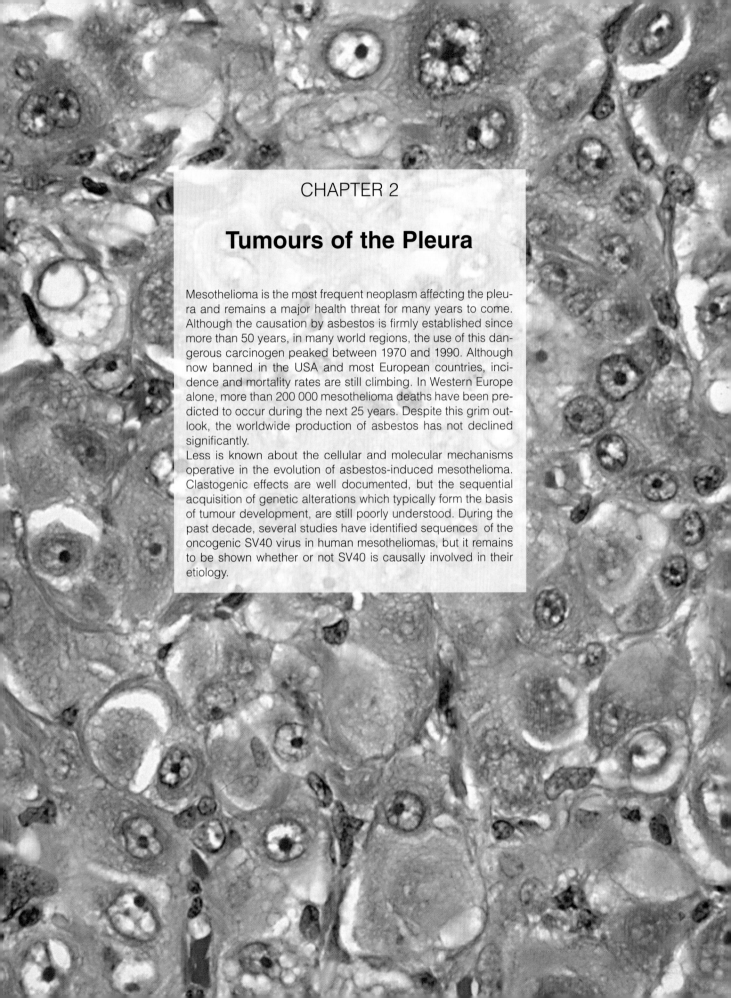

CHAPTER 2

Tumours of the Pleura

Mesothelioma is the most frequent neoplasm affecting the pleura and remains a major health threat for many years to come. Although the causation by asbestos is firmly established since more than 50 years, in many world regions, the use of this dangerous carcinogen peaked between 1970 and 1990. Although now banned in the USA and most European countries, incidence and mortality rates are still climbing. In Western Europe alone, more than 200 000 mesothelioma deaths have been predicted to occur during the next 25 years. Despite this grim outlook, the worldwide production of asbestos has not declined significantly.

Less is known about the cellular and molecular mechanisms operative in the evolution of asbestos-induced mesothelioma. Clastogenic effects are well documented, but the sequential acquisition of genetic alterations which typically form the basis of tumour development, are still poorly understood. During the past decade, several studies have identified sequences of the oncogenic SV40 virus in human mesotheliomas, but it remains to be shown whether or not SV40 is causally involved in their etiology.

WHO histological classification of tumours of the pleura

Mesothelial tumours
Diffuse malignant mesothelioma	9050/3
Epithelioid mesothelioma	9052/3
Sarcomatoid mesothelioma	9051/3
Desmoplastic mesothelioma	9051/3
Biphasic mesothelioma	9053/3
Localized malignant mesothelioma	9050/3
Other tumours of mesothelial origin	
Well differentiated papillary mesothelioma	9052/1
Adenomatoid tumour	9054/0

Lymphoproliferative disorders
Primary effusion lymphoma	9678/3
Pyothorax - associated lymphoma	

Mesenchymal tumours
Epithelioid hemangioendothelioma	9133/1
Angiosarcoma	9120/3
Synovial sarcoma	9040/3
Monophasic	9041/3
Biphasic	9043/3
Solitary fibrous tumour	8815/0
Calcifying tumour of the pleura	
Desmoplastic round cell tumour	8806/3

[1] Morphology code of the International Classification of Diseases for Oncology (ICD-O) {6} and the Systematized Nomenclature of Medicine (http://snomed.org). Behaviour is coded /0 for benign tumours, /3 for malignant tumours, and /1 for borderline or uncertain behaviour.

TNM classification of pleural mesothelioma

TNM classification [1,2]

T – Primary Tumour

TX   Primary tumour cannot be assessed

T0   No evidence of primary tumour

T1   Tumour involves ipsilateral parietal pleura, with or without focal involvement of visceral pleura

T1a Tumour involves ipsilateral parietal (mediastinal, diaphragmatic) pleura. No involvement of visceral pleura

T1b Tumour involves ipsilateral parietal (mediastinal, diaphragmatic) pleura, with focal involvement of the visceral pleura

T2   Tumour involves any ipsilateral pleural surfaces, with at least one of the following:
- confluent visceral pleural tumour (including the fissure)
- invasion of diaphragmatic muscle
- invasion of lung parenchyma

T3* Tumour involves any ipsilateral pleural surfaces, with at least one of the following:
- invasion of endothoracic fascia
- invasion into mediastinal fat
- solitary focus of tumour invading soft tissues of the chest wall
- non-transmural involvement of the pericardium

T4**Tumour involves any ipsilateral pleural surfaces, with at least one of the following:
- diffuse or multifocal invasion of soft tissues of chest wall
- any involvement of rib
- invasion through diaphragm to peritoneum
- invasion of any mediastinal organ(s)
- direct extension to contralateral pleura
- invasion into the spine
- extension to internal surface of pericardium
- pericardial effusion with positive cytology
- invasion of myocardium
- invasion of brachial plexus

Notes: *T3 describes locally advanced, but potentially resectable tumour
      **T4 describes locally advanced, technically unresectable tumour

N –   Regional Lymph Nodes [3]

NX   Regional lymph nodes cannot be assessed

N0   No regional lymph node metastasis

N1   Metastasis in ipsilateral bronchopulmonary and/or hilar lymph node(s)

N2   Metastasis in subcarinal lymph node(s) and/or ipsilateral internal mammary or mediastinal lymph node(s)

N3   Metastasis in contralateral mediastinal, internal mammary, or hilar node(s) and/or ipsilateral or contralateral supraclavicular or scalene lymph node(s)

M –   Distant Metastasis

MX   Distant metastasis cannot be assessed

M0   No distant metastasis

M1   Distant metastasis

Stage Grouping

Stage	T	N	M
Stage IA	T1a	N0	M0
Stage IB	T1b	N0	M0
Stage II	T2	N0	M0
Stage III	T1, T2	N1	M0
	T1, T2	N2	M0
	T3	N0, N1, N2	M0
Stage IV	T4	Any N	M0
	Any T	N3	M0
	Any T	Any N	M1

---

1 {738,2045}.
2 A help desk for specific questions about the TNM classification is available at http://www.uicc.org/tnm/.
3 The regional lymph nodes are the intrathoracic, internal mammary, scalene and supraclavicular nodes.

Mesothelioma

A. Churg
V. Roggli
F. Galateau-Salle
Ph.T. Cagle
A.R. Gibbs
Ph.S. Hasleton
D.W. Henderson
J.M. Vignaud

K. Inai
M. Praet
N.G. Ordonez
S.P. Hammar
J.R. Testa
A.F. Gazdar
R. Saracci
R. Pugatch

J.M. Samet
H. Weill
V. Rusch
T.V. Colby
P. Vogt
E. Brambilla
W.D. Travis

Definition

Diffuse malignant mesothelioma: a malignant tumour arising in the pleura from mesothelial cells, and showing a diffuse pattern of growth over the pleural surfaces.

ICD-O Codes

Epithelioid mesothelioma	9052/3
Sarcomatoid mesothelioma	9051/3
Desmoplastic mesothelioma	9051/3
Biphasic mesothelioma	9053/3

Synonyms

This tumour is properly referred to as "diffuse malignant mesothelioma", but is often abbreviated as "malignant mesothelioma" or just "mesothelioma." Care needs to be taken when using these terms, since localized mesothelial tumours exist in the pleura and have different behaviour.

Epidemiology

Pleural mesotheliomas are largely seen in patients over 60 years of age, but the age distribution is wide and occasional tumours are observed in children. In North America tumours in males outnumber those in females by approximately 9:1, but in other countries such as the UK, France and Australia this ratio is lower.

In North America the incidence of mesothelioma in females is about 2-3/million/yr and this number is essentially unchanged over the last 30 years {8}. In men the incidence is now about 20/million per year. The male incidence increased steadily until the early 1990's but appears to have peaked and there is a suggestion that the numbers are decreasing. The experience in North America is distinctly different from that in Australia, France and the UK, where the incidence is considerably higher and number continue to increase. For example, in Australia, the current incidence in 2000 was 60/million in men and 11/million in women {1156}. Within Europe, the mesothelioma burden varies coniderably. For practical purposes the mortality of pleural mesothelioma is 100%. It is possible that some very early stage tumours have been cured by so-called triple modality therapy: extrapleural pneumonectomy followed by chemotherapy and radiation therapy, but this remains to be proven and would only apply to a small number of cases.

Etiology

Asbestos

In most industrialized countries, greater than 90% of pleural mesotheliomas in men are related to prior asbestos exposure. In women in North America only about 20% of tumours are caused by asbestos {1862}. In other countries, particularly the UK and Australia, where extensive use was made of crocidolite, the proportion of mesotheliomas in women related to asbestos exposure is higher. The latency period is typically very long, with a mean of 30-40 years. Asbestos rarely if ever produces mesothelioma with a latency period less than 15 years. From past exposure, future mortality from mesothelioma has been estimated. In the UK, the number of death cases is expected to peak in 2015-2020, with more than 2000 per year {1588}. Another study postulated that in Western Europe approximately a quarter of a miilon people will die from asbestos-induced mesothelioma over the next 35 years, men born around 1945-1950 being at highest risk {1587}.

However, recent European incidence rates have already started to level off {1346,1347}.

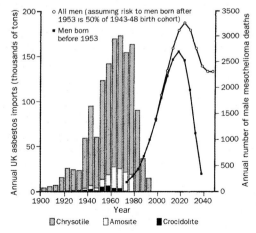

Fig. 2.01 Asbestos imports into the United Kingdom and predicted mesothelioma deaths. The mortality is expected to reach a maximum around the year 2020. From J. Peto et al. {1588}.

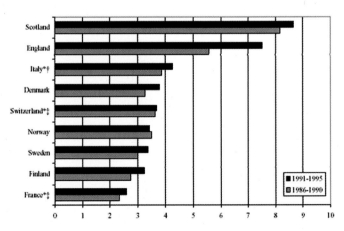

Fig. 2.02 European pleural mesothelioma incidence. Truncated (40-74) age-standardized rates per 100,000 person-years. From F. Montanaro et al. {1347}.

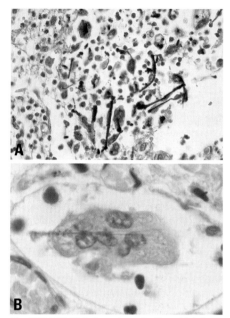

Fig. 2.03 A Multiple ferruginous bodies with inflammatory reaction. B A ferruginous body within a multinucleated macrophage.

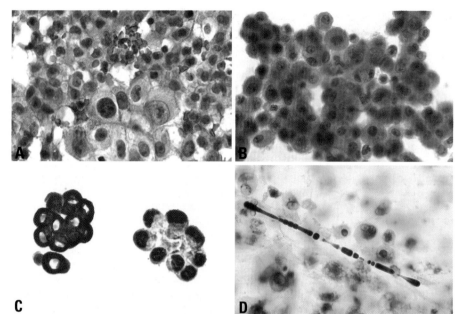

Fig. 2.04 Diffuse malignant mesothelioma - cytology. A Group of mesothelial cells with enlarged, slightly irregular nuclei and with multiple nucleoli in some cells. B Note bland mesothelial cell appearance of the malignant cells. C Immunostain for cytokeratin (left) stains strongly in the cytoplasm of this cluster of cells of diffuse malignant mesothelioma in a pleural effusion. Immunostain for calretinin (right) stains the nucleus of diffuse malignant mesothelioma cells in a pleura effusion. D Asbestos body in the sputum of an exposed individual.

Fibre types. There are distinct differences in the propensity of the different asbestos fibre types to cause mesothelioma. Amphibole (amosite and crocidolite) asbestos is considerably more potent than chrysotile, and crocidolite is more dangerous than amosite. The exact ratio among these 3 fibres depends upon the approach used to investigate the problem: a recent report of estimates of cohort, mean fibre exposure suggested a ratio of 500:100:1 (crocidolite:amosite:chrysotile) for relative risk {858}.

SV40

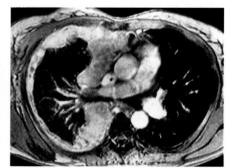

Fig. 2.05 Diffuse malignant mesothelioma. In this CT scan, the pleura shows marked diffuse thickening by mesothelioma, with resulting encasement of the lung.

Some polio vaccines used during 1955 and 1962 were contaminated with the Simian monkey virus 40 (SV40) and this infection has since spread to millions of people in several world regions, including North America and most European countries Several studies have shown, that some human neoplasms, in particular, mesothelioma, brain tumours, bone sarcomas and non-Hodgkin lymphomas frequently contain sequences of SV40, a highly oncogenic DNA virus in rodents {2085}. For mesotheliomas, this was first reported in 1994 {283} and has been confirmed in subsequent analyses {668}. SV40 induces DNA strand breaks in human mesothelial cells {253} and causes pleural mesotheliomas in hamsters {374}. The viral large T-antigen (Tag) inactivates the function of the tumour suppressor genes *TP53* and retinoblastoma *(RB)* and induces chromosomal aberrations {106,285}. The small t-antigen (tag) may contribute to transformationby binding to the protein phosphatase PP2A {106,668}.

Whether a latent SV40 infection is a causal factor in the development of mesothelioma, remains to be assessed. Epidemiological studies provided no evidence that populations which received the contaminated polio vaccine have an elevated cancer risk {542}.

Other causes

These include the non-asbestos fibre, erionite (seen only in Cappadocia, Turkey), therapeutic radiation, and possibly processes that lead to intense pleural scarring such as prior plombage therapy for tuberculosis.

Pathogenesis

A considerable fraction of inhaled asbestos fibers remain permanently entrapped in lung tissue. The majority of these fibers remain naked, without causing a tissue reaction: these are probably responsible for the clastogenic, and, eventually, carcinogenic effects. A minority of asbestos fibers induce an accumulation of monocytes and become surrounded and encapsulated by multinucleated macrophages. This process is associated with deposition of protein and of haemoglobin-derived iron, resulting in the formation of ferruginous bodies.

Clinical features

Signs and symptoms

The most common presenting symptoms in mesothelioma are dyspnoea, usually due to a large pleural effusion, and chest wall pain {796}. These may be associated with constitutional symptoms, especially weight loss and malaise. Additional clinical features include chills, sweats, weakness, fatigue, malaise and anorexia {18}. Unusual presentations include spontaneous pneumothorax {943}, mass lesions and/or segmental or lobar pulmonary collapse, and mediastinal invasion with laryngeal nerve palsy or superior vena caval obstruction. Myalgias, aphonia, dysphagia, abdominal distension, nausea and a bad taste in the mouth have also been reported {1189}.

Imaging
On a chest radiograph malignant mesothelioma often manifests as a large pleural effusion that may obscure an underlying pleural mass or thickening. It is not unusual to see associated pleural plaques. The pleural disease may take on a circumferential pattern of involvement with disease extending along the fissural, mediastinal and/or pericardial pleura. The ipsilateral hemithorax may appear contracted. CT scanning and MRI better define the extent of pleural disease, in particular chest wall, diaphragmatic, pericardial, mediastinal lymph node, or pulmonary involvement.

Relevant diagnostic procedures
Malignant pleural mesothelioma (MPM) is usually diagnosed by pleural biopsies obtained by videothoracoscopy (VATS). Occasionally, pleural fluid cytology will yield a sufficient sample for diagnosis although approximately 50% of patients will have cytologically negative fluid. In addition, VATS pleural biopsy provides samples for immunohistochemistry, which is usually required to support a definitive histological diagnosis. Thoracotomy is not required for diagnosis and should be avoided because it increases the risk of tumor implantation into the chest wall and therefore, may affect the technical feasibility of subsequent definitive resection. In patients whose pleural space is fused by locally advanced tumor, tissue can be obtained via a 5cm incision with very limited rib resection and direct pleural biopsy.

Computed tomography (CT) is the standard imaging study for the initial staging of MPM. However, it does not accurately predict the presence or absence of superficial chest wall invasion (i.e. involvement of the endothoracic fascia and intercostal muscles) or full thickness involvement of the diaphragm. Magnetic resonance imaging (MRI) may be slightly

more accurate than CT in these areas but not consistently enough to be used as a routine imaging modality. If transdiaphragmatic tumor extension is suspected on CT or MRI, this is best confirmed or disproved by laparoscopy. Positron emission tomography (PET) detects metastatic disease in approximately 10% of patients in whom this is not suspected clinically or seen by CT and is therefore used in some insitutions as a routine part of the initial staging evaluation. The maximum standard uptake value (SUVmax) on PET also appears to have prognostic significance. None of these imaging studies accurately predicts the presence or absence of mediastinal lymph node metastases, an important issue because these are known to have a prognostic impact on survival. Mediastinoscopy can identify some but not all lymph nodes metastases because approximately 25% of these occur in areas that are not accessible by mediastinoscopy (e.g. internal mammary lymph nodes).

Cytology
In industrialized countries, about 1% of malignant pleural effusions are caused by diffuse malignant mesothelioma. Mesothelioma cells in effusions are virtu-

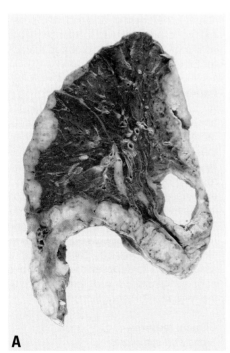 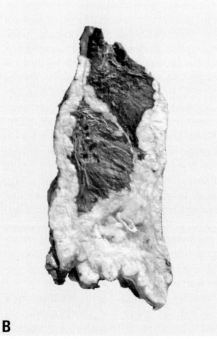

A   **B**

Fig. 2.06 Malignant mesothelioma. **A** Gross image of malignant mesothelioma at autopsy showing the typical appearance of the tumor encasing the lung, and, in this example, the pericardium. **B** Extensive mesothelioma growth with compression of residual lung tissue.

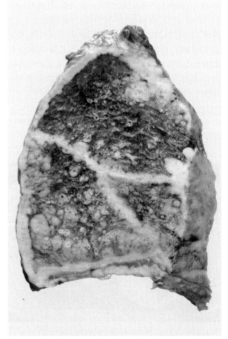

Fig. 2.07. Metastatic pleural adenocarcinoma (pseudomesothelioma). Note infiltration of lung tissue which is typically absent in mesothelioma.

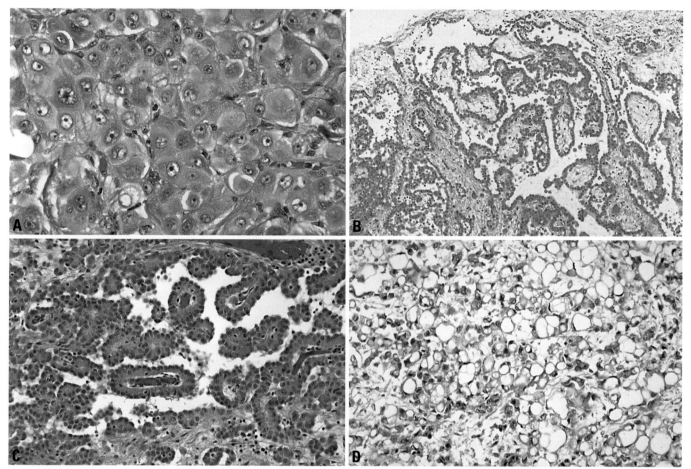

Fig. 2.08 Malignant mesothelioma, epithelioid type. **A** The tumour consists of a sheet of epithelioid cells with abundant eosinophilic cytoplasm and vesicular nuclear chromatin with prominent nucleoli. From Travis et al. {2024}. **B** Papillary proliferation of epithelioid cells. From Travis et al. {2024}. **C** Tubulopapillary pattern. From Travis et al. {2024}. **D** Microcystic (adenomatoid pattern). From Travis et al. {2024}.

ally always of epithelioid type, since cells of the sarcomatoid type are seldom shed into the fluid.

Mesothelioma cells in effusions may be arranged in sheets, clusters, morulae or papillae, sometimes with psammoma bodies. These cells show a range of cytological appearances from pleomorphic to bland, but frequently lack the significant atypia seen in carcinoma. On the other hand, benign mesothelial cells may exhibit features usually associated with malignancy, such as increased cellularity, pleomorphism and mitotic activity. Therefore, differentiation of mesothelioma from benign mesothelial hyperplasia with reactive atypia may be very difficult or impossible in cytologic specimens, since tissue invasion cannot be evaluated. Overall the accuracy of purely cytologic diagnoses, as opposed to tissue diagnoses, of malignant mesothelioma is fairly low. Immunostains of sections from paraffin-embedded cell blocks

may help to confirm the lineage of the cells.

Macroscopy and localization

In its early stages, mesothelioma presents as multiple small nodules on the parietal and sometimes visceral pleura. With progression the nodules become confluent with resulting fusion of the visceral and parietal pleurae and encasement and contraction of the lung. The tumour may reach several centimetres in thickness and range from firm to gelatinous in consistency. Loculated collections of fluid may occur within the tumour. Spread frequently occurs along the interlobar fissures, into the underlying lung, through the diaphragm, and into the chest wall. Mediastinal involvement with invasion of the pericardial sac and encirclement of other midline structures is also common, as is extension to the opposite pleural cavity. Mesotheliomas may metastasize to the pulmonary

parenchyma and to hilar and mediastinal lymph nodes. This appearance is not pathognomonic for mesothelioma, since a variety of primary and secondary pleural malignancies may spread in a similar fashion leading to the encasement of the lung.

Tumour spread and staging
Patterns of mesothelioma spread
Invasion of chest wall fat and muscle is characteristic, especially along needle tracks or surgical biopsy sites. Substantial displacement of the mediastinum to the contralateral hemithorax may occur. Spread through the diaphragm can result in seeding of the peritoneum and ascites, which is frequently found at autopsy and rarely causes uncertainty regarding the primary site.

Infiltration into alveolar spaces may produce a histologic pattern that resembles organising pneumonia, desquamative interstitial pneumonia, or bronchiolo-alveolar carcinoma {1476}. Peribronchial lymphovascular spread can occur, sometimes with miliary spread. Lymph node metastasis rarely is a presenting manifestation of mesothelioma {1906}. At autopsy, haematogenous metastases from pleural mesothelioma may be found in lung, liver, adrenals, bone, brain or kidney {815}. It is rare for mesothelioma to present clinically as metastatic disease {1415}. Staging is performed according to the TNM classification proposed by the International Mesothelioma panel and the UICC {738,2045}.

Histopathology

While the term "desmoplastic mesothelioma" is universally accepted for a particular subtype of highly aggressive sarcomatoid mesothelioma, there is no agreement on the nomenclature of other subtypes, particularly the numerous morphologic variants of epithelioid malignant mesothelioma. Recognition of these variants is important for diagnosis, but because they have no clear prognostic significance, we recommend that most epithelioid and sarcomatoid mesotheliomas be diagnosed with no further sub-classifiers beyond those shown at the beginning of this chapter.

Epithelioid mesothelioma

Epithelioid mesothelioma shows epithelioid cytomorphology. Most epithelioid mesotheliomas are remarkably bland, but more anaplastic forms are occasionally seen. Epithelioid mesotheliomas show a wide range of morphologic patterns. Sometimes one pattern predominates but several different patterns are commonly seen in the same tumour. In most tumours the cells have eosinophilic cytoplasm with bland relatively open nuclei. Mitoses are infrequent. In the poorer differentiated forms, the nuclei are coarser with prominent nucleoli, mitoses are frequent, and some multinucleate tumour giant cells occur; however, these tumours are uncommon and often difficult to separate from carcinomas.

The most frequent patterns encountered are tubulopapillary, adenomatoid (microglandular) and sheet-like. Less common patterns include small cell, clear cell and deciduoid. The tubulopapillary form exhibits varying combinations of tubules, papillae with connective tissue cores, clefts and trabeculae. The cells lining the tubules and papillae are flattened to low cuboidal and relatively bland. Psammoma bodies are occasionally observed. The adenomatoid form shows microcystic structures, with lace-like, adenoid cystic or signet ring

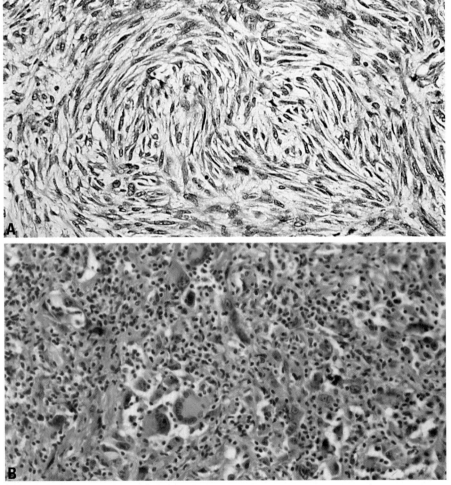

Fig. 2.09 Sarcomatoid mesothelioma. **A** Interlacing fascicles of spindle cells. From Travis et al., {2024}. **B** Sarcomatoid pleural mesothelioma with bizarre anaplastic tumor giant cells. Such an appearance closely mimics that of malignant fibrous histiocytoma.

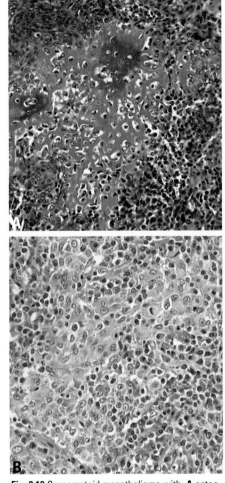

Fig. 2.10 Sarcomatoid mesothelioma with **A** osteosarcomatous differentiation. **B** Inflammatory lymphohistiocytic pattern. From Travis et al. {2024}.

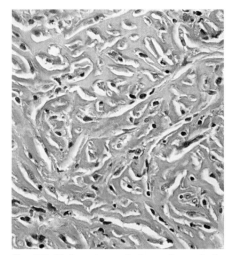

Fig. 2.11 Malignant mesothelioma, desmoplastic type. Haphazard arrangement of slit-like spaces. From Travis et al. {2024}.

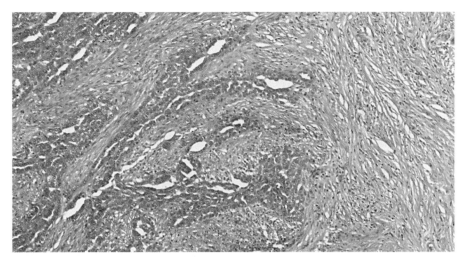

Fig. 2.12 Malignant mesothelioma, biphasic type. A combination of sarcomatoid and epithelioid patterns. From Travis et al. {2024}.

appearances, but does not stain for neutral mucin. Sheets and nests of cells are frequently seen in association with other patterns. Uncommonly, solid, monotonous, relatively non-cohesive sheets of polygonal cells occur, simulating large cell carcinoma or lymphoma. Tumours with anaplastic and/or tumour giant cells may be designated pleomorphic. Mesothelioma can mimic non-Hodgkin lymphoma (so-called lymphohistiocytoid mesothelioma, regarded by some as a form of sarcomatoid mesothelioma) and small cell carcinoma, but usually lacks karyorrhexis and haematoxyphylic staining of blood vessels of the latter tumour. Rarely large cells with clear cytoplasm are prominent, mimicking metastatic renal cell carcinoma. Small foci of cells with plump eosinophilic cytoplasm resembling deciduoid cells of pregnancy are frequently present in epithelioid mesothelioma and uncommonly predominate (so-called deciduoid mesothelioma). The fibrous stroma of epithelioid mesotheliomas can vary from relatively scanty to copious and can show varying degrees of cellularity from hyalinised acellular to highly cellular, merging with sarcomatoid. These tumours may be difficult to distinguish from a biphasic mesothelioma. Myxoid change may be conspicuous, with nests of epithelioid cells "floating" in the matrix; the matrix in such tumours is hyaluronate, and shows hyaluronidase-sensitive staining with Alcian blue.

Immunohistochemistry is an important adjunct to the diagnosis of malignant mesothelioma, particularly in distinguishing it from pulmonary adenocarcinoma. A combination of two or more positive mesothelial with two or more negative epithelial (carcinoma) markers is most useful, their choice to a large extent depending upon the experience of the laboratory. The most useful mesothelial markers appear to be cytokeratin 5/6, calretinin and Wilms tumour gene-1 (WT1). N-cadherin is promising but needs more study. The most useful epithelial markers appear to be CEA (monoclonal), CD15, Ber EP4, B72.3, MOC 31 and thyroid transcription factor 1 (TTF-1). The immunohistochemistry panel will require amendment where the differential diagnosis includes tumours other than pulmonary adenocarcinomas. A broad-spectrum keratin is useful to exclude rare cases of large cell lymphoma, metastatic malignant melanoma and epithelioid haemangioendothelioma. The use of immunohistochemical markers for the diagnosis of malignant versus reactive mesothelial lesions remains controversial.

Sarcomatoid mesothelioma

The sarcomatoid variant of pleural mesothelioma consists of spindle cells arranged in fascicles or having a haphazard distribution. The pattern most often resembles fibrosarcoma, but marked anaplasia and bizarre multinucleate tumour cells may result in a picture closely mimicking that of malignant fibrous histiocytoma. In a small percentage of cases, areas resembling osteosarcoma, chondrosarcoma or other sarcomas may be present.

Sarcomatoid mesotheliomas typically stain positively for cytokeratins when a broadspectrum antibody cocktail is used, although an absence of staining may be seen in occasional cases. Areas with chondrosarcomatous or osteosarcomatous differentiation often stain negatively for cytokeratins {2220}. Sarcomatoid mesotheliomas may stain positively for vimentin, actin, desmin, or S-100. Some cases may also show staining for calretinin {87}.

The differentiation from sarcomatoid (pleomorphic) carcinoma of the lung secondarily invading the pleura or metastatic sarcomatoid renal cell carcinoma can be exceedingly difficult. Immunostains do not reliably differentiate between these possibilities {271}. In such cases, gross and clinical features may be helpful.

Desmoplastic mesothelioma

Desmoplastic mesothelioma is characterized by dense collagenized tissue separated by atypical cells arranged in a storiform or "patternless" pattern, present in at least 50% of the tumour. These tumours can readily be confused with benign organizing pleuritis, especially on small biopsy specimens. Certain diagnostic criteria strongly suggest malignancy. These include frankly sarcomatoid areas, foci of bland collagen necrosis, invasion of adipose tissue, skeletal muscle, or lung, and distant metastases {1229}. Bone metastases from desmo-

Table 2.01
Differential diagnosis of diffuse malignant mesothelioma.

Metastases to the pleura*
- Carcinoma - Sarcoma - Lymphoma - Malignant Melanoma
Primary diffuse pleural sarcoma
- Angiosarcoma - Epithelioid haemangioendothelioma - Synovial sarcoma - Other sarcoma
Thymic tumours, primary or metastatic
Desmoplastic small round cell tumour and Ewing sarcoma family
Localized primary pleural tumours
- Localized malignant mesothelioma - Solitary fibrous tumour (benign and malignant forms) - Sarcomas - Well-differentiated papillary mesothelioma - Adenomatoid tumour - Calcifying fibrous pseudotumour - Nodular pleural plaque

*Metastasis to the pleura or reaching the pleura by direct spread from the lung or chest wall.

plastic mesothelioma {1219} are potentially liable to histological misdiagnosis as a primary benign fibrous tumour of bone.

Cytokeratin staining may be of greatest utility in highlighting invasion by keratin positive spindle cells into adipose tissue, skeletal muscle, or lung. The mere presence of keratin positive staining in the thickened pleura itself is of no particular benefit, since reactive processes often have keratin-positive spindle cells.

Biphasic mesothelioma

Mesotheliomas contain both epithelioid and sarcomatoid patterns in about 30% of cases. Any combination of the patterns noted above may be present. Each component should represent at least 10% of the tumour to warrant the term biphasic. The percentage of cases classified as biphasic will increase with more thorough tumour sampling.

Grading

Malignant mesotheliomas are not ordinarily graded. Epithelioid forms are often deceptively monotonous and can be remarkably bland in appearance. Mitoses are scarce in most epithelioid mesotheliomas. Sarcomatoid forms may be bland or fairly anaplastic. However, beyond the distinction between epithelioid and sarcomatoid forms, these histopathologic features do not correlate well with prognosis.

Differential diagnosis

The differential diagnosis of diffuse malignant mesothelioma is shown in Table 2.01. The most important differential is metastatic or locally invasive (from lung or chest wall) tumour that covers the pleural surface. However, various localized tumours also exist in the pleura and some mimic mesothelioma microscopically. For this reason, knowledge of the gross distribution of tumour, whether obtained from radiographic studies, the operator's description of the findings at thoracotomy or thoracoscopy, or from a resected or autopsy specimen, is crucial to making a proper diagnosis.

Postulated cell of origin

The exact cell of origin of malignant mesothelioma is unclear. Although the common belief is that these tumours arise from surface mesothelial cells, some experimental data suggest that they may arise from submesothelial cells that differentiate in a variety of directions.

Precursor lesions

It is likely that malignant mesothelioma develops through an in-situ stage. There are at present no reliable histologic criteria for separating lesions that might be *in situ* mesothelioma from atypical benign reactions. The use of the term 'atypical mesothelial hyperplasia' is recommended for purely surface mesothelial proliferations that might or might not be malignant.

Somatic genetics

Cytogenetics and CGH

Most studied cases appear to be epithelioid mesotheliomas, although some reports do not distinguish cell type. Karyotypic and comparative genomic hybridisation (CGH) analyses have demonstrated that most mesotheliomas have multiple chromosomal alterations.

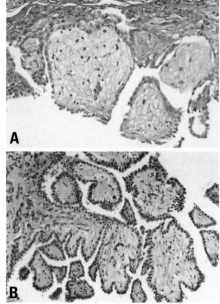

Fig. 2.13 A Well differentiated papillary mesothelioma. **B** Solitary papillary WDPM.

Although no single change is diagnostic, several recurrent sites of chromosomal loss have been identified. Deletions of 1p21-22, 3p21, 4q, 6q, 9p21, 13q13-14, and 14q have been repeatedly observed {103,177,178,1075,1942}. Monosomy 22 is the most frequent numerical change. Losses of 4p and proximal 15q have been reported in some CGH studies, and minimally deleted regions at 4p15 {1815} and 15q15 {457} have been documented. Recurrent losses of 17p12-pter, including the p53 locus, have been observed in some investigations {103, 1075}. Loss of heterozygosity (LOH) analysis has confirmed that each of the above sites is frequently deleted in mesothelioma and, for most of the affected chromosomes, has defined a single minimally deleted region (reviewed in {1997}). Allelic loss from chromosome 4 has been reported to occur at multiple locations, with the most frequent site being 4q33-34 {1815}. LOH in 6q occurs at several non-overlapping regions between 6q14 and 6q25 {142}. Similarly, multiple non-overlapping regions of allelic loss have been reported for chromosome 14, with 14q11.2-12 and 14q23-24 each being observed in two independent studies {179,458}. Chromosomal gains are less common than losses in mesothelioma, although recurrent gains of 1q, 5p, 7p, 8q22-24, and 15q22-25 have been described. These abnormalities reflect similarities and differences with carcinoma of the lung.

Molecular genetic alterations

Inactivation of the *CDKN2A/ARF* locus at 9p21 is a frequent finding in mesothelioma {345,2178}. *CDKN2A/ARF* encodes the tumour suppressor genes p16^{INK4a} and p14^{ARF}. Homozygous deletions of this locus are common, especially in cell lines, and inactivation by promoter methylation is also a recurrent finding {1071}. Immunohistochemical analysis suggests that loss of p16^{INK4a} expression is a frequent finding {839}. Deletions of *p14^{ARF}* are frequently observed. This mechanism of cell cycle control disruption is also common in non-small cell carcinomas. Unlike lung cancers, *TP53* mutations are relatively uncommon {417, 1020,1302}, possibly because SV40 Tag is expressed in some mesotheliomas and retains its ability to bind to and inactivate p53 {284}. Also in contrast to lung cancer, mutations of the *NF2* tumour suppressor gene, located at chromosome 22q12, have been reported frequently in mesothelioma {165,1778}. Biallelic inactivation of *NF2* occurs by combined point mutation and LOH {346}. The previously mentioned monosomy of chromosome 22 may reflect these findings. Another tumour suppressor gene, *GPC3*, is frequently down regulated due to aberrant promoter methylation {1413}.

Recurrent activation of oncogenes by point mutation or amplification has not been documented in mesothelioma {1020,1302}. However, asbestos induces mRNA expression of the c-*fos* and c-*jun* proto-oncogenes in mesothelial cells {810}, and asbestos-induced mesothelial cell transformation is linked to increases in AP-1 DNA binding complexes and the AP-1 component, Fra-1 {810,1639}. Other experimental evidence indicates that when SV40 infects mesothelial cells, it causes activation of the Met and notch-1 proto-oncogene products {185,267}. In contrast to lung cancers, relatively few genes are methylated in mesotheliomas. The gene most frequently methylated is the *RASSF1A* tumour suppressor gene {2018}.

Genetic susceptibility (Familial cancer syndromes)

Multiple cases of pleural mesothelioma have been reported from families with documented exposure to asbestos or other carcinogenic mineral fibres, such as erionite {81,1175,1697}. While investigation of members of one family with familial mesothelioma failed to identify germline mutations, the molecular changes in the tumours were similar to those found in sporadic mesothelioma {80}. One study {960} described an association at population level with HLA antigens B41, B58 and DR16. Specific genetic indicators of susceptibility to mesothelioma development have not yet been identified {1740}: currently available observations may reflect differential levels and duration of exposure to carcinogenic fibres among affected and non-affected members of a family, random sequences of events, or genuine variations in individual susceptibility.

Prognosis and predictive factors
Clinical criteria

Chest pain, dyspnoea and weight loss as presenting symptoms may be associated with a poorer prognosis {822,1708}. There was a trend towards pain being related to sarcomatoid differentiation {1711}. Good prognostic indicators are a young age at presentation, epithelioid subtype, stage of disease {1711} good performance status, lack of chest pain and female sex below the age of 50 years {1861}.

Histopathological criteria

Most series show that patients whose tumours have a purely epithelioid histology have the longest survival, those with a purely sarcomatoid histology the worst, and those with mixed patterns an intermediate survival. The differences in median survivals as a function of histologic subtype are only however, a matter of a few months. In the future, therapy may be influenced by histologic subtype, since no patient with a sarcomatoid pattern treated with trimodality therapy survived for 5 years {2235}.

Genetic predictive factors

While there are many similarities in the frequencies of various genomic imbalances between epithelioid and sarcomatoid mesotheliomas, several chromosomal locations (3p, 7q, 15q, 17p) show significant variations {1075}. For example, deletion at 3p21 is common in epithelioid tumours but rare in sarcomatoid and biphasic tumours. To date, cytogenetic prognostic factors have not been

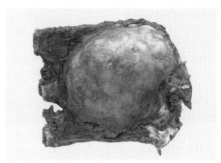

Fig. 2.14 Localized malignant pleural mesothelioma.

reported. Loss of 7q, which is associated with poor prognosis in other tumour types, was observed in ~20% of sarcomatoid tumours but was not observed in epithelioid cases {1075}. Moreover, the incidence of amplicons was 4-5-fold higher in sarcomatoid than in epithelioid tumours. Gene expression profiles in a small number of cases has been reported to predict outcome independent of histologic subtype {714}

Well differentiated papillary mesothelioma

Definition

Well differentiated papillary mesothelioma (WDPM) of the pleura represents a distinct tumour with a papillary architecture, bland cytologic features and a tendency toward superficial spread without invasion.

ICD-O code   9052/1

Epidemiology

WDPM is a rare pleural tumour, with fewer than 50 cases reported in the world literature {261,864,2204}. These tumours are considerably more common in the peritoneum, where they predominantly occur in women {444}. This sex predominance is not obvious in the pleural cases. The reported age range in pleural lesions is 31-79 with a median of 63 for both sexes {261,864,2204}.

Etiology

Asbestos exposure has been reported in some cases {261,656}, but this has not been established in epidemiologic studies.

Localization

These lesions may be localized or multifocal and widespread.

Clinical features

Patients present with dyspnoea and recurrent pleural effusion or as an incidental finding. They rarely present with pneumothorax or chest pain. Unilateral free-flowing pleural effusions may be seen, with or without nodular pleural thickening or fibrous hyaline plaques.

Macroscopy

These tumours may appear as solitary or multiple localized masses. The visceral or parietal pleura may be involved and may have a velvety appearance.

Histopathology

WDPM is characterized by papillae, consisting of predominantly stout myxoid fibrovascular cores covered by a single layer of bland flattened to cuboidal mesothelial cells, exuding from the pleural surface. Basal vacuoles may be present in the lining cells. Nucleoli are inconspicuous and mitotic figures absent. The surface cells stain positively for mesothelial markers.

In the strictest definition, invasion is not present in WDPM. However, some cases of otherwise typical WDPM may show limited invasion. Nevertheless, diffuse malignant mesotheliomas may have areas with a WDPM-like pattern and should not be designated as WDPM. Consequently, great caution should be employed in diagnosing WDPM in small biopsies.

Prognosis and predictive factors

These tumours are often indolent with prolonged survival. The development of invasion may herald a more aggressive clinical course. The occurrence of rapidly progressive disease suggests that the underlying disease is a diffuse malignant mesothelioma, a problem that may reflect sampling inadequacy.

Localized malignant mesothelioma

Definition

A rare tumour that grossly appears as a distinctly localized nodular lesion without

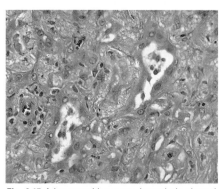

Fig. 2.15 Adenomatoid tumour. Irregularly shaped gland-like spaces are present within a fibrous stroma. From Travis et al. {2024}.

gross or microscopic evidence of diffuse pleural spread, but with the microscopic, histochemical, immunohistochemical and ultrastructural features of diffuse malignant mesothelioma.

ICD-O code: code according to the histologic subtype of mesothelioma.

Clinical features

Most reported cases have been incidental findings on chest x-ray or CT scan. Occasionally they present with pleural effusions.

Macroscopy

Localized malignant mesotheliomas are circumscribed nodular tumours that measure up to 10cm in diameter. They may be attached to the visceral or parietal pleura, are pedunculated or sessile, and can extend into the subjacent lung.

Histopathology

These tumours are histologically identical to diffuse malignant mesotheliomas and may be epithelioid, sarcomatoid, or biphasic (mixed). They show a pattern of immunohistochemical staining identical to diffuse malignant mesothelioma {425}.

Prognosis

Some localized malignant mesotheliomas are cured by surgical excision {425}. Recurrent tumours may metastasize like sarcomas and usually do not spread along the pleural surface.

Adenomatoid tumour

Definition

A rare solitary small pleural tumour with histological features identical to those seen in adenomatoid tumours in other locations.

ICD-O code   9054/0

Clinical features

The few reported cases have been incidental findings at gross examination of the pleura.

Macroscopy

The tumours appear as solitary distinctly nodular lesions.

Histopathology

The tumour cells are flattened to cuboidal and usually eosinophilic; they form glands and tubules, often with marked cytoplasmic vacuolisation {958}. They show a pattern of staining identical to that seen in diffuse malignant mesothelioma. Adenomatoid tumour must be separated from some diffuse epithelial mesotheliomas that may, in individual microscopic fields, show a similar pattern.

Prognosis and predictive factors

These neoplasms are identical to adenomatoid tumours in other locations and are benign.

Lymphomas

P.M. Banks
N.L. Harris
R.A. Warnke
Ph. Gaulard

Primary effusion lymphoma

Definition
A neoplasm of large B-cells presenting as serous effusions, usually without detectable tumour masses, universally associated with human herpes virus 8 (HHV8)/Kaposi sarcoma herpes virus (KSHV), and usually occurring in the setting of immunodeficiency.

ICD-O code   9678/3

Synonym
Body cavity-based lymphoma.

Epidemiology
The majority of cases arise in the setting of human immunodeficiency virus (HIV) infection {60,311,1421}. Most patients are young to middle aged homosexual males. This neoplasm is rare even in the setting of HIV infection. Cases have been reported in HIV negative allograft recipients, particularly after cardiac transplantation {512,561,937}. The disease has also been reported in the absence of immunodeficiency especially in elderly individuals   {282,380,821,1029,1422, 1995}.

Localization
The most common sites of involvement are the pleural, pericardial and peritoneal cavities. Typically only one body cavity is involved. One case has been reported arising in the artificial cavity of a breast implant {1721}. The most common extra-cavitary site of presentation is the gastrointestinal tract; the GI tract, mediastinal and retroperitoneal soft tissue and other extranodal sites may also be secondarily involved {130,209,415,479,877}.

Clinical features
Patients typically present with effusions in the absence of lymphadenopathy or organomegaly. Some patients, both HIV+ and HIV-, have pre-existent Kaposi sarcoma {60,937,1721}. Rare cases are associated with multicentric Castleman disease {380,1995}.

Etiology
The consistent presence of HHV8 in the neoplastic cells in all cases suggests a pathogenetic role for this virus in the development of the tumour {311}. There is consistent expression of viral IL-6 (vIL-6) in primary effusion lymphomas, suggesting that this and other cytokines may play a role in the pathogenesis of the tumours {62,514}. In one study of an EBV- HIV- case, HHV8 related transcripts including viral G-coupled protein receptor, viral Bcl2, viral cyclin D1, viral IL6 and viral MIP I and II were detected in tissue from a primary effusion lymphoma and an HHV8+ gastric lymphoma but only vIL6 was detected in a multicentric Castleman disease lesion from the same patient {1995}. Oncogenic genes encoding viral cyclin D, bcl2, G-protein coupled receptor IL-6, Flice inhibitory protein and others were also shown to be expressed in another EBV- PEL {379}. NF kappa-B is constitutively activated on HHV8+ PEL cell lines, and its inactivation leads to apoptosis, suggesting that, similarly to EBV, HHV8 may promote cell survival through this pathway {989}.

Although multicentric Castleman disease and primary effusion lymphoma may coexist in some patients, a clonal relationship between them has not been established {82}.

Most but not all cases are coinfected with EBV, but do not express the transforming proteins EBNA-2 and LMP1 and 2. Each case contains a single strain of clonal EBV, but there is considerable heterogeneity among cases; thus no specific role for EBV in the pathogenesis has been found {561,868}.

Histopathology
With Wright or May Grunwald Giemsa staining performed on cytocentrifuge preparations, the cells exhibit a range of appearances, from large immunoblastic or plasmablastic cells to cells with more anaplastic morphology. Nuclei are large, round or irregular in shape, with prominent nucleoli. The cytoplasm is typically very abundant and is deeply basophilic,

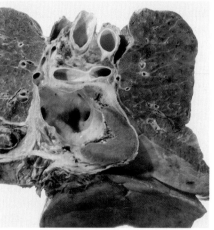

Fig. 2.16 Diffuse lymphoma of the pleura in a patient with AIDS.

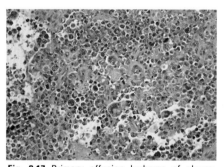

Fig. 2.17 Primary effusion lyphoma of pleura. Discohesive atypical lymphoid tumour cells with a few pleomorphic cells.

and vacuoles may be present in occasional cells. A paranuclear hole suggesting plasmacytoid differentiation may be seen. Binucleated or multinucleated cells may be present that can resemble Reed-Sternberg cells.

The cells often appear more uniform in histological sections than in cytospin preparations. They are large, with some pleomorphism, ranging from large cells with round or ovoid nuclei to very large cells with irregular nuclei and abundant cytoplasm; multinucleation can occur {60,311,1421}. Pleural biopsies show tumour cells adherent to the pleural surface, often embedded in fibrin and occasionally invading the pleura.

This disease should be distinguished from pyothorax-associated diffuse large

B-cell lymphoma, which usually presents with a pleural mass lesion. The cells of pyothorax-associated diffuse large B-cell lymphoma have the appearance of immunoblasts, and are EBV positive and HHV8 negative {1972}.

Immunoprofile
The neoplastic cells typically express leukocyte common antigen (CD45) but are usually negative for the pan-B-cell markers CD19, CD20 and CD79a {60, 1421}. Surface and cytoplasmic expression of immunoglobulin is likewise often absent. The B-cell specific transcriptional activator programme appears to be disrupted in primary effusion lymphoma, with decreased or absent expression of PU.1, Oct 2 and BOB.1, possibly accounting for the failure to produce immunoglobulin {72}. CD30 is typically positive. The cells lack germinal centre-associated markers CD10 and Bcl-6 and express MUM1/IRF4, associated with late germinal centre and post-germinal centre B cells {281}. Plasma cell-related markers such as CD38, and CD138 are typically expressed {650}. Aberrant cytoplasmic CD3 expression has been reported {130}, as well as CD7 and CD56 {1608}. Because of the markedly aberrant phenotype, it may be difficult to assign a lineage with immunophenotyping. Rare cases of HHV8+ primary effusion lymphoma that express only T-cell-associated antigens have been reported {1146,1720}.
The nuclei of the neoplastic cells are positive by immunohistochemistry for the HHV8/KSHV-associated latent protein {522,1555}, and this staining can be useful in confirming the diagnosis. EBV-positive cases have a Type I latency phenotype, expressing only EBNA-1; EBNA-2 and LMP-1 and 2 are not expressed at levels detectable by immunohistochemistry {278}.
Cell lines from primary effusion lymphomas have been shown to express both the Met tyrosine kinase receptor and its ligand, hepatocyte growth factor, similarly to myeloma cell lines {278}.

Histogenesis
Post-germinal center B-cell with differentiation towards plasma cells.

Somatic genetics
Immunoglobulin genes are rearranged and are mutated consistent with a post-germinal center B cell {1258}. The BCL6 gene is somatically mutated in most cases, consistent with a post-germinal center B cell {649}. Some cases also have rearrangement of T-cell receptor genes {865}. Most cases have multiple but non-recurring cytogenetic abnormalities {512}. Comparative genomic analysis has revealed gains in sequence of chromosomes 12 and X {1401}. HHV8 viral genomes are present in all cases. EBV is detected in most but not all cases by EBER *in-situ* hybridisation {60,209, 561,1421}. Cases in HIV- non-immunosuppressed patients appear to be more often EBV- {512}. Two cases with only T-cell antigen expression and rearrangement of the T-cell receptor gene have been reported {1146,1720}. The relationship of these cases to the more common B-cell neoplasm is unclear.
Gene expression analysis by DNA microarray technology has shown a distinctive profile for the cells of primary effusion lymphoma, including genes indicating differentiation towards plasma cells and a set of genes unique to this type of lymphoma {1027}.

Prognosis and predictive factors
The clinical behaviour is extremely aggressive, with most reported patients dead in less than one year. Recently a few cases have been reported to respond to antiviral therapy or combination chemotherapy or both with prolonged survival {209,1029}.

Pyothorax-associated lymphoma

Definition
Pyothorax-associated lymphoma (PAL) is a neoplasm of large B cells, typically with immunoblastic morphology, usually presenting as a pleural mass. It is strongly associated with Epstein-Barr virus (EBV). This rare type of primary pleural B-cell lymphoma occurs in patients with a clinical history of longstanding pyothorax resulting from pulmonary tuberculosis or tuberculous pleuritis.

Synonyms and historical annotation
Since its first recognition in 1987, it has been established that PAL belongs to the diffuse large B-cell lymphoma (DLBCL) category {915}. Although the recent WHO classification of Tumours of Haematopoietic and Lymphoid Tissues describes different clinical subtypes among DLBCL (i.e. mediastinal, intravascular, and primary effusion lymphoma) {919}, PAL has not been included as a distinct clinico-pathologic entity in this recent classification, probably in view of its rarity in most western countries. We include it in this classification of pleural tumours since it specifically occurs in this location.

Epidemiology
Pyothorax-associated lymphoma (PAL) occurs in adults, usually in the 5-8th decades with a median age around 65-70 years. It seems to affect males more often than females {1437,1586}. PAL develops in patients without overt systemic immunosuppression, but consistently after a history of pyothorax resulting from artificial pneumothorax for treatment of pulmonary tuberculosis or, more rarely, tuberculous pleuritis. The interval between the onset of pleuritis and initial symptoms of lymphoma ranges from 20—67 -years, with a 37-48 years median interval {1437,1586}. Most PALs have been reported in Japan, apart from several cases in France and Italy {63,79, 1250,1339,1437,1503,1586}.

Etiology
Strong association with Epstein-Barr virus (EBV) has been demonstrated {631, 1503,1743}. Depending on the series, EBV DNA or EBV-encoded RNA (EBERs) are demonstrated in lymphoma cells of 70-100% of cases. They also express latent infection genes, including EBV nuclear antigen 2 (EBNA-2) and latent membrane protein 1 (LMP-I), resulting in a latency III pattern of EBV expression, similar to that observed in lymphoproliferative disorders occurring in immuno-compromised patients. Although the pathogenesis is not clearly understood, previous findings {954} suggest a role for chronic inflammation at the local site in the proliferation of EBV-transformed B-cells by enabling them to escape the host immune-surveillance system and/or by providing local production of cytokines such as IL-6 and IL-10 {955, 956}.
There is no association with HIV, HTLV, or HHV8 infections.

Sites of involvement
In contrast to primary effusion lymphoma (PEL), PAL typically presents as a tumour

mass that involves the pleural cavity and shows direct invasion to adjacent structures such as the chest wall, lung and diaphragm in most cases, whereas pleural effusion is rarely observed. Extrathoracic/metastatic dissemination (bone marrow, liver, abdominal lymph nodes, etc) is only rarely observed at presentation {1437,1586}.

Clinical features

Patients typically present with symptoms related to a pleural tumour mass, with pains in the chest and/or back, or respiratory symptoms such as productive cough, often with haemoptysis or dyspnoea. Other common symptoms are fever and weight loss. A tumour swelling in the chest wall is present in 40% of the patients. Chest radiography and computed tomography reveals a tumour mass in most patients, which is located in the pleura (80%), pleura and lung (10%) and lung near pleura (7%) with a tendency to invade adjacent structures, mainly the chest wall, and is larger than 10 cm in about half of the patients {1437}. These features often suggest a diagnosis of lung cancer or pleural mesothelioma. About 70% of the patients have a Ann Arbor stage I-II localized disease. The serum lactate dehydrogenase (LDH) level is elevated in most patients {1437, 1586}. Due to the presence of several clinical prognostic factors (low performance status, age, elevated LDH level), the majority of patients belong to the intermediate group of the International Prognostic Index (IPI) score {2}.

Morphology

In tissue sections, there is a diffuse destructive proliferation of large cells. Despite a range of appearances, most cases show a predominant population of immunoblasts with round nuclei showing large single or multiple nucleoli. They may have features of plasmacytoid differentiation. Some cases are consistent with a centroblastic lymphoma and a few have been reported to have anaplastic features. PAL is characterized by a high proliferative rate with numerous mitotic figures and prominent apoptosis. Areas of necrosis and angiocentric or angioinvasive features have been reported, thus resembling features of lymphoproliferative disorders occurring in immunocompromised patients. The disease should be distinguished from primary effusion

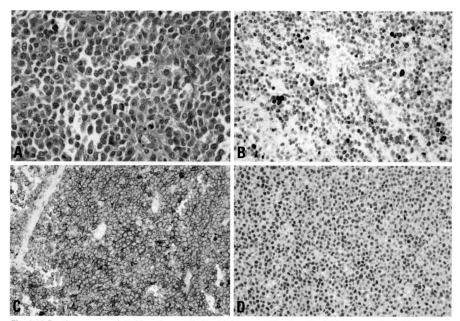

Fig. 2.18 Pyothorax associated lymphoma. **A** At a higher magnification, the infiltrate consists of large neoplastic cells, with immunoblasts and many cells showing a plasmacytoid differentiation with eccentric nuclei and abundant cytoplasm. **B** The neoplastic cells are strongly positive for CD79a. **C** However, in this case, they also show aberrant strong expression for CD2. **D** Immunostaining with the EBNA-2 antibody shows that virtually all neoplasic cells disclosed strong nuclear staining for EBNA-2.

lymphoma (PEL), which commonly presents as serous effusions without detectable tumour masses in patients with a setting of immunodeficiency, is characterized by a proliferation of large B-cells which are CD30, CD38 and CD138 positive but lack CD20 and CD79a B cell markers, and is constantly associated with HHV8 infection.

Immunophenotype

Typically, lymphoma cells are positive for CD79a and CD20 B-cell antigens. Cases with plasmacytoid differentiation, however, have been reported to lack CD20 or even CD79a. They may show weak heterogeneous expression of plasma cell related markers such as CD138. Cytoplasmic expression of immunoglobulins can be detected. CD30 activation marker can be expressed. Surprisingly, a number of cases may express at least one T-cell marker (CD2, CD3, CD4, and/or CD7), most frequently with a dual B/T phenotype {1380,1433,1437,1586, 2010}. A similar observation has been made in PAL cell lines {36,433}. Thus, in some PALs, because of a markedly aberrant phenotype – i.e., null-cell phenotype or expression of some T-cell markers – it is difficult to assign a lineage.
Based on CD20 negativity and expression of T-cell antigens, rare cases of

pyothorax-associated T-cell lymphoma have even been reported. However, one of these cases, investigated for genotypic studies, was demonstrated to contain a B-cell clone without clonal rearrangement of the T-cell receptor genes, thus indicating that such cases correspond to B-cell lymphomas with aberrant T-cell phenotype {2010}. Although the reason for such an aberrant phenotype in PAL is unknown, it is noteworthy that it has also been described in B-cell lines infected by EBV as well as in some EBV transformed B-cell lymphomas arising in immunosuppressed patients, and it has been suggested that EBV might promote this dual phenotype.
Recently, it has been shown that lymphoma cells in PAL express a uniform CD10-, BCL-6-, MUM1/IRF-4+ phenotype, in agreement with derivation from a late germinal centre/post-germinal centre B-cell {1586}.
Lymphoma cells are positive by immunohistochemistry for EBV in most cases, showing an EBNA-2+/LMP-1-/+ phenotype consistent with a type III latency. EBNA-2 is usually highly expressed in the nuclei of most tumour cells, whereas LMP-1 is found in a few neoplastic cells {1339,1586}. Demonstration of EBV is very useful in establishing a diagnosis.

Genetic features

Immunoglobulin genes are rearranged and are mutated {1333}. No characteristic chromosomal alterations have been identified. A high frequency of p53 mutations and of c-myc amplifications have been described {867,2191}. As seen above, EBV genomes are detected in virtually all cases by in situ hybridization with EBERs probes and lymphoma cells also express EBNA-2 and LMP-I viral proteins. By Southern blot, they carry monoclonal EBV genome {433,631} and chromosomal integration of EBV has been recently demonstrated in one cell line {433}. A small percentage of PAL are reported to be EBV-negative. However, EBV genomes have been found by using sensitive PCR techniques in at least a few cases that were scored as EBV-negative on the results of in situ hybridization and immunohistochemical studies {1503, 1586}. In contrast to PEL, HHV8 sequences and expression of HHV8 /ORF73 antigens are absent in PAL {1496,1586}.

Postulated normal counterpart

EBV-transformed late germinal centre/ post-germinal centre B-cell.

Prognostic features

Most series report a very poor prognosis with a median survival of less than one year. However, in a recent series, more than half of the patients showed a responsiveness to chemotherapy and/or radiotherapy and the patients who achieved complete remission after therapy had a 50% 5-year survival rate {1437}.

Mesenchymal tumours

W.D. Travis   H. Tazelaar
A. Churg   R. Pugatch
M.C. Aubry   T. Manabe
N.G. Ordonez   M. Miettinen

Epithelioid haemangio-endothelioma / angiosarcoma

Definition
Pleural epithelioid haemangioendothelioma (PEH) is a low to intermediate grade vascular tumour composed of short cords and nests of epithelioid endothelial cells embedded in a myxohyaline matrix. The tumours are distinctive for their epithelioid character, sharply defined cytoplasmic vacuoles, intraalveolar and intravascular growth and central hyaline necrosis. High-grade epithelioid vascular tumours are called epithelioid angiosarcomas.

ICD-O code
Epithelioid haemangioendothelioma
                              9133/1
Angiosarcoma   9120/3

Epidemiology
Most patients with PEH are Caucasian, 65-85% are men and the mean age is 52 years with a range of 34-85 years {424, 435,533,1184,2120}.

Clinical features
Patients usually present with diffuse pleural thickening, pleural effusion, and/or pleuritic chest pain. Some patients have both pulmonary as well as pleural involvement. {424,1184,510,536,1184, 1227,1453}.

Imaging
CT scans or chest x-rays characteristically demonstrate pleural thickening and pleural effusions may represent the primary manifestation {424,1184}, sometimes accompanied by pulmonary nodules.

Macroscopy and localization
Epithelioid haemangioendotheliomas may involve the pleura diffusely and mimic the gross appearance of diffuse malignant mesothelioma {424,1184, 2222,2239}.

Histopathology
The tumours often show a biphasic pattern with nests of epithelioid cells within a spindle cell stroma. The stroma is usually reactive, but may be neoplastic. It often shows a myxoid or chondroid appearance. A tubulopapillary pattern may be seen in about one third of cases. The epithelioid tumour cells show large round to oval nuclei with a vesicular chromatin pattern. Epithelioid angiosarcomas are high grade and typically show large nucleoli more frequent mitoses than the low to intermediate grade epithelioid haemangioendotheliomas. Intracytoplasmic vacuoles are common.

Immunohistochemistry
Most tumours stain with one or more endothelial markers including CD31, CD34, Fli1, and factor VIII (von Willebrand factor) {599,828,1184}. Cytokeratin is expressed in up to 50% of cases, causing some difficulty in differentiating it from carcinoma {424,1184, 1308}. However, the staining is usually weak to moderate and weaker than vimentin staining {424,1184}.

Electron microscopy
Electron microscopy reveals abundant intermediate filaments, micropinocytosis and Weibel- Palade bodies. An interrupted basal lamina surrounding the tumour cells is present and cytoplasmic lumina may be seen {1184}.

Differential diagnosis
The differential diagnosis includes chronic fibrous pleuritis, malignant mesothelioma, metastatic carcinoma and melanoma. Key to recognition of this tumour in the pleura is awareness of its morphologic and immunohistochemical characteristics, particularly that it may show a biphasic and papillary appearance. If keratin staining in an epithelioid tumour in the pleura is weak or negative, an epithelioid vascular tumour should be considered and immunohistochemistry for vascular markers should be performed.

Histogenesis
Epithelioid haemangioendotheliomas are derived from endothelial cells.

Prognostic factors
Epithelioid vascular tumours that present in the pleura have an aggressive clinical course. There is no known effective therapy for these patients.

Synovial sarcoma (SS)

Definition
Synovial sarcoma (SS) is a biphasic mesenchymal neoplasm with epithelial and spindle-cell components, or a monophasic tumour which consists purely of a spindle cell component. Both biphasic and monophasic types can occur in the pleura and they can be easily confused with malignant mesothelioma or pulmonary sarcomatoid carcinoma.

ICD-O codes
Synovial sarcoma   9040/3
Synovial sarcoma, spindle cell
                              9041/3
Synovial sarcoma, biphasic
                              9043/3

Synonyms
Synovial cell sarcoma, malignant synovioma, synovioblastic sarcoma

Etiology
There are no known etiological factors.

Clinical features
Patients with biphasic tumors may present at a younger age (mean 25 years, range 9-50 years) {644} than those with monophasic tumours (mean of 47 years (range 33-69 years) {89}. SS shows no gender predilection {89,644,1463}. chest pain is the most common presenting manifestation but pleural effusions, dyspnea, dysphagia or pneumothorax can occur {89,644}. Pleural SS can be aggressive with almost half of patients dead of disease (with a mean of 18 months).

Macroscopy and localisation
Pleural SS are usually localized, solid tumours, but they can present with diffuse pleural thickening like mesothelioma

{89,394,644,1463}. Some tumors have a pseudocapsule, causing them to be well demarcated from the surrounding tissues. The tumors may grow on a pedicle. They are usually large tumours with a mean size of 13 cm (range 4-21 cm). Cut surface of the tumour can show cystic degenerative changes and necrosis.

Tumour spread and staging
Pleural SS typically recurs within the pleural cavity and may invade the involving chest wall as well as adjacent structures including the pericardium, and diaphragm.

Histopathology
Histologic features of pleural SS are exactly the same as for those described in the lung (see lung chapter). While the monophasic type is most common within the lung, a high percentage of pleural tumors are biphasic {89,394,644,1463}. Mucin can be demonstrated in some biphasic tumors.

Immunohistochemistry of pleural SS typically shows focal positive staining for keratin and/or EMA with positive bcl-2, CD99 and vimentin. The glandular component of biphasic tumors may express BER-EP4 and CEA. Calretinin and S-100 may be focally positive, but desmin, smooth muscle actin and CD34 are usually negative.

Differential diagnosis
In the pleura, the most important differential diagnosis is malignant mesothe-

lioma, followed by sarcomatoid carcinoma, solitary fibrous tumour and metastatic synovial sarcoma {89,394,644,1463}. Compared to mesothelioma, pleural SS occur more often in younger patients, they are more likely to be localized, and tend to grow more rapidly. A pseudocapsule may be present in pleural SS, but this is typically absent in mesothelioma {644}. The spindle cells of SS tend to grow in long interweaving fascicles while in mesothelioma the cells grow in blunt short fascicles. Haemangioperi-cytomatous growth and hyaline fibrosis are common in SS and uncommon in mesothelioma. The presence of mucin in glands and expression of CEA and/or BER-EP4 favors biphasic SS, although BER-EP4 can be seen in some series in a high percentage of mesotheliomas up to 20% of mesotheliomas. Demonstration of the X:18 translocation is very helpful in confirming the diagnosis of SS.

Histogenesis
Remains unknown. It is thought to be a totipotential mesenchymal cell and it has not been proven to arise or differentiate from synovium.

Somatic genetics
Synovial sarcoma has the distinctive translocation t (X; 18)(p11; q11) that is not seen in the other tumors mentioned above in the differential diagnosis, most importantly mesothelioma and sarcomatoid carcinoma {89,694,850,957,1310, 1992}. Fortunately this can readily be

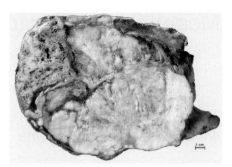
Fig. 2.19 Malignant fibrous tumour of the pleura.

demonstrated in formalin-fixed paraffin-embedded tissue. Other details about this translocation are summarized in the lung chapter.

Solitary fibrous tumour (SFT)
Definition
An uncommon spindle-cell mesenchymal tumour of probable fibroblastic derivation that often presents a prominent haemangiopericytoma-like vascular pattern, but may exhibit other histologic patterns. A morphologically identical tumour occurs in numerous other extrathoracic sites.

ICD-O code   8815/0

Synonyms
Also known as localized fibrous tumour, this lesion was once variously designated benign mesothelioma, localized fibrous mesothelioma, and submesothelial fibroma. The use of names that include 'mesothelioma' for this tumour is discouraged because of potential confusion with diffuse malignant mesothelioma.

Etiology
No etiologic agent has been identified; in particular there is no link with asbestos exposure.

Clinical features
Signs and symptoms
The most common symptoms at presentation are cough, chest pain, and dyspnoea. Some patients may present with hypertrophic osteoarthropathy and, on rare occasions, symptomatic hypoglycemia as a result of the production of an insulin-like growth factor {629}. Some tumours are incidental findings.

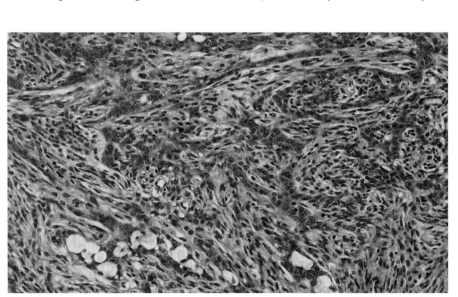
Fig. 2.20 Pleural synovial sarcoma. This biphasic tumour consists of glandular and spindle cells.

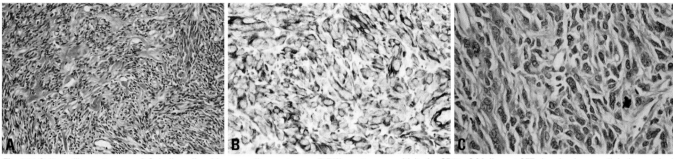

Fig. 2.21 Solitary fibrous tumour. **A** Spindle cells with ropy collagen stroma. **B** Diffuse strong positivity for CD34. **C** Malignant SFT showing hypercellularity, marked cellular atypia and high mitotic activity.

Imaging

Solitary fibrous tumours of the pleura present on chest radiographs as pleural-based soft tissue masses. The margins are well defined and there is no associated rib destruction or chest wall abnormality. A pleural effusion may be present. Tumours can vary in size from small lesions to very large masses that occupy most of the hemithorax. When large, they require CT or MR scanning to differentiate them from lung masses. The margin at which the lesion meets the chest wall is smooth. On CT scanning, they show a pattern of heterogeneous contrast enhancement and compress but do not invade the contiguous lung. Rarely, their attachment to the chest wall by a pedicle can be seen.

Macroscopy

Most tumours arise in the visceral pleura, but they may also originate in the lung parenchyma and mediastinum. They are well circumscribed and often pedunculated {544}. Rarely they may be multiple. The cut surface is usually firm and whitish, often with a whorled appearance. Myxoid change, haemorrhage, and necrosis may occasionally be seen and suggest that the tumour is malignant; large size also suggests malignancy. These features mandate extensive sampling.

Histopathology

SFT typically exhibits a patternless architecture characterized by the coexistence of hypo- and hypercellular areas separated by fibrous stroma having haemangiopericytoma-like branching blood vessels. The hypercellular areas are composed of bland spindle cells arranged in short intersecting fascicles, creating herringbone or storiform arrays. The hypocellular areas may be highly collagenized or, less frequently, present myxoid changes. Malignant SFTs (ICD-O 8815/3) are characterized by greater cellularity with an infiltrative growth pattern, moderate to marked cellular atypia and high mitotic activity (> 4 mitoses per 10 high-power fields) {544}.

Immunohistochemical studies are helpful in confirming the diagnosis of SFT. In contrast with sarcomatoid mesothelioma, these lesions tend to be positive for CD34, and bcl-2, and are always negative for cytokeratin {1519}. However, malignant SFT may not always express CD34 and bcl-2. The differential diagnosis of SFT in the pleura includes sarcomatoid mesothelioma, and a variety of benign and malignant soft tissue tumours, such as haemangiopericytoma, malignant fibrous histiocytoma, monophasic synovial sarcoma, thymoma, and peripheral nerve sheath tumours.

Somatic genetics

Only a few studies have reported cytogenetic findings in SFT. Reported abnormalities include: t(4;15)(q13;q26){436}; 46,XY,t(6;17) (p11.2;q23), ins (9;12) (q22;q15q24.1), inv (16) (p13.1q24) {508}. In the latter case the rearrangement of 12q13-15 is similar to that described in a subset of haemangiopericytomas of soft tissue and meninges {508}.

In one malignant SFT of the pleura successful karyotyping was obtained from the primary and recurrent tumours. The initial karyotype showed two abnormal clones: 48, XY; +8; +8; del(9)(q22; q32) [19] and 46, XY, t(1;16)(q25;p12) [7]. Culture of the recurrent tumour yielded one clone identical to the dominant clone of the initial karyotype {447}.

Comparative genomic hybridisation (CGH) of 12 SFT of pleura showed no chromosomal imbalances in 58 percent of cases. Losses on chromosome arms 13q (33%), 4q and 21q (17% each) were the most frequent abnormality. Significant gains were seen at chromosome 8 and at 15q in two cases each. There was no correlation between tumour size and molecular pathology findings {1073}. Another CGH study of one SFT revealed losses of 1p33—>pter, 17pter q21, entire copies of chromosomes 19 and 22, and gains of 1p21-p22, 2q23-q32.3, 3pl2-q13.2, 4p14-q28, 6p12-q21, 9p21—>pter and 13q21-q31. Further-more, there was loss of 20q, as was previously reported elsewhere in a case of benign and a case of malignant SFT {48}.

Calcifying tumour of the pleura

Definition

A rare slow growing plaque-like lesion occurring in the visceral pleura, composed of nearly acellular fibrous tissue, and associated with extensive dystrophic calcification (which may be psammomatous).

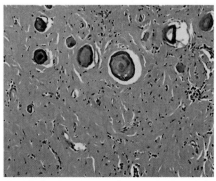

Fig. 2.22 Calcifying tumour. Psammoma-like calcifications within a dense fibrous stroma. From {2024}.

Synonyms and historical annotation

Calcifying fibrous pseudotumour, childhood fibrous tumour with psammoma bodies

Clinical features

Signs and symptoms

Rare examples of calcifying tumour of the pleura (CTP) are reported in the pleura {1599}, or mediastinum {929}, but these tumours more often occur in the soft tissues of the extremities, trunk, scrotum, groin, neck, or axilla {575}. Most cases occur in children and young adults with no sex predilection. Patients may present with chest pain or they may be asymptomatic.

Imaging

Chest radiographs or CT scans show a single pleural mass or multiple pleural-based nodular masses with central areas of increased attenuation due to calcification, which may be extensive.

Macroscopy and histopathology

The lesions consist of circumscribed, but unencapsulated masses of hyalinized collagenous fibrotic tissue interspersed with lymphoplasmacytic infiltrates and calcifications, often with psammomatous features The lesions are limited to the pleura and typically do not involve the underlying lung parenchyma. Multiple lesions may be seen {758}. The fibrous cells may be positive for vimentin and Factor XIIIa and CD68 {830}, but negative for actin, desmin, S100 protein, CD31, and usually, CD34 {2128}.

Differential diagnosis

The differential diagnosis includes other pleural lesions such as solitary fibrous tumour of pleura, calcified granulomas, calcified pleural plaques, and chronic fibrous pleuritis as well as intrapulmonary lesions such as hyalinizing granuloma, inflammatory pseudotumour, and amyloid.

Prognosis and predictive factors

As in the soft tissues, local excision appears adequate therapy for CFT of the pleura. If these lesions behave in a similar fashion to CFT of soft tissues, one might expect a low frequency of local recurrence.

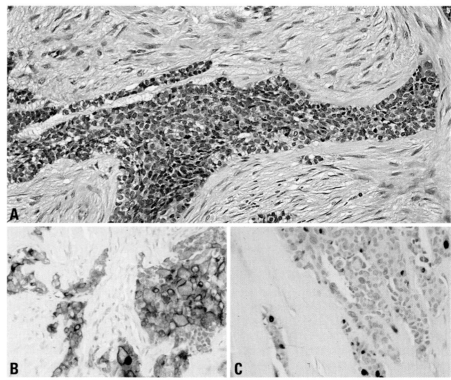

Fig. 2.23 Desmoplastic round cell tumour. **A** Cellular round cell component within a dense fibrous stroma From {2024}. The tumour cells stain positively for **B** keratin and, for **C** desmin with a dot-like pattern.

Desmoplastic small round cell tumour of the pleura

Definition

DRCT is a primitive polyphenotypic neoplasm typically occurring on the serous surfaces in the abdominal cavity and rarely in the pleura of young adult males. It possibly represents a primitive mesothelial-related lesion.

ICD-O code   8806/3

Clinical features

The reported six cases involving pleura {164,1524,1551,1739,1936} occurred in 4 men and 2 women aged 17-29 years (median age 23 years) and usually presented with chest pain and pleural effusion. Although this pleural tumour usually is fatal within 2 years, one patient lived over 5 years {1524}. DRCT can also present with an intrapulmonary mass {1936}.

Histopathology

Grossly the tumour typically forms multiple pleural-based nodular masses and can produce pulmonary encasement resembling that of malignant mesothelioma. Mediastinal involvement is typical of pleural-based tumours; bilateral pleural involvement and pulmonary parenchymal metastases may also occur. Histologically the tumour is composed of irregularly shaped islands or larger sheets of small round tumour cells in cellular desmoplastic stroma. Focal nuclear atypia can occur in the tumour cells, and the stroma may contain vascular proliferation.

Immunohistochemical profile

The typical features include expression of keratins, EMA, desmin (often in a perinuclear dot-like pattern), vimentin and Wilms tumour protein WT1 {677}. Since translocation splits the latter gene, antibodies to WT1 should be used that recognize the preserved carboxyterminus of the protein. NSE-positivity and expression of CD15 are also common.

Genetics

The presence of WT1-EWS gene fusion with the t(11;22) translocation are the key diagnostic features of this tumour {677}.

CHAPTER 3

Tumours of the Thymus

Tumours of the thymus account for less than 1% of all neoplasms and, therefore, do not contribute significantly to the
overall human cancer burden. However, their etiology is largely
unknown and the biology is complex. Thymomas often manifest clinically by causing autoimmune diseases, in particular
myasthenia gravis.

The histological typing of tumours of the thymus remains a
challenge for surgical pathologists. The Working Group
responsible for this volume largely followed the previous WHO
classification published in 1999. Some recently recognized
entities have been added, together with updated diagnostic
criteria.

WHO histological classification of tumours of the thymus

Epithelial tumours

Thymoma[1,2]	8580/1
Type A (spindle cell; medullary)	8581/1
Type AB (mixed)	8582/1
Type B1 (lymphocyte-rich; lymphocytic; predominantly cortical; organoid)	8583/1
Type B2 (cortical)	8584/1
Type B3 (epithelial; atypical; squamoid; well-differentiated thymic carcinoma)	8585/1
Micronodular thymoma	8580/1
Metaplastic thymoma	8580/1
Microscopic thymoma	8580/1
Sclerosing thymoma	8580/1
Lipofibroadenoma	

Thymic carcinoma (including neuroendocrine epithelial tumours of the thymus)	8586/3
Squamous cell carcinoma	8070/3
Basaloid carcinoma	8123/3
Mucoepidermoid carcinoma	8430/3
Lymphoepithelioma-like carcinoma	8082/3
Sarcomatoid carcinoma (carcinosarcoma)	8033/3
Clear cell carcinoma	8310/3
Adenocarcinoma	8140/3
Papillary adenocarcinoma	8260/3
Carcinoma with t(15;19) translocation	
Well-differentiated neuroendocrine carcinomas (carcinoid tumours)	
Typical carcinoid	8240/3
Atypical carcinoid	8249/3
Poorly differentiated neuroendocrine carcinomas	
Large cell neuroendocrine carcinoma	8013/3
Small cell carcinoma, neuroendocrine type	8041/3
Undifferentiated carcinoma	8020/3
Combined thymic epithelial tumours, including neuroendocrine carcinomas	

Germ cell tumours (GCT) of the mediastinum

GCTs of one histological type (pure GCTs)

Seminoma	9061/3
Embryonal carcinoma	9070/3
Yolk sac tumour	9071/3
Choriocarcinoma	9100/3
Teratoma, mature	9080/0
Teratoma, immature	9080/3

GCTs of more than one histological type (mixed GCT)	
Variant: Polyembryoma	9072/3
GCTs with somatic-type malignancy	
GCTs with associated haematologic malignancy	

Mediastinal lymphomas and haematopoietic neoplasms	
B-cell lymphoma	
Primary mediastinal large B-cell lymphoma	9679/3
Thymic extranodal marginal zone B-cell lymphoma of mucosa-associated lymphoid tissue (MALT)	9699/3
T-cell lymphoma	
Precursor T-lymphoblastic lymphoma	9729/3
Precursor T-lymphoblastic leukaemia	9837/3
[Precursor T-cell acute lymphoblastic leukaemia (ALL)/Precursor T-cell lymphoblastic lymphoma (LBL)]	
Anaplastic large cell lymphoma and other rare mature T- and NK-cell lymphomas of the mediastinum	9714/3
Hodgkin lymphoma of the mediastinum	9650/3
"Grey zone " between Hodgkin and Non-Hodgkin lymphoma	9596/3
Histiocytic and dendritic cell tumours	
Langerhans cell histiocytosis	9751/1
Langerhans cell sarcoma	9756/3
Histiocytic sarcoma	9755/3
Malignant histiocytosis	9750/3
Follicular dendritic cell tumour	9758/1
Follicular dendritic cell sarcoma	9758/3
Interdigitating dendritic cell tumour	9757/1
Interdigitating dendritic cell sarcoma	9757/3
Myeloid sarcoma and extramedullary acute myeloid leukaemia	9930/3

Mesenchymal tumours of the thymus and mediastinum	
Thymolipoma	8850/0
Lipoma of the mediastinum	8850/0
Liposarcoma of the mediastinum	8850/0
Solitary fibrous tumour	8815/0
Synovial sarcoma	9040/3
Vascular neoplasms	
Rhabdomyosarcoma	8900/3
Leiomyomatous tumours	
Tumours of peripheral nerves	

Rare tumours of the mediastinum

Ectopic tumours of the thymus

    Ectopic thyroid tumours

    Ectopic parathyroid tumours

Metastasis to thymus and anterior mediastinum

---

[1] Morphology code of the International Classification of Diseases for Oncology (ICD-O) {6} and the Systematized Nomenclature of Medicine (http://snomed.org). Behaviour is coded /0 for benign tumours, /3 for malignant tumours, and /1 for borderline or uncertain behaviour.
[2] For thymus, designated as malignant; change from /1 to /3

TNM classification of malignant thymic epithelial tumours

TNM classification [1,2,3]

T – Primary Tumour

TX	Primary tumour cannot be assessed
T0	No evidence of primary tumour
T1	Tumour completely encapsulated
T2	Tumour invades pericapsular connective tissue
T3	Tumour invades into neighbouring structures, such as pericardium, mediastinal pleura, thoracic wall, great vessels and lung
T4	Tumour with pleural or pericardial dissemination

N – Regional Lymph Nodes

NX	Regional lymph nodes cannot be assessed
N0	No regional lymph node metastasis
N1	Metastasis in anterior mediastinal lymph nodes
N2	Metastasis in other intrathoracic lymph nodes excluding anterior mediastinal lymph nodes
N3	Metastasis in scalene and/or supraclavicular lymph nodes

M – Distant Metastasis

MX	Distant metastasis cannot be assessed
M0	No distant metastasis
M1	Distant metastasis

Stage Grouping

Stage			
Stage I	T1	N0	M0
Stage II	T2	N0	M0
Stage III	T1	N1	M0
	T2	N1	M0
	T3	N0, 1	M0
Stage IV	T4	Any N	M0
	Any T	N2, 3	M0
	Any T	Any N	M1

---
[1] {899}
[2] A help desk for specific questions about the TNM classification is available at http://www.uicc.org
[3] This is not an official UICC TNM Classification.

TNM classification of thymic germ cell tumours

TNM classification [1,2,3]

T – Primary Tumour

TX	Primary tumour cannot be assessed
T0	No evidence of primary tumour
T1	Tumour confined to the organ of origin (thymus and mediastinal fat)
T1a	Tumour ≤ 5 cm
T1b	Tumour > 5 cm
T2	Tumour infiltrating contiguous organs or accompanied by malignant effusion
T2a	Tumour ≤ 5 cm
T2b	Tumour > 5 cm
T3	Tumour invades into neighbouring structures, such as pericardium, mediastinal pleura, thoracic wall, great vessels and lung
T4	Tumour with pleural or pericardial dissemination

N – Regional lymph nodes

NX	Regional lymph nodes cannot be assessed
N0	No regional lymph node metastasis
N1	Metastasis to regional lymph node present
N2	Metastasis in other intrathoracic lymph nodes excluding anterior mediastinal lymph nodes
N3	Metastasis in scalene and/or supraclavicular lymph nodes

M – Distant Metastasis

MX	Distant metastasis cannot be assessed
M0	No distant metastasis
M1	Distant metastasis present

Stage Grouping of the Pediatric Study Group [1,3]

Stage I	Locoregional tumour, non-metastatic, complete resection
Stage II	Locoregional tumour, non-metastatic, macroscopic complete resection but microscopic residual tumour
Stage III	Locoregional tumour, regional lymph nodes negative or positive; no distant metastasis; biopsy only or gross residual tumour after primary resection
Stage IV	Tumour with distant metastasis

---
[1] {167}
[2] A help desk for specific questions about the TNM classification is is available at http://www.uicc.org/tnm
[3] This is not an official UICC TNM Classification.

Tumours of the thymus: Introduction

H.K. Müller-Hermelink
P. Engel
T.T. Kuo
Ph. Ströbel
A. Marx
N.L. Harris

P. Möller
F. Menestrina
Y. Shimosato
H. Asamura
A. Masaoka
L.H. Sobin

Tumours of the thymus comprise neoplasms assumed to arise from or differentiate towards thymic cellular constituents, including thymic epithelial tumours (thymomas, thymic carcinomas, neuroendocrine tumours), germ cell tumours, lymphoid and haematopoietic neoplasms and mesenchymal tumours.

Histogenesis and differentiation

Thymoma. It has long been assumed that thymic epithelial cells originate from both the ectodermal and endodermal germ cell layers. However, a growing body of evidence suggests that the diverse thymic epithelial populations all develop from a common thymic epithelial stem cell of endodermal origin {181, 684}. This concept does not exclude the occurrence of more differentiated "committed stem cells" with medullary, cortical or other phenotypes {1671}. Tumours that we know as thymomas derive from thymic epithelium. In spite of morphological and immunological evidence for tumour differentiation towards a medullary or cortical epithelial phenotype, available data do not allow to unequivocally assign thymic tumours to defined functional and anatomical compartments of the normal thymus {1691}.

Neuroendocrine thymic tumours. Both a neural crest and thymic epithelial cell derivation have been considered {316, 471,1139,2116,2137}. The latter hypothesis is supported by combined (mixed) thymoma-neuroendocrine tumours and the occurrence of either thymomas or thymic neuroendocrine tumours in MEN1 syndrome patients {461,1535,1687, 2094}.

Lymphomas. The thymus is the site of the earliest stages of T-cell and natural killer (NK)-cell development. Precursors of dendritic cells, mature dendritic cells, and small numbers of B cells are also found in the normal thymus. Among thymic haematopoietic neoplasias, there is good evidence that T-lymphoblastic lymphomas arise from lymphoid progenitors, while mediastinal large B-cell lymphomas are of putative thymic B-cell ori-

gin. In addition, some histiocytic and myeloid neoplasias are of teratomatous derivation. By contrast, the origins of thymic MALT, NK-cell and Hodgkin lymphomas are less clear. The same holds true for many mesenchymal tumours.

Epidemiology

Tumours of the thymus are among the rarest human neoplasms, comprising <1% of all adult cancers, with an incidence rate of 1–5 / million population / year. Thymomas are the most frequent thymic tumours in adults, followed by mediastinal lymphomas, some of which

arise from mediastinal lymph nodes. In children, the mediastinum is the site of 1% of all tumours; most common are non-Hodgkin lymphomas, while thymomas are extremely rare.

Etiology

The etiology of thymic tumours is largely unknown. Some epidemiologic clustering of thymomas and neuroendocrine tumours has been observed among patients with multiple endocrine neoplasia (MEN1) syndrome {461,1687}. Epstein-Barr virus (EBV) infection may play a role in a minority of thymic carci-

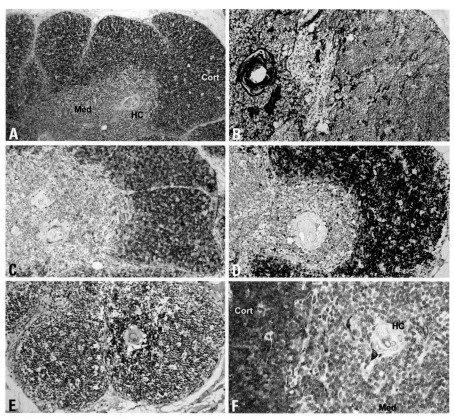

Fig. 3.01 Normal thymus. **A** Normal thymus in a child. Well developed cortical areas (Cort), thymic medulla (Med) and Hassall´s corpuscles (HC). The thymic cortex is divided by septa into lobules. The septa extend to the corticomedullary junction and harbour vessels. The space between these vessels and the subcapsular epithelial cells that delineate thymic lobules is called "perivascular space". **B** Identification of thymic epithelial cells by the pan-cytokeratin antibody KL1. **C** Identification of immature CD1a positive T-cells. **D** High Ki67 index in the cortex but not medulla. **E** The CD20+ B-cell compartment is largely confined to the thymic medulla. B-cells surround Hassall´s corpuscles. **F** Myoid cells as revealed by anti-desmin staining (brown) in the thymic medulla (Med), one of them directly adjacent to a Hassall´s corpuscle (HC).

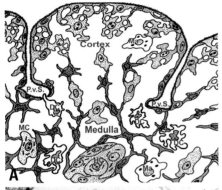

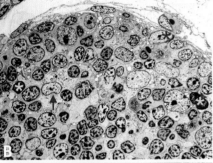

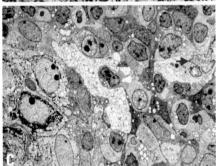

Fig. 3.02 A Cartoon of the non-lymphoid cellular components of the normal thymic cortex and medulla, including Hassall's corpuscle (HC). Various thymic epithelial cells, dendritic cells (DC), macrophages (MA), and myoid cells (MC). Subcapsular and medullary epithelial cells delineate septa and perivascular spaces (PvS) at the corticomedullary junction. **B** Electron micrograph showing cortical and subcortical thymic epithelial cells (TEC), apoptotic bodies, and macrophages. **C** Electron micrograph of thymic medulla, depicting a medullary epithelial cell —, a dendritic cell → and a Hassall's corpuscle (HC).

nomas, as well as some Hodgkin, rare non-Hodgkin and NK/T-cell lymphomas.

Clinical features

Patients may exhibit symptoms due to local complications (pain, superior vena cava syndrome, respiratory insufficiency or tachycardia because of pleural or pericardial implants and effusions), as well as systemic symptoms (fever or weight loss).

In addition, thymomas can cause a large variety of autoimmune diseases (Table 3.01) which are often typical for a specific tumour type and may precede or follow thymoma resection {987}. Type A, AB and B thymomas exhibit an unrivaled frequency and spectrum of autoimmune phenomena, comprising neuromuscular, haematopoietic, dermatologic, rheumatic/vasculitic, hepatic and renal diseases. Myasthenia gravis is by far the most frequent and preferentially associated with type AB and B2, B3 thymomas, while hypogammaglobulinaemia (Good syndrome) is more typical for type A thymoma. Pure red cell aplasia is also a rare complication of type A thymomas, though recent data find a less specific association with this thymoma subtype {1096}. Thymic carcinomas are not associated with myasthenia gravis or hypogammaglobulinaemia, but occasionally with other autoimmune diseases. Cytopenias and/or hypogammaglobulinaemia can result in serious bacterial and opportunistic infections. Lymphocytosis and thrombocytosis can occur. Whether the increased incidence of second cancers in thymoma patients is related to genetic or environmental etiologies or thymoma-induced immunodeficiency is unknown {1395,1537}.

Table 3.01
Autoimmune diseases associated with thymomas. Rare manifestations are indicated by an asterisk.

Neuromuscular Diseases
Myasthenia gravis
Neuromyotonia*, rippling muscle disease*, polymyositis/dermatomyositis*
Encephalitis* (limbic, cortical, and brainstem)
Intestinal pseudoobstruction*
Haematologic Autoimmune Diseases
Anaemia: pure red cell aplasia (in all thymoma subtypes) {168} pernicious anaemia, haemolytic anaemia, aplastic anaemia
Other isolated cytopenias, eg eosinophils, basophils, neutrophils
Immunodeficiencies: Hypogammaglobulinaemia +/- T-cell deficiencies (Good syndrome)
Dermatologic Diseases*
Pemphigus (foliaceus, paraneoplastic) Lichen planus
Alopecia areata
Endocrine Disorders
Addison disease, Cushing disease Graves disease
Renal and Hepatic Diseases
Glomerulonephritis, autoimmune hepatitis
Systemic Autoimmune Diseases*
SLE, Sjögren disease, systemic sclerosis Graft-versus-Host-Disease

Histopathological classification

Thymomas

Histological classification schemes for thymomas traditionally have been descriptive (predominantly spindle, predominantly lymphocytic, predominantly epithelial, mixed lymphoepithelial) {158, 1086,1134,1172,1732}, or were based on the combined consideration of morphology (spindle, polygonal, mixed tumour cells) and lymphocyte content {1086, 1808}. Except for the spindle cell type, these classifications largely lacked prognostic significance independent of stage {1172,1253,1808}.

The histogenetic or functional classification included terms (medullary, cortical) that reflected the normal differentiation of the major functional and anatomic com-

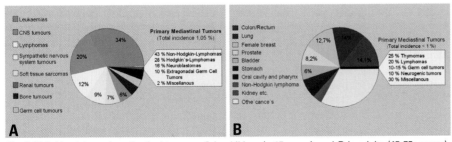

Fig. 3.03 Epidemiology of mediastinal tumours **A** in children (< 15 years), and **B** in adults (45-75+ years). Thymomas are exceedingly rare in children, while they are the most common mediastinal tumours in adults.

Table 3.02

Comparison of Masaoka tumour stages and corresponding TNM classification. Modified, from K. Koga et al. {1043}.

Masaoka stage	T	N	M
I	1	0	0
II	2	0	0
III	3	0	0
IVa	T4	0	0
IVb	any T	≥ N1 or ≥ M1	

partments of the thymus {1245,1404}. This classification proved to be of independent prognostic value {341,856, 1017,1540,1630} and was highly reproducible {378}. However, although some morphological and immunological studies have supported the histogenetic concept {235,859,1015,1086,1452,1510, 1886}, it has not been generally accepted {1058,1691,1917}.

In 1999, a WHO Working group suggested a non-committal terminology, preserving the distinct categories of the histogenetic classification, but using letters and numbers to designate tumour entities {1690}. The rationale for the concept to label thymomas as type A, AB, and B is derived from a growing body of morphological, functional and genetic evidence {235,859,896,1510,1631,2242}, suggesting that these thymoma subgroups form distinct entities both in morphological and clinical terms.

In recent years, this WHO classification {1690} has been well accepted and is largely retained in the current WHO classification as it provides an easy comparison of clinical, pathological and immunological studies {235,318,1196, 1511,1744,1886}.

Thymomas of type A, AB, and B exhibit organotypic (thymus-like) architectural features. These tumours have not been observed in organs other than the thymus, though they may arise from heterotopic thymic tissue in the head and neck region, anywhere in the mediastinum, pleura and lung {1691}. By contrast, the heterogeneous thymic carcinomas (called type C thymomas in the previous WHO classification) exhibit morphologies that are encountered also in organs other than the thymus.

Thymic carcinomas comprise malignant, usually invasive epithelial tumours with clear-cut atypia, largely absent organotypic features and a very diverse differ-

entiation, resembling carcinomas outside the thymus. This category includes neuroendocrine epithelial tumours.

Germ cell, lymphoid, haematopoietic and mesenchymal tumours
The classification of these tumours follows the WHO Classification of gonadal germ cell tumours {526}, tumours of haematopoietic and lymphoid tissues {919} and tumours of soft tissues and bone {590}.

Useful morphological terms
Encapsulated.
A thymoma completely surrounded by a fibrous capsule of varying thickness which is not infiltrated by tumour growth. Thymic tumours that infiltrate into, but not through, the capsule still belong in this category.

Minimally invasive.
A thymoma surrounded by a capsule which is focally infiltrated by tumour growth with invasion of the mediastinal fat. The capsular invasion needs to be complete in order for the tumour to be placed in this category. Minimally invasive thymomas are usually identifiable as such only after microscopic examination in so far as they generally appear to the surgeon indistinguishable from encapsulated thymomas at the time of excision.

Widely invasive.
A thymoma spreading by direct extension into adjacent structures such as pericardium, large vessels or lung. This type of thymoma usually appears invasive to the surgeon at the time of excision, which may be incomplete as a result.

Implants.
A thymoma in which tumour nodules separate from the main mass are found on the pericardial or pleural surface. These implants tend to be small and multiple and their microscopic appearance is usually, but not always, similar to that of the parent tumour.

Lymph node metastases.
A thymoma that involves one or more lymph nodes anatomically separate from the main mass. This excludes direct extension into the node by the tumour. The nodes most commonly involved by metastatic thymoma are mediastinal and supraclavicular. It is a rare event even in

long-standing cases. but may exceptionally be the first clinical manifestation of the tumour.

With distant metastases.
A thymoma with metastases to distant site(s), most commonly lung, liver, and skeletal system. This excludes metastases to lymph nodes and local extension into adjacent organs.

Grading of malignancy
Thymic epithelial tumours consist of several histological subtypes, i.e., thymoma types A, AB, B1, B2 and B3, and thymic carcinomas, in increasing order of malignancy {1691} Thymoma type A and AB generally behave like a benign tumour, type B1 as a low-grade malignant tumour (10-year survival rates of over 90%), type B2 has a greater degree of malignancy, and type B3 in the advanced stage shows a poor prognosis, just like thymic carcinoma and malignant tumours of other organs {1511}. Among the various subtypes of thymic carcinoma, squamous cell carcinoma, basaloid and mucoepidermoid carcinoma have a better prognosis than other histological subtypes. The malignancy grade of thymic neuroendocrine tumours (carcinoids) is intermediate between thymoma and thymic carcinoma. The rare small cell and large cell carcinomas tend to be highly malignant.

TNM Classification and stage grouping
The TNM Classification and stage-grouping has been applied to malignant tumours of many organs {2045}, but there is currently no authorized TNM system for thymic epithelial and neuroendocrine tumours. In the TNM Supplement 2nd edition {899}, a tentative classification of malignant thymomas appeared for testing. It is mainly based on the Masaoka system and its revised versions {1255,2036,2184}. While the tentative classification applies only to malignant thymic epithelial tumours {899}, it has in this chapter been extended to include neuroendocrine tumours.

Invasion
Crucial points in defining the T-categories are invasion through the capsule and invasion into neighbouring structures. Although invasive growth outside the thymus detected by the surgeon at

the time of thoracotomy has been repeatedly reported to have significant impact on the prognosis {693,1043}, the prognostic significance of minor degrees of invasion detected by histological examination remains controversial. Many reports on thymoma have shown little or no difference in survival between Masaoka stage I and stage II thymomas {693,1043,1130,1511,1579,1645}. Furthermore, some thymomas and most thymic carcinomas are devoid of a capsule entirely or in part, which makes the definition of "encapsulation" meaningless. Therefore, the current and proposed categories "T1 (completely encapsulated)" and "T2 (with invasion of pericapsular connective tissue)" may not be biologically meaningful and may be impossible for pathologists to use. Criteria for minimal invasion need to be better defined.

Tumour size

On the other hand, tumour size has been used as an important parameter to define T-categories; critical dimensions of 11 cm and 15 cm have been reported {183,1172}. Especially in Blumberg's report, tumour size was one of the significant parameters for survival by multivariate analysis {183}. Critical size may be quite different among thymoma and thymic carcinoma, including neuroendocrine tumours. This consideration of tumour size might also be necessary in a revised definition of the T-category.

Surgical resectability

The present T denominator includes tumours with different characteristics: one extreme is an easily resectable tumour with minimal invasion into the pericardium and a good prognosis and another extreme is a non-resectable tumour with invasive growth into multiple neighbouring organs. A further division of T3 tumours into potentially

Table 3.03
Malignant potential in terms of mortality, combining WHO histologic type and tumour stage, according to Shimosato et al. {1808}. Stage IV thymomas should be considered as tumours of high malignant potential, although metastatic type A or AB thymomas with long-term survival have been reported.

Histology	Tumour Stage	Malignant potential
Type A, AB, (B1) thymoma	I and II	None (very low)[1]
	III	Low
Type B2, B3 thymoma	I	Low
	II and III	Moderate
Thymic carcinoma:		
Low-grade squamous cell, basaloid or mucoepidermoid carcinoma, carcinoid	Stage I and II	Moderate
	Stage III	High
Other histological types	Any stage	High

[1]These tumours amount to 40-50% of all thymomas {341,1511,1631}.

resectable and curable ones and non-resectable ones with a poor prognosis is desirable, especially for planning treatment.

Lymph node metastasis

This is rare in thymoma, and the basis for the definition of stage IVB (Masaoka) for thymomas with lymph node metastasis {1255}. In the tentative TNM classification, N1 (metastasis to anterior mediastinal lymph nodes) is defined as stage III. However, the prognostic equivalence between T3 and N1 has not yet been assessed. The appropriateness of the nodal grouping N1 to N3 needs to be investigated further. Depending on the tumour location in the anterior mediastinum, the lymphatic pathway by which tumour cells spread might be different. Consequently, the sentinel lymph node might be located elsewhere other than the anterior mediastinum.

Stage-Grouping

The most important issue in stage-grouping is the definition of stages I and II. The survival curves of patients with thymomas of stages I and II are superimposed at around 100% at 5 and 10 years after surgery {693,1511}. In other reports, a minimal difference has repeatedly been reported {1043,1130,1579,1645}. If the definition of the T-category remains unchanged, the present stages I and II could be merged into a new stage I; however, no data are available on thymic carcinoma with respect to stages I and II. Stage III in the present tentative system, which is a heterogeneous group, is recommended to be divided into a potentially resectable group with a favourable prognosis and an unresectable group with a poor prognosis, respectively.

Thymomas

A. Marx
Ph. Ströbel
A. Zettl
J.K.C. Chan
H.K. Müller-Hermelink

N.L. Harris
T.T. Kuo
Y. Shimosato
P. Engel

Definitions

Thymomas (type A, AB, B thymomas) are neoplasms arising from or exhibiting differentiation towards thymic epithelial cells, regardless of the presence and relative numbers of non-neoplastic lymphocytes {1691}. Their malignant potential is either absent or low to moderate.

Thymic carcinomas are malignant epithelial tumours because of overt cytological atypia, almost invariable invasiveness and lack of "organotypic" (thymus-like) features.

Combined thymoma, combined thymoma/thymic carcinoma. These terms are used for a combination of thymoma subtypes and of thymomas with thymic carcinomas, including thymic neuroendocrine carcinomas, within one tumour mass.

Thymoma (type X) with anaplasia is the suggested diagnostic term for a very uncommon group of tumours with borderline morphological freatures between thymoma and thymic carcinoma.

Epidemiology

Thymomas and thymic carcinomas are uncommon tumours with an annual incidence of approximately 1-5 per million population. There are only very limited epidemiologic data, but cautious interpretation of data from the Danish National Board of Health suggests that the incidence has not changed significantly over the last three decades. Thymomas and thymic carcinomas occur at almost all ages (range 7-89 years) with a peak incidence between 55-65 years. They are exceedingly rare in children and adolescents {1577,1876}. There is no pronounced sex predilection {318,341,1016,1630}. Patients exhibit an increased incidence of second cancers irrespective of the histology of the thymic epithelial tumour {1537}.

Etiology

The etiology of thymomas is still largely unknown. They have been repeatedly observed in patients with MEN1 syndrome {461,1535,1644,1648,2094}.

Epstein-Barr virus appears to play an etiologic role in subsets of lymphoepithelioma-like, poorly differentiated squamous and undifferentiated thymic carcinomas both in Asian {343,1174,1265, 2174} and Western countries {785,894, 1234,1876}. There is no increased risk of developing thymomas in patients receiving radio-chemotherapy for mediastinal Hodgkin lymphoma {1455} or breast cancer {1498}.

Principles of thymoma classification

1. There are two major types of thymoma depending on whether the neoplastic epithelial cells and their nuclei have a spindle or oval shape, and are uniformly bland (Type A thymoma) or whether the cells have a predominantly round or polygonal appearance (Type B) {1691}.

2. Type B thymomas are further subdivided on the basis of the extent of the lymphocytic infiltrate and the degree of atypia of the neoplastic epithelial cells into three subtypes B1 (richest in lymphocytes), B2, and B3 (richest in epithelial cells).

3. Thymomas combining type A with B1-like or (rarely) B2-like features are designated type AB.

4. Thymic carcinomas are termed according to their differentiation (squamous cell, mucoepidermoid, etc.). In the 1999 WHO classification {1690}, the term WHO type C thymoma was the "headline designation" to stress their thymic epithelial origin. In the current classification, this term was eliminated since all non-organotypic malignant epithelial neoplasms other than germ cell tumours are designated thymic carcinomas.

5. Combined thymomas are specified by the WHO histology and approximate percentage contributed by each component of the combined thymoma.

6. Traditionally, the term "malignant thymoma" has been used for (i) thymomas with advanced stage, i.e. local invasiveness, pleural or pericardial implants or metastasis, irrespective of tumour histology or (ii) thymic epithelial tumours with marked atypia (thymic carcinomas), irrespective of tumour stage {1170,1691, 1841,1924}. The use of the term "malig-

Table 3.04
Differential diagnosis of thymomas types A, AB, B and thymic carcinomas

Feature	Thymomas	Thymic carcinomas
Organotypic (thymus-like) histological features	Almost always present (lobular pattern, perivascular spaces, immature, TdT+ / CD1a+ / CD99+ T-cells)	None or abortive
CD5, CD70 and CD117 expression in epithelial cells	No	Frequent (~ 60%)
Invasion	Variable	Almost always
Myasthenia gravis	Variable: 10–80%	No
Other autoimmune diseases	Common	Rare
Clinical behaviour	Often curable by surgery; metastases are rare.	Often unresectable {318}; metastases are frequent
	Usually long survival due to indolent clinical course	Often short survival due to progressive disease

nant thymoma" as a synonym for a locally invasive thymoma irrespective of the WHO histological type is discouraged, since it may not properly reflect the excellent prognosis of type A and AB thymomas of advanced stage {318,341, 1510,1511,1630}.

Prevalence of thymoma subtypes

The predominant histological subtypes in most published series are type B2 and AB thymomas (each 20-35% of all cases), while type B1 and type A thymomas count among the rare types (5-10% in most studies) {856,1510,1967}. The percentage of thymic carcinomas has been reported to be about 10–25% {318, 341,541,1404,1510}.

In children, type A, B1 and B2 thymomas have been observed, in addition to undifferentiated and EBV-positive lymphoepithelioma-like thymic carcinomas {274, 1577,1876}. The morphologically heterogeneous and rare carcinomas with t(15;19) translocation typically occur in children and young adults {1081,1148, 2072}.

Genetic features

Recurrent genetic alterations have so far been reported for type A and B3 thymomas as well as for thymic squamous cell carcinomas {896,1567,2238,2242}. Type A thymomas only show few genetic alterations, with deletions of chromosome 6p reported as a recurrent genetic alteration {437,2065,2238}. Type A areas in type AB thymomas are genetically distinct from type A thymoma {699,896}. Type B3 thymomas frequently show gains of chromosome 1q and losses of chromosomes

6 and 13q. Type B2 thymomas are genetically related to type B3 thymomas {896}. Thymic squamous cell carcinomas frequently show gains of chromosomes 1q, 17q and 18 and losses of chromosomes 3p, 6, 16q, and 17p {2238}. The shared genetic abnormalities underline the close relationship between type B3 thymomas and thymic squamous cell carcinomas.

Prognosis and predictive factors

The most relevant prognostic factors in thymoma are tumour stage {341,1511, 1630,1808}, WHO histologic type {341, 1511} and completeness of resection {318,1419}.

Type A and AB thymomas in stages I and II virtually always follow a favourable clinical course {341,476,1511}, and even at higher stages may not be fatal due to a very slowly progressive course {1808}. They are considered benign tumours {784,1404} or neoplasms of low malignant potential. Type B1 thymomas have a

very low malignant potential; rare local recurrences or late metastases may occur {318}. Type B2 and B3 thymomas and thymic carcinomas, are clear-cut malignant tumours. B2 and B3 thymomas and well differentiated squamous, basaloid and mucoepidermoid carcinomas follow a more favourable course than poorly differentiated squamous cell carcinomas and other thymic carcinomas {1924}. The prognosis of combined thymomas may be determined by the most malignant component {1093,1912}. Paraneoplastic pure red cell aplasia, other cytopenias, or hypogammaglobulinaemia (Good syndrome) have an adverse effect {987} whereas paraneoplastic myasthenia gravis had no or a positive factor on survival {318,341}.

Table 3.05
Genetic alterations reported for the different WHO histological thymoma subtypes.

WHO Type	Chromosomal Gains	Chromosomal Losses	Source
Type A	none	-6p	{437,1325,2065,2238, 2242}
Type AB	none	-5q21-22, -6q, -12p, -16q	{699,896,897}
Type B3	+1q	-6, -13q	{896,897,2238,2242}
Thymic squamous cell carcinoma	+1q, +17q, +18	-3p, -6, -13q,-16q, -17p	{896,897,1848,2238}

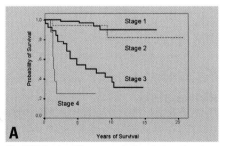
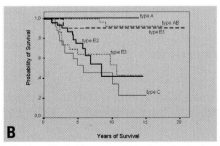
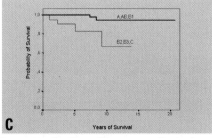

Fig. 3.04 Kaplan-Meyer survival statistics of patients with thymic epithelial tumours. **A** Survival of patients with thymomas or thymic carcinomas according to stage. Masaoka tumour stage is the most important and statistically most significant independent prognostic parameter for survival in almost all clinico-pathological studies. From G. Chen et al. {341}. **B** Survival of patients with thymomas or thymic carcinomas according to histological type. WHO-based histology was a statistically significant prognostic parameter for survival in most clinico-pathological studies. In some studies, B3 thymomas and thymic carcinomas had a significantly worse prognosis than B2 thymomas (L. Quintanilla-Martinez et al. {1631}; M.Okumura et al. {1511}), but not in others (G. Chen et al. {341}). **C** WHO-based histological subtype is an independant prognostic marker in patients with thymomas and thymic carcinomas infiltrating beyond the tumour capsule into the mediastinal fat (Masaoka stage II). A no/low-risk group of tumours (type A, AB, B1 thymomas) is distinguished from a moderate/high-risk group (B2 and B3 thymomas and thymic carcinomas). From G. Chen et al. {341}.

Type A thymoma

T.T. Kuo
K. Mukai
T. Eimoto
R.H. Laeng
K. Henry
J.K.C. Chan

Definition
Type A thymoma is an organotypic thymic epithelial neoplasm composed of bland spindle/oval epithelial tumour cells with few or no lymphocytes. The tumour cells can form a variety of histologic structures.

ICD-O code   8581/1

Synonyms
Spindle cell thymoma, medullary thymoma

Epidemiology
Type A thymoma is a relatively uncommon type of thymoma and accounts for 4-19% of all thymomas {541,1510,1511, 1808}. The age at manifestation ranges from 32 to 83 years, with a mean age of 61 years {1538,1540,1630}, which is higher than the mean age of 50 years of all thymoma patients {341,1095}. No consistent gender predilection has been reported {318,1511,1540,1630}.

Clinical features
Approximately 24% of type A thymomas are found in patients with myasthenia gravis {318,341,1511,1538,1540,1630}. Others are found because of local symptoms or incidentally discovered on imaging examination. Association with pure red cell aplasia may occur, but in contrast to earlier reports, pure red cell apla-

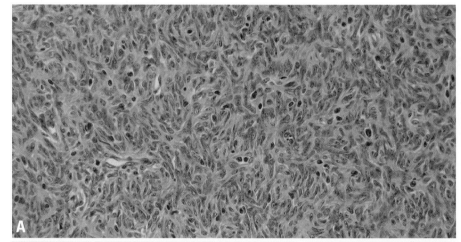
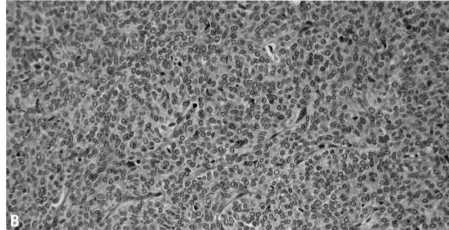

Fig. 3.06 Type A thymoma is composed of spindle cellls (**A**) or oval cells (**B**) with bland nuclei arranged in solid sheets without any particular pattern (**B**) or in a storiform patern (**A**).

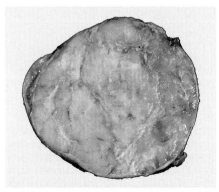

Fig. 3.05 A well encapsulated type A thymoma with vaguely lobulated appearance and thin white fibrous bands.

sia may also occur in other thymoma types {1096}.

Macroscopy
Grossly, type A thymoma is usually well circumscribed and encapsulated. The cut surface is tan white and shows vague lobulation with less distinct dissecting white fibrous bands than is seen in other types. Cystic change or calcification of the capsule may be seen. Average tumour size is 10.5 cm.

Tumour spread and staging
The majority of type A thymomas (80%) occurs as Masaoka stage I in the anterior mediastinum, followed by stage II

(17%) and rarely stage III (3%) {341,541, 1095,1510,1511,1538,1540,1630,1631,1 808}. Single exceptional cases of stage IV type A thymoma have been reported {1403}.

Histopathology
Histologically, the tumour has few or no lymphocytes and shows neither distinct lobules nor dissecting fibrous bands as seen in other types of thymoma. The tumour cells are spindle and/or oval-shaped with bland nuclei, dispersed chromatin and inconspicuous nucleoli; they are arranged in solid sheets without any particular pattern or in a storiform pattern {1403,1691}. Type A thymoma

cells can form cysts of various size, glandular structures, glomeruloid bodies, rosettes with or without a central lumen, Masson's haemangioma-like papillary projections in cystic spaces, or meningioma-like whorls {1086,1095,1403, 1538,1691,1808}. Extremely elongated fibroblast-like spindle cells may be seen focally. Vessels in the background may impart a haemangiopericytoma-like appearance {1538}. Perivascular spaces are less commonly seen than in other types of thymoma {318}. Although type A thymoma is a lymphocyte-poor tumour, spindle cell micronodules in a lymphoid stroma may be present at places {1981}. Most tumour cells are individually surrounded by reticulin fibers {1086,1691}. Cells in mitosis are seldom found, but lobular infarcts can occur. Rarely, thymic carcinoma can arise in type A thymoma. Areas of necrosis may be a clue to this phenomenon; examination of these areas reveals hyperchromatic anaplastic nuclei and/or mitotic figures indicating the presence of carcinoma {1093}.

Immunophenotype

The tumour cells are strongly positive for AE1-defined acidic cytokeratins (CKs), and negative for AE3-defined basic CKs. Other CKs of different molecular weights show variable expression except that CK20 is negative {1086}. In general, the cystic and glandular structures express stronger CK {1808}. CD20-positive tumour cells may be detected focally {354,1403, 1538}. There is no expression of CD5 {1538}, and BCL-2, CD57 and EMA are variable and usually only focally expressed {227,1631,1808,1872, 1981}. Most tumour cells are surrounded by basement membrane-like deposits as demonstrated by anti-laminin and anti-type IV collagen antibodies. TP53 protein and Ki-67 show only low or no expression {1539,1872, 1980,1981}. Two antigens, metallothionein and PE-35, found in normal thymic medullary cells are also expressed in type A thymoma cells {798,1087}. The few lymphocytes, if present, are T cells positive for CD3 and CD5. CD1a+ and CD99+ immature T cells may be present but comprise a minority of the T cells. CD20+ B cells are usually absent except in focal micronodular areas with a lymphoid stroma, if these are present.

Histogenesis

Type A thymoma has been postulated to derive from the normal thymic medullary epithelial cells {1403,1404}. Evidence in support of this postulate include their similar immunohistochemical expressions of CD20, cytokeratins, metallothionein, and PE-35 as well as the relative paucity of immature T cells {354,798, 1086,1087,1095,1452,1538,1631}.

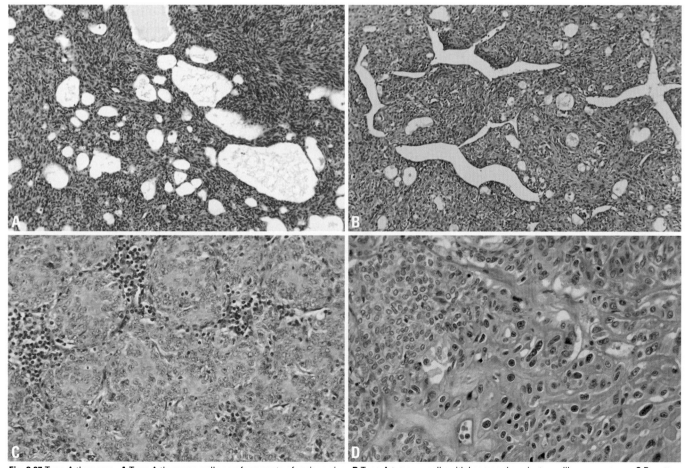

Fig. 3.07 Type A thymoma. **A** Type A thymoma cells can form cysts of various size. **B** Type A tymoma cells with haemangiopericytoma-like appearence. **C** Rosettes without a lumen. **D** Anaplastic malignant cells arising in type A thymoma.

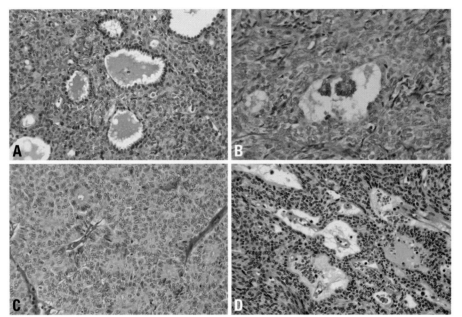

Fig. 3.10 Type A thymoma. CGH hybridization of a WHO type A thymoma shows loss of chromosome 6p21-pter revealed by an excess of red hybridization signal of normal DNA as compared to the green hybridization signal of tumour DNA (highlighted by the arrows).

Fig. 3.08 Different histological patterns in type A thymoma. **A** Glandular structures. **B** Glomeruloid bodies. **C** Rosettes with lumens. **D** Perivascular spaces.

Somatic genetics

Type A thymoma has been found to have t(15;22)(p11;q11) {438} or a partial loss of the short arm of chromosome 6 {2238}. Consistent loss of heterozygosity has been found only in the region 6q23.3-25.3, which is common to type A and B3 thymomas and squamous cell thymic carcinomas {897,2242}. Unlike type B3 thymomas and squamous cell thymic carcinoma, no aberrations in the APC, RB1, and TP53 gene loci or in regions 3p22-24.2 and 8q11.21-23 are found in type A thymoma {2242}, which could be the genetic basis for its generally benign clinical course.

Prognosis and predictive factors

The overall survival of patients with type A thymoma has been reported to reach 100% at 5 years and 10 years {1403, 1511}, even though approximately 20% of them have stage II or stage III tumours. Generally, type A thymoma is regarded as a benign tumour without having a risk of recurrence if the tumour can be completely removed surgically {1095,1403,1404}. However, exceptional case reports of local recurrence or distant metastasis have been documented {1043,1403, 1538}. Rarely, type A thymoma can undergo malignant transformation into thymic carcinoma {1093}. The association with myasthenia gravis has been reported to have either a better or no effect on prognosis {318,1511,1630}.

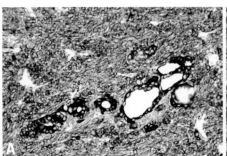
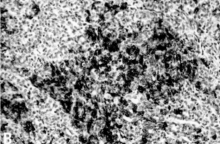
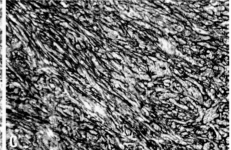

Fig. 3.09 Immunophenotype of type A thymoma. **A** Immunopositivity for AE1-defined acidic cytokeratins. Note the stronger expression of cytokeratin by the glandular structures. **B** Focal epithelial expression of CD20. **C** Tumour cells are surrounded by abundant type IV collagen as demonstrated by immunostaining.

Type AB thymoma

common subtype

T.T. Kuo
K. Mukai
T. Eimoto
R.H. Laeng
K. Henry
J.K.C. Chan

Definition
Type AB thymoma is an organotypical thymic epithelial neoplasm composed of a mixture of a lymphocyte-poor type A thymoma component and a more lymphocyte-rich type B-like component. The tumour cells in the type B-like component are composed predominantly of small polygonal epithelial cells with small round, oval or spindle pale nuclei showing dispersed chromatin and inconspicuous nucleoli, and are smaller and paler than those of B1 or B2 thymomas. Lymphocytes are more numerous than in the type A component, but may be less numerous than in B1 thymomas. There is a great variation in the proportion of the two components, and while usually both components are present in most sections, either type A or type B areas can be scanty.

ICD-O code   8582/1

Synonym
Mixed thymoma

Epidemiology
Type AB thymoma is either the most or the second most common type of thymoma and accounts for 15-43% of all thymomas {341,541,1095,1510,1511,1538, 1540,1631,1808}. The patients' ages range from 29-82 years with a slightly younger mean age of 55 years than type A thymoma {1538,1540,1630}. A slight male predominance has been noted in most reports {1511,1538,1540,1630}.

Clinical features
The clinical presentation is similar to that of type A thymoma. Approximately 14% of type AB thymomas are associated with myasthenia gravis {341,541,1510,1511, 1538,1540,1630,1808}. Paraneoplastic pure red cell aplasia has also been reported {1096}. Other tumours manifest by local symptoms or can be asymptomatic and are found incidentally upon imaging examination.

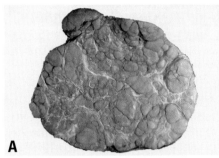
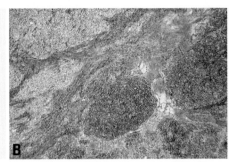

Fig. 3.11 A Macroscopic appearance of a type AB thymoma showing multiple nodules separated by fibrous bands. **B** Type AB thymoma composed of lymphocyte-associated type B nodules and diffuse lymphocyte-poor type A areas.

Macroscopy
Grossly, type AB thymoma is usually encapsulated and the cut surface shows multiple tan coloured nodules of various size separated by white fibrous bands. Average tumour size is 7.7 cm.

Tumour spread and staging
The majority of type AB thymoma (71.7%) occur in the anterior mediastinum as Masaoka stage I followed by stage II (21.6%) and stage III (5.6%) {341,437,1404,1510,1511,1539,1540, 1691}. Rare cases of stage IV type AB thymoma (1.1%) have been reported {1325,1404,1510,1539,1691}.

Histopathology
Histologically, type AB thymoma shows a nodular growth pattern with diffuse areas and is composed of a variable mixture of a lymphocyte-poor type A thymoma component and a more lymphocyte-rich type B component. All histological features of type A thymoma can be seen in the type A component. However, the type B areas are distinctive and different from either B1, B2, or B3 thymoma. The tumour cells in the type B component are composed predominantly of small polygonal epithelial cells with small round, oval or spindle pale nuclei showing dispersed chromatin and inconspicuous nucleoli {1086,1403,1691,1808}. The large, vesicular epithelial cells with nucleoli that are characteristic of B2 thymoma are only rarely seen {1086}. The type A and type B components either form discrete separate nodules or intermix together {1403,1691}. The type A component in the latter areas may form bundles of extremely elongated fibroblast-like spindle cells. Type B areas harbour lymphocytes in variable numbers and medullary differentiation is rarely observed. In particular, Hassall corpus-

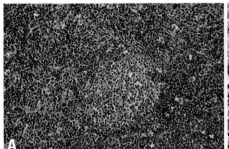
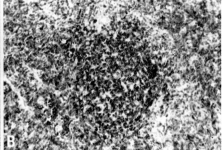

Fig. 3.12 Type AB thymoma. **A** Medullary differention in type B component. **B** The lymphocytes in the focus of medullary differentiation are distinctively CD5+ T cells.

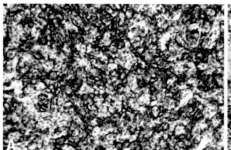
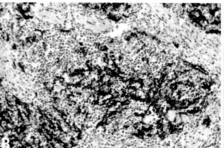
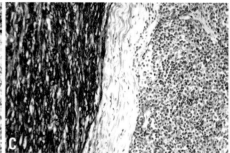

Fig. 3.13 Type AB thymoma. **A** Type B component cells are immunopositive for cytokeratin 14. **B** CD20+ tumour cells in type B component. **C** Abundant laminin production is seen in type A component (immunostained with anti-laminin antibody).

cles are absent. There is a great variation in the proportion of both components and in particular, type A areas can be extremely scanty to almost absent {1086,1403,1691}. Unlike type A thymoma areas, type B areas show reticulin fibers around tumour nodules rather than around individual tumour cells.

Immunophenotype

The patterns of cytokeratin (CK) expression of type AB thymoma are essentially similar to those of type A thymoma, except that the epithelial cells in type B areas are usually CK14+ {1086}. CD20+ tumour cells can be seen in both type A and type B areas, and the associated lymphocytes are T cells positive for CD3 and CD5, including varying proportions of CD1a+ CD99+ immature T cells. The lymphocytes in the foci of medullary differentiation are distinctively CD5+ T cells. B cells are usually absent. The fibroblast-like elongated type A cells are strongly positive for vimentin and EMA and may show weak CK staining. There is no expression of CD5. BCL-2 and

CD57 are variably and usually weakly expressed {227,1631,1808,1872,1981}. TP53 protein and Ki-67 are extremely low or absent {1539,1872,1980,1981}. In contrast to type A thymoma areas, the type B areas show less production of laminin and type IV collagen.

Histogenesis

The cellular origin of the type A component, like in type A thymoma, has been postulated to derive from or differentiate towards thymic medullary epithelial cells {798,1087,1403,1404}. The type B component ultrastructurally resembles epithelial cells at the corticomedullary junction {1017}, but is similar to thymic subcapsular epithelial cells in expression of CK14 {1086}; thus its normal counterpart is uncertain.

Somatic genetics

Deletion of chromosome 6 with or without formation of ring chromosome 6 has been found in type AB thymoma {437, 1043,1076,2065}. In addition, complex multiple chromosomal aberrations have

been described in individual cases {699}. Loss of heterozygosity at 5q21-22 (APC), as seen in type B thymoma, has been detected in a minority of type AB thymoma {897}.

Prognosis and predictive factors

The overall survival rate of patients with type AB thymoma is 80-100% at 5 years and 10 years {1403,1511}. Although type AB thymomas may present as stage II or stage III tumours, they can be usually cured by radical surgery {1095,1403, 1404}. Therefore, they are generally regarded as clinically benign tumours {1403,1404}. Recurrence and metastasis are exceptionally rare {1043,1403,1538}. An association with myasthenia gravis has been reported to have either a better or no effect on prognosis {318,1511, 1630}.

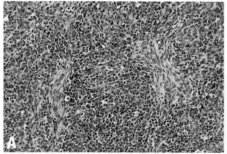
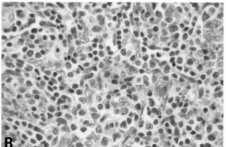
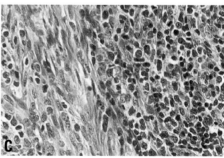

Fig. 3.14 Type AB thymoma. **A** The lymphocyte-associated type B component and the lymphocyte-poor type A component intermix together. The type A component cells appear as elongated fibroblast-like spindle cells. **B** The type B component is composed of predominantly small polygonal cells with small round or oval pale nuclei with pale chromatin and inconspicuous nucleoli. **C** Type A component is poor in lymphocytes (left), while type B component is lymphocyte-rich (right).

Type B1 thymoma

G. Palestro
R. Chiarle
A. Marx
H.K. Müller-Hermelink
I. Sng

Type B cells of AB ≠ Type B cells of B1, 2, 3

Definition
Type B1 thymoma is a tumour of thymic epithelial cells with a histological appearance practically indistinguishable from the normal thymus, composed predominantly of areas resembling cortex with epithelial cells scattered in a prominent population of immature lymphocytes, and areas of medullary differentiation, with or without Hassall's corpuscles, similar to normal thymic medulla.

ICD-O code   8583/1

Synonyms
Lymphocyte-rich thymoma; lymphocytic thymoma; organoid thymoma; predominantly cortical thymoma

Epidemiology
B1 thymoma is a relatively rare tumour of the adult age (mean of 41-47 years) with no significant difference in the distribution of genders {318,1511,1631}. B1 thymoma corresponds to 6% to 17% of all thymomas {318,341,1095,1405,1511, 1630,1631}.

Localization
B1 thymoma arises in the anterosuperior mediastinum, but rare localizations are described in the neck, pleura or lung {632,1238}.

Clinical features
B1 thymoma is often diagnosed because of associated immunological diseases such as myasthenia gravis (18-56% of the cases) {318,341,1511}, but local symptoms such as cough, dyspnoea and pain may occur. Rare associated syndromes are hypogammaglobulinemia and pure red cell aplasia {987,1088, 2000}. It can be detected by X-ray, CT or MRI imaging as an enlarged mediastinal area or mass.

Macroscopy
B1 thymoma is usually a well-defined or encapsulated greyish mass. Thick fibrous capsule and septa can be present, as well as cystic spaces or small haemorrhagic and necrotic areas.

Tumour spread and staging
B1 thymoma is considered to have a low-grade malignant potential being completely encapsulated (stage I) in about 53-58% of the cases or invading only the mediastinal fat (stage II) in another 24-27% of the cases {341,1511}. Less frequently it can invade the pleura, pericardium, great vessels or adjacent organs; metastases are exceedingly rare {318,341,1511,1631}. Staging is done according to the Masaoka Classification.

Histopathology
Type B1 thymoma has also been called predominantly cortical, organoid or lymphocyte-rich thymoma because it contains predominantly expanded areas closely resembling the normal functional thymic cortex. The neoplastic epithelial cells are scant, small, with very little atypia, and are surrounded by non-neoplastic T lymphocytes. B1 thymomas may grow in expansile sheets or more often display a highly organoid lobular architecture recapitulating the normal thymic cortex with prevalence of the lymphocyte-rich inner cortical zone. Lobules may be of varying size and separated by thin or thick acellular fibrous bands. The neoplastic epithelial component is relatively inconspicuous and appears as interspersed oval cells with pale round nuclei and small nucleoli, although some cells may be large and occasionally have conspicuous nucleoli. The epithelial cells are dispersed and do not form cellular groupings. The lymphoid component is a densely packed population of small lymphocytes, which have clumped chromatin. Tingible-body macrophages may be scattered throughout giving rise to a starry-sky appearance. Perivascular spaces are not as frequent as in the other B thymomas. Cystic spaces and areas of necrosis, when present, are usually small.

Pale areas of medullary differentiation are always present, composed of more loosely packed lymphocytes; Hassall's corpuscles may be seen but are less numerous than in normal medulla. They range from poorly formed epithelial groupings to large structures with prominent keratinised centres.

Differential diagnosis
Type B1 thymoma is distinguishable from the normal non-involuted thymus mainly based on architectural differences, including the large excess of cortical areas compared to small areas resembling the thymic medulla, fewer Hassall corpuscles, less regular lobulation and a thick fibrous capsule or irregular fibrous septa.

B1 thymoma must be distinguished from B2 thymoma.

B1 thymoma with a high predominance of T lymphocytes may simulate T lymphoblastic lymphoma. An infiltrative pattern of lymphocytes into septa and capsule would favour lymphoma. The presence of a prominent cytokeratin meshwork and low CDK6 expression in T lymphocytes favours B1 thymoma {355}.

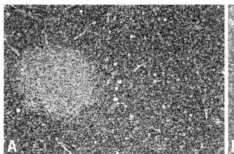
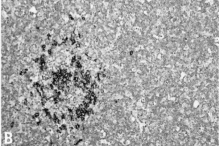

Fig. 3.15 Type B1 thymoma. **A** CD1a staining highlights immature T-cells in the cortex-like areas. **B** CD20 staining highlights B-cells in the medullary areas.

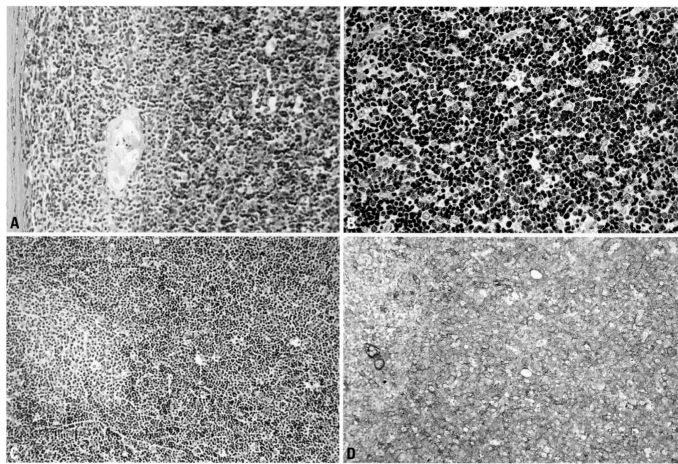

Fig. 3.16 Type B1 thymoma. **A** Medullary island (MI) showing Hassall corpuscles. The abnormal localization of MI adjacent to septa or the tumour capsule is very typical. **B** High-power of cortex-like areas in B1 thymoma showing a vast majority of lymphoid cells compared to few inconspicuous epithelial cells characterized by vesicular, clear nuclei and distinct but small nucleoli. **C** Small medullary island (light), that is devoid of Hassall corpuscles is surrounded by a predominant, cortex-like component rich in immature T-cells (dark). This patttern has been the rationale for labelling B1 thymoma as "organoid thymoma". **D** Cytokeratin 19 staining labels a network of epithelial cells which is more delicate than in B2 thymoma (compare with fig. 3.18D)

Immunophenotype

The neoplastic epithelial cells express a cytokeratin pattern similar to normal cortical epithelial cells (CD19 diffuse, CK7, CK14, CK18 focal positivity, CK20, CD5, CD20 and CD70 negative) {354, 851,854, 1086} and have a low fraction of growth {1290}. Admixed cortical T lymphocytes are CD1a+, CD4+, CD8+, CD5+, CD99+ and TdT+, with high proliferation rate, whereas lymphocytes in medullary islands are mostly mature T cells: CD3+, CD5+, CD1a-, CD99-, TdT- {355}.

Histogenesis

The postulated cell of origin is a thymic epithelial cell capable of differentiating towards both cortical and medullary type.

Prognosis and predictive factors

B1 thymoma is slightly more aggressive than A and AB thymomas, but less malignant than B2, B3 thymomas and thymic carcinomas. In B1 thymoma, complete surgical resection is possible in 91-94% of the cases {318,1511}, with less than 10% of recurrences {318,1511}.

Actuarial 10-year survival rates are more than 90% due to the frequent stage I or II presentation {318,341,1511}. Staging is the most important prognostic indicator, whereas age, gender and myasthenia gravis are not significant prognostic parameters {318,341,1511,1631}.

Type B2 thymoma

Common subtype

H.K. Müller-Hermelink   R.H. Laeng
I. Sng   N.L. Harris
G. Palestro   P.J. Zhang
T.J. Molina   A. Marx

Definition

Type B2 thymoma is an organotypical thymic epithelial neoplasm composed of large, polygonal tumour cells that are arranged in a loose network and exhibit large vesicular nuclei with prominent large nucleoli, closely resembling the predominant epithelial cells of the normal thymic cortex. A background population of immature T cells is always present and usually outnumbers the neoplastic epithelial cells.

ICD-O code   8584/1

Synonyms

Cortical thymoma; lymphocytic thymoma (obsolete); mixed lymphocytic and epithelial thymoma (obsolete)

Epidemiology

Type B2 thymoma accounts for 18-42% of all thymomas {318,341,776,1016, 1540,1630,1631,1967}. Differences in the prevalences of type B2 thymomas among different institutions reflect the strong correlation with myasthenia gravis (MG) rather than real demographic differences. Patients´ ages range from 13-79 years, with a mean of 47-50 years {318,1016,1631}. There is no consistent gender predominance {341,1016,1511, 1630}.

Localization

B2 thymomas are almost always located in the anterior mediastinum. Ectopic cases are on record, including cases with extensive pleural involvement ("pleural thymoma"). Similarly to all types of thymoma, they may arise ectopically in the head and neck region, pleura or lung {632,1238,1500}.

Clinical features

The most frequent manifestations are symptoms of MG (30-82% of cases) {318,341,1016,1511,1630}. Local symptoms (chest pain, dyspnoea, cough) occur in about 20% of cases. Rare complications are superior vena cava syndrome {1651}, pure red cell aplasia

{1088,1651}, hypogammaglobulinaemia (Good syndrome) {987} and other autoimmune phenomena .

Macroscopy

Grossly, type B2 thymomas are encapsulated or vaguely circumscribed and show a mean diameter of 6.3 cm {318, 1630}. They can invade mediastinal fat or adjacent organs. The cut surface is soft or firm and exhibits tan-coloured nodules separated by white fibrous septae. There may be cystic changes, haemorrhage, and fibrosis.

Tumour spread and staging

The majority of type B2 thymomas occur in the anterior mediastinum as Masaoka stage I (10-48%), stage II (13-53%) or stage III (19-49%) tumours. Metastatic stage IV B2 thymomas are less common (mean 8.9%) {318,341,1511,1630}, and distant metastases (stage IVB) are rare (up to 3%) {1511}.

Histopathology

There are usually large, coarse lobules of tumour with delicate septa, somewhat resembling the lobular architecture of the normal thymic cortex. Neoplastic cells are large and polygonal, and their large nuclei display an open chromatin pattern with prominent central nucleoli, similar to the appearance of normal cortical thymic epithelial cells. The neoplastic epithelial cells form a delicate loose network, forming palisades around perivascular spaces and along septa; large, confluent sheets of tumour cells are not a usual feature, but may occur. If such foci are present, they should be examined closely to make sure that the tumour cells are of B2 and not B3 type. Small epidermoid foci resembling abortive Hassall's corpuscles {1016} may occur in up to 25% of cases, but medullary islands are missing or inconspicuous, and typical Hassall´s corpuscles are exceptional find-

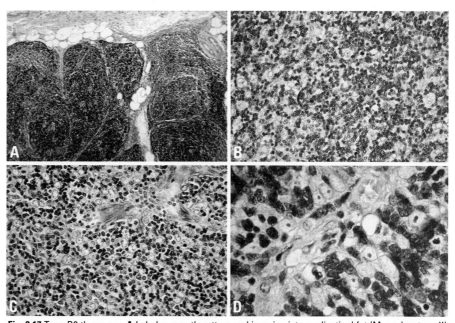

Fig. 3.17 Type B2 thymoma. **A** Lobular growth pattern and invasion into mediastinal fat (Masaoka stage II) **B** Medium power of B2 thymoma resembling B1 in terms of the very high number of lymphoid cells. However, the nuclei and nucleoli are larger and more conspicuous here than in B1 thymoma. **C** Medium power showing a relatively high number of large tumour cells among a slightly more numerous lymphoid component. Note inconspicuous cytoplasm but prominent large nuclei of tumour cells with prominent medium-sized nucleoli. **D** High magnification of the former illustration.

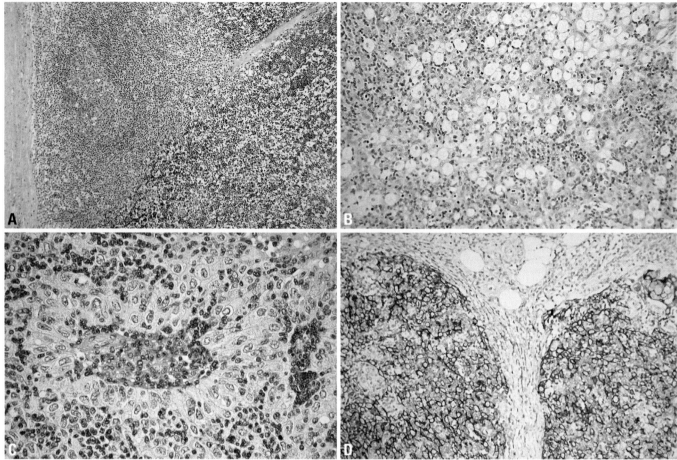

Fig. 3.18 Type B2 thymoma. **A** Lymphoid follicle with prominent subcapsular germinal centre, associated with myasthenia gravis. **B** Type B2 thymoma after massive corticosteroid treatment: paucity of lymphoid cells, shrinkage of tumour cell nuclei and prominent infiltration of macrophages. **C** Perivascular space with prominent palisading of elongated large tumour cells. High number of lymphoid cells in the perivascular space (center) and in an intraepithelial position (periphery of image). **D** Cytokeratin 19 immunoreactivity of neoplastic epithelial cells highlights the lobular growth pattern of B2 thymoma.

ings. Tumour cells are usually outnumbered by non-neoplastic lymphocytes.

Areas of B3 thymoma occur in association with B2 thymoma in 17-29% of the cases {341,541}. These are recognized as lymphocyte-poor areas in which the tumour cells are often smaller, with more nuclear irregularity, less conspicuous nucleoli, and distinct cell borders. If any component is of B3 type, it should be classified as combined B2/B3 thymoma.

Lymphoid follicles in perivascular spaces or septa are more frequent in MG-associated cases. Regressive changes, either spontaneous or induced by immunosuppressive treatment, include necrosis and lymphocyte depletion followed by collapse of the epithelial network and infiltrates of histiocytes and lipidized macrophages. A decreased tumour cell size is often apparent in condensed or sponge-like postnecrotic areas.

Immunophenotype
Immunophenotypically, neoplastic cells are cytokeratin (CK) 19+ (100%), CK5/6+ (90%), CK7+ (80%), CK20-, EMA-; antibodies AE1/3, Cam5.2 and Leu7 (anti-CD57) are almost always reactive {367,1016,1086,1631}. CD5, CD20, CD70 are not expressed by epithelial cells of B2 thymoma {354, 851,854}. Intraepithelial lymphocytes are predominantly immature T-cells: CD1a+, CD4+, CD8+, CD5+, CD99+, TdT+ with a high Ki67 index of 70-90%. Lymphocytes in rare medullary islands are mostly mature T-cells: CD3+, CD5+, CD1a-, CD99-, TdT-, and significantly less proliferative {327,355,1016,1631}.

Differential diagnosis
B1 thymoma is also lymphocyte-rich but epithelial cells are inconspicuous, smaller, and less numerous than in B2 thymomas. In addition, the nuclei and nucleoli are smaller and the medullary islands are more prominent than in B2 thymomas.

B3 thymoma, in contrast to B2 thymoma, is relatively lymphocyte-poor. Neoplastic epithelial cells form confluent sheets and solid areas with a small but distinctive population of intraepithelial immature T-cells. The neoplastic cells are usually slightly smaller than those of B2 thymoma, with irregular nuclear membranes, smaller nucleoli, nuclear grooves, and less vesicular chromatin. T-lymphoblastic lymphoma (T-LBL) may exhibit the same immunophenotype and proliferative activity of lymphoid cells as those of type B1 and B2 thymomas. However, the

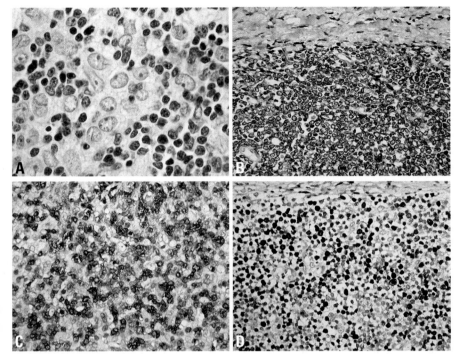

Fig. 3.19 Type B2 thymoma. **A** Relatively high number of tumour cells with medium-sized nucleoli among a majority of small lymphocytes. **B** Differential diagnosis B2 thymoma versus lymphoblastic lymphoma (T-LBL): CD1a expression in a rare initial T-LBL that is in a pre-infiltrative phase without infiltration of thymic septum (top of image). **C** CD1a-positive immature T-cells between B2 thymoma tumour cells with large clear nuclei and conspicuous nucleoli. **D** High Ki67 index. Note the non-infiltrated septum at top of image.

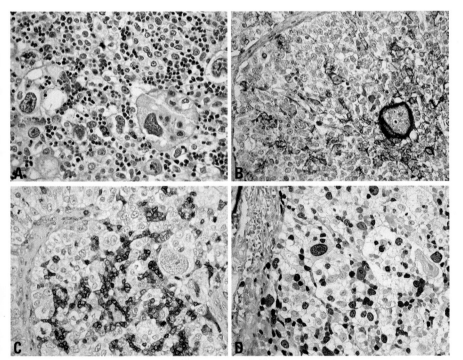

Fig. 3.20 Thymoma with anaplasia. **A** Anaplastic giant epithelial cells in a B2 thymoma with few intraepithelial lymphocytes. **B** Anaplastic giant cells are cytokeratin 19+ but not histiocytes. Note unusual down-regulation of cytokeratin 19 expression in many other neoplastic epithelial cells. **C** Anaplastic thymoma harbouring a significant population of CD1a+ immature T-cells like other thymomas but in contrast to thymic carcinomas. **D** Ki-67 immunohistochemistry showing proliferations of anaplastic giant cells.

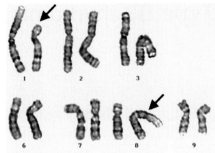

Fig. 3.21 Anaplastic thymoma (B2 thymoma with anaplasia). Metaphase with t(1;8)(p13;p11) translocation. G-banded karyotype showing 46, XY, t(1;8)(p13;p11).

epithelial network is destroyed in T-LBL, and lymphoblasts usually infiltrate beyond the epithelial compartment into thymic septa and mediastinal fat. Very high CDK6-expression is a distinguishing feature of T-LBL {355}.

Histogenesis
The postulated cell of origin is a thymic epithelial cell capable of differentiating towards cortical-type epithelial cells.

Somatic genetics
Recurrent genetic aberrations have not been reported. More than 80% of B2 thymomas are aneuploid {743}. In a single case with marked anaplasia and giant cell formation, a t(1;8)(p13;p11) translocation has been reported {1722}.

Prognostic and predictive factors
Type B2 thymoma is a tumour of moderate malignancy, with higher malignant potential than B1 thymoma, but appears to be slightly less aggressive than type B3 thymoma {1016,1511,1630}. It is often invasive, thus non-resectable at presentation in 5-15% of cases. Recurrences, even after complete resection, are reported in 5-9%, and metastases in up to 11% {341,1511,1630}. Recurrences typically occur after 1-7 years, but are compatible with long-term survival (>10 years) {1510}. The most relevant prognostic factors are tumour stage and resectability, while gender, age, and MG have no adverse effect on survival {318,341,1645}. Reported 10 year survival rates range between 50-100% {341,1511,1540,1630}.

Type B3 thymoma

H.K. Müller-Hermelink
K. Mukai
I. Sng
G. Palestro
A. Zettl

T.J. Molina
R. H. Laeng
N.L. Harris
A. Marx

Definition
Type B3 thymoma is an organotypic thymic epithelial tumour predominantly composed of medium–sized round or polygonal cells with slight atypia. The epithelial cells are mixed with a minor component of intraepithelial lymphocytes, resulting in a sheet-like growth of epithelial cells.

ICD-O code   8585/1

Synonyms
Well-differentiated thymic carcinoma (ICD-O code 8585/3); epithelial thymoma; squamoid thymoma

Epidemiology
Type B3 thymoma accounts for 7-25% of all thymomas {318,341,1016,1540,1630, 1967}. Patients´ age ranges from 14-78 years, with a mean age of 45-50 years {318,1016,1511}. There is no consistent sex predominance {341,1016,1511, 1630}.

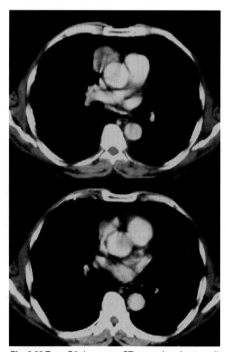

Fig. 3.22 Type B3 thymoma. CT scan showing a well circumscribed tumour in the anterior mediastinum

Clinical features
The most frequent manifestations are symptoms of myasthenia gravis (30-77% of cases) {318,341,1016,1511,1630}. Local symptoms like chest pain, dyspnoea or cough are common, while superior vena cava syndrome {1651}, pure red cell aplasia {1088,1651}, hypogammaglobulinaemia (Good syndrome) {987} or other autoimmune phenomena are rare.

Macroscopy
Grossly, type B3 thymomas are usually not encapsulated but show a vaguely infiltrative border with extension into mediastinal fat or adjacent organs. Diameters range from 2-13 cm (mean: 7.6 cm) {318,1016,1630}. The cut surface is typically firm and exhibits grey to white nodules separated by white fibrous septa. Soft yellow or red foci, cyst formation or hard calcified regions indicate regressive changes that are particularly frequent among large and, paradoxically, small (<3 cm), encapsulated or sclerotic type B3 thymomas {1085}.

Tumour spread and staging
The majority of type B3 thymomas occurs in the anterior mediastinum as Masaoka stage II (15-38%) or stage III tumours (38-66%), while stage I cases are rare (mean: 4.2%) {318,541,1016,1511,1540}. Stage IV type B3 thymomas, comprising cases with either pleural spread (stage IVA) or distant metastases (stage IVB), occur in 6-26% (mean: 15%) {318,341, 1016,1511,1630}. Distant metastases have been reported in up to 7% of cases {1511} and preferentially involved the same organs as in type B2 thymomas: lung, liver, bone and soft tissues.

Histopathology
Histologically, tumour cells form lobules that are separated by thick fibrous and hyalinized septa. A major diagnostic criterion is the paucity of intraepithelial lymphocytes, resulting in the formation of tumour cell sheets with a vaguely solid or epidermoid appearance. Intercellular

bridges are, however, not a feature of B3 thymoma. In the majority of cases, tumour cells are polygonal, medium-sized, and the round or elongated nuclei are often folded or grooved and characteristically smaller with less prominent nucleoli than in B2 thymomas. Palisades around perivascular spaces and along septa are often conspicuous. While medullary islands are usually absent, small foci of keratinization mimicking Hassall corpuscles may be present.

Variants
In a minority of cases, slightly more atypical, enlarged and hyperchromatic nuclei occur focally. Other rare variants show either polygonal cells with nuclei and nucleoli more similar to those in B2 thymomas (large cell variant) or partial clear cell changes with focal loss of interepithelial lymphocytes. Focal or extensive spindle cell formation may also occur.

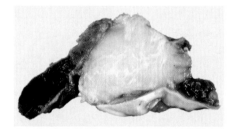

Fig. 3.23 Type B3 thymoma with invasion of pleura and pericardium.

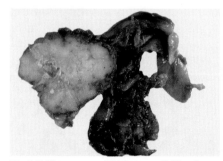

Fig. 3.24 Macroscopy of B3 thymoma (left) and remnant thymus (right). The cut surface of the tumour is white, lobulated and shows infiltration into the surrounding mediastinal fat. Focal regressive changes just left from the tumour centre.

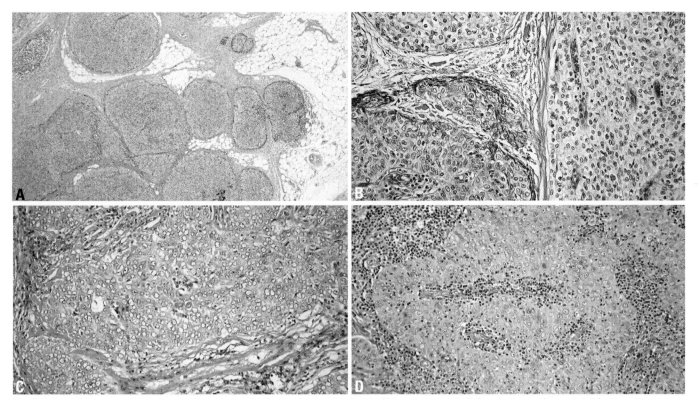

Fig. 3.25 Type B3 thymoma. **A** Lobular growth pattern and infiltration into mediastinal fat (Masaoka stage II). **B** Clear cell areas (top and right) adjacent to an area with a common histology (darker region in lower left part of image). **C** Ground glass appearance of tumour cells. Low number of intraepithelial lymphocytes. **D** Large cell variant with B2-like large nuclei and prominent nucleoli: by its atypia the case appears "borderline" to squamous cell carcinoma of the thymus.

None of these variants has been shown to affect the biological behaviour of type B3 thymomas.

Combined thymomas exhibiting B2 and B3 areas are common (17-29%) {341, 541}, while tumours combining features of type B3 thymoma and thymic carcinoma are rare (3%) {341}.

As in B2 thymomas, lymphoid follicles inside septa or perivascular spaces may occur particularly in myasthenia gravis-associated cases. Steroid treatment may produce a sponge-like appearance and accumulation of foam cells in intraepithelial microcysts {1016}. Anaplasia can occur in type B3 thymomas: a small group of tumours show a high degree of atypia with the maintenance of organotypic features that is characteristic of thymomas. "B3 Thymoma with anaplasia" is the suggested diagnostic terminology.

Immunophenotype

The epithelial cells are positive for cytokeratin (CK) 19, CK5/6, CK7, CK10, CK 8, as well as for AE1/3 and Leu7 (anti-CD57), while CK20 is not expressed {367,1016,1086,1631}. In contrast to type B2 thymomas, focal EMA positivity is a characteristic feature. CD5, CD20, CD70 {354,851,854} and TTF1 are not expressed in epithelial cells.

Most intraepithelial lymphocytes are immature T-cells: CD1a+, CD4+, CD8+, CD5+, CD99+ and TdT+.

Differential diagnosis

B2 thymoma, in contrast to B3 thymoma, is lymphocyte-rich. Neoplastic epithelial cells are scattered among lymphocytes and do not form confluent sheets or extensive solid areas. B2 thymomas do not express epithelial membrane antigen (EMA).

Low-grade squamous cell carcinoma of the thymus shows more pronounced epidermoid differentiation, usually with readily detectable intercellular bridges. Significant numbers of immature intraepithelial lymphocytes are absent.

Type A thymoma may resemble the spindle cell variant of B3 thymoma. In type A thymoma, there is usually a significant reticulin network around individual tumour cells, the degree of atypia is lower, and perivascular spaces with epithelial palisades are absent.

Histogenesis

The postulated cell of origin is a thymic epithelial cell capable of differentiating towards a less differentiated cortical-type epithelial cell than in B2 thymoma.

Somatic genetics

In a series of 16 B3 thymomas investigated by comparative genomic hybridization (CGH), all tumours showed genetic imbalances. Recurrent genetic gains were observed on chromosome 1q in 69%, recurrent losses on chromosome 6 in 38% of cases, and on chromosome 13q in 31% {2238}. In microsatellite analysis, two major pathways in the tumorigenesis of B3 thymoma were described, one characterized by losses of 6q (6q23.3-q25.3), the other by losses of chromosome 3p (3p22-p24.2; 3p14.2, FHIT locus), 5q (5q21, APC locus), 13q (13q14, RB1 locus) and 17p (17p13, TP53 locus) {896,2242}. Virtually 100% of B3 thymomas are aneuploid by DNA cytometry {743}.

Prognosis and predictive factors

B3 thymoma is a tumour of intermediate malignancy. It is almost always invasive,

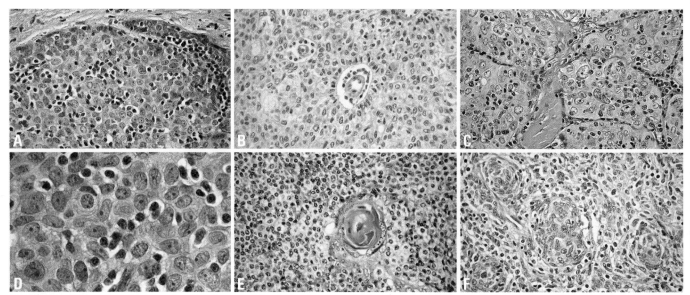

Fig. 3.26 Type B3 thymoma. **A** Large cell variant: large nuclei and conspicuous nucleoli and paucity of intraepithelial lymphocytes. **B** Typical perivascular spaces (PVS) with tumour cell palisading. **C** Large cell variant, lobular growth pattern; few intraepithelial lymphocytes. **D** High power of fig. 3.26C. **E** Hassall corpuscle in a B3 thymoma (usually rare). **F** Abortive formation of Hassall corpuscles and vague spindling of tumour cells.

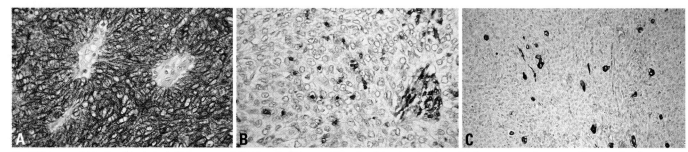

Fig. 3.27 Immunohistochemistry in type B3 thymoma. **A** Cytokeratin 19 immunohistochemistry showing the solid sheet pattern of tumour cells and palisading around perivascular spaces. **B** CD1a staining showing a low number of immature intraepithelial lymphocytes and immature lymphocytes in a perivascular space. Predominance of epithelial cells is obvious. **C** Type B3 thymoma with unusually high number of desmin and myoid cells.

shows frequent local recurrences (15-17% of cases) {1016,1630}, is often unresectable at presentation (17-47%) {318,1511,1630} and metastasizes in up to 20% of cases {341,1511}. Recurrences typically occur after 1-6 years, but late recurrences (after 14 years) have been reported {1016}. Some authors {1016,1511,1630} but not others {341, 1540} found B3 thymomas slightly more aggressive than B2 thymomas in terms of survival. The most relevant prognostic factors are tumour stage and resectability, while gender, age, and MG status have no adverse effect on survival {318,341,1645}. Reported 10 year survival rates range between 50-70% {341,1511,1540,1630}.

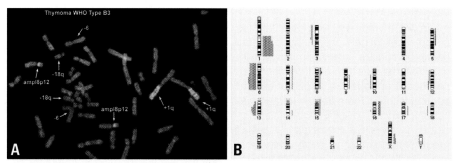

Fig. 3.28 A CGH hybridization of a type B3 thymoma shows gain of chromosome 1q and loss of chromosome 6 as the typical genetic alterations of this thymoma type (red hybridization signal corresponding to loss, green hybridization signal corresponding to gain of chromosomal material). This case in addition showed loss of chromosome 18q and a high-level amplification on chromosome 8p12 (white arrows). **B** Chromosomal ideogram showing gains and losses of chromosomal material in 23 cases of type B3 thymomas. The most frequent recurrent genetic imbalances in type B3 thymoma are gains of chromosome 1q (60%) and losses of chromosome 6 (43%) (Bars on the right side: gains of chromosomal material, bars on the left side: losses of chromosomal material).

Micronodular thymoma with lymphoid stroma

A. Marx
Ph. Ströbel
M. Marino
T. Eimoto
N.L. Harris
R.H. Laeng

Definition
Micronodular thymoma (MNT) is an organotypic thymic epithelial tumour characterized by multiple, discrete epithelial nodules separated by an abundant lymphocytic stroma that usually contains prominent germinal centres. The epithelial component is composed of bland, oval to spindle-shaped cells with few intraepithelial lymphocytes. The epithelial component is similar to type A thymomas.

ICD-O code   8580/1

Synonym
Micronodular thymoma with lymphoid B-cell hyperplasia

Epidemiology
MNT is a rare entity accounting for only about 1-5% of all thymomas. The age at diagnosis ranged between 45–95 years {1914}. While the mean age in a published series was 58 years {1914}, in a recent unpublished series of 33 cases it was 70 years. There was no sex predilection.

Localization
All published cases occurred in the anterior mediastinum. We have observed a single ectopic MNT in the lateral cervical region {1294}.

Clinical features
Clinical features usually are related to the size and local extention of the tumour. With very few exceptions (<5%) {1538},

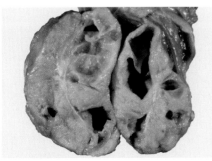

Fig. 3.29 Cystic micronodular thymoma.

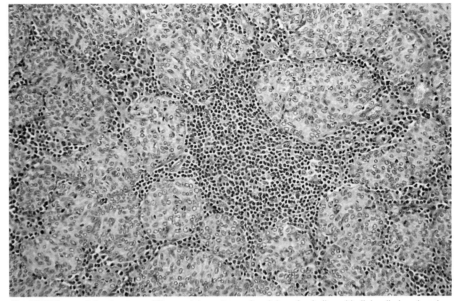

Fig. 3.30 Micronodular thymoma. Micronodular pattern of nodules of spindle epithelial cells in a lymphocyte-rich stroma but with few intraepithelial lymphocytes.

MNT is not associated with paraneoplastic myasthenia gravis. Other autoimmune phenomena that are common in other thymoma types have not been reported.

Macroscopy
Size of MNT varies between 3-15 cm in diameter. Cystic tumour areas of variable size are common macroscopic findings.

Tumour spread and staging
MNT is encapsulated (>90%) or minimally invasive {1914}. Local excision has been unproblematic and curative {1914}. In our own series, two advanced tumours with infiltration of the pericardium and pleura, respectively, were encountered. No tumour-associated deaths have been reported.

Histopathology
Microscopically, MNT is characterized by multiple, discrete or focally confluent epithelial nodules separated by an abundant lymphocytic stroma that may contain follicles with prominent germinal centres surrounded by mantle and enlarged marginal zones. There is a variable number of mature plasma cells. The epithelial nodules are composed of slender or plump spindle cells with bland looking oval nuclei and inconspicuous nucleoli. Rosette formation of epithelial cells may be seen. Nodules contain few interspersed lymphocytes. There are no Hassall corpuscles or perivascular spaces. Mitotic activity is absent or minimal. Micro- and macrocystic areas, particularly in subcapsular localization, are common.

Immunohistochemistry
The epithelial component in MNT stains positive for cytokeratins 5/6 and 19. CAM5.2 and CD57 are positive in about 60% each. CD20 is generally not expressed in the epithelium of MNT {1538}, in contrast to the epithelial component in about half of conventional type A and AB thymomas. Cysts in MNT stain positive for CK 5/6, 7, 8, 19, EMA, and CAM5.2.
The majority of the lymphocytes in MNT are CD20+ B-cells, but mature CD3+CD5+ T cells can outnumber B cells focally. Moreover, immature, Ki67+, CD1a+, CD10+, TdT+ and CD99+ thymocytes are almost always present

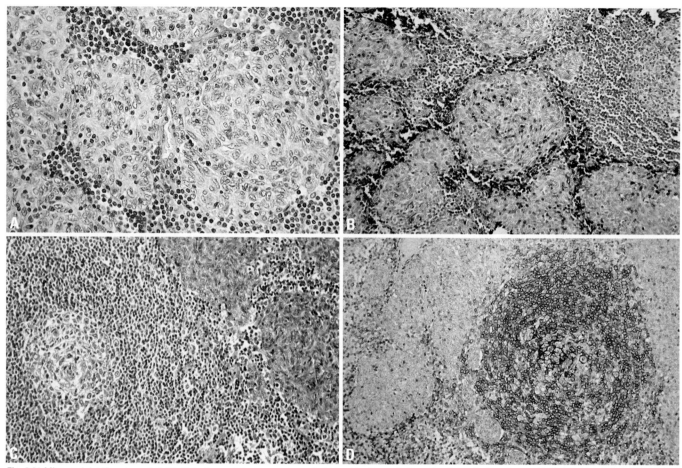

Fig. 3.31 Micronodular thymoma. **A** Epithelial micronodules are composed of bland looking spindle epithelial cells. Few intraepithelial lymphocytes but abundant lymphocytes around epithelial micronodules. **B** CD1a staining showing a few intraepithelial immature T-cells inside the epithelial nodules and in the direct periphery (outside) of the nodules. **C** Histoarchitectural hallmarks are cohesive micronodules of neoplastic epithelia surrounded by a lymphocytic stroma with hyperplastic lymph follicles. **D** CD20 staining of a lymphoid follicle between epithelial micronodules in a case of micronodular thymoma.

{1981} restricted to a narrow band surrounding the epithelial cell nodules, while intraepithelial lymphocytes are scarce.

B-cells frequently form follicles with or without germinal centres with a well developed network of follicular dendritic cells and a population of CD57+ T-cells. Germinal centre B-cells are CD10+ and bcl-2-. Mantle zones consist of IgD+ B-cells, while marginal zones are IgD- and CD23-. Plasma cells are usually polyclonal. In a recent series of 18 MNTs, expansion of monoclonal B cell populations was observed in 33% of cases, with half of them showing features of low grade lymphoma (MALT type and follicular lymphoma) {P. Ströbel et al., submitted}.

Differential diagnosis

MNT should be differentiated from conventional type AB thymomas, which in rare cases may also contain single lymphoid follicles. In contrast to type AB and other organotypic thymomas, the lymphocytic-rich areas in MNT do not contain epithelium. Of note, MNT may rarely (10%) occur together with an otherwise typical type A and AB thymoma {1538,1630}. Single combinations with B2 thymoma have been observed {452}.

Histogenesis

A medullary epithelial cell origin has been postulated {452}.

Prognosis and predictive factors

There have been no reports on recurrences, metastasis or tumour-related deaths.

Metaplastic thymoma

J.K.C. Chan
A. Zettl
M. Inoue
D. de Jong
S. Yoneda

Definition
Metaplastic thymoma is a circumscribed tumour of the thymus in which anastomosing islands of epithelial cells are intermingled with bland-looking spindle cells.

ICD-O code　　　　　8580/1

Synonyms
Metaplastic thymoma has been reported in the literature under the designations "thymoma with pseudosarcomatous stroma", "low grade metaplastic carcinoma" and "biphasic thymoma, mixed polygonal and spindle cell type" {1808,1919, 2210}.

Epidemiology
This rare tumour occurs in adult patients, with a median age of 53 years and mean age of 50.9 years. There is male predominance (M:F ratio 3:1) {1485,1919, 2210,2211}.

Localization
The tumour has not been described outside the thymus.

Clinical features
Most patients are asymptomatic, being incidentally found to have an anterior mediastinal mass, while some present with cough. None of the patients have myasthenia gravis or other paraneoplastic syndromes.

Macroscopy
The tumour is well circumscribed to encapsulated, but can exhibit invasive buds. The cut surfaces show homogeneous, rubbery, grey-white tumour. The reported maximum dimensions of the tumours range from 6-16 cm.

Tumour spread and staging
The Masaoka stage distribution at presentation is as follows: 75% stage I, 17% stage II, 8% stage III {1485,1919,2210, 2211}. Occasional tumours can show infiltration of adjacent tissues {2210} and may recur {2211}.

Histopathology
The tumour is well circumscribed, sometimes with a narrow rim of residual thymic tissue incorporated in its peripheral portion. Occasional cases can show invasion of the surrounding tissues. In contrast to conventional thymomas, it does not show a lobulated growth pattern. Typically, the tumour exhibits a biphasic architecture comprising epithelial islands intertwining with bundles of delicate spindle cells. The two components are present in highly variable proportions from area to area of a single tumour and from case to case.

The epithelial component takes the form of anastomosing islands to broad trabeculae, and often exhibits a squamoid quality or whorled configuration. The constituent cells are polygonal, ovoid or plump spindle, with oval vesicular nuclei, small distinct nucleoli and a moderate

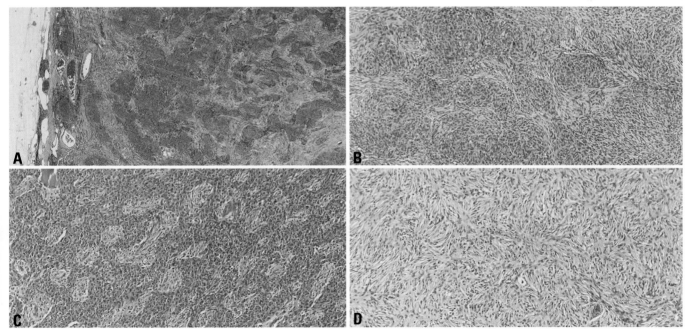

Fig. 3.32 Metaplastic thymoma. **A** The tumour is well circumscribed. A thin rim of residual thymic tissue is incorporated into the peripheral portion. **B** Anastomosing rounded islands of epithelial cells are disposed among spindle cells. **C** Broad trabeculae of epithelium are separated by narrow zones of spindle cells. **D** A storiform growth pattern is seen.

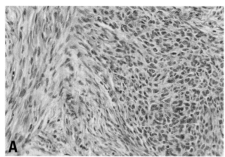
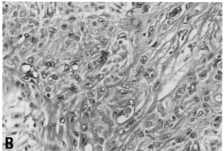

Fig. 3.33 Metaplastic thymoma. **A** The epithelial component (right field) is fairly well delineated from the spindle cell component. The latter comprises slender cells that are bland-looking. **B** The squamoid epithelial island shows enlarged atypical nuclei that are either hypochromatic or hyperchromatic. It is richly traversed by twigs of collagen fibrils.

amount of lightly eosinophilic cytoplasm. Some cells can exhibit large empty-looking nuclei, large hyperchromatic nuclei or nuclear pseudoinclusions. Despite the nuclear atypia, mitotic figures are rare. Twig-like hyaline or sclerotic material may be abundant around and within the epithelial islands.

The spindle cells show a short fascicular or storiform growth pattern. They are often separated by small amounts of loose tissue or delicate collagen fibrils. They are always bland-looking and often mitotically inactive, with fine nuclear chromatin and slender bipolar cell processes. They may show sharp delineation or gradual merging with the epithelial islands. In the rare recurrences, the spindle cells can show nuclear atypia and mitotic activity, associated with acquisition of additional genetic aberrations {2211}. Lymphocytes are usually sparse, but some cases can exhibit a light infiltrate of small lymphocytes and plasma cells. There can be scattered foci of stromal calcification.

While both the epithelial and spindle cell components are readily recognizable in most cases, some cases show marked predominance of one component to the exclusion of the other in some or most areas. A diagnosis of such cases can be difficult without extensive sampling to identify the typical biphasic pattern.

Immunophenotype
Epithelial cells show strong staining for cytokeratin and variable staining for epithelial membrane antigen, and they do not show cell membrane staining for CD5. The spindle cells show focal weak or negative staining for cytokeratin and epithelial membrane antigen, positive staining for vimentin, and inconsistent staining for actin. CD20 is negative. Proliferative fraction (Ki67 index) is low (<5%). The T lymphocytes within the tumour proper usually exhibit a mature immunophenotype (TdT negative). Ultrastructurally, the spindle cells may or may not show epithelial characteristics such as tonofilaments and cell junctions {1485,1919}.

Differential diagnosis
It is most important not to mistake metaplastic thymoma for the vastly more aggressive sarcomatoid carcinoma (car-

cinosarcoma). The latter often shows prominent coagulative necrosis, significant atypia in the spindle cells and readily identified mitotic figures.

Histogenesis
Biphasic metaplastic thymoma is a tumour of thymic epithelial cells. The spindle cell component probably arises as a metaplastic phenomenon, rather than a stromal reaction in view of its marked predominance and presence of genetic aberrations in a recurrent case. Tumour circumscription, relatively bland cytology and usually good prognosis suggest that the tumour is benign. However, lack of association with myasthenia gravis, tumour lobulation and perivascular spaces suggest some relation to thymic carcinoma. Molecular studies, however, favour interpretation of this tumour as a thymoma.

Somatic genetics
Comparative genomic hybridization and microsatellite studies on a limited number of cases have shown no or few genetic alterations, suggesting a closer relationship with type A or type AB thymoma than with thymic carcinoma or type B3 thymoma. Tumour recurrence is apparently associated with acquisition of multiple genetic aberrations.

Prognosis and predictive factors
Among 11 patients with follow-up information, 10 have remained well after surgical excision at 1.5-20 years (median 5 years) {1485,1919,2210,2211}. One patient developed local recurrence at 14 months, and died at 6 years {2211}.

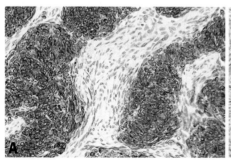
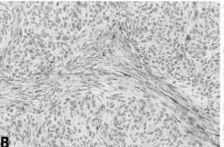
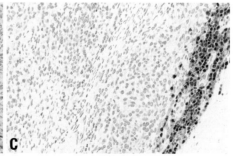

Fig. 3.34 Metaplastic thymoma. **A** Immunostaining for pan-cytokeratin shows strong staining of the epithelial islands. Very few spindle cells are positive. **B** Immunostaining for epithelial membrane antigen shows that the spindle cells are weakly positive, while the epithelial component is only focally positive. **C** Immunostaining for TdT highlights only the thin band of lymphocytes within the incorporated thymic tissue in the periphery. There are no TdT positive cells within the tumour proper.

Rare thymomas

A. Marx
G. Chen
Ph. Ströbel
T.T. Kuo
P.J. Zhang

Microscopic thymoma

ICD-O code   8580/1

Microscopic thymoma is the term applied to usually multifocal epithelial proliferations (<1 mm in diameter) that preferentially occur in myasthenia gravis-associated thymuses (15% of cases) without a macroscopically evident tumour {1580}. Respective epithelial nodules occur at lower frequency in 4% of non-myasthenic control thymuses {1626}. Microscopic thymoma may arise in cortical or medullary thymic compartments {1580}. Histologically, it shows marked heterogeneity and can be composed of bland-looking or more pleomorphic, polygonal or plump spindle cells, usually without intraepithelial immature T-cells. Though microscopic thymoma may occur adjacent to conventional thymoma, its role as a precursor lesion of "macroscopic thymoma" is unresolved {1580}.

Sclerosing thymoma

ICD-O code   8580/1

This is an exceedingly rare tumour (<1%) exhibiting the features of a conventional thymoma in terms of epithelial cell morphology and lymphocyte content, but with exuberant collagen-rich stroma. While some cases were small (<3 cm)

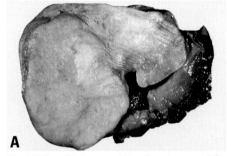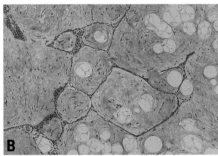

Fig. 3.35 Type B1 thymoma / Lipofibroadenoma. **A** Gross appearance of a composite thymic tumour. The left lower part is a B1 thymoma and the right upper attached mass is a lipofibroadenoma. Note the white yellow colour of the latter. The right lower piece is the thymus. **B** Lipofibroadenoma. A thymic lipofibroadenoma composed of interconnecting thin strands of epithelial cells forming animal-like figures in an abundant fibrous stroma with scattered fat cells.

and probably resulted from tumour regression {1085}, we observed a well circumscribed B2-like thymoma with a diameter of 18 cm exhibiting a collagenous, partially hyalinized stroma harbouring scant and bland looking fibroblasts. There was neither necrosis nor haemorrhage, suggesting that the stroma resulted from a fibrogenic stimulus delivered by thymoma epithelium. The 18-year-old male, non-myasthenic patient remained free of complications after complete resection.

Lipofibroadenoma

Lipofibroadenoma of the thymus is a recently described neoplasm that

occurred adjacent to a conventional type B1 thymoma in a patient with pure red cell aplasia {1096}. The tumour resembles fibroadenoma of the breast, taking the paucity of lymphocytes and the extended narrow strands of epithelial cells into account. With respect to the predominance of stroma over the epithelial component (including rare Hassall corpuscles), the tumour shares morphological features with thymolipoma. As with thymolipoma, it is unknown whether the epithelial, the fibrolipomatous or both components are neoplastic or whether the "lesion" is a hamartoma.

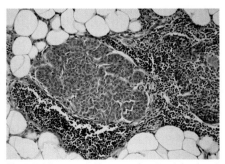

Fig. 3.36 Microscopic thymoma. Small nodule of oval and spindle epithelial cells in an atrophic thymus. There are almost no intraepithelial lymphocytes.

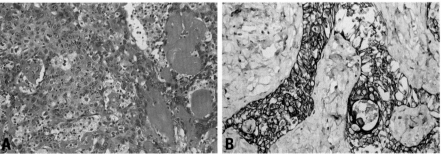

Fig. 3.37 Sclerosing thymoma. **A** Higher magnification shows a residual B3 thymoma in the center of a sclerosing thymoma. **B** Cytokeratin 19 immunoreactivity of epithelial tumour cells resembling a B1 thymoma.

Squamous cell carcinoma

M. Fukayama
T. Hishima
T. Fujii
A. Zettl
Y. Shimosato

Definition
Thymic squamous cell carcinoma is a type of thymic tumour with features of squamous cell carcinoma as seen in other organs, with or without clear-cut evidence of keratinization in routinely stained sections {1094,1691,1806,1808, 1841,1924, 2032,2143}. In contrast to thymomas of the A and/or B categories, thymic carcinomas lack immature T-lymphocytes {632,1748}.

ICD-O code   8070/3

Synonym
Epidermoid keratinizing and nonkeratinizing carcinoma.

Epidemiology
Thymic carcinomas are rare. The incidence of thymic carcinomas occurring in combination with a thymoma has been reportedly 10-20%. Squamous cell carcinoma is the most frequent subtype of thymic carcinoma, and the frequency is higher in Asia (90%) {1510,1808} than in the West (30%) {318,1094,1841, 1924, 2032,2143}. Most cases occur at middle age, and the male to female ratio varies from 1 to 2.3 {1808}.

Localization
Thymic squamous cell carcinoma exclusively presents as an anterior mediastinal tumour, and frequently invades the adjacent lung tissue.

Clinical features
The most frequent symptom is chest pain. Other symptoms are cough, fatigue, fever, anorexia, weight loss, and superior vena cava syndrome. There have been no reports on myasthenia gravis (MG) or pure red cell aplasia, but paraneoplastic polymyositis can occur. A few MG-associated thymomas have been reported to progress to thymic squamous cell carcinoma {1808}.
Thymic squamous cell carcinoma can be detected by imaging techniques. Cystic changes and calcium deposits are rare. A relatively larger size and the lack of septal or nodular structures within the tumour support the diagnosis of carcinoma rather than invasive thymoma {501, 946}.

Macroscopy
Squamous cell carcinomas usually lack encapsulation or internal fibrous septation that are common in thymomas. They are firm to hard with frequent foci of necrosis and haemorrhage.

Tumour spread and staging
Thymic squamous cell carcinomas frequently invade the lungs, pericardium, and major vessels. The most frequent sites of metastases are the lymph nodes (mediastinal, cervical, and axillary), followed by the bone, lung, liver and brain {1808}.

Most cases of thymic squamous cell carcinomas belong to Masaoka stage III and IV at the time of surgery.

Histopathology
There are two hallmarks for the diagnosis of thymic squamous cell carcinoma: the clear-cut cytological atypia in the large epithelial cells that are arranged in nests and cords, and the broad zone of fibro-hyaline-stroma separating the tumour cell nests {1094,1806,1808,1841,1924,

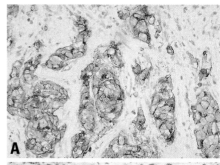
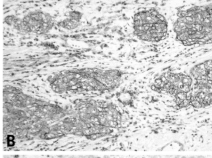
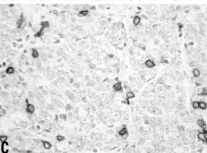

Fig. 3.39 Immunohistochemistry of squamous cell carcinoma of the thymus. **A** Diffuse immunostaining to CD70. **B** CD5 is also expressed in nearly all neoplastic cells. Note the immunolabelling of lymphocytes in the stroma. **C** Neuroendocrine differentiation in thymic squamous cell carcinoma. CD56-positive cells scattered in neoplastic cells.

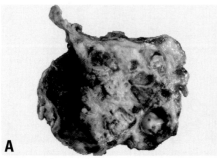
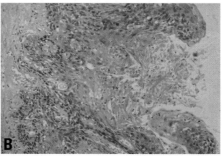

Fig. 3.38 **A** Squamous cell carcinoma occurring in multilocular thymic cysts. Papillary growth of the tumour in a large and haemorrhagic cyst. **B** Well differentiated squamous cell carcinoma, showing papillary growth in the cystic space and invasion of the underlying stroma.

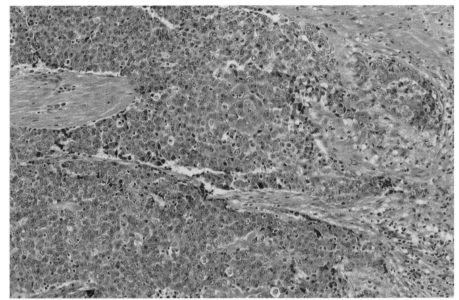

Fig. 3.40 Keratinizing squamous cell carcinoma of the thymus. Large polyhedral cells with cytological atypia, arranged in nests and cords, in fibrohyaline stroma.

2032,2143}. A lobular growth pattern and some remnant perivascular spaces may be recognized. Lymphocytes, when present, are mature and usually admixed with plasma cells.

Squamous cell carcinoma is composed of large polyhedral cells arranged in nests and cords, and shows evidence of keratinization and/or intercellular bridges. The nuclei are vesicular or hyperchromatic, and nucleoli are usually readily apparent. Cytoplasm is eosinophilic. The number of mitotic figures is variable. Foci of spontaneous necrosis are frequently seen, as is the invasion of intratumoural blood vessels.

Immunohistochemistry
The epithelial cells of most thymic squamous cell carcinomas are immunoreactive to CD5, CD70 and CD117 {151,511, 816,851,1059,1887,1978}. Thymomas are negative to CD5 except for some cases of type B3. Squamous cell carcinomas of other organs are negative to CD5 and CD70, and thus both markers are quite useful to confirm the thymic origin of squamous cell carcinomas in the anterior mediastinum. However, tumour cells in nasophayngeal carcinoma and Hodgkin lymphoma may be CD70+. Neuroendocrine markers (chromogranin, synaptophysin, GTP binding protein Go-alpha subunit, or CD56/NCAM) alone or in combination are positive in two-thirds of thymic squamous cell carcinomas in focal or dispersed distribution {852,853, 1139}. Some of these neuroendocrine cells show positivity for alpha-subunit of human chorionic gonadotropin or ACTH {630}.

Differential diagnosis
It is sometimes difficult to exclude the possibility of lung carcinoma showing a prominent extra-pulmonary growth. Palisading or radial arrangement of the cells at the borders of nests as often seen in squamous cell carcinoma of the lung and oesophagus, is not commonly observed. In addition, immunohistochemical evidence (CD5, CD70 and CD117 positivity) may support the thymic origin of the neoplastic squamous cells {632,854}. Infiltration of immature T-cells (CD1a+, TdT+, CD99+) as seen in thymoma is not observed in thymic carcinomas {327,632,1748}.

Well-differentiated squamous cell carcinoma may rarely occur in a thymic cyst {633,1161}. This type of carcinoma needs to be differentiated from the pseudopapillary growth found in the multilocular thymic cyst {1907}, and should be classified in a different category.

Precursor lesions
Some cases of thymic squamous cell carcinoma are thought to arise from pre-existing thymomas based on the observation of combined thymic epithelial tumours that harbour squamous cell carcinoma and conventional (usually B3) thymoma components {1093,1386, 1912}. The two components may be widely separated, or observed in admixture or in a gradual transition within the same tumour mass.

Histogenesis
Thymic squamous cell carcinomas may be derived from thymic epithelial stem cells.

Somatic genetics
Trisomy 8 and der(16)t(1;16) have been reported in a single case of thymic squamous cell carcinoma {1847}. Loss of

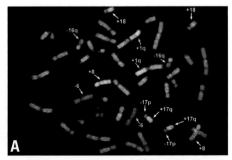
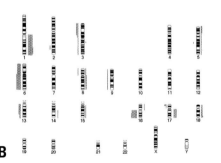

Fig. 3.41 Thymic carcinoma. **A** CGH hybridization of a thymic squamous cell carcinoma shows gain of chromosome 1q, loss of chromosome 6 and loss of chromosome 16q as the typical genetic alterations of this tumour type (highlighted by the yellow arrows; red hybridization signal corresponding to loss, green hybridization signal corresponding to gain of chromosomal material). This case in addition showed loss of chromosome 17p, and gain of chromosomes 8 and 17q (highlighted by the white arrows). **B** Chromosomal ideogram showing gains and losses of chromosomal material in 12 cases of thymic squamous cell carcinoma investigated by CGH. The most frequent recurrent genetic imbalances in thymic squamous cell carcinoma are losses of chromosome 16q (67%), gains of chromosome 1q (60%) and losses of chromosome 6 (50%). (Bars on the right side: gains of chromosomal material, bars on the left side: losses of chromosomal material).

chromosome 16q, 6, 3p, and 17p and gain of 1q, 17q and 18 are frequently observed by comparative genomic hybridization {2238}. Deletion of chromosome 6 {896} and gain of 1q are common alterations in type B3 thymomas, whereas alterations at 3p, 16q, 17p, 17q and 18 are characteristic of squamous cell carcinoma. TP53-overexpression has been observed in most of thymic carcinomas, but the frequency of TP53-overexpression in thymomas varies considerably {339,835,1980,2118}. TP53 gene mutation can be detected in 30% of thymic carcinomas {339}. Inactivation of p16 (CDKN2A) and methylation of promoter region of p16 are relatively more frequent in thymic carcinomas than in thymomas {835}. Bcl-2 expression is observed in nearly all thymic carcinomas, while it is absent in most thymomas except for type A {1979}.

Prognosis and predictive factors
The prognosis of squamous cell carcinoma is largely dependent on tumour stage and grade {1808}. They have a better prognosis than other types of thymic carcinomas with the exception of basaloid carcinoma.

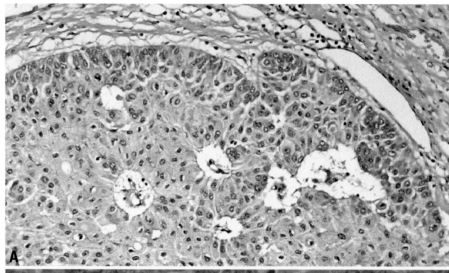

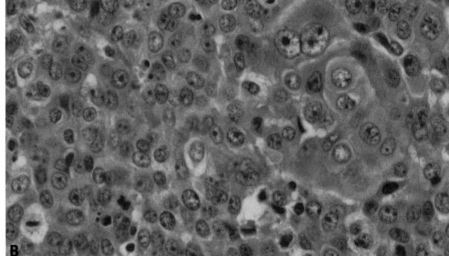

Fig. 3.42 A Thymic squamous cell carcinoma, nonkeratinizing type. In contrast to B3 thymoma, this tumour shows moderate atypia and lacks intraepithelial immature T-cells. The prominent perivascular spaces hint to to the thymic origin of this tumour. **B** Squamous cell carcinoma. Apparent evidence of keratinization, a squamous pearl, within the tumour nest.

Basaloid carcinoma

M.R. Wick
A. Zettl
A.S. Baur
H.K. Müller-Hermelink
A. Marx

Definition
Basaloid carcinoma is a thymic carcinoma composed of compact lobules of tumour cells with peripheral palisading and a basophilic staining pattern due to a high nuclear-cytoplasmatic ratio. Basaloid carcinoma shows a remarkable tendency to originate in multilocular thymic cysts.

ICD-O code   8123/3

Synonym
Basaloid squamous cell carcinoma of the thymus {1663}.

Epidemiology
A very rare variant of thymic carcinoma with only 10 cases reported in the literature so far {861,886,980,1266,1841, 1924,1974}. In a large series of thymic carcinomas, only 5% were basaloid carcinomas {1924}. Most cases occur in the 5th decade of life (reported age range 41 to 65), male and female partients are equally affected.

Clinical features
The symptoms are non-specific. Patients may show symptoms related to a mediastinal mass, e.g. chest pain or dyspnoea. In asymptomatic patients, the tumour may be detected by routine X-ray or during unrelated thoracotomy. No paraneoplastic autoimmune phenomena such as myasthenia gravis are observed.

Etiology
More than half of the reported cases of basaloid carcinoma were associated with a multilocular thymic cyst {886,980, 1841,1974}. Basaloid carcinoma of the thymus may thus incidentally arise within a preexisting multilocular thymic cyst or may induce cystic changes in the non-neoplastic thymus as a reactive response {886}.

Morphology
The tumour size ranges between 5 and 20 cm. Basaloid carcinomas are mostly well-circumscribed, grey to tan masses surounded by a thin fibrous capsule with focal haemorrhage and cyst formation. In about 60% of reported cases basaloid carcinomas were found as a mural nodule in a multilocular thymic cyst and/or showed cystic changes in the tumour.

Microscopically, basaloid carcinoma is composed of rather monotonous, small to medium-sized, columnar, round to oval, or vaguely spindled tumour cells with high nucleo-cytoplasmic ratios, hyperchromatic round to oval nuclei with inconspicious nucleoli, scant amount of amphophilic cytoplasm, and indistinct cytoplasmic borders. The cells are haphazardly arranged in trabeculae, anastomosing cords, islands and nests, and typically show prominent palisading at the periphery with the tumour cells being elongated and radially arranged similar to patterns seen in basal cell carcinoma of the skin. Perivascular spaces can be prominent. Mitoses are frequent. Occasionally, focal keratinization in the centre of the cell nests with concentric whorls of bland, metaplastic-appearing

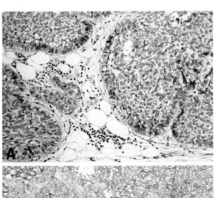
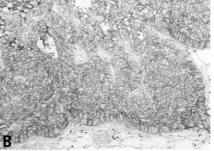

Fig. 3.43 Basaloid carcinoma of the thymus. **A** Sharply outlined islands of basophilic tumour cells showing peripheral pallisading. **B** Strong CD5 immunoreactivity in virtually all tumour cells.

squamous epithelium in continuity with the basaloid cells are noted {886,1924}. In some cases, globular eosinophilic deposits of basement membrane-like material is observed {1663}. There may be tumour areas with numerous poorly formed gland-like, cystic spaces lined by basaloid tumour cells and containing PAS-positive/mucicarmin negative stromal mucin {1663,1924}.

The multilocular thymic cyst frequently associated with basaloid carcinoma is lined by benign appearing squamous epithelium which may imperceptively blend with the basaloid tumour cells.

Immunohistochemistry
On immunohistochemistry, basaloid carcinomas express keratin and EMA. As other thymic carcinomas, they can express CD5 {511}. Basaloid carcinomas are negative for S-100, neurendocrine markers (NSE, chromogranin and synaptophysin) {886,980}.

Differential diagnosis
A mediastinal metastasis of a basaloid carcinoma of other primary location, particularly of the upper and lower respiratory tract needs to be excluded. Neuroendocrine carcinomas may histologically mimic basaloid carcinoma.

Genetics
CGH analysis of a single case of basaloid carcinoma of the thymus showed multiple gains and losses of chromosomal material, among them gain of chromosome 1q and losses of chromosomes 6 and 13. These abnormalities strongly overlap with those previously found in thymic squamous cell carcinomas {2238}.

Prognosis
Initially regarded as low-grade malignancy {1924}, metastasis to lung and liver have been reported in 30% of cases {1266,1841,1924}.

Mucoepidermoid carcinoma

M.R. Wick
A. Marx
H.K. Müller-Hermelink
Ph. Ströbel

Definition

Mucoepidermoid carcinoma of the thymus is a rare morphologic variant of primary thymic carcinoma characterized by the presence of squamous cells, mucus-producing cells and cells of intermediate type. Mucoepidermoid carcinoma of the thymus closely resembles mucoepidermoid carcinomas of other organs.

ICD-O code   8430/3

Epidemiology

This rare tumour comprises approximately 2% of published thymic carcinoma cases {785,1841,1924}. It tends to occur in aged individuals.

Clinical features

Mucoepidermoid carcinomas are not associated with myasthenia gravis and may be asymptomatic {1924}.

Morphology

On macroscopy, the cut surface of mucoepidermoid carcinomas is nodular with fibrous bands and a mucinous appearance {1663,1841}. On histology, the mucous tumour cells are polygonal, columnar or more goblet-like and form solid masses or line cysts {1663,1841}. Mucin-producing cells are strongly PAS-positive {1841}. Areas with squamous differentiation can be solid or form part of a cyst linings. The squamous epithelial cells show minimal to moderate atypia with rare mitoses. The intermediate cells are polygonal or spindle shaped with a moderate amount of eosinophilic cytoplasm and round to oval nucleolus with finely dispersed chromatin.

Postulated cell of origin

Pluripotent epithelial stem cells of endodermal origin have been postulated in the pathogenesis of mucoepidermoid carcinoma of the thymus by some authors {1841}.

Prognosis and predictive factors

Only single case reports on the clinical course have been published. Snover et

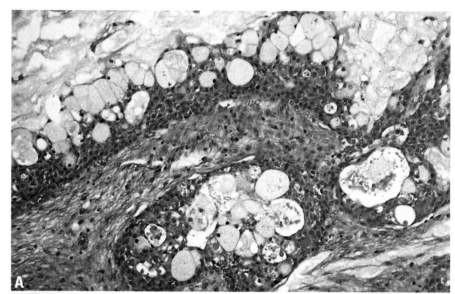
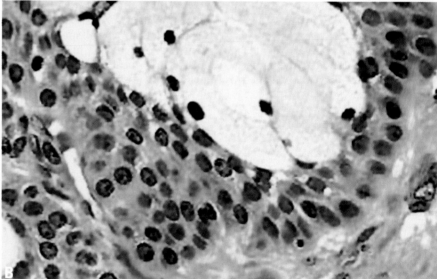

Fig. 3.44 Mucoepidermoid carcinoma of the thymus. **A** Admixture of mucin-producing and squamous cells in a predominantly cystic neoplasms. **B** Higher magnification showing mucin producing cells surrounded by squamous epithelial cells. From J. Rosai and L.H. Sobin {1690}.

al. {1841} described one case of mucoepidermoid carcinoma of the thymus with a "low grade morphology" that was completely resectable and the patient was alive after 28 months. However, a number of cases of "thymic adenosquamous carcinoma" with focal mucin production but a high grade morphology {1663} and unfavourable prognosis have been described {625,1094, 1264,1381,1946,1965,2009,2032,2098}. At the moment, it is not clear whether these cases represent poorly differentiated mucoepidermoid carcinomas or form a separate tumour entity.

Lymphoepithelioma-like carcinoma

T.T. Kuo
J.K.C. Chan
K. Mukai
T. Eimoto
H. Tateyama

Definition
Lymphoepithelioma-like carcinoma (LELC) of the thymus is a primary thymic carcinoma characterized by a syncytial growth of undifferentiated carcinoma cells accompanied by a lymphoplasmacytic infiltration similar to undifferentiated carcinoma of the nasopharynx. Thymic LELC may or may not be associated with Epstein-Barr virus (EBV). However, undifferentiated carcinoma in a dense fibrous stroma without a significant lymphoid infiltration but positive for EBV is tentatively included in this category.

ICD-O code   8082/3

Synonym
Lymphoepithelial carcinoma

Epidemiology
Thymic LELC is a rare tumour. It occurs twice more commonly in male than female patients. The patient's age ranges from 4-76 years with a median of 41 years and a bimodal peak age incidence at 14 years and 48 years {328,343, 785,873,885,889,1094,1472,1876,1924, 2143,2174}.

Localization
Thymic LELC occurs in the anterior mediastinum and usually extends into contiguous structures. Lymph node, lung,

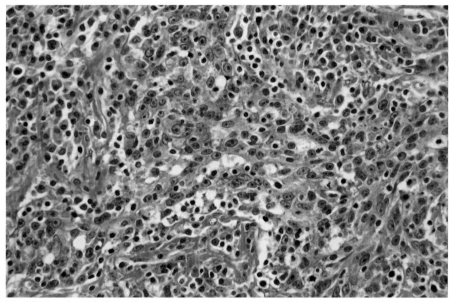

Fig. 3.46 Lymphoepithelioma-like carcinoma of the thymus. Syncytial tumour cells are characterized by large nuclei with open chromatin, prominent nucleoli, and indistinct cytoplasmic membrane. Note the heavy infiltrates of lymphoplasmacytic cells.

liver, and bone are frequent sites for metastasis {785,2143}.

Clinical features
The patients usually complain of dull chest pain, cough, or dyspnoea and constitutional symptoms, but some patients are asymptomatic and incidentally found to have an anterior mediastinal mass upon imaging examination {785,2143}. Superior vena cava syndrome is seen in patients with more advanced disease {785,873,889,2143}. There is no association with myasthenia gravis or other paraneoplastic syndromes, but hypertrophic pulmonary osteoarthropathy has been reported in children {491,873,889,1472}.

Macroscopy
Grossly, the tumour is solid and yellow white with areas of necrosis. It is usually incompletely encapsulated.

Histopathology
Histologically, the tumour is composed of nests or anastomosing cords of carcinoma cells in a lymphoplasmacytic stroma. Germinal centres, eosinophils, and gran-

ulomas may be seen. The tumour cells have large vesicular nuclei with open chromatin and one or more distinct eosinophilic nucleoli and show indistinct cytoplasmic membranes. The nuclei are unevenly crowded and may appear to be overlapping. Lymphocytes are not only present in the stroma, but are also intimately admixed with the carcinoma cells. Mitotic activity is variable but is often pronounced. Foci of tumour necrosis are usually observed. The histopathologic appearances of LELC may overlap with those of poorly differentiated squamous cell carcinoma with a lymphoplasmacytic stroma. Currently, with lack of molecular data on LELC and squamous cell carcinoma of the thymus to determine their relationship, if any, the diagnosis of thymic LELC should be restricted to tumours showing the typical histologic appearances similar to that of nasopharyngeal undifferentiated carcinoma (but allowing for presence of focal primitive squamous cell differentiation in the form of eosinophilic mildly keratinizing cytoplasm). Furthermore, since the so-called "undifferentiated carcinoma" has not

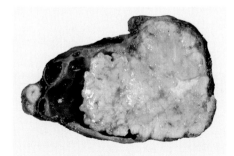

Fig. 3.45 Lymphoepithelioma-like carcinoma (LELC) of the thymus. A solid tumour with an irregular border and a yellow necrotic area. The tumour is growing into a multiloculated cyst on the left side.

been clearly defined for the thymus {1691}, cases that do not show all classical appearances of LELC should not be included under this category.

Immunohistochemistry
The tumour cells are strongly positive for AE1-defined acidic cytokeratins (CKs), and negative for AE3-defined basic CKs. CK7 and CK20 are also negative. CD5 may be expressed focally or not at all {511}. The carcinoma cells also commonly express BCL-2 {338}. The majority of lymphoid cells are CD3+, CD5+, CD1a-, CD99-, and TdT- mature T cells {327}. Smaller numbers of CD20+ B cells are present in the stroma and among the carcinoma cells. Plasma cells that are present are polyclonal.

Histogenesis
Thymic LELC presumably arises from thymic epithelial cells.

Somatic genetics
Overall, approximately 47% of cases of thymic LELC show association with EBV as demonstrated by EBER in situ hybridization or DNA analysis {328,343, 491,873,1472,1876,2174}. EBV is almost always positive in thymic LELC occurring in children and young adults, while EBV positivity rate is lower in adults over the age of 30 years. In two childhood cases studied, the latent membrane protein-1 gene of EBV did not have a 30-base pair deletion as seen in other EBV associated neoplasms {873,1089}. The association with EBV is not related to geographic or ethnic factors {885}. Based on the EBV status, LELCs can be designated as either EBV+ LELC or EBV- LELC pending clinicopathologic and further molecular genetic investigation for their differences. The rare lethal carcinoma with t(15;19) translocation {985,1876} occurring in the mediastinum and respiratory tract of young people may share histologic features of LELC, but it is not associated

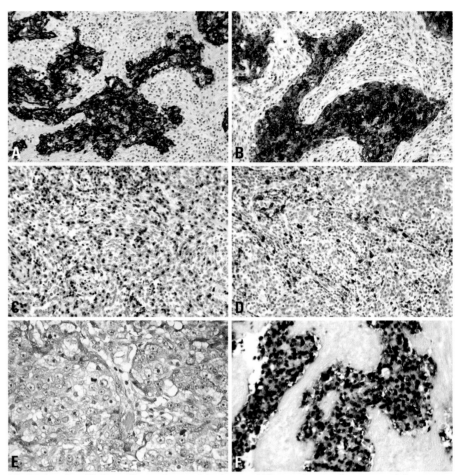

Fig. 3.47 Lymphoepithelioma-like carcinoma of the thymus. **A** The carcinoma cells are strongly immunopositive for AE1-defined acidic cytokeratins. **B** The neoplastic cells are immunopositive for BCL-2. **C** Abundant infiltrating lymphoid cells in lymphoepithelioma-like carcinoma are CD3+ mature T cells. **D** In contrast, only few CD20+ B cells are present. **E** LELC without prominent lymphoid stroma but a syncytial arrangement of large tumour cells with indistinct cell borders, large nuclei and conspicuous nucleoli. **F** Carcinoma cells showing strong nuclear signal of EBER (Epstein-Barr virus early RNA) by in-situ hybridization.

with EBV {616,985}. This unique neoplasm is believed to be a different entity, although no chromosomal genetic information is currently available for thymic LELC.

Prognosis
Thymic LELC is a highly malignant neoplasm with a poor prognosis. The esti-

mated average survival is 16 months in 88% of patients {885}. The presence or absence of EBV does not seem to have prognostic significance.

Sarcomatoid carcinoma

A.C.L. Chan
J. K. C. Chan
T. Eimoto
K. Mukai

Definition
Sarcomatoid carcinoma is a thymic carcinoma in which part or all of the tumour resembles soft tissue sarcoma morphologically.

ICD-O code   8033/3

Synonyms
Carcinosarcoma, spindle cell thymic carcinoma

Epidemiology
Sarcomatoid carcinoma is uncommon and accounts for only up to 7% of all thymic carcinomas {1924}. It is a tumour of late adulthood, predominantly fourth to eighth decades.

Localization
The tumour is located predominantly in the anterior mediastinum, with frequent invasion of the adjacent structures.

Clinical features
The patients present with cough, dyspnoea, dysphagia, chest pain, weight loss, or superior vena cava syndrome {1478,1897,2143}. Imaging studies reveal the presence of a large anterior mediastinal mass.

Macroscopy
Grossly, the tumour is unencapsulated, often with infiltrative borders. The cut surfaces show whitish or greyish fleshy tumour with variable extent of necrosis and haemorrhage. Microcysts may be present.

Tumour spread and staging
The tumour is locally invasive, with frequent invasion of the adjacent pleura, lung and pericardium, and encroachment on the major blood vessels in the mediastinum. Metastases to mediastinal lymph nodes and parenchymal organs (especially the lungs) are common.

Histopathology
Sarcomatoid carcinoma is an infiltrative tumour often with large areas of coagulative necrosis. It shows intimate intermingling of carcinomatous and sarcomatoid components, but the carcinomatous component can be subtle or demonstrable only by immunohistochemistry or electron microscopy in some cases. The carcinomatous component usually comprises cohesive clusters and sheets of poorly differentiated epithelial cells with significant nuclear pleomorphism, and some cases may show obvious squamous differentiation. The sarcomatoid component frequently comprises fascicles and storiform arrays of discohesive spindle tumour cells with pleomorphic nuclei, coarse chromatin, distinct nucleoli and frequent mitotic figures. Heterologous elements may be observed, most commonly rhabdomyosarcomatous and occasionally osteosarcomatous; the term 'carcinosarcoma' is sometimes applied for such cases {534,1478,1509,1841,1897}. In the rhabdomyosarcomatous areas, spindle cells with cross striations and large cells with abundant eosinophilic fibrillary cytoplasm are found. In the osteosarcomatous component, osteoid production by tumour cells is seen.

Immunohistochemically, the carcinomatous component expresses epithelial markers such as cytokeratin and epithe-

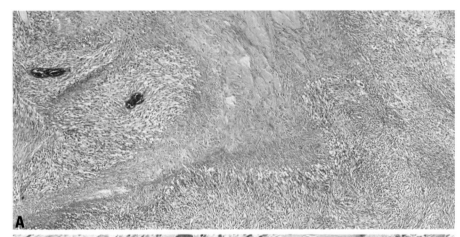
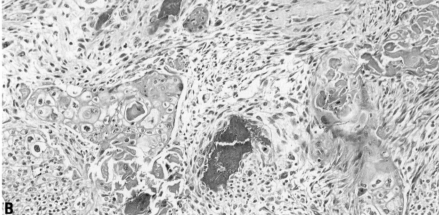

Fig. 3.48 Sarcomatoid carcinoma of the thymus. **A** Usually spindle cells predominate, and there are areas of geographic necrosis. **B** A biphasic pattern is obvious in this case. The carcinomatous component takes the form of a squamous cell carcinoma, and it gradually merges into a spindle cell (sarcomatoid) component.

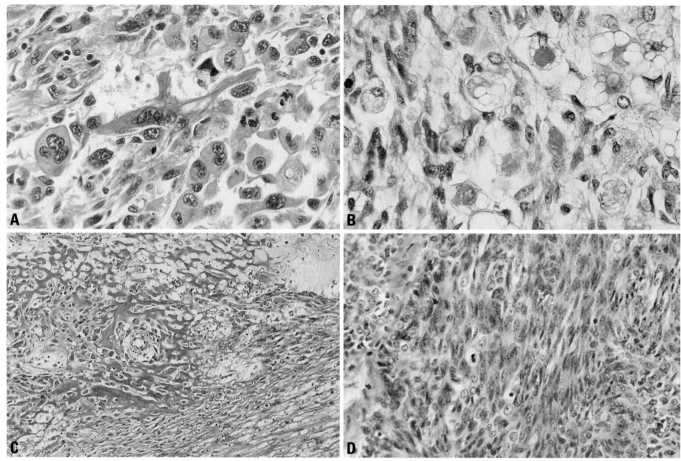

Fig. 3.49 Sarcomatoid carcinoma of the thymus. **A** An elongated rhabdomyoblast with cross-striations is seen among polygonal carcinoma cells with pleomorphic nuclei. **B** Skeletal muscle differentiation characterized by rounded rhabdomyoblasts with vacuolated cytoplasm are interspersed among the spindle sarcomatoid cells. **C** Osteoid formation. **D** So-called spindle cell thymic carcinoma. The tumour comprises sheets and islands of compact atypical spindle cells.

lial membrane antigen. In the sarcomatoid areas, cytokeratin-positive tumour cells range from abundant to scanty or even absent {534,1093,1478,1509,1841, 1897,1916}. Variable expression of myoid markers (e.g. desmin, actin, myogenin, myoD1, myoglobin) is seen in the rhabdomyosarcomatous component {534,1478,1509,1841,1897}. The cases studied for CD5 have been negative for this marker {1093,1916}. Only rare tumours have been examined ultrastructurally, but desmosome-like junctions have been described in the spindle cell area of one case {534}.

Immunohistochemistry
In a tumour where only sarcomatoid component is identified despite extensive sampling, distinction from a sarcoma depends on the demonstration of epithelial differentiation in at least some tumour cells by immunohistochemistry

(e.g. cytokeratin, epithelial membrane antigen) or electron microscopy. Sarcomatoid carcinoma predominated by rhabdomyosarcomatous component may have been confused with mediastinal rhabdomyosarcoma in the literature. The latter sarcoma more commonly affects children and young adults. Although rhabdomyosarcoma can express cytokeratin, the positive tumour cells coexpress myoid markers, whereas at least some tumour cells in sarcomatoid carcinoma express cytokeratin only {534,1509}.
The entity reported as "spindle cell thymic carcinoma" comprises lobules and compact sheets of atypical spindle cells, and is probably an unusual form of sarcomatoid carcinoma. There is frequent transition with thymoma with spindle cell (type A) morphology. The spindle cells show epithelial characteristics and no evidence of true mesenchymal differ-

entiation on immunohistochemical evaluation {1509,1916}.

Differential diagnosis
Sarcomatoid carcinoma has to be distinguished from biphasic metaplastic thymoma, which differs in showing good circumscription of the tumour and bland-looking spindle cells, even though the interspersed squamoid epithelial islands may sometimes show nuclear pleomorphism {1919,2210}.Spindle cell carcinoid can be distinguished from sarcomatoid carcinoma by the presence of delicate fibrovascular septa, granular cytoplasm, generally less striking nuclear pleomorphism, and usually presence of a conventional carcinoid component in some foci; the diagnosis can be further confirmed by positive immunostaining for neuroendocrine markers.
The biphasic pattern of sarcomatoid carcinoma may raise the differential diag-

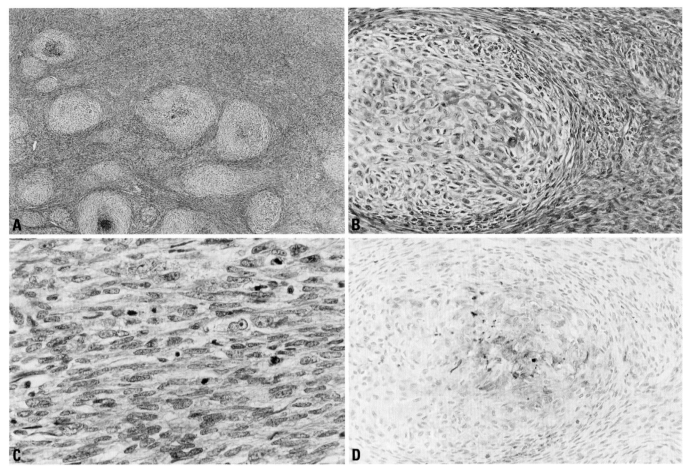

Fig. 3.50 Sarcomatoid carcinoma of the thymus. **A** In this example, pale-staining nodules are disposed among spindle cells. **B** The pale-staining nodules represent areas with subtle epithelial differentiation. This field shows some resemblance to metaplastic thymoma. **C** The sarcomatoid component comprises closely packed spindle cells with moderate nuclear atypia and frequent mitotic figures. **D** Immunostaining for EMA highlights nodular structures.

noses of synovial sarcoma and mesothelioma. Synovial sarcoma differs in showing more monotonous and uniform spindle cells and glandular differentiation in the epithelial component. The diagnosis can be further confirmed by the identification of t(X;18)(p11.2;q11.2) or SYT-SSX1 or SYT-SSX2 gene fusion. Mesothelioma differs in being pleural or pericardial-based, showing papillary-glandular formation in the epithelial component, expressing mesothelial-associated markers (e.g. calretinin), and showing mesothelial differentiation ultrastructurally (e.g. bushy microvilli).

Precursor lesions
Some cases show an identifiable component of thymoma, most commonly with spindle cell (type A) morphology, suggesting transformation from an underlying thymoma {1093,1897,1916}.

Histogenesis
The sarcomatoid component may arise from metaplasia of the carcinomatous component, wherein the tumour cells often gradually lose epithelial characteristics and simultaneously acquire mesenchymal or mesenchymal-like features. Alternatively, the tumour is derived from primitive cells with multidirectional differentiation.

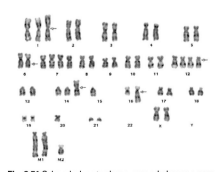

Fig. 3.51 G-banded metaphase spread shows a complex karyotype, including der(16)t(1;16)(q12;q12.1).

Somatic genetics
Only one case has been studied by cytogenetics, with identification of a complex chromosomal abnormality including der(16)t(1;16)(q12;q12.1) {534}. Interestingly, this chromosomal translocation has also been previously reported in a case of thymic squamous cell carcinoma {1847}, suggesting a pathogenetic relationship with thymic squamous cell carcinoma in at least some cases.

Prognosis and predictive factors
Sarcomatoid carcinoma is an aggressive tumour, with most patients dying of disease within three years of diagnosis despite aggressive multi-modality therapy.

Clear cell carcinoma

M.R. Wick
A. Zettl
T.T. Kuo
J.K.C. Chan
A. Marx

Definition
Clear cell carcinoma is a thymic carcinoma predominantly or exclusively composed of cells with optically clear cytoplasm. Thymomas with clear cell features are not included in this group.

ICD-O code   8310/3

Synonym
Carcinoma of the thymus with clear-cell features {797}

Epidemiology
This is a very rare variant of thymic carcinoma, with only 13 "pure" cases reported to date {797,1094,1877,1924,2032, 2166}. Clear cell carcinomas constitute only 3% of all thymic carcinomas {1924}. Clear cell carcinoma has also been reported as a high-grade component in a combined thymoma/thymic carcinoma that, in addition, showed areas of spindle cell (WHO Type A) thymoma, squamous cell carcinoma and undifferentiated carcinoma {1093}. The age range of the reported cases is 33 to 84 years, and the tumour tends to prevail in men (male : female ratio 1.6) {797, 1663}.

Clinical features
Patients may show symptoms related to a mediastinal mass, e.g. chest pain or dyspnoea. Some patients are asymptomatic, with the tumour being detected by routine X-ray or during unrelated thoracotomy. There are no associated paraneoplastic autoimmune phenomena gravis.

Macroscopy
Macroscopically, the reported tumour size ranges between 4 and 12 cm (average 9 cm). The tumours may appear encapsulated and non-infiltrative, or may extensively infiltrate the surrounding tissues. The cut-surface shows solid or cystic tumour with or without haemorrhage and focal necrosis.

Histopathology
Microscopically, clear cell carcinomas of the thymus often show rather bland cellular features which contrast their clinical aggressiveness. Tumour cells are rather monotonous and polyhedral, and usually display slight cellular pleomorphism with round to oval, vesicular nuclei, moderate nuclear atypia, finely dispersed chromatin, and small discernible nucleoli. They have abundant lucent, mostly clear to granular, sometimes faintly eosinophilic, cytoplasm which mostly, but not always is due to accumulation of glycogen. Clear cell carcinomas commonly show a lobulated architecture with nests, lobules or sheets of tumour cells being surrounded by a dense fibrous stroma, and lack the sinusoidal vasculature characteristic of metastatic clear cell carcinoma of the kidney. Rarely, few scattered intratumoral lymphocytes, minute foci of squamous differentiation or focal necrosis are observed. The tumour commonly exhibits an infiltrative growth, with tumour extending into the surrounding mediastinal fat and remnant thymus, even in cases which macroscopically appear well-delineated.

Special studies
Tumour cells usually show strong cytoplasmic diastase-labile PAS positivity, but PAS negative cases have also been reported {1877}. Clear cell carcinomas are keratin positive (cytokeratin 7 expression may be absent), EMA is expressed in 20% of cases studied {797}. As in other types of thymic carcinomas, a subgroup of clear cell carcinomas may

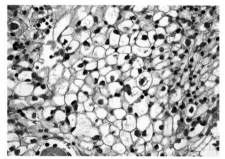

Fig. 3.52 Clear cell carcinoma. Tumour cells have abundant, optically clear cytoplasm and well defined cell membranes {1690}.

express CD5 {511,1093}. They are negative for PLAP, vimentin, CEA and S-100 {797}, and do not contain a population of immature (CD1a- or CD99-positive) T-lymphocytes.

Differential diagnosis
When making the diagnosis of thymic clear cell carcinoma, metastatic clear cell epithelial malignancies, particularly renal, pulmonary and thyroid clear cell carcinoma have to be excluded. Other differential diagnoses include mediastinal diffuse large B-cell lymphoma, mediastinal seminoma, mediastinal parathyroid neoplasms, metastatic clear cell sarcoma or melanoma, glycogen-rich alveolar rhabdomyosarcoma, and clear cell paraganglioma. Furthermore, thymoma with clear cell features must be differentiated from clear cell carcinoma and from combined thymoma/thymic clear cell carcinoma {1093}. Clear cell features are common only in WHO Type B3 thymomas and they are almost always focal {797,2032}. Most tumours show a predominance of conventional B3 areas that exhibit gradual transitions to foci of bland-looking clear cells. While the conventional B3 areas harbour at least few CD1a+ and CD99+ immature T-cells, they may be absent in the clear cell areas. Significant PAS-positivity, necrosis, increased proliferative activity, desmoplastic stroma or TP53 overerexpression are typically absent in clear cell foci of WHO B3 thymomas. By contrast, the clear cell carcinoma (with squamoid features) arising in a WHO Type A thymoma (combined thymoma/thymic carcinoma) was PAS+, showed extensive necrosis, cyst formation and a desmoplastic stromal reaction {1093}.

Prognosis
Clear cell carcinomas are highly malignant, aggressive mediastinal neoplasms with frequent local recurrences and metastases. Most reported patients died of the disease. Deaths are related to metastatic disease or local infiltration of organs in recurrence {797}.

Papillary adenocarcinoma

Y. Matsuno
J. Rosai
Y. Shimosato

Definition

Papillary adenocarcinoma is a rare type of primary thymic carcinoma, characterized by a prominent papillary pattern of growth. Although reports of this tumour are rare, it may be the source of some metastatic papillary carcinomas with psammoma bodies in the cervical lymph nodes of patients without tumours in the thyroid gland.

ICD-O code   8260/3

Synonym

Papillary carcinoma

Epidemiology

Papillary adenocarcinoma of the thymus is a rare neoplasm, and only five cases have been reported {1263}. It affects elderly individuals in their sixth to seventh decades of life. Males and females appear to be equally affected.

Clinical features

Papillary adenocarcinoma generally presents as an enlarging anterior mediastinal mass. The tumour may appear cystic. Paraneoplastic symptoms such as myasthenia gravis or pure red cell aplasia have not been described.

Macroscopy

The tumours are more or less encapsulated, and usually large (measuring 5-10 cm). The cut surface is irregularly lobulated, white and firm. Prominent cyst formation containing serohaemorrhagic fluid may be seen. Adhesion or direct invasion to the adjacent lung, pleura or pericardium is observed in most cases. Pleural implants may be found.

Histopathology

The tumour shows a tubulopapillary proliferation of uniform cuboidal to columnar cells, mainly lying in a monolayer, but occasionally showing a glomeruloid arrangement. The tumour cells have eosinophilic or clear cytoplasm. Their nuclei are round to ovoid, with coarsely condensed chromatin, and a few small but prominent nucleoli. Psammoma bodies may be present. Areas of coagulation necrosis, sometimes massive, are scattered throughout the tumour. Invasion into the adhesive extrathymic tissues accompanied by a dense collagenous stroma may be seen. A small number of tumour cells show positive staining for mucin. The mitotic count may vary from 1 to 7/10 HPF among cases. Permeation of tumour cells into lymphatics such as the subpleural or intrapulmonary perivascular lymphatics may be extensive. In the majority of cases, type A thymoma is found as a component within the tumour mass; one case showed high-grade histology and a predominantly solid and sheet-like growth accompanied by well-developed papillary structures, high-grade atypia and high mitotic rate. In contrast to the other four cases, there was no evidence of a type A thymoma component.

Immunophenotype

Papillary adenocarcinoma shows variable degrees of staining for LeuM1 and BerEP4. CEA and CD5 may also be positive, but CD20, thyroglobulin, pulmonary surfactant apoprotein and calretinin are negative. In addition, CD99-positive lymphocytes are absent, but may be found in the coexisting thymoma portion.

Differential diagnosis

Differential diagnosis of this rare type of thymic carcinoma includes mediastinal thyroid neoplasm (i.e. papillary carcinoma), malignant mesothelioma, germ cell tumour, metastatic adenocarcinoma, and adenocarcinoma of foregut cyst origin {1915}.

Histogenesis

It has been suggested that papillary adenocarcinoma originates from type A thymoma as an expression of malignant transformation {1263}. This is based not only on the morphological similarities between the tubuloglandular or papillotubular structures sometimes seen in type A thymomas and those of the carcinoma, but also the occasional coexistence of a type A thymoma component within the tumour.

Prognosis and predictive factors

Since the number of reported cases is limited, specific information on the histopathologic prognostic factors of papillary carcinoma of the thymus is not available.

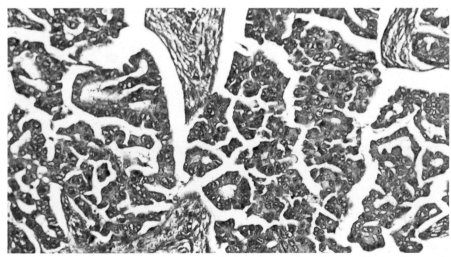

Fig. 3.53 Papillary adenocarcinoma of the thymus. Highly papillary configuration resembling papillary carcinoma of the thyroid {1690}.

Non-papillary adenocarcinomas

H.K. Müller-Hermelink
A. Marx
T.T. Kuo
M. Kurrer
G. Chen
Y. Shimosato

There have been rare reports about non-papillary adenocarcinomas in the thymus. Among them are: an adenocarcinoma with glandular differentiation arising in a thymic cyst {98}, as is also typical for papillary carcinoma {541}; an adenoid cystic carcinoma equivalent to the analogous salivary gland carcinoma {1841}; and a mucinous (colloid) carcinoma of the thymus {360}. The latter case arose in a 15 year old boy and was CD5-negative by immunohistochemistry.

An exceptional tumour in the thymus exhibiting features of a hepatoid carcinoma was observed in a 78 year-old female without an extrathymic neoplasm. The tumour had a diameter of 10 cm, was not encapsulated and virtually devoid of fibrous or inflammatory stroma. Respiratory distress was the only clinical symptom. The tumour recurred locally two years after surgery and responded to radiotherapy. Considering the female sex and protracted clinical course, lack of a yolk sac component and absence of alpha-fetoprotein in the tumour and the patient's serum, a diagnosis of hepatoid carcinoma of thymus appears more likely than a "monophasic" variant of hepatoid yolk sac tumour of the mediastinum {606,1349,1355}.

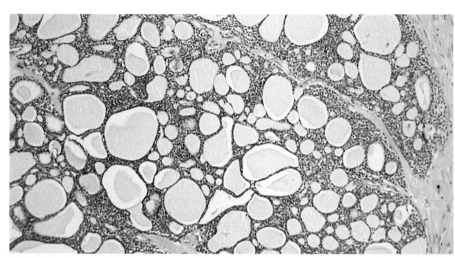

Fig. 3.54 Thymic adenoid cystic carcinoma. This salivary gland-type thymic carcinoma shows a glandular and cribriform pattern.

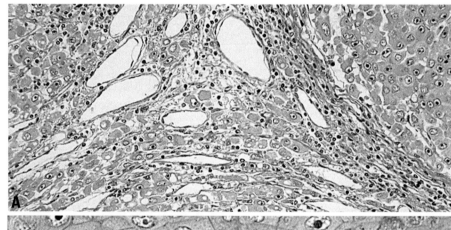

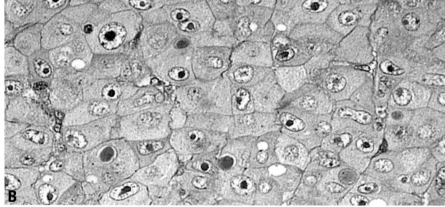

Fig. 3.55 Thymic hepatoid carcinoma. **A** Tumour nodules composed of large polygonal tumour cells resembling activated hepatocytes. No hepatic sinuses, no portal structures and absence of a tumour stroma. **B** Large polygonal cells with abundant eosinophilic cytoplasm. PAS+ globules (immunorecative for alpha-1-antitrypsin, not shown) occurred inside the cytoplasm and in between epithelial cells.

Carcinoma with t(15;19) translocation

A. Marx
C.A. French
J.A. Fletcher

Definition
Carcinoma with translocation t(15;19)(q13:p13.1) is a rare, aggressive and lethal carcinoma of unknown histogenesis arising in the mediastinum and other midline organs of young people.

Synonyms
Aggressive t(15;19)-positive carcinoma, midline lethal carcinoma

Epidemiology
Six cases of t(15;19)-positive carcinoma have been reported {439,616,985, 1081,1148,2072}. All occurred in children or young adults (age range: 5-34 years), particularly females (F : M ratio = 5:1).

Etiology
The etiology of t(15;19)-positive carcinoma is unknown. Epstein-Barr virus does not play a role {985,2072} .

Localization
Translocation t(15;19)-positive carcinoma has been reported to arise in supradiaphragmatic midline organs. Three of 6 cases arose adjacent to the thymus in the mediastinum {985,1081,1148}. Other primary locations were epiglottis {2072}, sinonasal region {616}, lung {439}, and bladder (unpublished findings (C.A.F., J.A.F.)).

Clinical features
Aggressive local invasiveness is characteristic. Intracranial extension occurred in a sinonasal case. Pleural effusions and superior vena cava syndrome are common in thoracic cases. Metastases are common and may involve lymph nodes, lung, bone, skin and subcutaneous soft tissue {2027}.

Histopathology
The presence of undifferentiated, intermediate sized, vigorously mitotic cells is characteristic. Commonly seen are sheets of undifferentiated cells forming syncytia with inter-epithelial lymphocytes, a pattern indistinguishable from

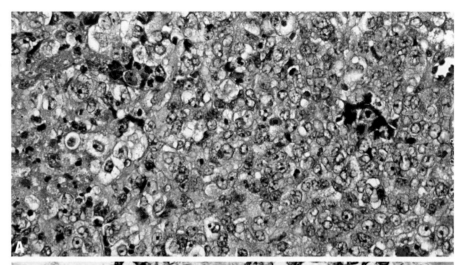

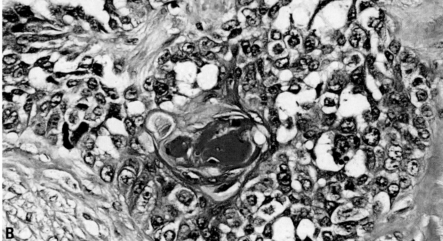

Fig. 3.56 Aggressive carcinoma with t(15;19) translocation. **A** The typical undifferentiated morphology of the tumour may mimic lymphoepithelioma or large cell lymphoma. **B** Focal squamous differentiation can be difficult to find, but is often present either histologically or ultrastructurally.

lymphoepithelioma {616}. Focal squamous differentiation is common {616, 1081,1148}, but not always seen, whereas glandular differentiation (mucoepidermoid carcinoma) {1148}) has only been reported once. Electron microscopy revealed squamous differentiation (rare desmosomes {1081,1148,2072}, tonofilaments {1148,2072}) in three cases. Care must be taken not to confuse the discohesive, undifferentiated round cells of t(15;19)-positive carcinoma with large cell lymphoma or germ cell tumour {616, 985,1081}.

Immunophenotype
The tumours consistently react, at least focally, with pan-cytokeratin markers {616,2072}. Inconsistent and usually focal positivity occurs for vimentin, EMA, and carcino-embryonic antigen (CEA) {985,2072}. CD30, CD45, PLAP, HMB45, S100, and neuroendocrine markers are negative.

Differential diagnosis
This lesion must be distinguished from large cell lymphoma, germ cell tumour, and t(15;19)-negative carcinomas, par-

ticularly lymphoepithelioma-like, poorly differentiated squamous cell, mucoepidermoid, and undifferentiated carcinoma.

Histogenesis

Despite various considerations {616,985, 1081,1148,2072}, derivation of this tumour is unknown.

Somatic genetics

The specific t(15;19)(q13;p13.1) translocation, which generates the 6.4-kb BRD4-NUT fusion oncogenes, is often the only demonstrable cytogenetic aberration. The translocation fuses the 5′ 10 exons of the ubiquitously expressed BRD4 bromodomain gene on chromosome 19 with nearly the entire transcript of the 15q13 gene NUT (nuclear protein in testis), that is normally exclusively expressed in testis {617}. Cytogenetics, fluorescence in situ hybridization (FISH), Southern blotting and RT-PCR studies can identify the translocation {616,617}. Additional chromosomal aberrations are rare {2027}.

Prognosis and predictive factors

All cases reported so far followed an extremely aggressive clinical course (average survival 18 weeks; range 8-38 weeks) {616}.

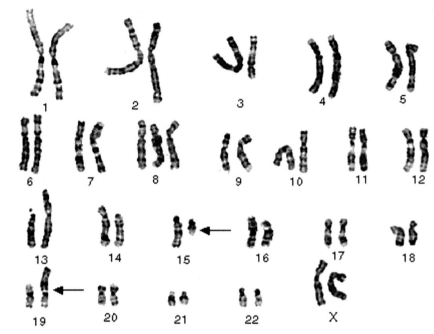

Fig. 3.57 Aggressive carcinoma with t(15;19) translocation. Karyotype from a teenage girl with the t(15;19) carcinoma. A reciprocal translocation involving chromosomes 15q13 and 19p13.1 has occurred. The der (19) contains the functional fusion oncogene.

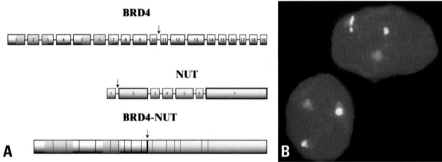

Fig. 3.58 Aggressive carcinoma with t(15;19) translocation. **A** Schematic of the BRD4 and NUT genes disrupted in the t(15;19)(q13;p13.1) chromosomal translocation. Exons are represented by horizontal bars, and introns by connecting lines. All characterized breakpoints (N=2), represented by vertical arrows, occur in intron 10 of BRD4 (gray), and intron 1 of NUT (green), splitting BRD4 roughly in half, and fusing to it nearly the entire NUT transcript. Both bromodomains (pink) of BRD4 are preserved in the fusion oncogene. The oncogenic mechanism is believed, at least in part, to result from unscheduled expression of NUT (normally expressed only in testis) driven by the promoter of BRD4, which is ubiquitously expressed. **B** Fluorescent in situ hybridization (FISH) depicting the t(15;19)(q13;p13.1) in a paraffin section. The red-green probe doublet, which normally flanks the NUT gene on chromosome 15, is split apart by the translocation.

Undifferentiated carcinoma
of the thymus

A. Marx
Ph. Ströbel
J.K.C. Chan
G. Chen
H.K. Muller-Hermelink

Definition
A thymic carcinoma growing in a solid, undifferentiated fashion but without sarcomatoid (spindle cell, pleomorphic, metaplastic) features {1924}.

ICD-O code
8020/3

The diagnosis of this rare type of thymic carcinoma is one of exclusion. Defining its epithelial nature usually requires immunohistochemistry. In children and young adults, carcinoma with t(15;19) translocation should be excluded by cytogenetics or RT-PCR {617,1081}. The most important differential diagnosis in adults is large cell carcinoma in the lung extending or metastasizing to the mediastinum.

Small cell carcinoma without (immunohistochemically) recognizable differentiation is traditionally classified among the neuroendocrine carcinomas of the thymus.

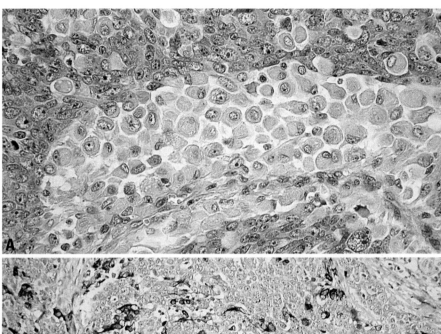
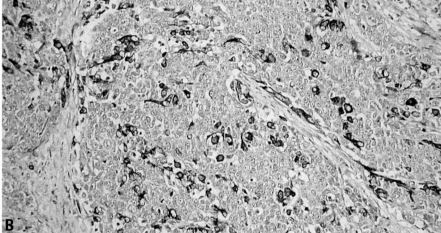

Fig. 3.59 Undifferentiated thymic carcinoma. **A** A solid growth pattern composed of large polygonal to round tumour cells, large nuclei and a slightly basophilic cytoplasm. No keratinization, no intercellular bridges, no glandular differentiation, no sarcomatoid features and no EBER expression by in situ hybridization. The prominent population of bland looking myoid cells with round inconspicuous nuclei and eosinophilic cytoplasm unequivocally identifies this carcinoma as a tumour of thymic differentiation. Myoid cells show no significant proliferative activity (in contrast to rhabdomyosarcoma cells). **B** Desmin staining demonstrates intratumorous myoid cells.

Thymic neuroendocrine tumours

A. Marx
Y. Shimosato
T.T. Kuo
J.K.C. Chan
W.D. Travis
M.R. Wick

Definitions

Thymic epithelial tumours that are predominantly or exclusively composed of neuroendocrine cells are classified as neuroendocrine carcinomas (NECs) of the thymus {1691}. They have to be distinguished 1) from otherwise typical thymic carcinomas, which may contain scattered or groups of neuroendocrine cells {853,1091,1139}, and 2) from non-epithelial neurogenic tumours, particularly paragangliomas

Neuroendocrine differentiation can be demonstrated by immunohistochemistry (positivity for chromogranin, synaptophysin, neuron-specific enolase, CD56) and/ or by ultrastructural identification of neurosecretory granules.

Neoplasms combining features of NEC and either thymoma or thymic carcinoma are included in the category of "combined thymic epithelial tumours"

Since the seminal work of Rosai and Higa, thymic neuroendocrine tumours that are "related to carcinoid tumours" have been distinguished from thymomas {1686,1688,2144}. The epithelial neuroendocrine tumours of the thymus comprise typical and atypical carcinoids, as well as large and small cell carcinomas.

Well differentiated neuroendocrine carcinomas

In line with the nomenclature of neuroendocrine tumours occurring in other sites of the body, it is proposed that thymic carcinoids be termed *well differentiated neuroendocrine carcinomas of the thymus* {349,1691}. The rationale for considering all these tumours as carcinomas {1691} is the observation that even "innocent" looking and encapsulated carcinoids bear a significant risk for recurrence, metastasis and tumour-associated death {628,1845,2140}. The carcinoids are further subdivided into typical and atypical carcinoids.

ICD-O codes

Typical carcinoid	8240/3
Atypical carcinoid	8249/3

Typical and atypical carcinoids

Following the introduction of the term "atypical carcinoid" by Arrigoni et al. in 1972 for a subgroup of moderately aggressive neuroendocrine neoplasms of the lung {75}, it became clear that the vast majority of carcinoids in the thymus correspond to atypical carcinoids when the same criteria are applied as in the lung {450,628,723,1361,1688,1808, 2062,2140}. As a group, atypical carcinoids more often show a diffuse growth pattern, advanced stage disease, and a higher degree of cytologic atypia {723, 1362,1691,1808,2062}.

Since virtually all thymic carcinoids are atypical carcinoids (see epidemiology), most studies report thymic carcinoids to have a worse prognosis compared with bronchial carcinoids {628,1361,1808, 2136}. However, varying criteria have been used for definition of atypical carcinoids of the thymus in these series {628, 1361,1845,2062}. In fact, the only clinico-pathological study applying WHO-defined criteria to classify atypical thymic carcinoids {723} challenged the view that thymic atypical carcinoids are clinically more aggressive than morphologically identical carcinoids of the lung. A better prognosis of atypical thymic carcinoids as compared to pulmonary carcinoids was even suggested by a recent study {1049} (5-year and 10-year survival rates of 84% and 75% respectively, compared with 87% and 87% for pulmonary typical carcinoids and 56% and 35% for pulmonary atypical carcinoids {2028}).

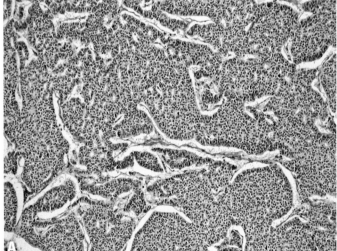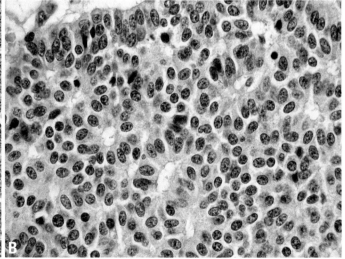

Fig. 3.60 Typical carcinoid. **A** Solid and trabecular growth pattern. Note absence of necrosis and mitoses. **B** On high magnification, rosettes, and bland cytology can be seen, but no mitoses.

Table 3.06
Classification of thymic neuroendocrine tumours (Neuroendocrine carcinomas, NECs) {1691}.

Neuroendocrine Carcinomas (NECs)			
Well-differentiated NEC		Poorly differentiated NEC	
Typical Carcinoid	*Atypical Carcinoid*	*LCNEC**	*SCC***
No necrosis; <2 mitoses per 2 mm^2 (10HPF)	Necrosis present and/or 2-10 mitoses per 2 mm^2 (10 HPF)	Non-small cell NEC with >10 mitoses per 2 mm^2 (10 HPF)	Small cell cytology
Morphological Variants Spindle cell type Pigmented type With amyloid (extrathyroidal medullary carcinoma) Oncocytic/oxyphilic type Mucinous Angiomatoid type Combinations of the above variants			*Variants* SCNEC combined with Non-NECs
Thymic NECs with shared features of (atypical) carcinoid and LCNEC/SCC Carcinoid with sarcomatous change ("metaplastic NEC")			

*LCNEC, large cell neuroendocrine carcinoma;
**SCC, small cell carcinoma; HPF, high power field

Poorly differentiated neuroendocrine carcinomas

Small cell carcinoma (SCC, neuroendocrine type) and large cell neuroendocrine carcinoma (LCNEC) of the thymus are considered *poorly differentiated neuroendocrine carcinomas of the thymus.*

ICD-O codes
Large cell neuroendocrine
carcinoma   8013/3
Small cell carcinoma,
neuroendocrine type   8041/3

Definitions
Four major categories of thymic neuroendocrine neoplasms are recognized:
Typical (classic) carcinoid. A carcinoid tumour comprised of polygonal cells with granular cytoplasm arranged in ribbons, festoons, solid nests and rosette-like glands. Tumours have less than 2 mitoses per 2 mm^2 (10 HPF) and necrosis is absent.
Atypical carcinoid. A carcinoid tumour with architectural features of the classic type but exhibiting a greater degree of mitotic activity and/or foci of necrosis (including comedonecrosis).

Small cell carcinoma, neuroendocrine type. A high-grade thymic tumour consisting of small cells with scant cytoplasm, ill-defined cell borders, finely granular nuclear chromatin, and absent or inconspicuous nucleoli. The cells are round, oval or spindle-shaped, and nuclear molding is prominent. The mitotic count is high. The morphologic features are indistinguishable from those of small cell carcinoma arising in the lung. Variant: Combined small cell carcinoma: A small cell carcinoma that also contains a component of non-small cell carcinoma such as squamous cell carcinoma or adenocarcinoma.
Large cell neuroendocrine carcinoma: A high-grade thymic tumour composed of large cells with neuroendocrine morphology such as palisading, trabeculae, nesting or rosette-like features; necrosis that is usually extensive; a high mitotic rate; and either neurosecretory granules by electron microscopy or positive neuroendocrine immunohistochemical markers.

Basis of the classification
Considering the paucity of data on clinicopathological correlations in thymic NECs {723,1361,1845} as compared to the statistically better analyzed pulmonary NECs {128,218,2023,2026}, the first edition of the WHO classification of tumours of the thymus {1691} suggested thymic neuroendocrine tumours to be classified using the same criteria applied for NECs of the lung {218}. Although this approach was not based on sufficient statistical data, it was meant to provide a morphological basis from which prospective and retrospective clinical studies

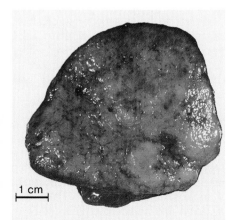

Fig. 3.61 Atypical carcinoid. Macroscopy of a well circumscribed tumour.

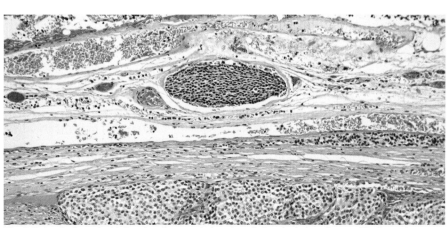

Fig. 3.62 Atypical carcinoid. Despite circumscription, there is lymphatic invasion outside the main tumour mass.

are launched to generate statistical data. This approach is maintained in the present edition of the WHO classification.

Epidemiology

Thymic NECs are rare, constituting 2-5% of thymic epithelial tumours {723,1361, 1808,2062}. In contrast to the lung {218, 1128,2023}, the great majority of cases are represented by atypical carcinoid. MEN-1-associated thymic NECs have all been carcinoids and occurred almost only in male adults (31-66 years; mean 44 years) {1987,1989}.

Epidemiological data on typical carcinoids are lacking. Atypical carcinoids are mainly tumours of adults (18–82 years; mean 48-55 years in both males and females) {723,1361,1845,2062}, but have also been rarely observed in children (8-16 years of age) {666,1185}. There is a male preponderance (M:F = 1:2-7) {528,723,1361,1845}.

By contrast, small cell carcinomas show no gender predilection and the patients on average are slightly younger {1094, 2032,2143}. The case of thymic large cell neuroendocrine carcinoma reported by Chetty occurred in a 68 year-old male patient {349}.

Etiology

About 25% of patients with thymic carcinoids have a positive family history of MEN-1 {1989}. Conversely, among MEN-1 patients, thymic carcinoids were found in 8% of cases {681}. Since thymic NECs cluster with only a minority of MEN-1 families, exhibit diverse mutations and are not associated with loss of heterozygosity (LOH) at the 11q13 (*MEN-1*) locus, it appears that genetic alterations in addition to *MEN-1* abnormalities (possibly involving a tumour suppressor gene(s) on chromosome 1p) are required for thymic carcinoids to develop {1988, 1989}. The role of a MEN-2 genetic background for the development of thymic carcinoids is less clear {1239}.

Localization

Thymic neuroendocrine carcinomas occur in the anterior mediastinum. A single case occurring in an ectopic thymus adjacent to the thyroid has also been published {900}.

Clinical features

Most poorly differentiated neuroendocrine carcinomas and about 50% of

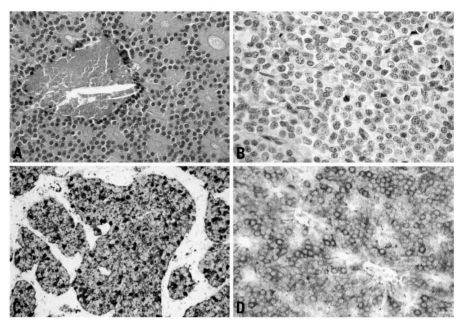

Fig. 3.63 Atypical carcinoid. **A** Striking rosette formation and a "punctate" area of necrosis (comedonecrosis). **B** Mitotic figures are seen. **C** Cytokeratin expression (Cam5.2; immunoperoxidase). **D** Strong chromogranin A staining.

well differentiated neuroendocrine carcinomas exhibit local symptoms (chest pain, cough, dyspnoea, or superior vena cava syndrome) {723,1361,1845}.

Carcinoid syndrome is exceedingly rare (<1%) {1845}. On the other hand, 17-30% of adult and >50% of childhood carcinoids of the thymus are associated with Cushing syndrome due to ACTH production {456,1845,1918}. In fact, 10% of all cases of "ectopic ACTH syndrome" are due to thymic carcinoids {162,2095}. Cutaneous hyperpigmentation due to tumour-derived alpha-MSH frequently accompanies and, rarely, precedes Cushing syndrome {666}. Cushing syndrome is exceptionally rare in thymic SCC {812}.

Acromegaly (due to tumour-derived GHRH) {924}, and inappropriate production of antidiuretic hormone or atrial natriuretic peptide {1507} are uncommon.

Hypercalcaemia/hypophosphataemia in thymic carcinoid patients may result either from tumour production of PTHrP {2214} or from primary hyperparathyroidism in the context of the MEN-1 syndrome {1989}.

MEN-1-associated thymic NECs are typically insidious tumours (carcinoids) that manifest by local symptoms, metastases, disturbances of calcium/phosphate metabolism or, rarely, with acromegaly {196}, while Cushing syndrome has not been reported {1988,1989}. Paraneo-plastic

autoimmune disorders, such as the Lambert-Eaton myasthenic syndrome, are very rare.

Macroscopy

Thymic carcinoids and poorly differentiated thymic NECs are virtually identical macroscopically. The majority are unencapsulated and can appear either circumscribed or grossly invasive. The size ranges from 2–20 cm (mean 8 -10 cm) {450,1361}. Cases associated with Cushing syndrome tend to be smaller (3-5 cm) due to earlier detection. They are grey-white and firm on cut section, can have a gritty consistency, and usually lack the characteristic lobulated growth pattern of thymomas. Oncocytic/ oxyphilic variants may show a tan or brown cut surface. Foci of haemorrhage and necrosis are apparent in 70% of cases {2137}. Calcifications are frequent in thymic NECs (30%) compared with extrathymic NECs {924}.

Tumour spread and staging

Locally restricted atypical carcinoids (encapsulated pT1 or infiltrating the mediastinal fat or thymus pT2) make up 40-50% of cases, but half of them exhibit local metastasis (pN1) {723,2062}. Invasion into adjacent organs (40-50%, pT3) or pleural or pericardial cavity (10%, pT4) is common {723,2062}.

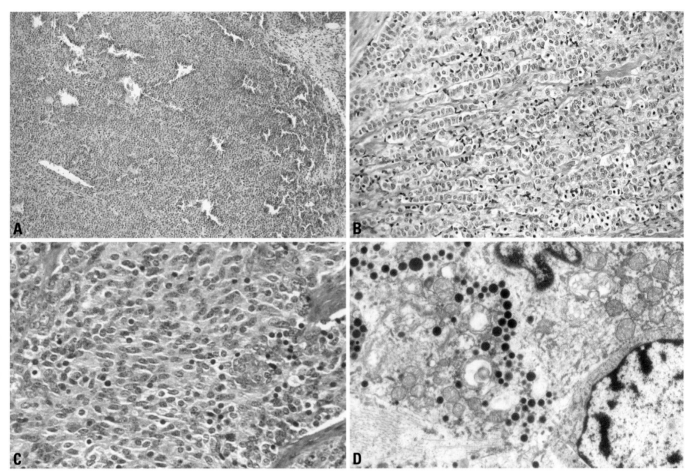

Fig. 3.64 Atypical carcinoid. **A** Solid growth pattern. **B** Trabecular growth pattern. **C** Spindle cell variant of carcinoid. **D** Spindle cell carcinoid. Transmission electron microscopy showing distinct electron dense neurosecretory granules of variable size in the cytoplasm of a tumour cell.

Metastases are present in 30-50% of cases {723,1845}. Lymph node metastases can involve mediastinal, cervical and supraclavicular lymph nodes {924} or they can be systemic {723}. Haematogenous metastasis to bone, liver, skin, brain, kidney, heart, adrenals and soft tissues have been reported {723,1013, 1845,2143}. Pericardial and pleural cavities can be sites of late NEC recurrences (up to 9 years after resection) {2035}.

Only very few cases of stage II *SCC* have been reported {1808,1841}, one with distant metastases {1841}. The vast majority of SCC are in stage III or IV {812,1094, 1841,2143}, and about half of them show lymph node or haematogenous metastases {1094,2032}.

Histopathology of well differentiated neuroendocrine carcinomas

Typical carcinoids

By definition, these are devoid of necrotic areas and exhibit a low mitotic rate (<2 mitoses per 2 mm² or 10 HPF using certain microscopes). The "classic" carcinoid can show a variety of "organoid" features: ribbons (trabeculae), festoons, solid nests, rosettes, glandular structures, and nuclear palisades, accompanied by a richly vascularized stroma. The trabecular and rosette patterns are the commonest, being found in over 50% of cases. The tumour cells are uniform and polygonal, with relatively small nuclei, finely granular chromatin, and eosinophilic granular cytoplasm. Lymphovascular invasion is common.

Atypical carcinoids

These show (1) areas of necrosis and a maximum of 10 mitoses per 2 mm² (10 HPF) of non-necrotic tumour area or (2) absence of necrosis but a proliferation rate of 2-10 mitoses/2 mm² or 10HPF. All architectural features of typical carcinoids can occur. Even small "punctate" area of necrosis (comedonecrosis) in an otherwise typical carcinoid justifies a diagnosis of "atypical carcinoid". Compared to typical carcinoids, atypical carcinoids more frequently show some degree of nuclear pleomorphism including rare "anaplastic" cells {723}, a focal diffuse growth pattern (so-called "lymphoma-like") {723,1361,1845,2062} or extensive desmoplastic stroma with Indian filing of tumour cells {2136}. Calcifications are also more characteristic of atypical carcinoids (up to 30% of cases) {924}.

Variants of thymic carcinoids

The morphologic variants should be assessed as being "typical" or "atypical" using the criteria listed above. Among the reported cases, almost all are classifiable as atypical carcinoids.

Spindle cell carcinoid

This is the commonest thymic carcinoid variant, being predominantly or totally composed of spindle cells often arranged in fascicles. Occasionally, spin-

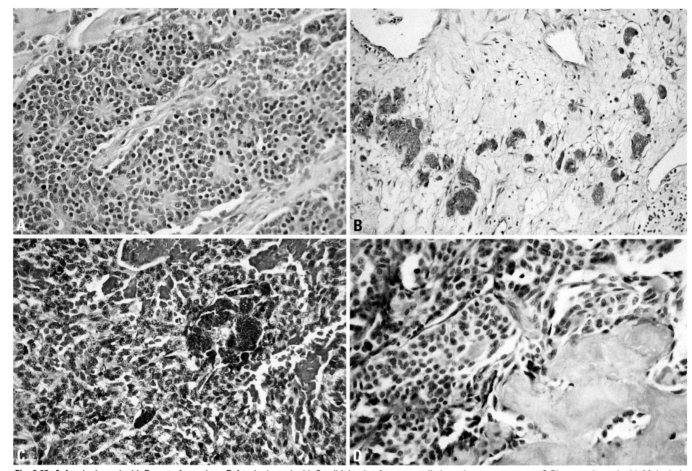

Fig. 3.65 A Atypical carcinoid. Rosette formation. **B** Atypical carcinoid. Small islands of tumour cells in oedematous stroma. **C** Pigmented carcinoid. Melanin is present in the cytoplasm of some tumour cells. **D** Carcinoid with amyloid. Tumour cells are accompanied by deposits of extracellular amyloid.

dle cell carcinoid can be admixed with a classic carcinoid {1169,1691,2141}.

Pigmented carcinoid
This variant of thymic carcinoid is characterized by presence of intracytoplasmic melanin (neuromelanin) in a variable number of tumour cells. Melanosomes can be detected by electron microscopy. There can be admixed melanophages containing phagocytosed melanin granules with a coarser appearance. Pigmented tumour cells can exhibit an otherwise classic or spindle cell morphology. This variant has also been reported to be associated with Cushing syndrome {857,1028,1114}.

Carcinoid with amyloid
This variant is accompanied by amyloid deposition in the stroma that can be identified by Congo stain {2141}. The tumour cells are usually spindle shaped and immunorective for calcitonin, so that the tumour is indistinguishable from medullary carcinoma of the thyroid

("extrathyroidal medullary carcinoma"). The histogenesis of this tumour is unclear. A derivation from extra-thyroidal C-cells or a thymic epithelial origin has been postulated {1691}.

Oncocytic/oxyphilic carcinoid
This is a rare variant that is composed of polygonal, large tumour cells with oxyphilic cytoplasm due to accumulation of mitochondria {1362,2183}. Oncocytic carcinoid is rarely associated with MEN-1 or Cushing syndrome {1362,2183}.

Mucinous carcinoid
This is a very rare variant that exhibits an alcian blue-positive mucinous stroma {1501,1911}. The tumours are often large (>8 cm) and can resemble metastatic mucinous carcinoma, such as from the gastrointestinal tract or breast. The stromal mucin is believed to result from regressive changes rather than production by the tumour cells. There can be a focal component of classic carcinoid.

The few reported cases have not been associated with Cushing syndrome.

Angiomatoid carcinoid
This rare variant resembles haemangioma macroscopically and microscopically due to the presence of large blood-filled cystic spaces. However, closer scrutiny shows that the spaces are lined by polygonal tumour cells but not endothelial cells {1360}.

Carcinoid with sarcomatous change
Carcinoids in combination with a sarcomatous tumour areas have been described rarely, and have pursued a highly aggressive clinical course {1090, 1557}. The sarcomatous component shows fibrosarcomatous, myoid, osseous or chondroid differentiation. The cases have been interpreted as examples of dedifferentiation or divergent development from a common precursor rather than collision of two clonally unrelated tumours.

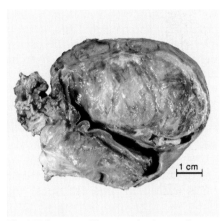

Fig. 3.66 Sarcomatoid neuroendocrine carcinoma.

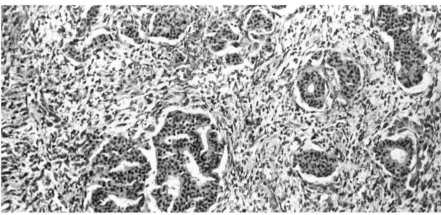

Fig. 3.67 Sarcomatoid neuroendocrine carcinoma. Sarcomatoid neuroendocrine carcinoma exhibiting a well differentiated and a sarcomatoid spindle cell components.

Carcinoids as components in other combined tumours

Carcinoids can be admixed with thymic small cell carcinoma (see below), and with thymoma or thymic carcinoma, particularly squamous cell carcinoma, adenosquamous carcinoma or undifferentiated carcinoma {1094,1783, 1913}.

Three examples of carcinoid (including one goblet cell carcinoid {1124}) have been reported as components of mature cystic teratomas of the thymus {1124, 1707,1787}. Two of the three patients (age: 43–63 years) were females. The reported outcome was favourable after complete surgical removal, but follow-up time was short.

Poorly differentiated neuroendocrine thymic carcinomas

Large cell neuroendocrine carcinoma (LCNEC)

LCNECs of the thymus are non-small cell NECs with a mitotic rate of > 10 per 10 HPF {1691}. Necrosis is almost always present and often extensive. The higher mitotic rate is the essential differentiating feature of this tumour from atypical carcinoid. In addition, large tumour cell size, including frankly anaplastic giant cells, are more common than in atypical carcinoids {349,723,1361}. Neuroendocrine-type architectural features, such as nesting, cribriform, trabecular, and rosetting, may occur but are often less well developed compared with atypical carcinoids {1691}.

LCNEC of the thymus cannot be distinguished from its pulmonary counterpart by morphology alone. Careful clinico-pathological correlation is essential to distinguish between primary thymic LCNEC and metastasis of an extrathymic LCNEC to the mediastinum.

Small cell carcinoma (SCC, neuroendocrine type) of the thymus

In contrast to carcinoids and LCNEC, the tumour cells of SCC are small (usually <3x diameter of a lymphocyte) and cytoplasm is very scant. Mitotic activity is usually higher than in other types of NEC. Nuclei can be round, oval or spindly, the chromatin is finely granular, and nucleoli are inconspicuous. Apoptotic bodies are often numerous. Evidence of neuroendocrine differentiation is usually supported by immunohistochemistry (chromogranin; synaptophysin; NCAM/CD56). Clinical imaging studies SCC are important for distinction between primary thymic origin and mediastinal metastasis, which is much more frequent than thymic SCC.

Immunophenotype

NECs are virtually all immunoreactive for broad spectrum cytokeratins (AE1/3, CAM5.2), often showing a dot-like staining. In contrast to Merkel cell carcinoma, cytokeratin 20 is not expressed in small cell carcinomas of neuroendocrine type (SCNECs) {326}.

Endocrine differentiation is revealed by reactivity with antibodies to neuroendocrine markers: synaptophysin, chromogranin, neuron-specific enolase (NSE) and NCAM/CD56. NCAM and NSE are slightly more sensitive (about >90% each) {1808} than chromogranin (70-90%) {1362,1845}, and synaptophysin (70%) {1362}. Most *carcinoids* and prob-ably also *LCNEC* express at least two of these markers in >50% of tumour cells {853,1362,1845,2062}.

Hormones can be detected in most thymic NECs in a variable (and sometimes very low) number of tumour cells. Expression of ACTH, HCG (alpha-subunit more than beta-subunit {853}), somatostatin, beta-endorphin, cholecystokinin, neurotensin, calcitonin {820, 1808,2062,2140}, is quite common, while serotonin, gastrin, and parathormone are uncommon {1845,1953}. Multihormonal tumours appear to be frequent {820, 853,1953}. Of note, there is no close correlation between the hormones detected by immunohistochemistry and the clinical symptoms {820}.

Nuclear expression of TTF-1 is absent in the vast majority of thymic carcinoids {1513} and LCNEC (our experience), though more cases need to be studied under defined conditions. TTF-1 data on thymic SCC are limited; three cases studied have been negative {351,975}.

Postulated cell of origin

Not definitively known. The relatively common occurrence of mixed NECs, squamous cell carcinomas of the thymus and the rare occurrence of neuroendocrine carcinoma associated with thymom argue in favour for a common thymic epithelial precursor as the progenitor of thymic NECs {2137}.

Somatic genetics and genetic susceptibiliy

Classical cytogenetic or comparative genomic hybridization data on sporadic thymic NECs have not been published. In a small series of MEN-1-associated

NECs, 2 of 7 cases show losses in the 1p region, while LOH at the MEN-1 locus at 11q13 is consistently absent {1989}. Therefore, a tumour suppressor gene on 1p, in addition to MEN-1 mutations, has been considered a candidate playing a role in the oncogenesis of thymic NECs. In one study of atypical carcinoids, DNA cytometry revealed aneuploidy in only 1 of 12 cases {723}. This aneuploid case was extensively metastatic (as were 3 euploid cases).

Differential diagnosis

NECs of the thymus are difficult to distinguish from the much more frequent mediastinal metastasis of pulmonary NECs {2137}. Immunohistochemical detection of TTF-1 expression might be helpful in distinguishing carcinoids and LCNEC of the lung from their thymic counterparts, since most thymic carcinoids {1513} and LCNECs are TTF-1 negative, while pulmonary NECs are TTF-1 positive in 50–75% of cases {272, 600,975}, although the TTF-1 expression status in pulmonary carcinoids has been questioned recently {1894}. Of note, TTF-1 negativity of a carcinoid in the mediastinum does not exclude metastasis from a gastrointestinal or pancreatic primary, since carcinoids in these locations are generally TTF-1 negative {272}. Whether TTF-1 is a useful marker to distinguish thymic SCNEC from the metastasis of small cell carcinoma of lung cancer is unclear {27,351,975}.

Otherwise typical thymic carcinomas with endocrine cells have to be distinguished from thymic NECs. The latter typically express neuroendocrine markers in a diffuse manner in >50% of tumour cells, while reactivity is restricted to scattered cells in thymic carcinomas {853,1139}.

Spindle cell carcinoids can resemble other spindle cell tumours of the thymus, including type A thymoma and synovial sarcoma, which are also cytokeratin-positive but lack finely granular chromatin pattern and neuroendocrine features. Nerve sheath tumours can be positive for NCAM/CD56, but lack cytokeratin and more specific neuroendocrine markers like chromogranin or synaptophysin.

Paragangliomas can closely mimic carcinoids by virtue of the similar architecture, high vascularity, strong expression of neuroendocrine markers, possible pigmentation, and possible association with Cushing syndrome {857,1028,1092, 1114,1350,1548}. In addition, carcinoids can occasionally show S100 positive sustentacular cells around nests of tumours cells {109,450}. The distinguishing features of carcinoids include: trabecular growth pattern, if present, and expression of cytokeratins. In morphologically equivocal cytokeratin-positive neuroendocrine tumours, ultrastructural analysis may be helpful {2140}.

Prognosis and predictive factors

Tumour stage has been found in most studies to be an important prognostic factor {528,628,723,1845,2144}. Atypical carcinoids are clearly aggressive, with 5-year and 10-year survival rates of 50-82% and 30%, respectively {628,723, 1845,2141}. Among atypical carcinoids, a lower mitotic rate (<3/10 HPF), minimal atypia, and lack of necrosis {1361,1362} are associated with a more favourable prognosis. Sarcomatoid differentiation may denote highly malignant clinical behaviour {1090}. It appears that the prognosis of LCNEC is worse than that of atypical carcinoid. Thymic SCNEC are more aggressive than atypical carcinoids (median survival: 25–36 months) {1094,1841,2032,2143}, although they are said to have a slightly better prognosis than their pulmonary counterparts {1808}. The poorly differentiated thymic NECs (small and large cell types) and NECs with combined features of carcinoid plus SCC are similarly highly aggressive, with patients dying of disease within 1 to 4 years {1361,1363}.

Early and late recurrences (local or systemic) are common (1–10 years) {528, 1902,2035} and appear to be associated with a bad prognosis {628,723,1362, 1845}. Local progression or local recurrence is observed in the majority of patients that finally die {349,450,1094, 1841,2032,2136}. Since the thymic NECs exhibit a poor response to chemo- and radiotherapy, radical resection of the primary tumour (together with local lymph nodes) must be a major therapeutic goal {450,628,723}.

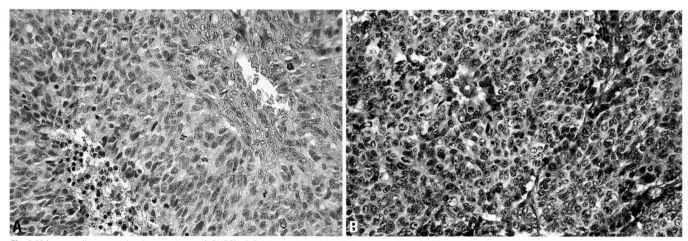

Fig. 3.68 Large cell neuroendocrine carcinoma (LCNEC). **A** Brisk mitotic activity distinguishes this LCNEC from atypical carcinoid, while the degree of necrosis and cytologic atypia is not different. **B** Note cytological details on this high power magnification.

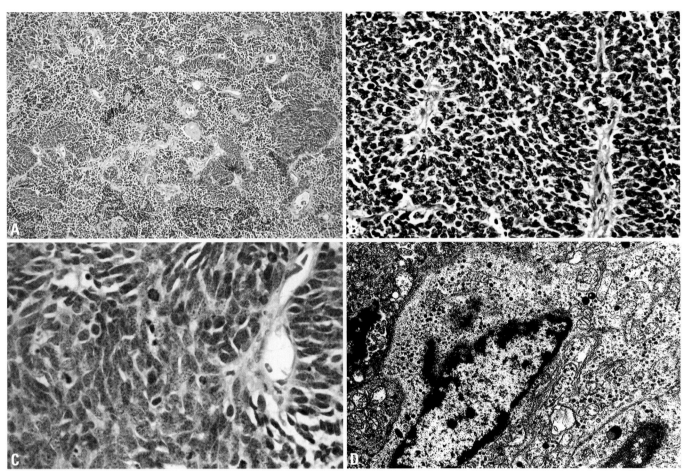

Fig. 3.69 Small cell carcinoma of the thymus. **A** Poorly differentiated neuroendocrine carcinoma: small cell carcinoma showing focal crush artifacts (low power). **B** Photomicrograph of primary small-cell neuroendocrine carcinoma of the thymus. **C** Cytological details: cellular crowding, elongated nuclei with salt and pepper chromatin structure, without recognizable nucleoli, scant cytoplasm, and high mitotic activity(high power). **D** Dense core granules are numerous in the cytoplasm of the tumour cells.

Combined thymic epithelial tumours

H.K. Müller-Hermelink
Ph. Ströbel
A. Zettl
A. Marx

Definition

Combined thymic epithelial tumours are neoplasms with at least two distinct areas each corresponding to one of the histological thymoma and thymic carcinoma types, including neuroendocrine carcinomas. The approximate percentage of each component should be specified in the diagnosis. Type AB thymoma is a separate entity by definition and does not fall under this category.

ICD-O code: Code the most aggressive component.

Synonyms

Composite thymomas; Composite thymoma-thymic carcinoma; Mixed neuroendocrine carcinoma-thymoma.

Epidemiology

Combined thymic epithelial tumours showing either A or AB thymoma areas combined with one of the type B thymoma subtypes or thymic carcinoma components are exceptionally rare (<1%). Likewise, combined neuroendocrine carcinoma-thymoma, and combined neuroendocrine/non-neuroendocrine thymic carcinomas are exceedingly seldom (<1%), while combined B3 thymoma-thymic squamous cell carcinomas are a bit more common (~1%). By contrast, various combinations of the type B thymoma subtypes B1, B2 and B3 account for 10-15% of all cases in large series {341,541}. Combined B2/B3 thymoma is by far the most common comined thymoma (8-12%), in accordance with the close morphologic and genetic relationship between B2 and B3 thymomas {897}.

Combined thymomas are not different from the respective individual thymomas in terms of age and sex association. Combined neuroendocrine thymic carcinoma-thymoma are tumours of adults, with most cases reported at age 50-60. There is a male predominance.

Etiology

The etiology of these tumours remains enigmatic. Unpublished genetic studies suggest that combined thymic epithelial tumours can arise by dedifferentiation of thymoma/ thymic carcinoma or by biphasic differentiation of a multipotential thymic epithelial precursor. The concept of tumour collision awaits genetic evidence {1841}.

Localization

Almost all cases were observed in the anterior mediastinum

Clinical features

There are no differences in the clinical manifestations of combined thymomas as compared to the individual components. Myasthenia gravis (MG) is by far the most common paraneoplastic manifestation (60-72%). One patient in our series of 107 combined thymic epithelial tumours presented with sarcoidosis, another patient with amyotrophic lateral sclerosis in addition to MG.

In combined neuroendocrine thymic carcinoma-thymoma myasthenia gravis, pure red cell aplasia {358,1336} and the carcinoid syndrome {1557} may occur.

Macroscopy

The size of combined tumours does not differ from that of the respective non-combined individual components.

Tumour spread and staging

All reported cases occurred in the anterior mediastinum as Masaoka stage I (6%), stage II (45%), stage III (29%), or stage IV (19%) tumours with intrathoracic metastases to pleura, lung and lymph nodes.

Histopathology

Among thymomas and thymic carcinomas, over 80% of combined tumours have clearly distinguishable, circumscribed areas showing typical B2 and B3 differentiation. Other common combinations are those of B1 and B2 (10%) or of B3 and non-neuroendocrine thymic carcinoma (5-7%). The carcinoma component in most cases is a squamous cell carcinoma. Lymphoepithelioma-like, sarcomatoid/anaplastic or undifferentiated carcinomas are uncommon. Rare cases of combined AB and B2 thymoma {341,1912}, and spindle cell (type A) thymomas in combination with thymic squamous cell {1912}, papillary {541,1263}, sarcomatoid or undifferentiated carcinoma have been observed, implying emergence of thymic carcinoma from a benign thymoma subtype.

Among neuroendocrine carcinomas (NECs), tumours composed of a (usually

Table 3.07
Combined neuroendocrine carcinoma–thymoma/thymic carcinomas reported in the literature.

Type of thymoma: descriptive terms	Corresponding WHO Classification	Corresponding neuroendocrine tumour	Source
Spindle cell thymoma	AB (?)	Thymic carcinoid	{358}
Lymphocyte-rich thymoma	B2	Thymic carcinoid	{1336}
Epithelial cell predominant thymoma	B3	Thymic carcinoid	{1808}
Undifferentiated thymic carcinoma	C	Thymic carcinoid	{1783}
Sarcomatoid thymic carcinoma	C	Thymic carcinoid	{1557}
Squamous cell carcinoma	C	Small cell carcinoma	{1841}
Adenosquamous carcinoma	C	Small cell carcinoma	{1094}

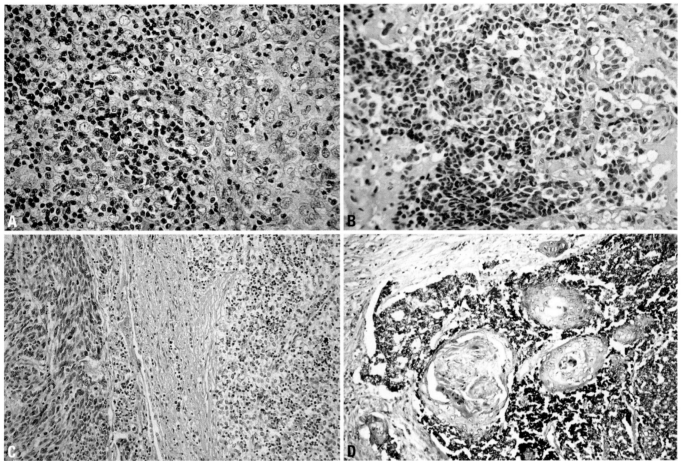

Fig. 3.70 Combined thymic epithelial tumours. **A** Combined B2 + B3 thymoma. Lymphocyte-rich B2 component (left) adjacent to lymphocyte-poor B3 component (right). **B** Combined carcinoid and small cell carcinoma. Combined neuroendocrine carcinoma: carcinoid (right) and small cell carcinoma (left). **C** Combined neuroendocrine carcinoma/thymoma. Type B3 thymoma (right) adjacent to poorly differentiated (spindle cell) neuroendocrine carcinoma of the thymus (left). **D** Combined small cell and keratinizing squamous cell carcinoma. Sharp segregation between foci of small cell carcinoma and the round clusters of keratinizing squamous cell carcinoma.

atypical) carcinoid component and a poorly differentiated NEC (small cell carcinoma or large cell neuroendocrine carcinoma) component have been reported {1362,1363,2142}.

To be designated combined neuroendocrine carcinoma–thymoma/thymic carcinoma, both tumour components should make up such a proportion of the tumour that both components can be readily recognized on H&E staining. By immunohistochemical or ultrastructural studies, scattered epithelial cells or small epithelial cell clusters with neuroendocrine features can be detected in rare conventional thymomas and many thymic carcinomas {39,853,1091,1139}. The term mixed neuroendocrine carcinoma – thymoma should not be used for these cases.

Somatic genetics

Genetic data have not been published. CGH studies on single cases of combined B2 and B3 thymomas or B3 and thymic carcinoma components suggest that the genetic alterations in these tumours are identical to those of their non-combined counterparts {896,2238, 2242} and that the individual components are clonally related. In one case of combined B3 thymoma and large cell neuroendocrine carcinoma, shared genetic alterations were observed, suggesting a common clonal origin of both tumour components.

Prognosis and predictive factors

Available data on combined thymomas suggest that the most aggressive component determines the clinical outcome {341,1912}. In one case of combined WHO Type B3 thymoma and thymic large cell neuroendocrine carcinoma, the patient died of widespread metastasis of the neuroendocrine carcinoma component.

Germ cell tumours of the mediastinum

M.R. Wick
E.J. Perlman
A. Orazi
H.K. Müller-Hermelink

A. Zettl
U. Göbel
C. Bokemeyer
J.T. Hartmann
A. Marx

The mediastinum is among the compartments of the body most frequently affected by germ cell tumours (GCT), second only to the gonads and ahead of other extragonadal GCT (EGGCT) that affect the retroperitoneum, sacrococcygeal region and central nervous system. Like their gonadal counterparts, mediastinal GCT can contain more than one histologic type of GCT and have been categorized for therapeutic purposes into pure seminomas, malignant non-seminomatous germ cell tumours (NSGCT, including embryonal carcinoma, yolk sac tumour, choriocarcinoma, and mixed GCTs), and teratomas. Mixed GCTs account for 34% of all mediastinal GCT and are, therefore, relatively less frequent than gonadal mixed GCTs.

As with the testicular germ cell tumours, there is a separate group of mediastinal germ cell tumours that present in infancy and early childhood that are comprised solely of teratomatous and yolk sac tumour components.

The preference of germ cell tumours (GCT) for the mediastinum has been explained by the distribution of fetal germ cell precursors (primordial germ cells) that migrate from the yolk sac to paired midline structures called germinal ridges which during very early development extend virtually throughout the axial dimension of the body during fetal development {1204}. If arrested during migration, some germ cell precursors may survive and serve as cells of origin for subsequent GCT development. Although mediastinal NSGCTs exhibit a worse prognosis than their gonadal counterparts {199} and can show virtually unique biological features (like clonally related haematologic neoplasms {315,1461, 2246}), recent genetic and epigenetic data support the concept that most gonadal and mediastinal GCTs share a common primordial germ cell ancestry {257,316,1764-1766}. However, since thymic epithelial stem cells and their plasticity have only partially been characterized {181}, a somatic stem cell derivation of at least some mediastinal GCTs

has not been excluded to date {860,2116}.

Basis of the classification

The terminology recommended for mediastinal GCT is the same as for germ cell tumours of the gonads {526}. The close embryologic relationship and generally similar morphological, genetic, clinical and biological features of GCTs support this concept. However, GCTs associated with haematologic malignancies are virtually unique to mediastinal GCTs, while monodermal teratomas, which are well known in the gonads, have not been observed in the mediastinum.

Epidemiology

Mediastinal germ cell tumours are rare neoplasms, representing less than 1% of all malignancies and 3-4% of all germ cell tumours in both adults and children {1033,1764}. Mediastinal GCT account for up to 16% of mediastinal neoplasms in adults and for 19-25% of mediastinal tumours in children {1356,1954}. Although annual incidence rates for testical GCT are strikingly different between Caucasians (~10/100.000) and Africans and Asians (1-2/100.000) similar incidence rates for mediastinal GCTs of about 0.1-0.2 per 100.000 can be calculated from Japanese {1955} and European nation-wide data {674}.

Mediastinal GCTs occur at all ages (0–79 years), though there is a bimodal age distribution, with a distinct peak in infancy {1356}. Children and adolescents (<18 years) account for 16-25% of all cases {1356,1954}. These can be divided into post-pubertal mediastinal germ cell tumours (which simply represent the lower end of the age distribution of adult GCT) and prepubertal mediastinal GCT {1764}. This bimodal age distribution corresponds to differences in genetic aberrations, sex predilection, and clinical outcome.

Post-pubertal mediastinal GCT account for 1-3% of all GCTs {721}. The mean age of affected adults is 33 years for seminoma patients and 28 years for patients

with an NSGCT {199,721,790}. The distribution of the histologic types varies from study to study. In some studies, mature teratoma is the most common single entity, while seminoma represents the largest histologic subentity among malignant mediastinal GCTs {1954}. In other studies, seminoma is the leading entity overall {721,1033}. In adults, mature teratomas {1356} and malignant mediastinal germ cell tumours for all practical purposes are restricted to males {1691}, though rare exceptions occur {411}, including germinomas in females {229, 1805,1954,2116}.

In children (including adolescents), mediastinal GCT account for 4% of all paediatric GCTs {1764}. Among extragonadal germ cell tumours mediastinal cases are third only to sacrococcygeal and central nervous system GCTs {721,1763}. In prepubertal children (<8 years), teratoma and yolk sac tumours are most prevalent, and other malignant histologic subtypes are virtually nonexistent {1764,1955}. The majority of these lesions present in infancy and early childhood. In prepubertal patients, teratomas have no sex predilection, whereas yolk sac tumours demonstrate a female predominance in young children with a 4:1 F: M ratio {1763}.

Etiology

The etiology of mediastinal germ cell tumours is unknown. The only established risk factor for mediastinal non-seminomatous GCT development is Klinefelter (KF) syndrome (reported risk 50 to several hundred-fold) {793,795}. The underlying pathogenetic mechanisms are, however, not understood. In KF patients, NSGCT develop from early adolescence to the age of 30. The increased frequency of GCTs is linked to the 47, XXY genotype, while men with mosaic KF syndrome (46, XXY) have no significantly increased risk {480,793}. Of note, testicular GCTs are not increased in patients with Klinefelter syndrome {793}, suggesting a unique oncogenic pathway for mediastinal non-seminomatous germ

Table 3.08
Clinical categorization of mediastinal germ cell tumours helps to guide the decision about neoadjuvant chemotherapy before radical resection and complete histological work-up. Clinical categories are derived from the synopsis of (i) the patological diagnosis that is usually based on fine needle biopsies, (ii) serum tumour marker levels (AFP, beta-hCG) and (iii) imaging studies.

Clinical category	Therapeutic implication
Seminoma[1,2]	Chemotherapy and/or irradiation

Malignant "non-seminomatous GCTs"
    Embryonal carcinoma
    Yolk sac tumours
    Choriocarcinoma
    Mixed germ cell tumours
	Chemotherapy, followed by resection of tumour remnants (irrespective of the histology)

Mature teratoma[1]	Resection
Immature teratoma[1]	Children: resection Adults: depending on tumour stage

[1] If patients with "pure" seminomas or "pure" teratomas as defined by fine needle biopsy exhibit elevated, age-adjusted tumour marker levels {696}, tumours are included in the "non-seminomatous" category. Sampling error is the most likely explanation for the discrepancy between histopathological diagnosis and clinical category.
[2] Elevated beta-hCG levels <100 IU/L (in adults) and <25 IU/L (in children) are compatible with a fine needle biopsy-based diagnosis of "pure" seminoma {197,696,1764}.

cell tumour (NSGCT) development in KF patients.

Apart from the well established association between haematologic malignancies and mediastinal NSGCTs, the frequency of other neoplasms is not increased {788} in patients with mediastinal GCT, arguing against a role of common cancer susceptibility genes in the development of mediastinal GCTs.

Site of involvement
The large majority of primary mediastinal GCTs arise within or adjacent to the thymus, but teratomas and yolk sac tumours {123} have also been described in the posterior mediastinum {1955}, in an intrapericardial location {172,1129, 1293}, and sometimes even within the myocardium {1764}.

Clinical features
Signs and symptoms
Mature teratomas are incidental findings in 50% of children and 66% of adults, while only 38% and 10% of patients with seminoma and malignant NSGCT, respectively, are asymptomatic {1954}. Presenting symptoms of GCTs are related to the local mass lesion and comprise chest pain (52%), respiratory distress (48%), cough (24%), hoarseness (14%) and the superior vena cava syndrome (14%) {1954}.

Respiratory compromise is more common in neonates and children than in adults, usually due to the extreme size of the lesion {1785,1954}, while the superior vena cava syndrome is more frequent in adults than children. Hydrops fetalis is a typical complication of pericardial teratoma {1129,1834}.
Fever and formation of multilocular thymic cysts result from local inflammatory reactions that frequently accompany GCTs and are most prominent in seminomas.
Precocious puberty due to increased beta-hCG levels can accompany mediastinal NSGCTs or mixed GCT {1769}. Children with Klinefelter syndrome and mediastinal NSGCTs have a particularly high frequency of precocious puberty {795,1106}.
Metastasis. Clinical symptoms related to metastatic spread may dominate. Most often symptoms are related to metastasis to the bone, liver, brain {518}, retroperitoneum and heart {40}.
Paraneoplastic autoimmune diseases, particularly myasthenia gravis, are virtually non-existant.
Haematologic proliferations associated with mediastinal GCT. An almost unique complication of mediastinal NSGCTs as compared to other extragonadal or testicular {1243} GCTs is the development of acute leukaemias {199,1132}, malignant

or benign {2246}) histiocytosis {83,129, 474,1112,1461}, myelodysplastic syndromes (MDS) or myeloproliferative diseases and haemophagocytic syndromes {83,1450,2055}. These haematologic proliferations occur in 2-6% of NSGCTs {199,789}, are clonally related to the GCTs {315,1113,1461} and develop independently of chemotherapy {474, 1461}. The NSGCT are most often yolk sac tumours or harbour a yolk sac component {83,315,1112,1461}, and can be associated with Klinefelter syndrome {129,490, 1461}.
Secondary MDS and AML that are related to etoposide chemotherapy in patients with mediastinal GCTs {100, 1047} must be distinguished from clonally-related haematologic malignancies. Secondary MDS and AML occurred in ~1.0% of cases in a large series {1047}. Chemotherapy-related AMLs usually manifest later (25–60 months after chemotherapy) than GCT-related AMLs (median time to onset 6 months, range 0–122) {789,1461}.

Metachronous testicular cancers in mediastinal GCTs. The risk for the development of metachronous testicular cancer (MTC) is low in mediastinal GCTs (10-year cumulative risk ~6%) {199,787}. MTCs are seminomas in ~70% of cases, although the underlying extragonadal GCT usually is a NSGCT {787}. Intratubular germ cell neoplasia of the testis is a rare accompanying finding in mediastinal GCTs {757}.

Imaging
Pure seminomas, with few exceptions {1810}, form uncalcified, homogeneous masses indistinguishable from lymphoma {1888}. By contrast, NSGCTs are usually heterogeneous masses, exhibiting central attenuation and a frond-like periphery {1888}. Since multilocular thymic cyst formation is a stereotypic response of the thymus to inflammatory stimuli, multilocular cystic lesions are not only typical for mature teratomas but accompany many other mediastinal GCT (particularly seminoma), thymomas, thymic carcinomas, Hodgkin or non-Hodgkin lymphomas or metastasis to the mediastinum.
A diagnosis of primary mediastinal GCT requires absence of a testicular or ovarian tumour on physical examination, high resolution ultrasonography, or MRI scan {198}. A bilateral testicular biopsy is not

mandatory for diagnosis of mediastinal GCTs.

Tumour markers
In patients with mature teratomas, tumour markers are almost always negative in the serum. By contrast, a-fetoprotein (AFP) and/or beta-human chorionic gonadotropin (beta-hCG) are elevated in 80-90% of malignant GCTs {1764}. AFP-positivity is more frequent (~73%) than increased serum levels of beta-hCG (~27%) {1955}. In adults, tumour marker levels at first presentation are citeria for the risk grouping (good, intermediate, poor) of GCT according to the IGCCCG system {4} as given in Table 3.09. In addition, unsatisfactory decline of AFP and/or beta-hCG levels during the early phase of chemotherapy appears to herald lack of tumour responsiveness and is therefore associated with a worse outcome {1273}. On the other hand, decline of tumour markers in spite of persistence or enlargement of a mediastinal GCT on repeated imaging can be due to the "growing teratoma syndrome" or somatic-type malignancy accompanying a chemosensitive GCT.

Tumour spread and staging
When all mediastinal GCT are considered, metastasis has been observed in ~20% of cases {1356,1359}. While mature teratomas do not metastasize, mediastinal seminomas show metastasis in up to 41% of cases {197,199}. In mediastinal NSGCT, metastasis to at least one site is present in 85-95% of patients at presentation, and hematogenous metastasis is the predominant type of dissemination. In contrast, lymph node metastasis is particularly common in seminomas. Haematogenous metastases typically involve lung (38%), bone, liver, brain {518}, retroperitoneum and heart {40}. Metastasis is a major criterion for staging and is an adverse prognostic factor in seminomas {790} and NSGCT {199, 790}.
A modification of the TNM classification of soft tissue tumours is recommended for staging of mediastinal GCTs.

Genetics
As indicated above, most GCT at extragonadal sites have been demonstrated to arise in primordial germ cells that have undergone erasure of imprinting prior to migration {1766}. The factors responsible

Table 3.09
IGCCCG criteria for the prognostic factor-based clinical "risk grouping" of malignant GCT in adults {4}. The criteria are not applicable to children before puberty.

IGCCCG Group	Criteria
Good	*Seminoma*: No non-pulmonary visceral metastases AND normal AFP, any HCG, any LDH *Non-Seminoma*: no patients classified as good prognosis
Intermediate	*Seminoma*: non-pulmonary visceral metastases AND normal AFP, any HCG, any LDH *Non-Seminoma*: no patients classified as intermediate prognosis
Poor	*Seminoma*: no patients classified as poor prognosis *Non-Seminoma*: all patients with mediastinal Non-Seminoma are classified as poor prognosis
IGCCCG= International Germ Cell Cancer Collaborative Group	

for the aberrant migration pathways and the ability of the germ cells to survive at the extragonadal sites are largely unknown. However, primordial germ cell migration has been shown to be determined by the ckit, stem cell factor receptor ligand pair. Abnormalities in expression of either the receptor or the ligand at any site in this pathway may result in abnormal migration or survival {1004}. The genetic changes that have been documented in primary mediastinal germ cell tumours vary with age at presentation and parallel the genetic changes found in germ cell tumours arising at gonadal sites in comparable age groups. This results in three categories of genetic changes within mediastinal germ cell tumours:

Malignant mediastinal germ cell tumours in infants and young children almost exclusively show yolk sac tumour histology. These tumours may be diploid or near-tetraploid and are uncommonly aneuploid {1517,1765}. Cytogenetic and comparative genomic hybridization (CGH) analysis of such tumours demonstrate gain of chromosomes 1q, 3, and 20q and loss of chromosomes 1p, 4q, and 6q {1765}. The same genetic changes have been identified in infantile yolk sac tumours of the sacral region and testis {1572,1573}. The two loci that have received additional attention and study are loss of distal 1p and loss of distal 6q {874,1574,1881}. Loss of distal 1p has been identified in 80% of infantile YST and is particularly intriguing due to its established role in another embryonal tumour of infancy, neuroblastoma. While candidate tumour suppressor genes

have been identified at this site, these have not been substantiated or confirmed. Loss of distal 6q is of interest due to the location of the potential tumour suppressor gene insulin growth factor type II receptor. IGF2R has multiple activities, one of which is to degrade IGF2, a potent growth promoter. Specific deletions, mutations, or imprinting abnormalities of IGF2R have not been documented.

Malignant mediastinal germ cell tumours in adolescents and adults demonstrate ploidy and genetic features similar to those described in their gonadal counterparts. In contrast to the tumours of young children, tumours in this category are usually aneuploid and demonstrate gain of chromosome 12p, regardless of the histologic subtype {316,1765}. This observation correlates with the presence of an isochromosome 12p {1057,1392, 2230}, which has been found in 84% of 25 malignant mediastinal germ cell tumours in adults reported to date {316}. The isochromosome 12p is formed by the duplication and centromeric fusion of the short arm of one chromosome, and loss of the long arm. In other patients amplification of fragment of the chromosome 12p (double minutes, homogeneously staning regions) can be observed. In testicular malignant GCTs, comparative genomic hybridization has been successful in identifying a small region of high level amplification at 12p11.2-12.1, providing an important clue to the localization of candidate proto-oncogenes on 12p. Additional recurrent changes seen in this category of germ cell tumours include loss of chromosome 13 and gain of chromosome 21

{1765}, findings also reported in malignant testicular GCT {1057,1673}.

Pure mediastinal teratomas (immature and mature) arising in all ages have demonstrated no genetic gains or losses {258,860,1765}. This observation is similar to those described in mature teratomas of the ovary, the infant testis, and other extragonadal sites in infants. However, it is distinctly different from genetic reports of mature teratomas in the adult testis, in which aneuploidy and the isochromosome 12p have been identified. Therefore, due to the extreme rarity of mature mediastinal teratomas in post-puberty males, caution is recommended prior to assuming a benign clinical behaviour in such cases. Supporting this is evidence provided by tumours that contain a mixture of teratoma and malignant germ cell histologies. In those cases for which it was possible to analyze the teratoma component separately from the malignant component, these tumours demonstrated similar abnormal CGH profiles within both the teratomatous and the malignant components {1765}. Similar findings have been reported at other sites {1205}.

In addition to the above changes, post-pubertal malignant mediastinal GCTs have long been associated with Klinefelter syndrome {480,793,795,1459, 2246}. The majority of adolescent and adult mediastinal malignant germ cell tumours arise in males {1359}, and up to half of these patients show an additional X chromosome within their peripheral blood lymphocytes {258,1765}. Therefore, adolescent males presenting with malignant mediastinal GCT should be evaluated for Klinefelter syndrome. No genetic differences between mediastinal GCT in individuals with and without Klinefelter syndrome have been described, and the underlying cause of the increased frequency of GCT in patients with Klinefelter syndrome is unknown. Constitutional sex chromosomal abnormalities have not been identified in mediastinal germ cell tumours of young children.

Prognostic factors

In the era of cisplatin-based chemotherapy for malignant GCTs, the most important "natural" prognostic factors in extragonadal GCTs are histology and localization of the primary tumour {997, 1461,1955}.

In NSGCTs, mediastinal localization is associated with a worse prognosis compared to their counterparts at other extragonadal and gonadal sites {105, 790,1159,1233,1764}. However, recent neoadjuvant strategies achieved dramatically improved outcomes also in NSGCTs of children {1764} and adults {198,199, 588}.

Initial AFP levels >10.000 ng/ml indicate a worse prognosis in children {105} while elevated beta-hCG is an independent adverse prognostic factor for survival in adults {199}.

Seminomas show a favourable response to radiotherapy and cisplatin-based chemotherapies, and their excellent prognosis (~90% survival) is not different from the prognosis of seminomas in other locations {198,199,790,1159,1955}. Adverse prognostic parameters in seminomas are liver metastasis or metastases to multiple other sites {790}.

Mature mediastinal teratomas have an excellent prognosis after complete resection in all age groups. In infants, tumours may be quite large and associated with developmental abnormalities due to compression of adjacent structures during development. Tumour-related deaths almost never occur when the tumour is able to be resected {721, 1159,1955}.

Following preoperative cisplatin-based chemotherapies of malignant GCTs, completeness of resection {786,787, 1764} less than 10% viable cells {588} and low-risk features according to the IGCCCG grouping system {4} are favourable prognostic factors. Decreased survival is associated with failure to respond to cisplatin and higher rates of relapses {790}. Unsatisfactory decline of AFP and/or beta-hCG levels during the early phase of chemotherapy appears to herald a worse outcome {1273}. Treatment failure is among the worst prognostic factors and is more common in mediastinal than other GCTs and is significantly associated with non-seminomatous histology and metastasis to liver, lung and brain {790}.

Table 3.10.
Interrelationship of age, tumour type, clinical behaviour and genetic alterations in mediastinal germ cell tumours. Data are derived from conventional cytogenetics, CGH studies and DNA ploidy analysis.

Age at clinical presentation	Histology	Sex predilection	Clinical behaviour	Recurrent genetic aberrations
Prepubertal	Teratoma (mature and immature)	M=F	Benign if resectable	None
	Yolk sac tumour	F>M	Malignant (80% survival)	del(6q), del(1p), gain 20q, gain 1p diploidy or tetraploidy
Adolescents and Adults	Teratoma (mature and immature)	M>>F	Benign	None
	Malignant GCT (all histologic subtypes)	M>>F	Malignant (50% survival)	i(12p), gain 21, loss 13, loss of Y, +Xc*, aneuploidy

* +Xc, constitutional gain of the X-chromosome (Klinefelter syndrome)

Seminoma

M.R. Wick
A. Zettl
J.K.C. Chan
C. Bokemeyer
J.T. Hartmann
E.J. Perlman
A. Marx

Definition

A primitive germ cell tumour composed of fairly uniform cells with clear or eosinophilic, glycogen-rich cytoplasm, distinct cell borders, and a round nucleus with one or more nucleoli, resembling primordial germ cells. Mediastinal seminomas are morphologically indistinguishable from their gonadal counterparts.

ICD-O code   9061/3

Epidemiology

Seminomas are rare mediastinal germ cell tumours first described in 1955 {2170}. Only 2 to 5% of all adult germ cell tumours arise in the mediastinum. Among extragonadal germ cell tumours, primary mediastinal seminomas account for 8% of cases {197,198}. In a large series reported from Japan, only 1.6% of primary mediastinal neoplasms are pure seminomas {1955}. The reported frequency of pure seminomas among primary mediastinal germ cell tumours ranges from 9% to 39% {520,1356,1371, 1955}, ranking seminoma second in frequency following teratoma {520,1356, 1371}.

With the exception of single cases {229,520,1955}, almost all reported mediastinal seminomas have occurred in men {520,1356,1371,1955}. The age ranges from 13 to 79 years {520,1356, 1371,1955}, with approximately two-thirds of the cases occurring in the 3rd and 4th decade {197,1371}.

Clinical features

Mediastinal seminomas typically arise in the anterior mediastinum, although a few cases have been reported to arise in the posterior mediastinum {1955}. Clinical symptoms are non-specific. Patients may present with symptoms related to a mediastinal mass, e.g. chest pain, dyspnoea, cough, superior vena cava syndrome. Some patients are asymptomatic, with the tumour being detected by routine X-ray or during unrelated thoracotomy {1371}. The size of the tumour may be rather large due to slow constant growth with overall little clinical symptoms. Moderate serum beta-hCG elevation (≤100 IU/L in adults and ≤25IU/L in children) may be found in up to one third of patients and is still compatible with the diagnosis of pure seminoma {197,696}.

At the time of diagnosis, the majority of mediastinal seminomas are localized, circumscribed masses without macroscopic or microscopic evidence of invasion into neighbouring organs such as pleura, pericardium, and great vessels {1371}. The preferential sites of distant spread, if present, are the lung, chest wall, brain, pleura, liver, adrenal gland, and bone {1349,1356}. Lymph node metastases most commonly occur in cervical and abdominal lymph nodes (in one series in 25% and 8%, respectively) {197}.

Etiology

The cellular origin of mediastinal seminomas is controversial {316}. Apart from gonads, seminomas may occur at other sites in the human body along the midline, such as the pineal gland, retroperitoneum, or the sacral area. During embryogenesis, migratory primordial germ cells may become misplaced along the midline on their way from the yolk sac to the embryonic gonadal ridge {293,1356}. A derivation from thymic myoid cells or from occult testicular intratubular germ cell tumour has been discussed {316,1689}. Yet, in contrast to patients with retroperitoneal seminomas, no testicular intraepithelial neoplasia is observed patients with mediastinal germ cell tumours {193,440, 441}.

The histogenetic relationship between mediastinal and gonadal seminoma is controversial. Genetic analysis of mediastinal seminomas have shown similar patterns of non-random chromosomal changes, in particular the presence of i(12p), as in gonadal seminoma {314, 316}, suggesting a very close pathogenetic relationship between seminomas at either sites. However, other studies

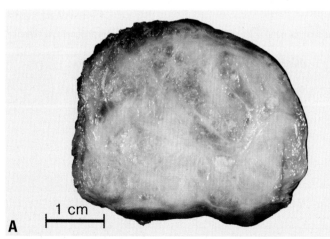
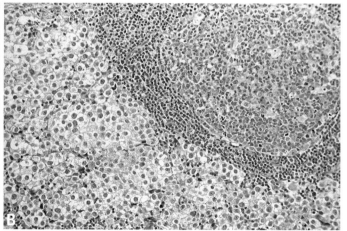

Fig. 3.71 Seminona. **A** Macroscopy of mediastinal seminoma. **B** Seminoma containing lymphoid follicle with prominent germinal center.

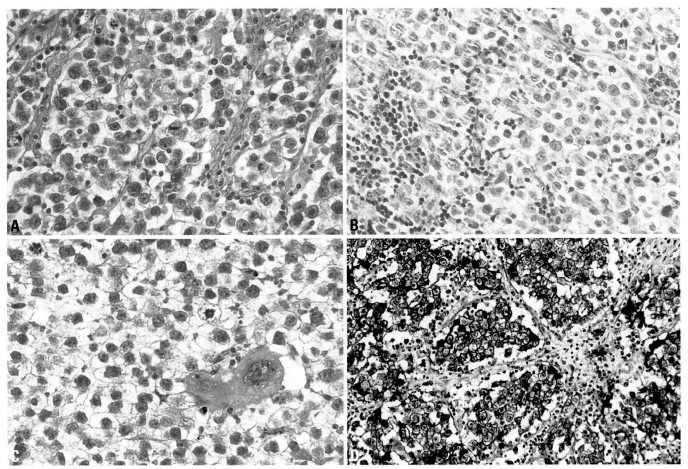

Fig. 3.72 Seminoma. **A** Large tumour cells with broad clear cytoplasm, large nuclei and conspicuous nucleoli. A light infiltrate of lymphocytes is present among the tumour cells and in the septa. **B** Mediastinal seminoma accompanied by lymphocytes and epithelioid cells including multinucleated giant cells. **C** Syncytiotrophoblast in mediastinal seminoma. **D** Immunoreactivity for CD117 in thymic seminoma.

report significant differences between the two. Compared with testicular seminomas, in one series, mediastinal seminomas are reported to more frequently express CAM5.2 (80% vs 21%), keratin (68% vs 0%), PLAP (93% vs 50%) and vimentin (70% vs 46%), possibly reflecting a more mature degree of tumour cell differentiation in the latter {1920}. *KIT* mutational analysis showed a different mutational pattern in mediastinal seminoma compared with testicular seminoma {1623}.

While Klinefelter syndrome is a risk factor for nonseminomatous mediastinal germ cell tumours, seminomas have not been observed {794}.

Morphology

Mediastinal seminomas are morphologically identical to their gonadal counterparts. Macroscopically, they are mostly well-circumscribed, fleshy tumours with a homogeneous, slightly lobulated to multinodular, tan-grey or pale cut surfaces. Punctate focal hemorrhage and yellowish foci of necrosis may be observed. The tumour size ranges from 1 to 20 cm (median size 4.6 cm) {197, 1371}.

Microscopically, mediastinal seminomas are composed of round to polygonal, fairly uniform tumour cells with round to oval, central, slightly squared, non-overlapping nuclei and one or more large central nucleoli. The tumour cells commonly have abundant glycogen-rich, clear to lightly eosinophilic cytoplasm and distinct cell membranes. Rarely, the tumour cells may show a dense eosinophilic cytoplasm or a greater degree of cellular pleomorphism. The tumour cells grow in confluent multinodular clusters, sheets, cords, strands or irregular lobules displaying a nesting pattern. Between the tumour cell aggregates, delicate fibrous septa are often observed.

Frequently, there is a prominent inflammatory cellular background infiltrate of small mature lymphocytes, plasma cells and occasional eosinophils. The infiltrate is typically most dense in and around the fibrous septa, but is also intermingled with the tumour cells. A granulomatous reaction ranging from ill-defined clusters of epithelioid histiocytes to well-defined epithelioid granulomas with Langhans giant cells may be present. Occasionally, germinal centers are present. The brisk inflammatory, granulomatous reaction and scar formation may obscure the underlying seminoma {1354,1371}.

In some cases, large syncytiotrophoblastic cells are scattered throughout the tumour, often in close proximity to capillaries and/or focal microhaemorrhage. These giant cells are multinucleated, with abundant basophilic cytoplasm and occasional intracytoplasmic lacunae. However, there are no cytotrophoblast cells or confluent nodules as in choriocarcinoma.

In a quarter of cases, remnants of thymic tissue can be found within or at the periphery {1356,1371}. In 10%, the thymic remnants undergo prominent cystic changes similar to multilocular thymic cysts, probably reflecting cystic transformation of remnant thymic epithelium induced by seminoma cells {1354}. In some cases, the thymic epithelium undergoes hyperplasia, and may lead to a misdiagnosis of thymic epithelial tumour.

Seminoma can also occur as a component in mixed germ cell tumours. Spermatocytic seminomas have not been described in the mediastinum.

Mediastinal seminomas commonly show diastase-labile PAS staining due to the presence of abundant glycogen.

Immunohistochemistry

Immunohistochemically, 80-90% of mediastinal seminomas are reported to be positive for PLAP, and 70% show vimentin positivity. CD117 positivity in a cell membrane or paranuclear Golgi pattern is common {1623}. Although up to 70% of cases show staining for pankeratin, the staining is often only focal, weak, and paranuclear. Immunostaining for beta-hCG highlights the scattered syncytiotrophoblastic cells, if present, and also isolated seminoma cells in about 5% of cases. CEA, EMA, and AFP are negative {1356,1371,1920}.

While it is prudent to rule out metastatic disease from a primary gonadal seminoma, mediastinal metastases are rare in gonadal seminomas, in particular in the absence of retroperitoneal lymph node metastasis {996}. Other differential diagnoses include metastatic melanoma, lymphoma, thymoma, thymic carcinoma, and in particular clear cell carcinoma (primary or metastatic).

Genetics

The genetic changes that have been described in mediastinal seminomas are the same as those reported in testicular seminomas, with 69% demonstrating the isochromosome i(12p) characteristic of post-pubertal malignant germ cell tumours at all sites. Mediastinal seminomas are most commonly aneuploid, with a minority having near-tetraploid DNA content.

Prognosis

Compared with mediastinal nonseminomatous germ cell tumours, pure mediastinal seminomas are associated with a favourable prognosis. A 5-year survival rate of 90% can be achieved with cisplatin-based combination chemotherapy which has largely replaced radiotherapy as the initial treatment in patients with mediastinal seminoma {197,198}. Primary radiotherapy seems to be asso-

ciated with a higher recurrence rate, but most patients have been salvaged with subsequent chemotherapy {197}. After completion of chemotherapy residual lesions detectable by radiographic studies frequently persist, in most cases consisting of necrotic masses that will ultimately shrink over time. In contrast to mediastinal nonseminomatous germ cell tumours, surgical resection is usually not indicated. Investigation by positron emission tomography (PET) is helpful in distinguishing viable from necrotic tumour residuals in seminoma patients {460}. In a large international study on mediastinal seminomas, liver metastases, two or more metastatic sites, and the presence of non-pulmonary visceral metastases have been identified as negative prognostic factors. Metachronous testicular germ cell tumours in patients with mediastinal seminoma are exceedingly rare {198}.

Embryonal carcinoma

M.R. Wick
E.J. Perlman
A. Zettl
F. Mayer
J.C.K. Chan
A. Marx

Definition

A germ cell tumour (GCT) composed of large primitive cells of epithelial appearance with abundant clear or granular cytoplasm, resembling cells of the embryonic germ disk and growing in solid, papillary and glandular patterns.

IDC-O code   9070/3

Synonym

Malignant teratoma, undifferentiated

Epidemiology

Embryonal carcinoma (EC) of the mediastinum is a tumour of young males (M/F ratio, >10:1) {1033,1955}. It occurs in pure form or as a component in mixed germ cell tumours at about equal frequencies {1033,1369,1955}. ECs (pure or mixed) account for up to 12% of all mediastinal GCTs {1033,1356} and for 30-65% of all NSGCT {997,1356,1955}. The mean age of adult patients is 27 years (range: 18-67 years) {1032,1955}. In the literature, EC in childhood is very rare before the age of 1 year and peaks (usually as part of a mixed GCT) between 1 and 4 years of age and again after the age of 14 years {1764}. However, as the pathologic features of solid yolk sac tumour (YST), and its distinction from EC is increasingly recognized, it is evident that the vast majority, if not all, the tumours in prepubertal patients previously classified as EC are better classified as YST.

In *adults*, EC as a component of mixed GCTs accounts for 9% of all mediastinal GCTs and for 75% of all NSGCT {1955}. EC is commonly associated with teratoma (56%), choriocarcinoma (22%) or seminoma (22%) {1032,1954}. The association with yolk sac tumour is very rare in adults {1955} but more common in adolescents {1369}.

In *adolescents*, combined EC accounts for 15% of all GCT {1764} and for 27-33% {1111,1764} or even more {1111} of the non-seminomatous subgroup. EC in this group is a component of most mixed GCT (77%) {1111,1764}. The association

with seminoma is equally frequent in children after puberty and adults (20-30%) {1764,1955}.

Clincal features

Patients present with thoracic or shoulder pain (60%), respiratory distress (40%), hoarseness, cough or fever (<10%), or superior vena cava syndrome (12%) {1955}. Gynaecomastia is uncommon and asymptomatic patients are rare {1808}. A quarter of patients have pulmonary metastasis at presentation and virtually all patients exhibit increased serum AFP levels, while ßHGG levels are elevated in cases with a choriocarcinoma component {1955}. Imaging findings are not specifically different from those reported for other NSGCT {1684}. A minority of patients show features of Klinefelter syndrome {150,1290}.

Etiology

The etiology of EC is unknown. The rare association with Klinefelter syndrome {150,1290} suggests a similar (but unresolved) etiology as in other mediastinal NSGCT. A single reported familial case {34} might indicate a fortuitous coincidence rather than a genetic predisposition. Risk factors for testicular GCTs {1204} appear largely irrelevant for the development of mediastinal GCTs {793}.

Tumour spread

Local tumour spread is common and can lead to compression and infiltration of the lung. About 25% of pure or combined ECs already show pulmonary metastasis at presentation {1955}. Further specific information on tumour spread in mediastinal EC is not available. However, since pure or combined ECs are among the most frequent malignant mediastinal GCTs, it is reasonable to assume that spread of ECs is similar to that of the whole NSGCT group, in that there is a high rate (~50%) of haematogenous metastasis (to lung, liver, brain and bones), while lymphogenous metastasis is apparently much rarer {199}.

Macroscopy

ECs are described as large tumours with invasion of the surrounding organs and structures. Grossly, the cut surface often reveals large areas of necrosis and haemorrhage. Viable tumour tissue is soft, fleshy, grey or white to pink or tan. In mixed GCT cystic spaces may be conspicuous.

Histopathology

Pure ECs show a more solid growth pattern than other NSGCTs. ECs form sheets, tubules or vague papillary structures composed of large polygonal or

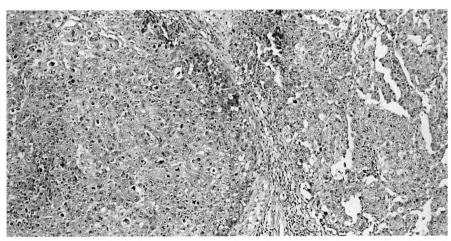

Fig. 3.73 Embryonal carcinoma. Low power showing solid growth pattern on the left side and poorly formed glands on the right side.

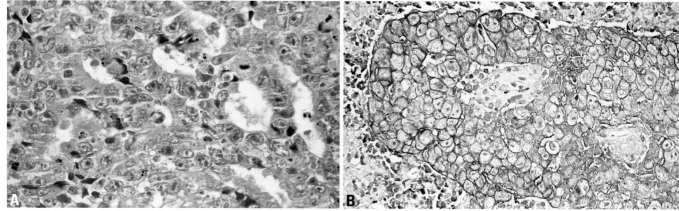

Fig. 3.74 Embryonal carcinoma. **A** High power. Cytological details of a tumour with glandular growth pattern. **B** Strong membranous CD30 staining.

columnar cells. The nuclei are large, round or oval, often vesicular, and can be hyperchromatic or have a light chromatin. They can be crowded and over-lapping. Prominent single or multiple nucleoli are common. The cell borders are often indistinct, especially in the solid areas. The cytoplasm is often amphophilic, but can be basophilic, eosinophilic, pale or clear {1808}. As in seminoma, scattered single or small groups of syncytiotrophoblasts can occur in EC. Mitoses are numerous and often atypical. Extensive necrosis can occur, and is particularly prominent in ECs combined with yolk sac tumour. The stroma is usually scant in viable tumour areas, but fibrotic adjacent to areas with regressive changes. Scattered lympho-cytes and a granulomatous reaction are uncommon.

In mixed GCTs, the EC component may be combined with a yolk sac tumour, teratoma, seminoma, choriocarcinoma, or combinations of these GCTs, and uncommonly somatic-type malignancies {1230}.

Immunohistochemistry
CD30 (Ki-1) is expressed in 85-100% of pure EC or EC components of mixed germ cell tumours {1135,1534}, while other germ cell tumours (with the excep-tion of rare cases of seminomas and yolk sac tumours {855,1369}) and other non-haematopoietic neoplasms are CD30-negative {1534}. There is distinct cell membrane staining with variable cyto-plasmic positivity.

In addition, ECs are uniformly and strongly reactive with antibodies to low-molecular weight cytokeratins, while EMA, carcinoembryonic antigen (CEA), and vimentin are usually negative. Alpha-fetoprotein (AFP) {1369,1920} and pla-cental alkaline phospatase (PLAP) {1808,1920} can occur in scattered tumour cells or small foci in about 30% of cases. One third of cases show beta-hCG expression in scattered syncytiotro-phoblastic cells.

Differential diagnosis
When syncytial areas are extensive, EC can mimic choriocarcinoma {1369}. However, a biphasic plexiform pattern produced by a mixture of syncytiotro-phoblasts and cytotrophoblasts is lack-ing, and pure ECs lack the extensive beta-hCG immunoreactivity of choriocar-cinoma {1369}. Yolk sac tumours can be distinguished from EC by a more varied growth pattern (most commonly micro-cystic and reticular), smaller cell size, presence of Schiller-Duval bodies, and lack of CD30 expression. EC can be dis-tinguished from seminoma by showing a greater degree of nuclear pleomorphism, at least focal definite epithelial character-istics (such as gland formation), uniform strong staining for cytokeratin, frequent CD30 expression, and usual lack of CD117 expression {1920}.

Mediastinal metastasis from large cell carcinoma of the lung can be a morpho-logic mimic {1369}. The young age of most EC patients, CD30 expression, and the tumour markers in the serum (such as

AFP and beta-hCG) are distinguishing features.

Metastasis to the mediastinum from a testicular EC or mixed GCT {932,996} has to be excluded.

Genetics
The genetic changes that have been described in mediastinal EC are the same as those reported in their testicular counterparts and demonstrate the isochromosome 12p characteristic of post-pubertal malignant germ cell tumours at all sites. Mediastinal EC is rarely associated with Klinefelter syn-drome {150,1290}. A single familial case {34} cannot be taken as evidence for a genetic predisposition.

Prognostic factors
There are no reports focussing on the prognostic factors of mediastinal EC. However, since EC histology has not been shown to be an adverse prognostic factor in several large clinical studies {199,237,1462}, it is likely that the prog-nostic factors described for NSGCT apply to EC. This conclusion is support-ed by a recent study: the long-term sur-vival rate of ~50% in adult patients with mediastinal EC after cisplatin-based chemotherapy {1955} was very similar to the rates published for large series of adult NSGCT. Similar conclusions appear justified for children with EC, although 5-year survival rates are signifi-cantly better (>80%) than for adults {1764}.

Yolk sac tumour

E.J. Perlman
A. Marx
C. Bokemeyer
M.R. Wick

Definition
A tumour characterized by numerous patterns that recapitulate the yolk sac, allantois and extra-embryonic mesenchyme.

ICD-O code   9071/3

Synonym
Endodermal sinus tumour

Epidemiology
Mediastinal yolk sac tumours (YST) present in two distinct age groups. In infants and young children, YST is virtually the only malignant germ cell tumour histologic subtype seen and there is a strong predominance of females (F:M, 4:1) {1765}. In these patients it is usually the sole histologic subtype, however it may occasionally be accompanied by teratomatous elements. The age at presentation ranges from the newborn period to 7 years of age, with over 75% of these patients presenting within the first three years of life {1764}. In contrast, in postpubertal patients YST is identified as the sole histologic element in approximately 10% of mediastinal tumours {1356,1369}. This is a much higher frequency than is seen in testicular sites, which may be due to the different cellular environments in which the tumours develop {316}. In addition, YSTs are often seen as one element within a mixed germ cell tumour {1369,1765,1955}. Like other mediastinal malignant GCT in post-pubertal patients, YST presents exclusively in males. The age at presentation ranges from 14 to 63 years {1369,1955}.

Clinical features
Patients with mediastinal YST often present with chest pain, dyspnoea, chills, fever, and superior vena cava syndrome {1369,1955}. The site of involvement is almost invariably the anterior mediastinum. Regardless of the age, alpha fetoprotein (AFP) levels are elevated in over 90 percent of cases.

Macroscopy
Macroscopically, pure YSTs are solid, soft, and the cut surface is typically pale grey or grey-white and somewhat gelatinous or mucoid. Large tumours often show haemorrhage and necrosis.

Histopathology
The histology of YST is the same regardless of the age of the patient or the site of presentation. For detailed discussions of the protean manifestations of endodermal sinus tumour, several excellent reviews are available {1102,1963,2050}. Cytologically, YSTs are composed of small pale cells with scant cytoplasm and round to oval nuclei with small nucleoli. Uncommonly, the cells may be larger with prominent nucleoli, and may therefore be difficult to distinguish from embryonal carcinoma or germinoma. The virtual nonexistence of the latter two histologic subtypes in young children lessens this diagnostic difficulty in this setting.

A number of different histologic patterns have been described; microcystic (reticular), macrocystic, glandular-alveolar, endodermal sinus (pseudopapillary), myxomatous, hepatoid, enteric, polyvesicular vitelline, and solid {1102, 1963,1990}. The majority of yolk sac tumours show more than one histologic subtype, and the different subtypes often merge subtly from one to another. These many different histologic types have not been shown to have prognostic or biologic significance, but aid in the recognition of unusual YSTs.

The *reticular or microcystic* variant is the most common histologic subtype, and is characterized by a loose network of spaces and channels with small cystic spaces lined by flattened or cuboidal cells with scant cytoplasm. A variant of the microcystic pattern is the *myxomatous pattern* in which the epithelial-like cells are separated by abundant myxomatous stroma. The *endodermal sinus pattern* has a pseudopapillary appearance and typically shows numerous Schiller-Duval bodies. These are glomeruloid structures with a central blood vessel covered by an inner rim of tumour cells, surrounded by a capsule lined by an outer (parietal) rim of tumour cells. The *polyvesicular vitelline pattern* is composed of compact connective tissue stroma containing cysts lined by cuboidal to flat tumour cells. The *solid pattern* is uncommon, and is usually

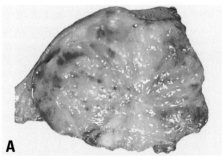
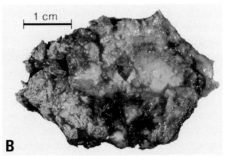

Fig. 3.75 Mediastinal yolk sac tumour (YST). **A** Macroscopy of pure mediastinal YST, showing a grey-white and gelatinous cut surface. No haemorrhage, no necrosis. **B** Macroscopy of a YST with a variegated cut surface including areas of necrosis and haemorrhage.

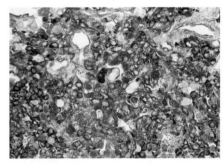

Fig. 3.76 Mediastinal yolk sac tumour with strong expression of AFP.

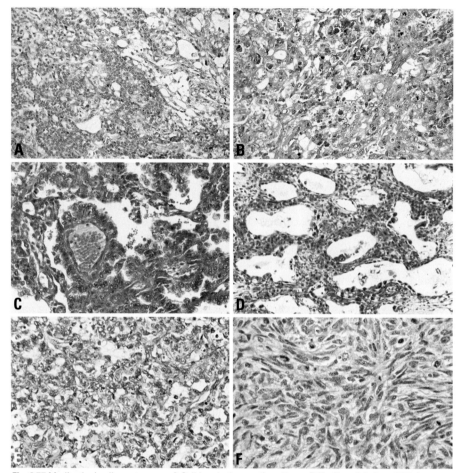

Fig. 3.77 Mediastinal yolk sac tumour. **A** Solid and microcystic pattern. **B** Hyaline globules. **C** High power showing Schiller-Duval bodies. **D** Polyvesicular/vitelline pattern. **E** Endodermal sinus pattern. **F** Focus with marked spindling of tumour cells.

Special studies

Strong positivity for AFP is helpful in diagnosis of YST. However, the reaction may also be variable. Therefore, negative staining does not exclude the diagnosis. YST also shows strong positive immuno-cytochemical staining with low molecular weight cytokeratin. Vimentin may show focal positivity in a minority of YSTs, but is negative in embryonal carcinoma {1369}.

Genetics

The genetic changes identified in YST depends on the age at presentation. Prepubertal YST demonstrate the same recurrent genetic abnormalities described in infantile sacral and testicular YST, including loss of the short arm of chromosome 1 (in particular the 1p36 region), loss of the long arm of chromosome 6, and gain of the long arm of chromosomes 1, and 20, and the complete chromosome 22 {671,1956}. In contrast, mediastinal YST following puberty are aneuploid and often demonstrate the isochromosome 12p characteristic of testicular malignant germ cell tumours in the same age group.

Prognosis and predictive factors

It is difficult to accurately provide prognostic information due to the rarity of these lesions, the variability in staging parameters utilized, and the variability in the chemotherapy provided. However, the most important predictive factor of both pre- and post-pubertal YST is the resectability of the primary lesion. This is more often possible in prepubertal patients due to a greater frequency of presentation at earlier stages. With cisplatin based chemotherapy these children have an overall survival of over 90% {1765}. In contrast, over half of postpubertal mediastinal YST have metastatic disease at presentation and the majority of these die of their disease; stage 1 and 2 patients are uncommon but often survive, particularly following aggressive chemotherapy {1369}.

seen only in small foci. This pattern may be difficult to distinguish from embryonal carcinoma or germinoma, however, the cells of yolk sac tumour are smaller and less pleomorphic. Unfortunately, these foci may be negative or only weakly positive for cytokeratin but usually retain their AFP positivity. *Hepatoid and enteric variants* are other less common forms of yolk sac tumour {2050}. The hepatoid pattern contains cells with abundant eosinophilic cytoplasm resembling fetal or adult liver {1614}. The enteric and endometroid patterns show glandular features resembling the fetal human gut and endometrial glands, respectively {377,386}. If these patterns are seen within an immature teratoma it may be difficult to determine whether they represent immature fetal tissue or YST. Fortunately, these unusual patterns of YST are usually accompanied by other more common patterns.

Schiller-Duvall bodies are present in only 50 to 75% of YST, and are seen predominantly in the microcystic and endodermal sinus patterns. Therefore, these are not required for the diagnosis. Hyaline droplets are commonly present in YST. However, these may also be found in a minority of embryonal carcinomas, as well as in some other epithelial tumours. These are composed of a variety of proteins, and are PAS positive, resistant to diastase digestion. The droplets may be positive for AFP as well as alpha-1-anti-trypsin, but often are not {1536}.

A spindle cell lesion has been described in YST-containing mediastinal germ cell tumours in post-pubertal men. Histologically, these tumours are composed predominantly of atypical spindle cells admixed with areas of classic YST. Immunohistochemical analysis demonstrates positive staining for keratin and AFP in both the spindle cell and reticular components of the tumour {1358}.

Choriocarcinoma

M.R. Wick
A. Zettl
J.K.C. Chan
C. Bokemeyer
E.J. Perlman
A. Marx

Definition
Choriocarcinoma is a highly malignant neoplasm displaying trophoblastic differentiation. It is composed of syncytiotrophoblast, cytotrophoblast and variably intermediate trophoblast cells. Mediastinal choriocarcinomas are morphologically indistinguishable from their gonadal or uterine counterparts.

ICD-O code   9100/3

Epidemiology
Pure mediastinal choriocarcinomas are exceedingly rare and virtually non-existent in children. Only 2.5 to 5% of mediastinal germ cell tumours are pure choriocarcinomas {997,1033,1356}. Pure choriocarcinoma constitute 9% of malignant mediastinal nonseminomatous germ cell tumours, and 4.3% of nonteratomatous germ cell tumours {1033,1349, 1356}.

Clinical features
The patients` ages range from 17 to 63 (most commonly the 3rd decade of life), and almost all reported cases were male patients {520,1821,1955}. At diagnosis, mediastinal choriocarcinomas are mostly large anterior mediastinal masses (average size 10 cm) {1357}. Primary chorio-

carcinomas have also been observed in the posterior mediastinum {1357}.
The patients present with symptoms due to the mediastinal mass, such as chest pain, dyspnoea, cough, superior vena cava syndrome. Patients may show gynecomastia due to elevated beta-hCG levels {1356,1821}. Mediastinal choriocarcinomas are highly aggressive neoplasms with early haematogeneous dissemination. In a series of 8 cases, metastases were observed in the lungs (88%), liver (50%), kidney (38%) and spleen (25%). Metastatic disease to the brain, heart, adrenals and bone has also been observed. {1033,1357,1821}.

Morphology
Mediastinal choriocarcinomas are large tumours with soft consistency and extensive hemorrhage and necrosis. Microscopically, they are composed of syncytiotrophoblast, cytotrophoblast and intermediate trophoblastic cells. Syncytiotrophoblasts are large multinucleated cells with numerous, pleomorphic, dark-staining nuclei, distinct nucleoli, and abundant densely eosinophilic cytoplasm which may contain cytoplasmic lacunae. Cytotrophoblasts are uniform, polygonal cells with round nuclei, prominent nucleoli, and clear cytoplasm.

Syncytiotrophoblasts and cytotrophoblasts may grow intermingled in a bilaminar plexiform pattern or in disordered sheets. Occasionally, scattered clusters of syncytiotrophoblasts cap cytotrophoblast nodules. Atypical mitosis and cellular atypia are common. There can be sheets of nondescript mononuclear cells that resemble intermediate trophoblast. Choriocarcinomas are typically intimately associated with dilated vascular sinusoids. Partial or complete replacement of the walls of blood vessels are common. There are often vast areas of haemorrhage and necrosis.
Mediastinal choriocarcinoma cannot be distinguished morphologically from metastatic choriocarcinoma. Since gonadal choriocarcinoma often displays extensive regressive alterations but still may give rise to widespread metastasis, the exclusion of a primary gonadal choriocarcinoma is particularly difficult, although mediastinal metastasis of gonadal choriocarcinoma seem to be very rare {997,1356}.
Trophoblastic neoplasms other than choriocarcinoma, such as monophasic choriocarcinoma and placental site trophoblastic tumour have not been reported in the mediastinum.

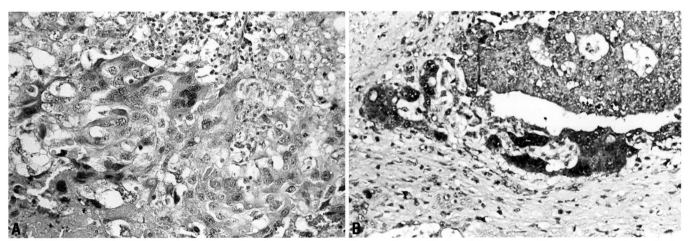

Fig. 3.78 Choriocarcinoma. **A** High power showing multinucleated and eosinophilic syncytiotrophoblastic cells intertwined with mononuclear cytotrophoblastic cells. **B** beta-hCG staining of syncytiotrophoblastic cells.

Immunohistochemistry

Syncytiotrophoblasts and cytotrophoblasts react with pankeratin markers and CAM5.2, whereas they are negative for PLAP, AFP, CEA, CD30 and vimentin. The syncytiotrophoblasts additionally express beta-hCG, while the cytotrophoblasts are variably positive for human placental lactogen {1357,1920}.

Apart from metastasis of an extramediastinal choriocarcinoma, the differential diagnoses include mediastinal mixed germ cell tumour (in which a further germ cell tumour component is found), sarcomatous component in teratoma, and mediastinal metastasis from a carcinoma with choriocarcinoma-like features/dedifferentiation.

Genetics

The genetic changes that have been described in mediastinal choriocarcinoma are the same as those reported in the testis and demonstrate the isochromosome i(12p) characteristic of postpubertal malignant germ cell tumours at all sites {316}. Such tumours are most commonly aneuploid, with a minority having near-tetraploid DNA content.

Prognosis

In most of the reported cases, patients died of disseminated disease shortly after diagnosis (average survival time 1 to 2 months) {520,1357,1821}. However, treament with cisplatin-based chemotherapy may improve the prognosis {1955}.

Teratoma

M.R. Wick
E.J. Perlman
U. Göbel
D. T. Schneider

P. Ströbel
J.C.K. Chan
A. Marx

Definitions

A germ cell tumour (GCT) that is composed of several types of organoid mature and/or immature somatic tissues derived from two or three germinal layers (ectoderm, endoderm and mesoderm).

Mature teratomas are tumours composed exclusively of mature, adult-type tissues. *Dermoid cyst* is a variant consisting of one or more cysts lined predominantly by keratinizing squamous epithelium with skin appendages. Monodermal teratomas analogous to struma ovarii have not been described in the mediastinum.

Immature teratomas contain immature, embryonic or fetal tissues exclusively or in addition to mature tissues. Mature and most immature mediastinal teratomas are benign tumours {1053,1244,1764, 1808}.

Teratomatous component is the term used to describe differentiated somatic tissues associated with a seminoma, embryonal carcinoma, yolk sac tumour or choriocarcinoma. The teratomatous component of mixed GCTs is very often immature {1808}.

Teratoma with somatic-type malignancy is a teratoma containing one or more components of non-germ cell malignant tumour, which may be a sarcoma or a carcinoma (ICD-O code 9084/3).

ICD-O codes

Mature teratoma	9080/0
Immature teratoma	9080/3

Epidemiology

Mediastinal teratomas account for 7-9.3% of mediastinal tumours {708,1171} and 50–70% of all mediastinal germ cell tumours {466,520,759,1356,1458, 1888,2116} Among teratomas of all sites, up to 27% occur in the mediastinum in adults, and 4-13% in children {708,1053,1763}.

Overall, there is an equal sex distribution {1171} or a slight female preponderance (M:F =1:1.4) {1808}, but immature teratomas occur almost exclusively in males {1808}.

The mean age of adults is 28 years (range 18–60) {1171}. In children, teratoma is the predominant mediastinal tumour during the first year and has been detected in fetuses as young as 28 weeks of gestation {708}. The proportion of immature teratomas (up to 40%) is much higher in the first year of life than at older age (~4-6%) {1053,1356,2116}. Mature teratoma can be associated with classical (47, XXY) and very rarely, mosaic Klinefelter syndrome {480}.

Clinical signs and symptoms

30-59% of mediastinal mature teratomas, particularly those in adults {1955}, are asymptomatic {708,1171, 1337}. Other cases can be associated

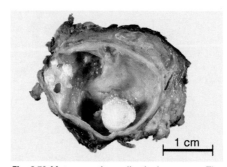

Fig. 3.79 Mature cystic mediastinal teratoma. The yellow areas represent mature fat.

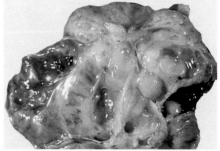

Fig. 3.80 Immature mediastinal teratoma with a variegated cut surface. Cystic areas are less prominent than in mature teratoma.

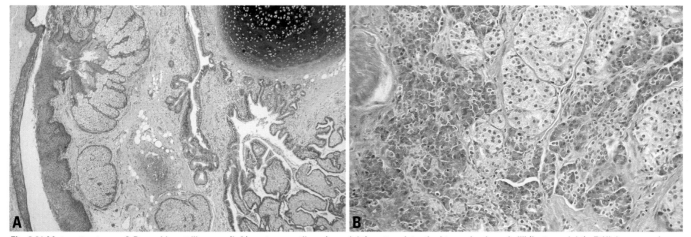

Fig. 3.81 Mature teratoma. A Dermoid cyst-like area (left), mature cartilage (top, right), mature intestinal type glands and villi (bottom, right). B High power of pancreatic tissue, including islets.

with chest, back or shoulder pain, dyspnoea, cough, and fever due to chronic pneumonia {708,1764}. Rare symptoms include superior vena cava syndrome, erosion of bronchi or vessels, Horner syndrome, or pneumothorax {696,708, 1764,1808}. Due to the occurrence of exocrine pancreatic tissue, rupture is more common in mediastinal teratomas than teratomas of other sites {1808,2038} and can result in pleural effusions or cardiac tamponade. Endocrine pancreatic component can cause hyperinsulinism and hypoglycaemia {1808}. Hydrops fetalis is a complication of congenital intra- and extrapericardial mediastinal teratoma {708}.

Imaging
Mature teratomas show multilocular cystic structures in almost 90% of cases {1888}. Attenuation is heterogeneous with varying combinations of soft tissue, fluid, fat and calcium {1337}. Calcifications occur in in 26% {1171} to 53% {1337}. A shell-like tumour wall calcification or identifiable bone and teeth occur in up to 8% each {1171, 1337}. Immature teratomas appear more often solid {1888}. With rare exceptions {1244}, the usual serum tumour markers (AFP; beta-hCG) are not elevated.

Site of involvement
More than 80% of mature teratomas occur in the anterior mediastinum, 3-8% in the posterior mediastinum and 2% in the middle mediastinum, while 13-15% involve multiple mediastinal compartments {963,1337,1829}. Teratomas can extend deeply into one or both thoracic cavities and elicit atelectasis.

Macroscopy
Mature mediastinal teratomas are usually encapsulated masses with a mean dia-

meter of 10 cm (range 3-25 cm) {1655, 2008,2116}. There can be adhesions to the surrounding lung or great vessels. The cut surface is variegated, showing cystic spaces with fluid or grumous materials, hair, fat, flecks of cartilage, and rarely teeth or bone {1808,1888}. Immature teratomas are often very large (up to 40 cm) {1975} and solid. They exhibit a soft to fleshy consistency or are extensively fibrous or cartilaginous {1808}. Haemorrhage and necrosis can be present.

Histology
Mature teratomas
These are characterized by a haphazard admixture of organoid mature tissues derived from 2 or 3 germinal layers. Skin and cutaneous appendages are consistent constituents and form cyst linings. Bronchial, neural, gastrointestinal, smooth muscle and adipose tissue com-

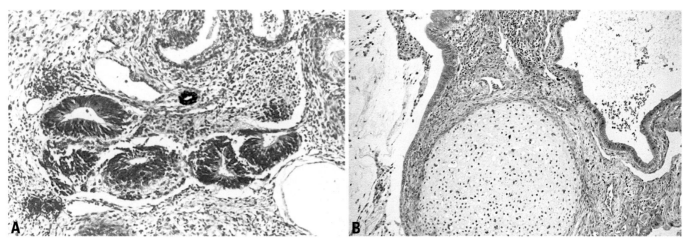

Fig. 3.82 Immature teratoma. A Immature neural tissue forming tubes. B Immature cartilage.

ponents are very frequent (>80%), while skeletal muscle, bone and cartilage are less common {708,1808}. Salivary gland, prostate, liver and melanocytes are even less frequent; thyroid tissue has not been reported {1808}. Pancreatic tissue is typical of mediastinal teratomas and found in up to 60% of cases, but is rare or absent in teratomas of other sites {521, 1808}.

Regressive changes, such as rupture of cystic structures, can be accompanied by a granulomatous inflammation {1808, 2116}. Remnant thymic tissue is found outside the capsule in 75% of mature teratomas {708}.

Immature teratoma

These lesions are characterized by embryonic or fetal tissues derived from the various germinal layers, such as immature glands lined by tall columnar epithelial cells, fetal lung, immature cartilage and bone, rhabdomyoblasts, blastema-like stromal cells. The most common immature components are neuroectodermal tissues, with neuroepithelial cells forming tubules, rosettes or retinal anlage {708,1808,2116}. By definition, pure immature teratoma should not harbour a morphologically malignant component.

Immunohistochemistry

The main role of immunohistochemistry in teratomas is: (i) to define the nature of immature components, such as rhab

domyoblasts (desmin, myogenin), neural components (S100; NSE) or immature cartilage (S100; GFAP) {1490}, and (ii) to exclude other germ cell or somatic malignancies. Pure teratomas are negative for PLAP, beta-hCG and CD30. AFP is usually negative, although liver cells and immature neuroepithelium in teratomas may express AFP.

Grading of immature teratoma

There are insufficient data to support a particular grading system for immature teratomas of the mediastinum. Grading according to Gonzalez-Crussi {708} was of no prognostic significance in children {696,1244,1764,1808}. However, it is important to realize the following: 1) the more immaturity is present in a teratoma, the higher the risk to find a yolk sac tumour component; 2) immaturity in a teratoma in an adolescent male is highly suspicious of a malignant i(12p)-containing germ cell tumour. Therefore, the pathologist should communicate clearly in the report the quantity (rough percentage) of immaturity.

Genetics

The pure mature and immature teratomas analyzed and reported to date do not show recurrent genetic gains and losses. This is in contrast to malignant germ cell tumours {1765}. Mature teratoma can be associated with classical and very rarely mosaic Klinefelter syndrome {480}.

Differential diagnosis

The main differential diagnosis is mixed germ cell tumour with a teratomatous component. Immature teratoma may be difficult to distinguish from teratoma with somatic type malignancy; the latter usually shows frank cytologic atypia and invasiveness that are absent in pure immature teratomas.

Prognostic factors

Mature teratoma is a benign tumour irrespective of the patient´s age. The prognosis of pure immature teratoma is age-dependent. In children, pure immature teratoma has an excellent prognosis with no risk of recurrence and metastasis {1244,1764}. The presence of an admixed malignant germ cell tumour component (detected in up 30% of immature teratomas after extensive sampling {1244}, and most commonly yolk sac tumour) is associated with a recurrence rate of 25%. In children, such mixed GCTs have a good prognosis after cisplatin-based chemotherapy (>80% 3-years-survival) {695,1244}.

In adults, the prognosis of pure immature teratoma is more guarded but experience is limited {2116}. Apparently pure immature teratomas with pulmonary metastases have been reported in adults, with only the metastasis showing a germ cell and/or somatic type malignancy {1808}.

Mixed germ cell tumours

M.R. Wick
E.J. Perlman
U. Göbel
D.T. Schneider

F. Mayer
Ph. Ströbel
J.K.C. Chan
A. Marx

Definition

A neoplasm composed of two or more types of germ cell tumours (GCTs). The diagnosis should be complemented by listing each component and its approximate proportion.

Polyembryoma represents a variant with a unique growth pattern that is characterized by the predominance of embryoid body-like structures. Embryonal carcinoma, yolk sac tumour, syncytiotrophoblastic cells and teratomatous components can usually be recognized in polyembryoma.

Embryonal carcinomas or seminomas containing scattered syncytiotrophoblastic cells do not qualify as mixed GCTs, but are classified as the respective "pure" GCTs.

ICD-O code

Polyembryoma   9072/3

Synonyms

Malignant teratoma intermediate, teratocarcinoma. The use of terms that do not precisely qualify the type and quantity of tumour components is discouraged.

Epidemiology

In adults, mixed GCTs account for 13-25% of all mediastinal GCTs {466,520, 1005,1033,2116}, second only to teratomas (40-60%) and as common as seminomas (15-20%) {520,1005,1356, 1808,2116}. Virtually all patients are male {1005,1356}.

In children, mixed GCTs account for about 20% of cases, and yolk sac tumour with mature or immature teratoma is the characteristic constellation. Other types of mixed GCTs are virtually nonexistent during the first four years of life {1764}. Among children <8 years of age, some authors {1005,1765} but not others {167} see a preponderance of females, while almost all adolescent patients > 8 years are males {1765}.

After the onset of puberty, mixed germ cell tumours can be associated with Klinefelter syndrome {150,795,1106, 1290,1765}.

Clinical features

Only ~10% of mixed GCTs are asymptomatic at diagnosis {1955}. Most patients present with general and local symptoms identical to those in other mediastinal GCT: chest pain, cough, dyspnoea, hoarseness, superior vena cava syndrome and cardiac tamponade {757, 1955}. Precocious puberty and gynecomastia are rare in polyembryoma {150} and other mixed GCTs {1106,1808}. In some cases, endocrinologic symptoms induced by beta-hCG production may precede tumour diagnosis by years {1769}.

A minority of patients present with symptoms attributable to metastases {709, 757,1955}. Clonally related leukaemias are rare (~2%) {40,729,789,1518}.

Imaging studies typically show a large inhomogeneous mass with necrosis, hemorrhage and infiltration of adjacent structures. Cystic spaces or adipose tissue hint to the presence of a teratomatous component {757,1888}.

Most cases (~90%) show elevated serum tumour marker levels {1005}. Raised AFP (~80%) is strongly correlated with a yolk sac tumour component, although teratomatous hepatoid cells and teratomatous neuroepithelium can also produce small amounts of AFP. Increased beta-hCG (~30%) levels occur in mixed GCTs with a choriocarcinoma component or with syncytiotrophoblast cells {2169}.

Post-chemotherapy findings, including the Growing Teratoma Syndrome

During or following chemotherapy, patients with GCT can alternatively show {2169}: (1) Normalization of tumour markers and resolution of the tumour mass (10%), (2) persistence of elevated tumour markers and the tumour mass due to resistance to chemotherapy (10%), or (3) normalization of tumour markers with residual tumour mass (80%).

In the latter group, 10-20% of patients exhibit tumour enlargement. This phenomenon can be due to a) chemotherapy-resistant GCT components that do not secrete AFP or beta-hCG; b) development of somatic-type malignancies; c) the "growing teratoma syndrome" (GTS). GTS is a rare complication of mixed GCTs {24} and defined by 1) an increase in tumour size during or after chemotherapy; 2) normalization of serum tumour markers; 3) identification exclusively of mature teratoma on histological analysis of the resected tumour specimen {1199}. The growing mediastinal mass is usually asymptomatic but can be accompanied by fever and dyspnoea {24,1256}. Lymphatic spread can involve mediastinal and supraclavicular lymph nodes {56}. Late GTS complications are local or metastatic development of malignant non-seminomatous GCTs and development of GCT-related sarcomas, carcinomas or leukaemias {56,1256}. The pathogenesis of GTS is largely unknown.

Tumour spread

Most mixed GCT exhibit extensive infiltration into mediastinal structures and adjacent organs. Rates of metastasis at time of diagnosis vary widely in different reports, from 20-36% {520,1356,1764, 1955} up to >80% {997,2169}. Metastasis to lung, pleura, lymph node, liver, bone and brain have been reported {156,1005,1765,1955}. Metastases to supraclavicular lymph nodes and lung due to occult mediastinal mixed GCTs are rare {708}.

Macroscopy

The tumours are often poorly circumscribed or frankly infiltrative, and show a heterogeneous cut surface with solid areas, haemorrhage and necrosis. Cystic spaces usually indicate presence of a teratomatous component. The size ranges between 3 and 20 cm (mean 10 cm) {908}. Tumours in the context of the "growing teratoma syndrome" measure up to 28 cm {24}.

Histopathology

Various types of GCTs can occur in any combination in mediastinal mixed GCTs. Their morphologies are identical to those of pure GCTs. The reported frequencies of the various GCT subtypes vary widely in the literature, but the following conclusions can be drawn:

In *adults*, the two most frequent components are teratoma (50-73%; mean 65%) and embryonal carcinoma (22–100%; mean 66%) {237,520,1005,1356,1955}. Less common are yolk sac tumour (0-83%; mean 48%), seminoma (22-50%, mean 38%), and choriocarcinoma (10–67%, mean 28%) {520,1005,1033, 1356,1955}. The teratoma components are more often immature than mature {17, 1033,1808}. The most common combination is teratoma and embryonal carcinoma (previously called teratocarcinoma), encounterd in 15-56% of cases (mean 40%) {237,1005,1808,1955}.

In *children*, a yolk sac tumour component occurs in most (>90%) mixed GCTs, followed by teratoma (~30%), and, in adolescents, seminoma, choriocarcinoma and embryonal carcinoma (~20% each) {709,1764}. In contrast to adults, the teratoma components in paediatric mixed GCTs are more often mature than immature {167,1725,1765}.

Polyembryomas {150} show a unique growth pattern mimicking embryoid bodies. These GCTs are composed of EC, YST, syncytiotrophoblast cells and teratoma. Adult, but not childhood, mediastinal mixed GCTs are frequently associated with non-germ cell malignancies (sarcomas, carcinomas, and/or leukaemias).

Histology of metastasis
The histology of metastases usually reflects the histology of the primary GCT or one of its components {17} but other GCT histologies and somatic type malignancies may occur, particularly after chemotherapy {56,406,1230,1256,2046}.

Postchemotherapy histology
After chemotherapy, viable non-teratomatous tumour occurs in up to 50% of cases even after normalization of serum tumour markers {1808,2049}. In the remaining cases, areas of necrosis, teratoma structures, inflammatory infiltrates including xanthogranulomatous reactions, and fibrosis can be encountered. Chemotherapy may unmask a previously overlooked somatic-type tumour or a teratomatous component. Metastases do not necessarily reflect the histology of remnant viable tumour cells in the primary location {56,1256}.

Immunohistochemistry
The immunohistochemical profiles reflect those of the various germ cell tumour components contributing to a given mixed GCT. AFP is expressed in virtually all mixed GCTs, at least focally, due to the frequent occurrence of yolk sac tumour components.

Genetics
In adults and children > 8 years old, gain of 12p and sex chromosomal abnormalities (often associated with Klinefelter syndrome) are the most common recurrent abnormalities of mediastinal mixed GCTs {258,1765}, including polyembryoma {150}. Additional recurrent changes include gain of chromosome 21 and loss of chromosome 13. These abnormalities are also encountered in the mature teratoma component and/or somatic-type malignant components of mixed GCTs, while pure teratomas are typically devoid of genetic imbalances {1394,1765}.

In children < 8 years old, i(12p) does not occur {1765}, and gain of the X chromosome and trisomy 21 {258,1765} are rare findings. Instead, gain of 1q, 3, and 20q and loss of 1p, 4q, and 6q are common {258,1765} in yolk sac tumour; teratomatous elements show no chromosomal abnormalities.

Postulated cell of origin
Toti- or pluripotent primordial germ cell.

Differential diagnosis
Embryonal carcinoma components may be difficult to recognize against a background of yolk sac tumour due to the heterogeneity of yolk sac tumour growth patterns. CD30 staining is a helpful diagnostic adjunct to resolve this differential. Due to the lack of cytotrophoblastic cells, scattered syncytiotrophoblasts in "pure" seminomas and embryonal carcinomas can be distinguished from the choriocarcinoma components of mixed GCTs.

Prognostic factors
In adults, mixed GCTs exhibit a long-term survival rate of 40-45% {1359} and there appears to be no significant difference between mixed and pure NSGCTs {1955}. Therefore, tumour stage, particularly metastasis to brain, liver, lung, and bone, and elevated beta-hCG levels might be major risk factors for mixed GCTs as for NSGCTs {199,790}. Modern

cisplatin-based chemotherapies and resection are the treatment of choice {199,236,1462,2172}.

In children, mixed GCTs usually harbour only yolk sac tumour and teratomatous components and their prognosis is not different from the prognosis of pure yolk sac tumour {1764}, suggesting that 5-year overall survival rates of >80% can be achieved with modern therapies {1764}. Local stage, distant metastasis and AFP levels have not been shown to be of prognostic significance in a recent paediatric series of NSGCTs that includes 24% mixed GCTs {1764}. In young children, mixed GCTs exhibiting microscopically small foci of NSGCTs in teratomas have a good prognosis after complete resection and chemotherapy {1244}.

Small series suggest that histology, specifically an extensive seminoma component of mixed GCTs, has a beneficial impact on survival {1349,1359}, while a choriocarcinoma component might indicate a more aggressive clinical course {466,2116}.

Postchemotherapy prognostic factors
Postchemotherapy findings are the most important prognostic factors in the era of multimodality treatments. Primary complete response, i.e. normalization of tumour marker levels and disappearance of the mediastinal mass after chemotherapy occurs in 10% of NSGCT patients and is associated with 80% long-term survival {587}. 20% of such patients relapse usually within 2 years after chemotherapy and may be amenable to salvage therapy after early detection of the relapse {2169}.

Among patients that show normalization of tumour markers and a residual tumour mass (80% of cases) {587,588,2169, 2172}, completeness of resection is the most important prognostic factor in adults {199} and children {11,1764}: salvage rates after incomplete resection are <10% in adults and <50% in children.

In addition, postchemotherapy histology has a bearing on prognosis {660,1655}: complete lack of viable tumour cells is associated with a 90% disease-free survival rate, while the rate drops to 60% if viable teratoma, including the growing teratoma syndrome, is encountered. Viable non-teratomatous GCT tumour or somatic-type malignant cells are associated with a 30% and <10% survival rate, respectively.

Patients with persistently elevated tumour markers have a worse prognosis than patients with normalization of tumour markers, although viable tumour cells are detectable in only half of the respective resection specimens {997}. Relapses after chemotherapy and surgery and primary resistance to chemotherapy are poor prognostic factors due to low salvage rates {199}.

Germal cell tumours with somatic-type malignancy

M.R. Wick
E.J. Perlman
Ph. Ströbel
J.K.C. Chan
A. Marx

Definition

A germ cell tumour (GCT) accompanied by a somatic-type malignant component of sarcoma, carcinoma or both. Leukaemias or lymphomas are also somatic-type neoplasms that can accompany mediastinal GCTs

Synonyms

Teratoma with malignant transformation {1394}; Malignant teratoma with nongerminal malignant tumour {1808}; Teratoma with non-germ cell malignancy.

Comments

Tumours included in this category have been collectively called "*Teratomas with malignant components*" etc. in the literature. However, since somatic-type malignancies are more common in mixed germ cell tumours than in teratomas {709,1230,1515,1808,2046} and can also occur in pure yolk sac tumours {2048} and seminomas {879,2047}, the germ cell tumour component that accompanies the somatic malignancy should be specified accordingly.

A minimum size of one low-power field has been suggested as the threshold for the diagnosis of somatic-type malignancy in GCTs {1655,2047}. However, this size criterion is arbitary. More important is the independent growth pattern demonstrated by the somatic-type malignancy. It would be helpful to estimate the size and percentage areas occupied by the somatic malignancy and give this information in the patholgy report.

Epidemiology

GCTs with somatic-type malignancies are rare (~ 2% of all male GCTs) {30}. About 25-30% of cases occur in the mediastinum {2047}. They account for up to 29% of all mediastinal GCTs of adults {40,199,1230,1394,1450,1808,1955}, but are almost non-existent in children {277,406,428,1005,1232,1764}. With few exceptions {277,428,1033}, the tumours occur in males. The age range is from 4-66 years {277,406,1005,1033,1230, 1356,1385}, with most cases occurring between 20-40 years.

The somatic-type malignancies may arise in the mediastinum or only in the metastases {277,1394,1808}. They are more common after chemotherapy and in tumours of late recurences {1665}. After removal of apparently mature teratomas, metastases with pure sarcomatous features have been rarely reported {277,1808}.

Clinical features

Signs and symptoms

The tumours show the same local symptoms as other mediastinal GCTs, but they are more frequently symptomatic (~90%) than pure teratomas (~50%) {1808}. Symptoms due to metastatic disease may accompany or follow local symptoms {1394}.

Most but not all cases show elevated AFP and/or beta-hCG levels in the serum. Other tumour markers (e.g. carcinoembyonic antigen [CEA] or neuronspecific enolase [NSE]) may be elevated according to the malignant components that are present.

Imaging studies typically reveal a solid mass (representing the sacoma or carcinoma component) associated either with a cystic teratomatous structure or with a lesion showing heterogeneous attenuation, predominant areas of enhancing soft tisuue elements, calcifications and massive necrosis {1888}.

Tumour spread

Sarcoma and carcinoma components can infiltrate into the mediastinal structures and the lung {1230}. Metastases have been reported in the majority of cases {1230,1505} and can be composed either of the somatic-type tumour {406,1230}, the GCT or one of its components {1230}, or of both somatic-type and germ cell tumour {1230,2046}. Metastatic spread may involve lung {406,1394}, regional lymph nodes {40,997}, bone {1515,2186}, brain {2046,2186}, liver {40,2046} and spleen {1394,2046}.

Table 3.11
Mediastinal germ cell tumours and associated somatic-type malignancies.

Germ cell tumour component	Frequency[1]	Somatic-type malignancies[2]

Teratoma (mature; immature)	~ 10-20%	Sarcomas/Neurogenic Tumours
		  Rhabdomyosarcoma
		  Angiosarcoma
		  Neuroblastoma
		  Liposarcoma
		  Leiomyosarcoma

Non-teratomatous GCT of one histological type (most commonly seminoma or yolk sac tumour)	< 5%	Osteo-, Chondrosarcoma, Ewing sarcoma/PNET[3] Malignant fibrous histiocytoma MPNST[4] Glioblastoma

Mixed germ cell tumours (almost all cases contain teratoma components)	> 75%	Epithelial Malignancies
		  Adenocarcinoma
		  Adenosquamous carcinoma
		  Squamous cell carcinoma
		  Undifferentiated carcinoma
		Haematological malignancies

[1]Percentage of all mediastinal GCTs with somatic-type malignancies
[2]More than one type of sarcoma and/or carcinoma can occur in a single GCT, and haematologic neoplasias can accompany sarcomas {1394}
[3]PNET, primitive neuroectodermal tumour; [4] MPNST, malignant peripheral nerve sheath tumour

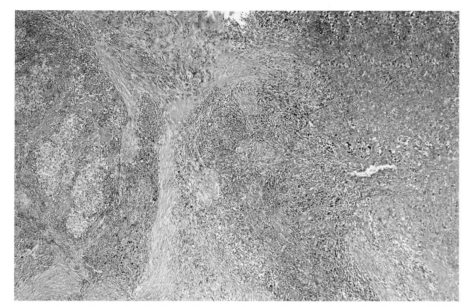

Fig. 3.83 Germ cell tumour (GCT) with somatic-type malignancy: Seminoma (left) and angiosarcoma (right).

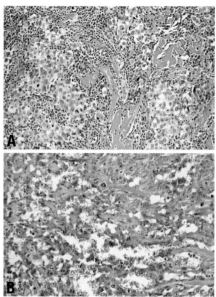

Fig. 3.85 GCT with somatic-type malignancy (STM): A Seminoma and B epithelioid angiosarcoma.

Macroscopy

The tumours range in size from 6 to 30 cm {1230,1356}. They usually exhibit a partially cystic and often variegated cut surface with focally necrotic areas. The carcinoma or sarcoma areas are firm and gray or haemorrhagic (e.g. angiosarcoma) and often adherent to adjacent mediastinal structures {2046}.

Histopathology

Mature {277,428,1033,1385} and immature {520,1195,1505,2186} teratomas, in addition to seminomas, yolk sac tumours or mixed germ cell tumours can be asso-ciated with various sarcomas (63% of cases) {428,2046,2047}, carcinomas (37%) {1385,1808}, combinations of both {1033,1808,2047} or carcinosarcoma {1808}. The somatic malignancy can be intimately intermingled with the GCT component, or forms an expansile nodular proliferation of atypical cells, often with increased mitotic rate and necrosis. Embryonal rhabdomyosarcoma {428,1230,1450} is the single most frequent somatic-type malignancy. Angiosarcoma {1230,2046}, leiomyosarcoma {1450} and neuroblastoma {397,1505} are also common. Any other type of sarcoma or combinations {1230} may occur, including chondrosarcoma, osteosarcoma, malignant fibrous histiocytoma, malignant peripheral nerve sheath tumour, glioblastoma {1808}, and liposarcoma {1359}.

The non-mesenchymal component can be adenocarcinoma (usually of colonic type) {1385,1394,1808,2047}, adenosquamous carcinoma {2047}, squamous cell carcinoma {1655} or primitive neuroectodermal tumours (PNET) {1655}. Melanocytic neuroectodermal tumours {49} and carcinoids {1707} are rare.

Immunohistochemistry

Somatic-type malignancies stain like their counterparts occurring elsewhere in the body. PLAP, AFP, beta-hCG, and CD30 are generally not expressed, while they can be detected in "pure" GCTs and the respective components of mixed GCTs. One should keep in mind that rhabdomyoblasts, embryonal rhabdomyosarcomas and leiomyosarcomas can express PLAP {700} and that hepatoid carcinomas can be AFP-positive.

Genetics

An isochromosome i(12p) genotype shared by the somatic-type neoplasia and the associated germ cell tumour component is typical {789,1113,1394}. In a case of teratoma-associated rhabdomyosarcoma, an add(2)q35-q37 genetic abnormality that is characteristic

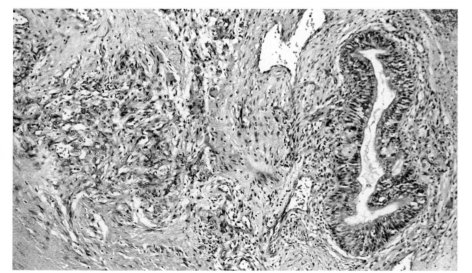

Fig. 3.84 Germ cell tumour with somatic-type malignancy. Immature teratoma and angiosarcoma.

for rhabdomyosarcoma was detected in the sarcoma but not the germ cell component {1394}. Thus, tissue-specific secondary chromosomal aberrations may be necessary for the development of somatic-type tumour components in GCTs. Klinefelter syndrome has been reported in association with GCT with somatic-type malignancy {2186}.

Postulated cell of origin

Malignant transformation of mature teratoma cells or divergent differentiation of a pluri- or totipotent primordial germ cell towards a germ cell tumour and the somatic-type malignancy have been suggested {314}. The latter hypothesis is favoured by the finding that "pure" mature mediastinal teratomas show no chromosome 12 abnormalities {1765} while a shared i(12p) abnormality is characteristic of teratomas that are clonally related with somatic type malignancies, including leukaemias {1394}.

Differential diagnosis

Immature teratoma may be difficult to distinguish from teratoma with somatic-type malignancy. Frank atypia and infiltrative growth favour the latter interpretation. Likewise, chemotherapy-induced atypia is usually diffusely distributed throughout the tumour, while somatic-type malignancy is a focal process often forming a recognizable mass and invading adjacent structures {1888}.
Scattered rhabdomyoblasts are a frequent feature of mature and immature teratomas and do not justify a diagnosis of rhabdomyosarcoma unless they show nodular tumour formation and/or infiltration of adjacent structures.
Rhabdomyoblasts can rarely occur in thymic carcinomas. The thymic carcino-

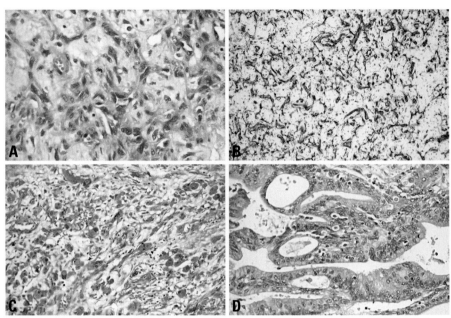

Fig. 3.86 Germ cell tumour with somatic-type malignancy. **A** Angiosarcoma component of the case shown in Fig. 3.85. **B** CD31 expression of the same case. **C** Immature teratoma and rhabdomyosarcoma. **D** Adenocarcinoma component in immature teratoma.

ma is morphologically different form GCT and commonly expresses CD5, while the rhabdomyoblasts are devoid of atypia and proliferative activity.

Prognostic factors

Presence of somatic-type malignancy in a GCT confers a dismal prognosis {406,520,709,997,1005,1230,1394,1515, 1655,2047}. There is no response to chemotherapy used for treatment of germ cell tumours. Only a minority of patients will survive after chemotherapy and complete surgical removal of mediastinal tumour remnants {879,1394, 2047}. Advanced local infiltration, metastatic disease, and incomplete resection are bad prognostic factors {997,1230,

2047}, while the type of somatic malignancy in the primary biopsy has no major impact on survival {1394}. Persistence of viable tumour after chemotherapy heralds an unfavourable outcome {660, 997,2169}. The median survival is only approximately 9 months {406,520, 709, 997,1005,1230,1394,1515,1655, 2047}.

Germ cell tumours with associated haematologic malignancies

A. Orazi
M.R. Wick
J.T. Hartmann
A. Marx

Definition

Germ cell tumours associated with haematologic malignances that are clonally related to the underlying GCTs. The association represents a variant of somatic-type malignancy that is unique to *mediastinal* GCTs. The haematologic malignancies can involve the mediastinum or present as infiltration of bone marrow or lymphatic organs, leukaemia or myelosarcoma. Haematopoietic malignancies that arise due to chemotherapy are not included in this category.

Historical annotation

The association between mediastinal GCTs and hematologic malignancies has been recognized since the 1970s {2599,2477}. Derivation from a GCT-derived pluripotent cell {2592,1681, 1698} and independence from previous radio-chemotherapy {1681,1698} were suggested since the 1980s. Genetic studies {1698,1735,1737} demonstrated chromosomal aberrations that were shared between GCTs and associated haematologic malignancies, providing evidence for a clonal relationship. Extramedullary haematopoiesis in a subgroup of mediastinal GCTs {1310} suggests that committed haematopoietic precursors can be an alternative origin. The predilection of the syndrome for mediastinal GCTs has remained unexplained.

Epidemiology

Haematologic malignancies develop in 2-6% of malignant nonseminomatous mediastinal GCTs {789, 1450} (i.e. 0.5–1,5% of all mediastinal GCTs) but virtually never in GCTs of other sites {1243}. Patients are typically adolescents or young adults (age range 9–48 years) and virtually all are males {315, 474,1461}. About 10-20% of cases have been associated with Klinefelter syndrome {129, 490,1461}.

Clinical signs and findings

In a series of 17 patients the most common clinical features at the diagnosis of the haematologic disorder include pancy- topenia, spleno-/hepatomegaly, or thrombocytopenia in a range of 20 to 35% each. Bleeding complications and infections arise due to cytopenias in myelodysplastic syndromes and acute leukaemias are also common events. Thrombo-embolic complications due to thrombocytosis and megakaryocytic hyperplasia {1461}, and mediastinal mass formation due to myelosarcoma is rare {1723}. Other clinical signs are leukaemic skin lesions, and flushing {789}, and the development of haemo-phagocytic syndromes {2055}. Haematological complications can accompany, follow {199,2055,2087} or precede local symptoms. Leukaemias most commonly become apparent within the first year after the diagnosis of GCTs (range 0–122 months; median 6 months) {474,789,1394,1461,1518}. There is no increased overall risk for other second tumours in mediastinal GCT patients {199,788}.

Etiology and pathogenesis

The etiology is unresolved. It has been speculated that expression of haematopoietic growth and differentiation factors in some mediastinal GCTs could drive differentiation of primordial germ cells into haematopoietic progeny. The profile of differentiation factors expressed may also underlie the preferred commitment of transformed precursors to the megakaryocytic and monocytic lineage {1450, 1518}. Concommittant mediastinal and extramediastinal leukaemias show a comparable immunophenotype and genotype, suggesting spread of haematopoietic tumour cells from GCTs to blood, bone marrow, and extra-medullary sites {1113,1394}.

Macroscopy

Gross findings are identical to those of non-seminomatous malignant GCTs.

Histopathology

The GCTs underlying the haematologic malignancies typically are non-seminomatous malignant GCT, most often yolk sac tumours or mixed germ cell neo- plasias with a yolk sac component, though immature teratomas and mixed germ cell tumours with somatic-type sarcomas have been observed {83,315, 1112,1394,1461}. In a series of 287 patients with nonseminomatous mediastinal germ cell tumours, yolk sac and teratocarcinoma histology have been significantly associated with the occurrence of haematologic neoplasias {789}. Categories of haematological malignancies reported are: acute leukemias {199,1132}, malignant (and rarely benign {2246}) histiocytosis {83,129,474,1112, 1461}, myelodysplastic syndromes {1450, 1846,2087}, myeloproliferative diseases {315,1113,1461}, and mastocytosis {335}. Among acute leukaemias, acute megakaryoblastic leukaemia (AML M7) and "malignant histiocytosis" (including AML M4 {729,1113} and M5 {2074}) are most common and account for about half of the cases {199,1461,1518}. In addition, AML M2 {2087}, M6 {1450,1729}, acute undifferentiated leukemia (AUL) {1461}, and acute lymphoblastic leukaemia {1132, 1461} have been described.

Myelodysplastic syndromes (MDSs) include refractory anaemia with excess blasts {1846} or cases with megakaryocytic hyperplasia {1460}, suggesting the 5q- syndrome {1394}. Myelodysplasia can precede AMLs {2087}.

Essential thrombocytemia and chronic idiopathic myelofibrosis are the characteristic myeloproliferative disorders encountered in association with mediastinal GCTs {663,814,1461}.

Leukaemias may diffusely or focally infiltrate the underlying GCT {1518} or can form tumorous lesions (granulocytic sarcomas) in the mediastinum {1723}. Extramediastinal manifestations (organomegaly, leukaemia) can occur in the presence or absence of detectable haematopoietic malignancy in the mediastinal GCT {1518}.

Immunohistochemistry

Interpretation of cytochemical findings in blood or bone marrow smears, and immunophenotypic profiles follows the

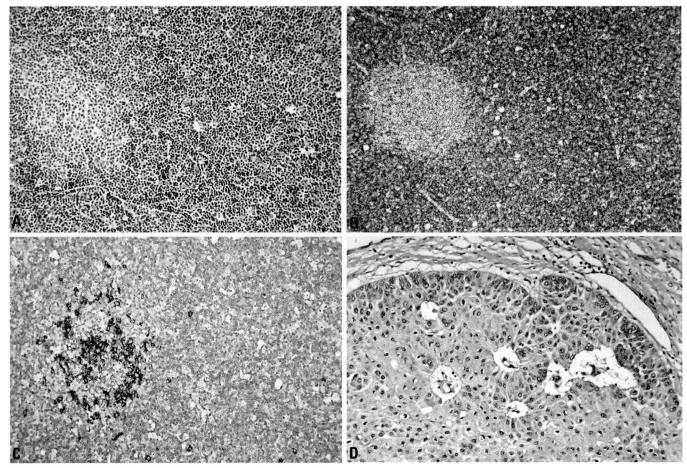

Fig. 3.86a A-D Case of a mediastinal germ cell tumour with haematopoietic component. **A, B** Note the haematopoietic component in the yolk sac tumour blood vessels. **C** Poorly differentiated myeloid precursors showing focal myleoid peroxidase immunoreactivity. Myeloblasts were also positive for CD34 (not shown). **D** Subsequent bone marrow biopsy shows acute myeloid leukaemia.

criteria of the WHO classification of tumours of haematopoietic and lymphoid tissues {919}. Useful immunohistochemical stainigs include myeloperoxidase (MPO), lysozyme, CD10, CD20, CD34, CD68, CD61, CD117, TdT, and glycophorin.

Genetics

Isochromosome 12 [i(12p)] is the most specific and most common chromosomal marker shared by GCTs and the associated haematologic malignancies {315, 1394,1461}. In addition, the haematologic malignancies can harbour genetic alterations that are typical for specific haematologic malignancies in general (del(5q); trisomy 8), suggesting that GCT-unspecific aberrations determine the phenotype of the associated haematologic malignancy {1394}.

Postulated cell of origin

Toti- or pluripotent primordial germ cell. Alternatively, the detection of non-neoplastic extramedullary haemotopoiesis in the yolk sac tumour component of some GCTs suggests that some haematologic malignancies can arise from more committed, somatic-type haematopoietic cells by malignant transformation {1518}.

Differential diagnosis

Clonally-related haematologic malignancies must be distinguished from secondary MDSs and AMLs that are related to salvage chemotherapy regimens including etoposide in patients with mediastinal GCT {100,1047}. Secondary MDSs ocurred in 0.7%, and AMLs in 1.3 % of cases in a large series {1047}. Chemotherapy-related AMLs do not show i(12p) and usually manifest later (25–60

months after chemotherapy) than germ cell-related AMLs (median time to onset 6 months, range 0–122) {789, 1461}.

Prognostic factors

The occurrence of a clonally related acute leukaemia in a patient with mediastinal GCT is among the most adverse prognostic factors. In a recent series, none of the reported patients has survived for more than 2 years after the onset of leukemia (median survival time: 6 months) {789}. These leukaemias appear to be refractory to current treatment protocols including aggressive induction chemotherapy and allogenic bone marrow transplantation. However, the clinical course in patients with myeloproliferative diseases may be more protracted {663,814}.

Mediastinal lymphomas and haematopoietic neoplasms: Introduction

E.S. Jaffe
N.L. Harris

Principles of classification

The classification of haematological malignancies has undergone significant reappraisal in recent years. These changes have resulted from insights gained through the application of immunological and genetic techniques, as well a better understanding of the clinical aspects of lymphoid and myeloid neoplasms through advances in diagnosis, staging and treatment. A multifaceted approach to both disease definition and diagnosis, as proposed by the Revised European and American Lymphoma (REAL) classification {783} and updated in the WHO classification {919}, is now considered the state of the art.

While morphology is still the starting point for pathologic diagnosis, immunologic and genetic techniques have been crucial in defining disease entities, and are often useful in differential diagnosis. The pathologist must also be cognizant of the clinical history, as the site of presentation and other clinical parameters are an important aspect of both disease definition and diagnosis. Finally, in many instances, lymphoid and myeloid neoplasms can be related to a normal cellular counterpart in the haematopoietic and lymphoid systems.

Mediastinal lymphomas arise in either mediastinal lymph nodes or the thymus gland. Thymic lymphomas are unique in many respects, as they reflect the function of the thymus gland as an organ involved in T-cell generation and differentiation {1863}. Precursor T-lymphoblastic lymphoma/leukaemia presents as a mediastinal mass in 85% of cases, and the immunophenotype of the neoplastic cells reflects the stages of cortical thymocyte differentiation {157,1604}. There are also rare reports of natural killer (NK)-cell tumours with an immature phenotype arising in the thymus gland {1046}, and the fetal thymus is one site of NK-cell development {1863}. B-cell lymphomas of the thymus gland are relatively rare. The most common of these is mediastinal large B-cell lymphoma (PMLBCL), of proposed origin from specialized thymic B-cells found in the medullary perivascular space {22,906}. Classical Hodgkin lymphoma, nodular sclerosis type, (HLNS) also arises in the thymus gland, and is genotypically of B-cell origin, although B-cell markers may be absent. Lymphomas of mucosa-associated lymphoid tissue (MALT)-type may arise in the thymus gland, as well as in other mucosal or epithelial sites, and reflect the intimate functional relationship between epithelial and lymphoid components in the thymus gland {891}. A functionally related lesion is the multilocular thymic cyst seen in autoimmune disease and HIV-infection {1051,1326,1923}. Lymphomas involving the mediastinal lymph nodes reflect to some extent the spectrum of systemic nodal lymphomas. However, because of its inaccessibility as a biopsy site, the primary diagnosis of lymphoma is uncommonly made in mediastinal lymph nodes. Myeloid neoplasms rarely have primary presentations in the mediastinum. A recently described entity, precursor T-lymphoblastic lymphoma with eosinophilia and t(8;13) typically presents with a mediastinal tumour with the immunophenotype of T-LBL, but is associated with development of acute myeloid leukaemia in the bone marrow {2179}. Acute myeloid leukaemias, often with megakaryoblastic differentiation may develop in the mediastinum and bone marrow in association with non-seminomatous germ cell tumours with an i(12)p {159,315,474,506,729,1113,1460, 1461,1723}.

Histiocytic and dendritic cell tumours are rare tumours that occasionally may present in mediastinal lymph nodes and the thymus gland. However, as with myeloid neoplasms, most histiocytic neoplasms presenting in the mediastinum are related to teratomatous germ cell tumours, indicative of the capacity of germ cell neoplasms to differentiate along many cell lines {159,729,1052,1518,1723}.

Epidemiology

The epidemiology of haematopoietic and lymphoid neoplasms of the mediastinum and thymus gland is heterogeneous, reflecting the diversity of disease entities presenting in this site. Precursor T-cell and NK-cell neoplasms are for the most part diseases of children and young adults, with an increased male: female ratio. Mediastinal large B-cell lymphoma and nodular sclerosis Hodgkin lymphoma share many epidemiological features, including prevalence in young adult females, and propensity to present with localized disease. This observation, plus the fact that synchronous and metachronous instances of mediastinal large B-cell lymphoma and nodular sclerosis Hodgkin lymphoma may be encountered, has suggested that these neoplasms may share a common cell of origin {710,1575}. In addition, there are rare grey zone lymphomas with features intermediate between both entities {1270,1704}.

Clinical features

With the exception of the relatively rare MALT-type lymphomas, most mediastinal lymphomas and haematopoietic neoplasms are clinically aggressive; patients typically present with symptoms related to a large mediastinal mass, or with pericardial or pleural effusions in lymphoblastic lymphoma. Other clinical features vary with the type of lymphoma.

Genetic features

The genetic features of these neoplasms for the most part are similar to their counterparts presenting in other sites. One exception is mediastinal large B-cell lymphoma, which has genetic features distinct from that of other diffuse large B-cell lymphomas {148,404,1756}.

Primary mediastinal large B-cell lymphoma

F. Menestrina
N.L. Harris
P. Möller

Definition
Primary mediastinal large B-cell lymphoma (PMLBCL) is a type of diffuse large B-cell lymphoma arising in the mediastinum, of putative thymic B-cell origin, with distinctive clinical, immunophenotypic and genotypic features.

ICD-O code   9679/3

Synonyms
Primary mediastinal clear cell lymphoma of B-cell type {1341}, mediastinal large-cell lymphoma of B-type with sclerosis {1296}. *REAL*: Primary mediastinal (thymic) large B-cell lymphoma {783}

Epidemiology
It accounts for about 2-3% of non-Hodgkin lymphomas and occurs predominantly in young adults (third and fourth decade), with a slight female predominance {3,305,783,1143}. Both of these factors distinguish PMLBCL from other types of diffuse large B-cell lymphoma, which have a median age in the 7th decade and a male predominance.

Etiology
It is unrelated to EBV or other known tumour viruses {1340,2034}. It might be driven by a still elusive oncogene, probably located on chromosome 9p {941}.

Localization
At presentation, the disease affects the antero-superior area of the mediastinum without superficial lymphadenopathy or hepato-splenomegaly. The thymus is typically involved and rare cases of lymphoma confined to the thymus have been reported, suggesting that the tumour arises in the thymus and secondarily involves mediastinal lymph nodes {918,1121}. The mass is often "bulky" (>10 cm in diameter) and is often locally invasive, infiltrating lung, pleura, thoracic wall and pericardium. Supraclavicular extension is sometimes observed {22, 1296,1341}. At progression, PMLBCL disseminates predominantly to extranodal sites, including lung and extrathoracic organs {305}: liver, kidney, and adrenal are the most frequent sites of parenchymal involvement; gastro-intestinal tract, ovary, CNS, and pancreas {171} are other reported sites. Bone marrow involvement is extremely rare.

Clinical features
Signs and symptoms are related to the mediastinal mass: superior vena cava syndrome (most frequently), airway obstruction, pleural and/or pericardial effusion. B symptoms may be present {1143}. Traditional or more sophisticated imaging techniques are important in detecting the mass, in documenting the involvement of other intra-thoracic structures and in deciding on the best approach to obtain a diagnostic biopsy.

Macroscopy
Radical surgery or debulking is rarely performed, because the mass is typical-

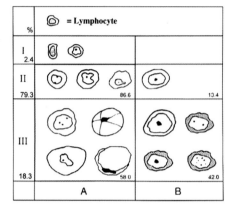

Fig. 3.87 Summary of the cytological variants encountered in a series of 109 mediastinal large B-cell lymphomas (PMLBCL). From Paulli et al. {1558}.

ly widely infiltrative at the time of the diagnosis. In resected specimens, the cut surface has a fleshy appearance, often with necrotic areas. Thymic cysts may be present. Diagnostic features may be lacking in small (e.g., trans-thoracic needle) biopsies when only sclerosing and/or necrotic tissue is obtained.

Tumour spread and staging
PMLBCL most probably arises intrathymically {22} and then aggressively invades adjacent structures and tissues, including regional lymph nodes, whereas distant lymph nodes are rarely affected. Leukaemia is never observed; however, haematogenous dissemination occurs during progression, as evidenced by distant organ involvement {305}. Staging procedures must exclude a secondary mediastinal involvement by a systemic diffuse large B-cell lymphoma; extrathoracic lymph nodes or bone marrow involvement would suggest this diagnosis.

Histopathology
The growth pattern is diffuse. PMLBCL has a broad range of cytomorphology; however, individual cases tend to be monomorphic. The cells range from

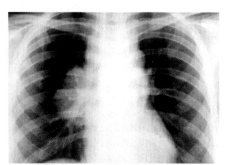

Fig. 3.88 Chest X-ray of a bulky mediastinal large B-cell lymphoma (PMLBCL).

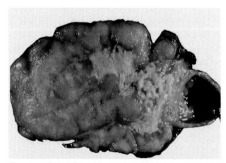

Fig. 3.89 PMLBCL with fleshy, whitish tumour tissue, containing necrotic and pseudocystic areas.

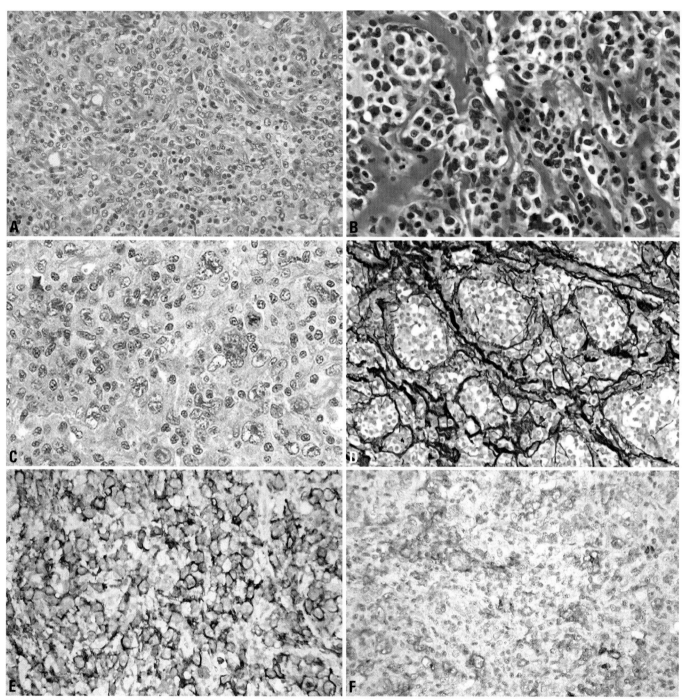

Fig. 3.90 Mediastinal large B-cell lymphoma. **A** High power view of mediastinal large B-cell lymphoma. **B** Note the clear cytoplasm and the very irregular nuclei with inconspicuous nucleoli. **C** Polymorphic tumour cells including Hodgkin-like cells. **D** Silver stain highlights the pseudoalveolar compartmentalization of the neoplastic tissue by collagen fibrils and fibers. **E** CD20 expression. **F** CD30 expression.

medium-sized to large (2-5 times the size of a small lymphocyte), have abundant, frequently clear cytoplasm and irregularly round or ovoid (occasionally multilobated) nuclei, usually with small nucleoli {1558}. Some cases may have more pleomorphic nuclei and abundant amphophilic cytoplasm and may resemble Hodgkin lymphoma or nonlymphoid tumours. Mitotic activity is high, similar to other large cell lymphomas. The centre of the lesion contains predominantly neoplastic cells. However, at periphery of the mass, a variable number of reactive cells such as lymphocytes, macrophages and granulocytes may be present. A frequent but not consistent feature is a distinctive fibrosis made up of irregular collagen bands compartmentalizing cellular areas of varying size {1296,1341,1558,2224}. The combination of different architectural patterns and cellular morphology might raise the differential diagnosis of thymoma, seminoma or Hodgkin lymphoma.

Depending on the surgical approach and specimen size, thymic remnants can be observed, usually better highlighted by immunohistology. Cystic change may be present in the thymic remnant. Lung, pleura and pericardium can be included. Rare cases of composite PMLBCL and Hodgkin lymphoma are reported {1704}.

Immunophenotype

PMLBCL expresses B-cell lineage-specific surface molecules such as CD19, CD20, CD22 {1344}, and the immunoglobulin-associated CD79a {1595} molecule, but not lineage-restricted T-cell antigens, except for MAL {404}, which is regarded as T-cell restricted and is not observed in other diffuse large B-cell lymphomas. CD10 has been detected in some studies in 20-25%, similar to its frequency in other large B-cell lymphomas {448,1595}, but has not been detected in other studies {1343,1344}. CD15 and CD21 are always negative. BCL6 protein may be detected by immunohistochemistry in 50-60% of the cases. Molecules often found in/on PMLBCL cells like CD38, PC-1, MUM1 and PAX5 {1595} in the absence of CD138 favour a post-germinal centre stage of maturation. The majority of PMLBCL do not express Ig {1296,1341}. In fact, the discrepancy between the lack of Ig and the constitutive CD79a {953} is characteristic of this disease. The lack of Ig expression is likely not related to a defect in the Ig transcriptional machinery since the Ig transcription factors Oct2 and BoB.1 are expressed {1595}. Furthermore, there is frequently a defect of HLA class I and/or II molecule expression {1342}.

CD30 expression, often weak and restricted to a subset of the tumour cells, is often observed in PMLBCL, especially when antigen retrieval techniques are used {829}. CD30 expression is typically low compared with the strong CD30 expression in neoplastic cells of classic Hodgkin lymphoma (HL) or in diffuse large B-cell lymphoma (DLBCL) of anaplastic type. This may result in differential diagnostic problems between PMLBCL, Hodgkin disease, and the so-called "grey zone" lymphomas of the mediastinum, which have features intermediate between HL and DLBCL {1704}.

Histogenesis

Histologically, PMLBCL has been attributed to the asteroid variant of thymic

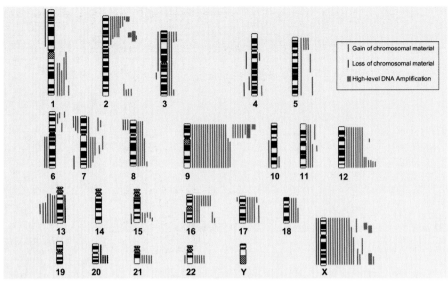

Fig. 3.91 Mediastinal large B-cell lymphoma. This tableau summarizes the data of the comparative genomic hybridization (CGH) of 44 cases of PMLBCL. From M. Bentz et al. {148}.

medullary B-cells {862}. Genetically, PMLBCL seems to be derived from B-cells that have been activated by a specific antigen, passed through the germinal centre and have shut down their mutational machinery before neoplastic transformation is completed {1158}. Immunophenotypically, PMLBCL are at post-germinal centre stage {1158,1344, 1595}.

Somatic genetics

Antigen receptor genes and BCL6. As in other diffuse large B-cell lymphomas, Ig heavy-chain and light-chain genes are rearranged and have high loads of mutations {872,1098,1158,1753}. Further, the vast majority of heavy-chain V genes are potentially functional by showing evidence of selection for a functional antibody. No bias towards particular gene families (such as VH4) were observed, so selection by an autoantigen or superantigen is unlikely. Intraclonal variation was not detected in the PMLBCL cases analysed so far, indicating that continuing mutational activity is not a prominent feature {1158}. The data on frequencies of *BCL-6* mutations in PMLBCL are conflicting, ranging from 6-50% {448,1532, 1595,2034}.

Genetic abnormalities. BCL-2 is germline, suggesting that the regular expression of bcl-2 protein in PMLBCL is regulatory {1595,2034}. *BCL-1* and *N-ras* are not altered while *p16, c-MYC,* and *TP53* occasionally carry mutations {1595,1754, 1755}. Different genetic

approaches, including comparative genomic hybridi-zation, FISH, arbitrarily primed PCR fingerprinting and classical cytogenetics have yielded a highly characteristic pattern of genomic alterations in PMLBCL: chromosomal gains (2p, 6p, 7q, 9p, 12, and X) are much more frequent than losses {941,1661,1756}. Most important is gain of chromosome arm 9p (9p+), which is detectable in up to 75% of cases {148}. This aberration is a chromosomal marker in PMLBCL, since 9+ is very rare in other nodal and extranodal B-cell lymphomas but, interestingly, is detectable in about 25% of classic Hodgkin disease {940}. In both tumours, the consensus region of the recurrent aberrations on 9p is subtelomeric. A second essential genomic region in PMLB-CL is the long arm of chromosome X. Aberrations of Xq, including high levels of DNA amplification, are present in up to 87% of cases of PMLBCL {148}. Recent molecular studies applying gene expression profiling show that classical Hodgkin lymphoma and PMLBCL are closely related {1694,1752}.

Prognosis and predictive factors

There are no histological {1558}, immunophenotypic or genotypic features that have prognostic potential. Similarly to other DLBCL, response to initial therapy is a good marker for prognosis. The survival with aggressive therapy is similar to that of other localized DLBCL {305,918,1143}.

Thymic extranodal marginal zone B-cell lymphoma of mucosa-associated lymphoid tissue (MALT)

A.C.L. Chan
J.K.C. Chan
H. Inagaki
S. Nakamura
P. Möller

Definition
Primary thymic extranodal marginal zone B-cell lymphoma of mucosa-associated lymphoid tissue is a lymphoma consisting predominantly of small B-cells with a centrocyte-like or monocytoid appearance, which surround reactive follicles and infiltrate the thymic epithelium to produce lymphoepithelial lesions.

ICD-O code   9699/3

Synonyms
Mucosa-associated lymphoid tissue (MALT) lymphoma; MALToma

Epidemiology
Primary thymic extranodal marginal zone B-cell lymphoma is rare, with less than 30 cases having been reported in the literature {493,778,891,905,1209,1279,1426, 1556,1700,1945,2188}. Most patients are in the fifth and sixth decades. There is female predominance (M:F = 1:3), and >60% of the reported cases are Asians.

Etiology
Primary thymic extranodal marginal zone B-cell lymphoma is strongly associated with autoimmune disease (>50% of the cases), especially Sjögren syndrome {891}. The autoimmune disease-associated reactive lymphoid hyperplasia may provide a fertile ground for emergence of the lymphoma. There is no association with Epstein Barr virus {891}. There is

currently no evidence for a histogenetic link with mediastinal large B-cell lymphoma.

Localization
The bulk of the disease is in the anterior mediastinum, but the regional lymph nodes and other extranodal sites (e.g. stomach, salivary gland, lung) may be involved concurrently.

Clinical features
Patients are usually asymptomatic, with the mediastinal tumour being discovered incidentally on chest radiograph. A minority of patients present with chest pain, shortness of breath, haemoptysis or back pain. In patients associated with autoimmune disease, the time interval between the onset of autoimmune disease and the discovery of the thymic tumour ranges from 2-25 years {891}. Monoclonal gammopathy (frequently IgA, occasionally IgG or IgM) is common, and may sometimes result in hyperviscosity syndrome {891,1209}. An association with Sjögren disease is frequently observed.

Macroscopy
Grossly, the tumour is often encapsulated and comprises solid greyish-white fleshy tissue commonly interspersed with multiple variable-sized cysts. Invasion into the adjacent pericardium and pleura is sometimes found.

Tumour spread and staging
Most tumours (>75%) are of low stage (Stage I/II) at presentation {891}. Concurrent extranodal marginal zone B-cell lymphoma in other MALT sites (e.g. salivary gland, stomach, lung) occurs in about 20% of cases, probably related to the homing characteristics of extranodal marginal zone B-cell lymphomas {891}.

Histopathology
The normal thymic lobular architecture is effaced by an abnormal dense lymphoid infiltrate, but residual Hassall corpuscles can still be identified. There are common-

ly many interspersed epithelium-lined cystic spaces. Reactive lymphoid follicles are scattered within the lymphoid infiltrate. There is a proliferation of small lymphocytes and centrocyte-like cells around and between these follicles. The centrocyte-like cells have small to medium-sized irregular nuclei, indistinct nucleoli, and a moderate amount of pale cytoplasm. They show extensive invasion of the Hassall corpuscles or the thymic epithelium lining the cystic spaces, forming lymphoepithelial lesions. The lymphoid cells within and immediately around the epithelial structures usually possess an even greater amount of clear cytoplasm, reminiscent of monocytoid B-cells. There are often interspersed aggregates of plasma cells, which are shown on immunohistochemical staining to be

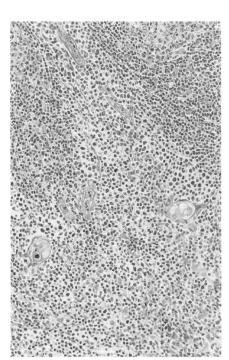

Fig. 3.93 Primary extranodal marginal zone B-cell lymphoma of the thymus. Part of a reactive lymphoid follicle is seen at the top. The lower field shows thymic epithelium (including Hassall corpuscles), heavily infiltrated by lymphoma cells. The cells within and immediately around the epithelial unit have abundant clear cytoplasm, resembling monocytoid B cells.

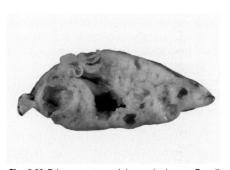

Fig. 3.92 Primary extranodal marginal zone B-cell lymphoma of the thymus. The cut surface shows fleshy, tan-coloured tumour tissue interspersed with multiple cystic spaces.

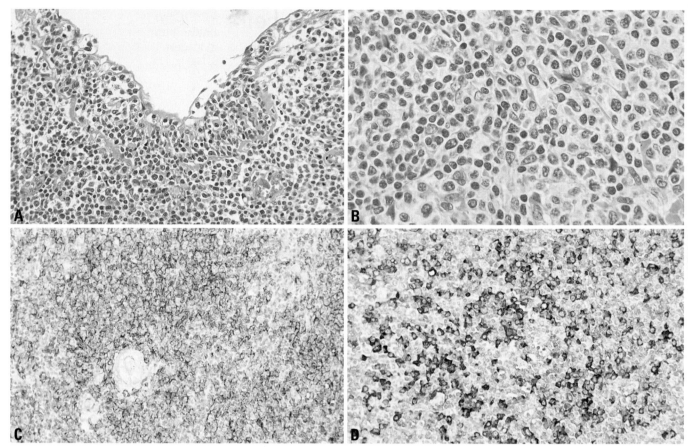

Fig. 3.94 Primary extranodal marginal zone B-cell lymphoma of the thymus. **A** The thymic epithelium lining the cysts is extensively infiltrated by the lymphoma cells. Note also the presence of small clusters of plasma cells. **B** The lymphomatous infiltrate comprises small lymphocytes, centrocyte-like cells and cells resembling monocytoid B cells. **C** Immunostaining for CD20 shows sheets of positive cells, confirming the B-cell lineage of the lymphoma. A residual Hassall corpuscle is seen in the left middle field. Note that plasma cells do not react. **D** Many plasma cells are highlighted by immunostaining for immunoglobulin (lambda light chain in this case).

part of the neoplastic clone. Scattered centroblast-like cells or immunoblasts are frequently found. Transformation to diffuse large B-cell lymphoma has only been rarely reported {1209}.

Immunophenotype
Immunohistochemically, the tumour cells express B-cell specific markers, such as CD20 and CD79a. They are negative for CD3, CD5, CD10, CD23, CD43, and cyclin D1. They commonly express BCL2. More than 75% of the cases express IgA {891}.

Differential diagnosis
The main differential diagnosis is reactive lymphoid hyperplasia of the thymus. In reactive lymphoid hyperplasia, which is most frequently associated with myasthenia gravis, the thymic lobular architecture is preserved, and there is no band-like or sheet-like proliferation of centro-

cyte-like cells and monocytoid cells {1556}.

Histogenesis
This lymphoma is derived from post-germinal centre marginal zone B-cells.

Somatic genetics
Immunoglobulin genes are clonally rearranged {950}. Although *API2-MALT1* fusion resulting from t(11;18) is present in up to 50% of extranodal marginal zone B-cell lymphomas in general, this chromosomal translocation is not detected in thymic extranodal marginal zone B-cell lymphomas {891}. Only one case has been studied by cytogenetics, with the finding of 46,X,dup(X)(p11p22) {778}.

Genetic susceptibility
There is no known genetic susceptibility. It remains unclear whether this lymphoma type shows a predilection for Asians.

Prognosis and predictive factors
Thymic extranodal marginal zone B-cell lymphoma is associated with an excellent outcome. Only one documented tumour-related death has been reported {891}. High tumour stage at presentation or concurrent involvement of other MALT sites is not necessarily associated with a poor prognosis. Most patients have undergone surgical resection both for diagnosis and treatment of low stage disease. Chemotherapy and radiotherapy have also resulted in complete remission in some cases.

Precursor T-lymphoblastic lymphoma / leukaemia

N. L. Harris
M. Borowitz
E.S. Jaffe
J. Vardiman

Definition
Precursor T-lymphoblastic lymphoma/ leukaemia is a neoplasm of lymphoblasts committed to the T-cell lineage, typically composed of small to medium-sized blast cells with scant cytoplasm, moderately condensed to dispersed chromatin and indistinct nucleoli, variably involving bone marrow and blood (precursor T-cell acute lymphoblastic leukaemia), thymus and/or lymph nodes (precursor T-cell lymphoblastic lymphoma).

ICD-O code
Precursor T-lymphoblastic lymphoma
               9729/3
Precursor T-lymphoblastic leukaemia
               9837/3

Synonyms
Precursor T-cell acute lymphoblastic leukaemia (ALL) / Precursor T-cell lymphoblastic lymphoma (LBL); T-cell lymphoblastic lymphoma; T-cell acute lymphoblastic leukaemia; convoluted lymphocytic lymphoma (Lukes-Collins); lymphoblastic lymphoma, convoluted cell type (Kiel, Working formulation); poorly-differentiated lymphocytic lymphoma (Rappaport); leukosarcoma (Sternberg sarcoma) (historical term) {1878}

Epidemiology
Precursor T-cell neoplasms occur most frequently in late childhood, adolescence, and young adulthood, with a male predominance. Fifteen percent of child-

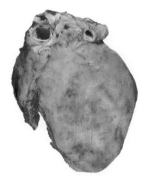

Fig. 3.95 Infiltration of the heart by a T-lymphoblastic lymphoma.

hood and 25% of adult ALL are of precursor T-cell type {206}. Cases presenting without bone marrow and peripheral blood involvement (lymphoblastic lymphoma) comprise 85% of lymphoblastic lymphomas, 25-30% of childhood non-Hodgkin lymphomas and only 2% of adult non-Hodgkin lymphomas worldwide {3}. Some studies indicate an increased prevalence of precursor T-cell neoplasia in underdeveloped countries, while precursor B-cell neoplasms are more common in industrialized countries {2016}.

Etiology
The etiology is unknown. No association with viruses or immune status has been demonstrated. Patients with ataxia telangiectasia are at increased risk for development of T-ALL, but the ATM gene has not been implicated in sporadic T-precursor neoplasia {1959}. In early childhood T-ALL, the neoplastic clone can be detected at birth by clone-specific T-cell receptor gene rearrangement, suggesting that the transforming event occurs in utero {559}.

Localization
The tumour typically involves the mediastinum, specifically the thymus, and often mediastinal lymph nodes. Supradiaphragmatic lymph nodes may also be involved, and tumour cells are often shed into the pleural fluid. The bone marrow and peripheral blood are involved in the majority of the cases. Central nervous system involvement is also common. Clinically, a case is defined as lymphoma if there is a mediastinal or other mass and <25% blasts in the bone marrow, and as leukaemia if there are >25% bone marrow blasts, with or without a mass. This is an arbitrary distinction and should be regarded as staging rather than classification.

Clinical features
Patients typically present acutely with symptoms related to a large mediastinal mass, often with pleural or pericardial

effusions. Airway compromise is common, and the presentation is often as a medical emergency

Histopathology
The thymus and mediastinal soft tissue as well as adjacent lymph nodes are involved. The epithelial meshwork is destroyed, septa are effaced, and the tumour cells spread through the capsule into adjacent mediastinal tissue. In tissue sections, the cells are small to medium-sized, with scant cytoplasm, round, oval, or convoluted nuclei, with fine chromatin and indistinct or small nucleoli. Occasional cases have larger cells. In lymph nodes the pattern is infiltrative rather than destructive, often with partial preservation of the subcapsular sinus and germinal centres. A starry-sky pattern may be present, but is usually less prominent than in Burkitt lymphoma. Pleural or pericardial fluid may be the initial diagnostic specimen. On smears, lymphoblasts vary from small cells with

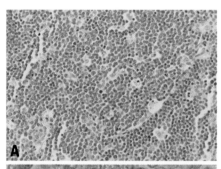

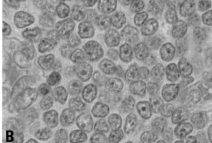

Fig. 3.96 Precursor T-lymphoblastic lymphoma **A** Monomorphous infiltrate with a starry-sky pattern. **B** Tumour cells have dispersed chromatin, small nucleoli, and scant cytoplasm, such that the nuclei appear to overlap.

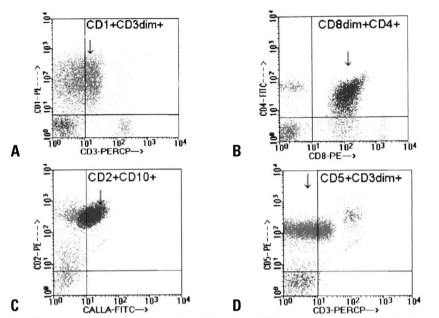

Fig. 3.97 Precursor T-cell acute lymphoblastic leukaemia (T-ALL). Flow cytometry of peripheral blood from an adolescent male with a mediastinal mass. **A** Cells are positive for CD1 and dimly for surface CD3. **B** Cells express both CD4 and CD8. **C** The cells express CD2 and CD10. **D** They are positive for CD5 and dimly for CD3.

scant cytoplasm, condensed nuclear chromatin, and indistinct nucleoli to larger cells with a moderate amount of cytoplasm, dispersed chromatin, and multiple nucleoli. Azurophilic granules may be present.

Recently, cases of mediastinal precursor T-cell lymphomas with increased tissue and bone marrow eosinophils have been described. Patients typically developed acute leukaemia with myeloid antigen expression. These cases were found to have a translocation t(8;13) in both the myeloid and lymphoid cells, indicating a true biphenotypic malignancy {2179}.

Immunophenotype
The lymphoblasts are positive for terminal deoxynucleotidyl transferase (TdT) in virtually all cases, and variably express CD2, CD7, surface or cytoplasmic CD3, CD5, CD1a, CD4 and/or CD8. Only surface CD3 is considered lineage-specific. Minimal criteria for classification as T-LBL are CD7+ and cytoplasmic CD3+. The constellation of antigens defines stages of differentiation, ranging from early or pro-T (CD2, CD7 and cytoplasmic CD3), to "common" thymocyte (CD1a, sCD3, CD4 and CD8), to late thymocyte (CD4 or CD8).

Although there is some correlation with presentation and differentiation stage (cases with bone marrow and blood presentation may show earlier differentiation stage than cases with thymic presentation {157,725}) there is overlap {1632}. Among cases that express T-cell receptor proteins, the majority are of the alpha/beta type and a minority express gamma/delta type; the latter appear to have a more immature phenotype {1938}. Rare cases of lymphoblastic lymphoma presenting in the mediastinum have the immunophenotype of immature natural killer (NK) cells {325,1046,1795}.

Differential diagnosis
On biopsy specimens, the differential diagnosis may include thymoma with a prominent immature T-cell population (B1 or B2 thymoma). The immunophenotype of T-LBL and of the normal precursor T-cells in thymoma can be identical. The infiltrative growth of the lymphoblasts with destruction of the epithelium and demonstration of clonality by molecular genetic analysis can be helpful in confirming the diagnosis of lymphoma.
In a patient with a mediastinal mass and lymphocytosis, a diagnosis of peripheral T-cell lymphocytosis associated with thymoma has to be included among the differential diagnoses {116,445}.

Histogenesis
Precursor T lymphoblasts at varying stages of differentiation.

Somatic genetics
Rearrangement of antigen receptor genes is variable in lymphoblastic neoplasms, and may not be lineage-specific; thus, precursor T-cell neoplasms may have either or both T-cell receptor (TCR) beta or gamma chain gene rearrangements and immunoglobulin heavy chain gene rearrangements {1939}. The majority have T-cell receptor gamma chain rearrangements, with either beta or delta rearrangements in the majority of the cases {1938}.

Chromosomal translocations involving the TCR alpha and delta loci at chromosome 14q11 and beta and gamma loci at 7q34 are present in about one-third of the cases {998,2044}; the partner genes are variable and include the transcription factors c-MYC (8q24), TAL1/SCL (1p32), RBTN1 (11p35), RBTN2 (11q13), and HOX11 (10q24) and the cytoplasmic tyrosine kinase LCK (1p34). In an additional 25%, the TAL1 locus at 1p32 has deletions in the 5' regulatory region {136}. Deletions of 9p involving deletion of the p16^{ink4a} tumour suppressor gene (CDK4 inhibitor) is also seen in T-lymphoblastic neoplasms {901,1601}.

Cases associated with eosinophilia and myeloid neoplasia have a t(8;13) involving the fibroblast growth factor receptor gene on chromosome 8 and a novel zinc-finger gene on chromosome 13 {2179}.

Analysis by gene expression array has shown that acute leukaemias of lymphoid and myeloid types can be distinguished, as can precursor T and precursor B-cell lymphoblastic leukaemias. The utility of these studies in diagnosis remains to be determined, however, some differentially expressed genes, such as TAL1/SCL can be detected by immunohistochemistry and may provide a marker for T-precursor neoplasia {552,706}

Prognostic factors
The prognosis with aggressive therapy is similar to that of precursor B-cell neoplasms, and is not affected by immunophenotype or genetic abnormalities. In children, treatment is generally more aggressive than that for precursor B-ALL, and is typically the same for lymphomatous and leukemic presentations {1361}. The median disease-free survival in one recent study of adult T-ALL was 28 months {206,2044}.

Anaplastic large-cell lymphoma and mature T and NK cell lymphomas of the mediastinum

S. Nakamura
T. Rüdiger
A. Marx

Definition
Mature T-cell and NK-cell neoplasms are derived from mature or post-thymic T cells and NK cells, respectively. Because they share some immunophenotypic and functional properties, these two classes of neoplasms are considered together.

ICD-O code
Anaplastic large-cell lymphoma
9714/3

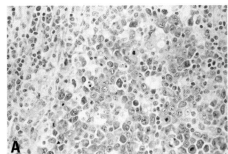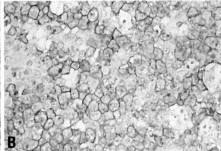

Fig. 3.98 Anaplastic large-cell lymphoma. **A** Hallmark cells with embryoform or kidney shaped nuclei, broad cytoplasm, and pale staining Golgi region; numerous apoptotic bodies and mitoses. **B** CD30 expression in the membrane and Golgi region.

Anaplastic large-cell lymphoma (ALCL)

ALCL mainly occurs in children and young adults, involving a variety of sites. The incidence of a mass presentation in the thymus and/or mediastinum varies from 8-39% with or without lymphadenopathy {231,1775,1930}. The higher figure of 39% likely results from inclusion in some series of "Hodgkin-like" ALCL, which is now thought to be a variant of Hodgkin lymphoma in most cases {919}. ALCL involving the thymus may be associated with cyst formation, evident on gross or microscopic examination. ALCL usually shows a cohesive growth pattern and cytologic features as follows: the cells are large, with round or indented nuclei, often described as reniform, embryo-, and horseshoe-shaped, multiple nucleoli that vary in size, and abundant cytoplasm. The so-called "hallmark cell" has an indented nucleus with a paranuclear, eosinophilic region corresponding to the Golgi region. Reactive cells may be numerous in rare cases, usually histiocytes or neutrophils; eosinophils are not common.

The tumour cells are strongly and consistently positive for CD30. Although they show T-cell receptor gene rearrangement on a molecular level, phenotypically their derivation from the T-cell lineage may be difficult to prove. CD2 and CD4 are the markers most frequently positive. CD3 is often but not always positive. Most cases express cytotoxic molecules such as

granzyme B and TIA-1. They also may exhibit positivity for other T-cell markers (CD43, CD45R0), EMA, while CD5 and CD7 are frequently negative. Anaplastic lymphoma kinase (ALK) is expressed in 40-70% of ALCL in various series. It may be nuclear and cytoplasmic or cytoplasmic only, depending on the translocation; it is more commonly expressed in pediatric cases, and is associated with an excellent prognosis {919}.

ALCL may pose differential diagnostic problems from carcinoma, mediastinal large B-cell lymphoma or Hodgkin lymphoma. Immunophenotyping for CD15, CD30, pan-B and pan-T antigens, cytotoxic molecules, EMA, keratin, and ALK protein may be essential for their exact diagnosis.

Somatic genetics
ALCL is associated with characteristic chromosome translocations involving the ALK gene on chromosome 2, with the partner being the NPM gene on chromosome 5 in most cases, and other genes in a minority of the cases {919}.

Mature T cell lymphomas

Mature T-cell neoplasms are very rare in the thymus, despite the importance of the thymus in T-cell ontogeny {1402, 1610,1827,2195}. Only 0.2% of peripheral T-cell lymphomas are diagnosed from mediastinal biopsies. Although there is no documented case of mature NK cell

lymphoma primarily affecting the thymus, 5 of 142 cases registered in the NK Cell Tumour Study Group in Japan showed mediastinal involvement (unpublished). In a patient with a mediastinal mass and lymphocytosis, a diagnosis of peripheral T-cell lymphocytosis associated with thymoma has to be included among the differential diagnoses {116,445}.

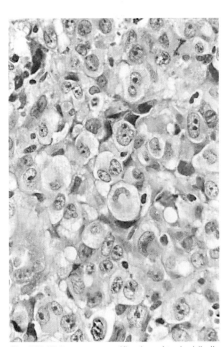

Fig. 3.99 High power magnification of typical 'hallmark' cells in ALCL.

Hodgkin lymphoma of the mediastinum

H.K. Müller-Hermelink
T. Rüdiger
N.L. Harris
E.S. Jaffe
A. Rosenwald
J.K.C. Chan

Definition

Hodgkin lymphoma (HL) is a neoplasm derived from B-cells in most cases, characterized by large tumour cells scattered in a characteristic inflammatory background. It encompasses two entities distinguishable by their phenotype and clinical presentation, namely nodular lymphocyte predominant Hodgkin lymphoma (NLPHL) and classical Hodgkin lymphoma (cHL) {50,496}.

Since HLs other than nodular sclerosis are exceedingly rare in biopsies from the mediastinum, these should be referred to in the WHO Classification of Tumours of Haematopoietic and Lymphoid Tissues {919}.

ICD-O code

Hodgkin lymphoma, nodular sclerosis
9650/3

Synonyms

In older publications, thymic HL was often designated as granulomatous thymoma {968}. Since the tumour cells are of lymphoid origin, the term Hodgkin lymphoma is preferred over Hodgkin's disease.

Epidemiology

Nodular sclerosis Hodgkin lymphoma (NSHL) is especially predominant in industrialized countries, in high socio-economic groups and in urban areas {782}. The age distribution shows a peak at the third decade, and probably also a second smaller peak in late life. The disease more commonly affects women than men. Patients with a history of infectious mononucleosis have a slightly higher incidence of HL. Both familial and geographical clustering have been described {1270}.

Localization

NSHL of the anterior mediastinum often takes origin from the thymus or mediastinal lymph nodes, or both may be involved {988,1080}.

Clinical features

The patients present with symptoms due to the presence of a large anterior mediastinal mass, such as chest discomfort or dyspnoea, or occasionally are asymptomatic, being incidentally found to have a mass lesion on chest radiograph. Some patients have simultaneous involvement of supraclavicular or lower cervical lymph nodes. A proportion of patients also have systemic symptoms. Myasthenia gravis has been described in one case of thymic HL {1494}.

Macroscopy

The thymus or mediastinal lymph nodes involved by NSHL show multiple firm greyish-white nodules, with or without visible fibrous bands. The thymus commonly exhibits interspersed cystic spaces {988}.

Tumour spread and staging

Hodgkin lymphoma typically spreads to contiguous lymph node regions, rather than showing discontinuous dissemination. Mediastinal Hodgkin lymphoma may be restricted to the mediastinum (stage I), associated with extension to adjacent lung (stage IE [E=extension]), or may involve cervical or other lymph nodes (stage II [2 nodal groups on the same side of the diaphragm] or III [nodal groups on both sides of the diaphragm]), and rarely spleen (stage III), bone marrow, or nonlymphoid organs such as liver (stage IV).

Histopathology

The architecture of the lymph node or the thymus is effaced by a nodular infiltrate that comprises variable numbers of

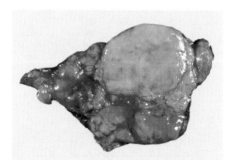

Fig. 3.100 A 31 year-old female with cough and a circumscribed thymic mass thought to be a thymoma. Cut surface shows a lobulated, firm, yellow-tan mass. Microscopical examination disclosed NSHL.

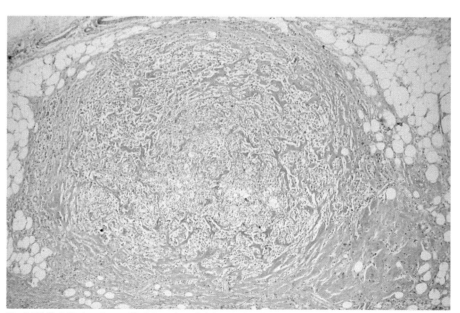

Fig. 3.101 Hodgkin lymphoma. Nodular sclerosis (classical Hodgkin lymphoma) of the thymus. Fibrous collagen bands completely surround a cellular nodule in the mediastinal fat.

Hodgkin and Reed-Sternberg cells associated with a rich inflammatory background. Classical Reed-Sternberg cells are large cells with apparently double or multiple nuclei and abundant eosinophilic or amphophilic cytoplasm. The nuclei are often rounded in contour, with thick nuclear membrane, pale chromatin, at least 2 eosinophilic nucleoli in 2 separate lobes, and perinucleolar clearing. Mononuclear variants are termed Hodgkin cells. Some tumour cells may have condensed cytoplasm and pyknotic nuclei, and are known as mummified cells. The lacunar variant of Reed-Sternberg cells is characterised by relatively small, lobated nuclei, often with small nucleoli, and abundant, pale cytoplasm that is retracted in formalin-fixed tissues.

NSHL invariably shows sclerosis, which in lymph nodes begins in the capsule, and divides the tumour into nodules of varying size. At least one fibrous band encapsulating a tumour nodule is considered to be the minimal criterion for the nodular sclerosis subtype. The inflammatory background of NSHL comprises lymphocytes, plasma cells, and granulocytes, especially eosinophils. Geographic necrosis is common, frequently accompanied by neutrophil infiltration and concentration of tumour cells around the necrotic areas.

Involvement of the thymus by cHL often results in cystic changes, and pseudo-epithelial hyperplasia of thymic epithelium mimicking thymoma on small biopsies. The cysts are lined by flat epithelium which is frequently non-keratinizing-squamous, but may be columnar, ciliated or mucus producing {988,1080}. Tumour may be detected within cyst walls, sometimes producing bulges into the lumen. Similar cystic changes can also occur in the thymus not involved by the lymphoma itself.

In small biopsies, both the characteristic pattern and tumour cells may be difficult to identify. To establish the primary diagnosis of cHL, either classical multinucleated Reed-Sternberg cells or lacunar cells showing the typical immunophenotype should be identified, and this may require examination of multiple levels of the biopsy. If fibrous bands cannot be identified, the case may be classified as cHL not further classified, with a note that the small specimen size precludes definitive subclassification.

Composite lymphomas with CHL and diffuse large B cell lymphoma infiltrates side by side are rare.

Immunohistochemistry

In cHL, tumour cells strongly and consistently express CD30. CD15 is detectable in more than 85% of the cases, although sometimes only focally {2090}. CD20 may be expressed in up to 20% of cHL {1760,2090,2248}, but it is usually weaker than in accompanying B-cells and staining intensity varies among tumour cells {1705}. CD79a is negative in the majority of cases. EBV is expressed in about 20% of NSHL, and may be detected by immunohistochemistry for its latent

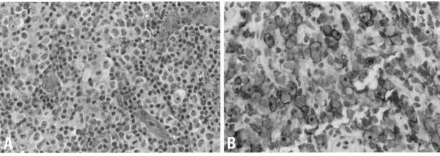

Fig. 3.102 Hodgkin lymphoma. **A** Hodgkin lymphoma, nodular sclerosis, BNLI Grade 2. A scalene lymph node biopsy from a 20 year-old female with a mediastinal mass shows a confluent infiltrate of large neoplastic cells with pleomorphic nuclei and pale cytoplasm, typical of lacunar variants of Reed-Sternberg cells. **B** CD30 shows strong membrane and Golgi region staining of the neoplastic cells. The cells express CD15 in a similar pattern but lack T and B-cell associated antigens.

Table 3.12
Synopsis of mediastinal Hodgkin lymphomas

Classification of Hodgkin lymphomas	Abbreviation	Frequency diagnosed from mediastinal biopsies with HL*	ICD-O code
Nodular lymphocyte predominant Hodgkin lymphoma	NLPHL	1%	9659/3
Classical Hodgkin lymphoma	CHL	99%	9650/3
Nodular sclerosis classical Hodgkin lymphoma	NSHL	80%	9663/3
Mixed cellularity classical Hodgkin lymphoma	MCHL	18%	9652/3
Lymphocyte-rich classical Hodgkin lymphoma	LRCHL	0%	9651/3
Lymphocyte-depleted classical Hodgkin lymphoma	LDHL	1%	9653/3

* German Hodgkin Study Group data based on 169 mediastinal biopsies, unpublished data.

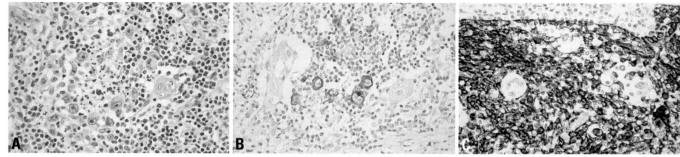

Fig. 3.103 Classical Hodgkin lymphoma of the thymus. **A** Hodgkin cells and granulocytes in thymic medullary region around Hassall corpuscle. **B** Strong CD30 expression in tumour cells. **C** CK19 staining reveals pseudoepitheliomatous hyperplasia around Hodgkin and Reed-Sternberg cells; this is frequently accompanied by thymic cyst formation. When tumour cells are less conspicuous than here, epithelial hyperplasia can be mistaken for thymoma on small biopsies.

membrane antigen or EBER probes {692}, while EBNA2 is not expressed {1991}. The incidence of EBV association in NSHL is generally lower than in other subtypes and varies geographically {692,782}. Vimentin {1705} and fascin {1600} are generally expressed in cHL, but rare in large B-cell lymphomas. The reactive background contains variable numbers of B- and T-lymphocytes, with the latter forming rosettes around individual tumour cells.

Histogenesis
Post germinal center activated B cells are the presumed cells of origin.
Somatic genetics

On a single cell level, rearrangement of the immunoglobulin genes can be demonstrated in almost all cases, indicating B cell derivation of the Reed-Sternberg cells and variants {1096A}. In cHL, the rearranged immunoglobulin gene is not transcribed, either due to non-functional mutations in the immunoglobulin genes {1099,1873} or due to a lack in essential transcription factors (such as *OCT-2, BOB-1*) {1874}. Rare cases with rearranged T-cell receptor genes have been observed {1414, 1776}.
In CGH-analysis, gains on the short arms of chromosomes 2 and 9, and on the long arm of chromosome 12 are fre-

quently detected. An overrepresentation of the *REL*-protooncogene (2p15-p16) and the *JAK/STAT* signal transduction pathway may play a major role in the pathogenesis {115,939,940,1249}.
Recent molecular studies applying gene expression profiling show that classical Hodgkin lymphoma and PMLBCL are closely related {1694,1752}.

Prognostic factors
Patients are usually treated with chemotherapy with or without radiotherapy, adapted to clinical stage. Stage is the single most important prognostic factor. The various subtypes of cHL do not differ in their prognosis, which has greatly improved with recent protocols {495}. In one study, cases that lacked CD15 expression had a worse prognosis than CD15+ cases {2090}. Grading systems for nodular sclerosis have been shown in some studies, but not others, to predict prognosis {574,825,1221,2069,2091}.

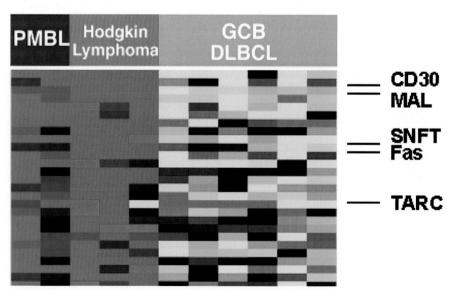

Fig. 3.104 Gene expression patterns shared between primary mediastinal large B-cell lymphoma (PMBL) and Hodgkin lymphoma (HL). Several genes, including CD30, MAL, SNFT, Fas and TARC show expression in PMBL and HL, in contrast to their low expression in the germinal center B-cell type of diffuse large B-cell lymphoma (GC, DLBCL). From A. Rosenwald et al. {1694}.

Grey zone between Hodgkin lymphoma and non-Hodgkin lymphomas (NHL)

H.K. Müller-Hermelink
T. Rüdiger
A. Rosenwald
N.L. Harris
E.S. Jaffe
J.K.C. Chan

Definitions

The term grey zone lymphoma has been assigned to neoplasms exhibiting indeterminate features between classical Hodgkin lymphoma (cHL) and large cell non-Hodgkin lymphoma (NHL), such that a definitive classification as cHL or NHL is not possible.

Composite lymphomas exhibit clearly separable lymphoma infiltrates with typical features of cHL and NHL side by side. They may or may not be clonally related. The different components and their proportions should be stated in the diagnsosis.

ICD-O code

Composite Hodgkin and
non-Hodgkin lymphoma   9596/3
This code may also be used for grey zone lymphomas.

Some tumours can exhibit indeterminate features of both cHL and large B cell lymphoma, such that definitive classification as cHL or NHL is impossible even after extensive immunophenotypic and molecular studies {1270,1704}. These lymphomas are termed grey zone lymphomas. Their occurrence is not surprising. Since Hodgkin lymphoma is a lymphoid malignancy derived from B-cells in nearly all cases {1097,1099,1237}, its interface to B-cell NHL may not always be clear-cut. The interface between NSHL and primary mediastinal large B-cell lymphoma (PMLBCL) is currently felt to comprise a biological transition: apart from their frequent mediastinal presentation, both tumours frequently lack functional expression of HLA class I and immunoglobulin genes. CHL is always CD30 positive, and primary mediastinal large B cell lymphoma is also frequently CD30 positive. CGH studies suggest that they share an overrepresentation of genomic material on the short arms of chromosomes 2 and 9 {148,1752}.

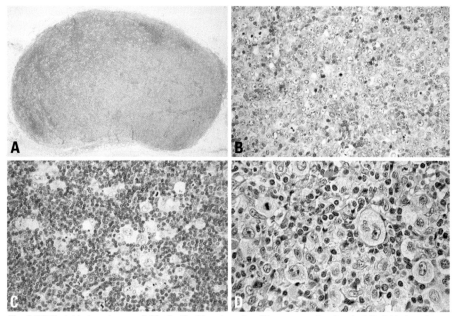

Fig. 3.105 Hodgkin lymphoma. **A** Mediastinal lymph node with a composite classical Hodgkin lymphoma (dark staining areas on upper and left side of the lymph node) and PMLBCL (pale area in the lower, middle and right side). Giemsa stain. **B** Pale area of the lymph node shown in A. PMLBCL, immunoblastic variant. Effacement of lymph node architecture by sheets of quite uniform medium-sized to large blasts showing prominent nucleoli. Giemsa stain. **C** Dark-staining area of the lymph node shown in A. Classical Hodgkin lymphoma, mixed cellularity subtype. Note the absence of fibrous bands. Hodgkin cells are surrounded by reactive lymphocytes and plasma cells. Note rosettes. Giemsa stain. **D** PMLBCL in mediastinal lymph node. Presence of scattered Hodgkin-like cells among B-blasts is insufficient for a diagnosis of composite Hodgkin and Non-Hodgkin lymphoma. Note absence of a reactive infiltrate of lymphocytes, plasma cells and eosinophils around the Hodgkin-like cells. Giemsa stain.

Finally, microarray-based studies have documented largely overlapping gene expression profiles in cHL and PMLBCL, stressing their close keenship {1694, 1752}. However, as HL is treated differently than NHL, it is important to distinguish between them, if possible.
NSHL and large B-cell lymphoma may occur metachronously {2233}, or synchronously (composite lymphoma) {710, 1575}.

Histopathology.

Grey zone lymphomas, by definition, have no specific morphology. They may manifest a vaguely nodular infiltrate with focal fibrosis. There are sheets of malignant cells, some of which resemble Reed-Sternberg cells or lacunar variants. The inflammatory background may be sparse or absent. The tumor cells typically all express CD20, and in addition strongly express CD30. CD79a and CD15 may be variably expressed. Retrospective clinical data suggest that the mostly male patients respond poorly to radiotherapy alone, and relapses in abdominal and extranodal locations are common {1704}.

Histiocytic tumours

J.K.C. Chan
T. Grogan
S.A. Pileri
E.S. Jaffe

Histiocytic tumours rarely occur as a primary tumour in the mediastinum. Details are available in the WHO Classification of Tumours of Haematopoietic and Lymphoid Tissues {919}. This section focuses on cases located in the thymus or mediastinum. Exceptionally, Rosai-Dorfman disease (Sinus Histiocytosis with Massive Lymphadenopathy, SHML) can also involve these sites.

Langerhans cell histiocytosis and sarcoma

Definitions
Langerhans cell histiocytosis is a neoplastic proliferation of Langerhans cells, with expression of CD1a, S100 protein, and the presence of Birbeck granules by ultrastructural examination.
Langerhans cell sarcoma differs from Langerhans cell histiocytosis in showing overtly malignant cytologic features; it can present *de novo* or progress from antecedent Langerhans cell histiocytosis.

ICD-O codes
Langerhans cell histiocytosis
                9751/1
Langerhans cell sarcoma
                9756/3

Synonym
Langerhans cell sarcoma was previously termed malignant histiocytosis X.

Epidemiology and clinical features
Involvement of the thymus or mediastinal lymph node by Langerhans cell histiocytosis or Langerhans cell sarcoma is rare {1181}. It usually occurs in the setting of disseminated disease {143,210,945, 1596,1761}.
Rare cases of Langerhans cell histiocytosis presenting with thymic involvement have been reported {219,683,1491, 1578,2096}. In children, the thymus is often markedly enlarged and extensively infiltrated by Langerhans cells; there can be invasion of the surrounding mediasti-

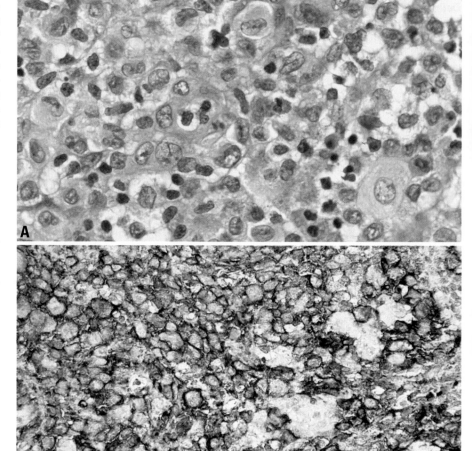

Fig. 3.106 Langerhans cell histiocytosis (LCH). **A** LCH presenting as a thymic mass. There is a diffuse infiltrate of cells with grooved nuclei and delicate nuclear membrane. Note some admixed eosinophils. **B** LCH with CD1a expression in tumour cells. Macrophages are spared.

nal structures. In adults, the thymic involvement is usually subtle, and is discovered incidentally in thymus removed primarily for another indication; thus the reported association with myasthenia gravis is probably fortuitous {219,683, 1578,2096}.

Histopathology
The key histologic feature of Langerhans cell histiocytosis is a diffuse infiltrate of non-cohesive Langerhans cells with grooved or markedly contorted nuclei, thin nuclear membranes, fine chromatin and eosinophilic cytoplasm. There are commonly admixed multinucleated giant cells and eosinophils. Necrosis can be present. The Langerhans cells typically express S-100 protein and CD1a.
The thymus can be involved diffusely or focally. The involved areas show destruction of the normal thymic parenchyma, damage to Hassall corpuscles, interlobular connective tissue infiltration, and scattered calcospherites {1761,1823}. Localized thymic involvement in adults often takes the form of scattered small nodular aggregates of Langerhans cells.

This can be accompanied by reactive lymphoid hyperplasia or multilocular thymic cyst {2096}.

Differential diagnosis
An important differential diagnosis is histioeosinophilic granuloma of the mediastinum, which is a reactive lesion resulting from iatrogenic pneumomediastinum, akin to reactive eosinophilic pleuritis {762,1304}. Although both histioeosinophilic granuloma and Langerhans cell histiocytes feature histiocytes and eosinophils, the histiocytes in the former are confined to the capsule or septa of the thymus with sparing of the parenchyma, the nuclei are uncommonly grooved, and S-100 protein and CD1a immunostains are negative.

Somatic genetics
In contrast to pulmonary eosinophilic granuloma, which in most cases is a non-neoplastic, reactive process in smokers, most cases of Langerhans cell histiocytosis occurring in non-pulmonary sites are believed to be clonal neoplasms, as demonstrated by X-chromosome inactivation {2149}. Thymic cases have not, however, been specifically studied.

Histiocytic sarcoma and malignant histiocytosis

Definition
Histiocytic sarcoma is a malignant proliferation of cells showing morphologic and immunophenotypic features similar to those of mature tissue histiocytes. There is expression of one or more histiocytic markers without accessory/dendritic cell markers. Tumourous masses of acute monocytic leukaemia are excluded. The term 'malignant histiocytosis' is sometimes applied for histiocytic sarcoma showing systemic disease, often with liver, spleen and bone marrow involvement.

ICD-O code
Histiocytic sarcoma   9755/3
Malignant histiocytosis   9750/3

Synonyms
True histiocytic lymphoma, histiocytic medullary reticulosis (obsolete)

Epidemiology
Among the recent series on histiocytic sarcoma diagnosed using strict criteria

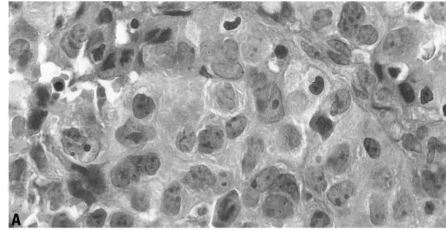
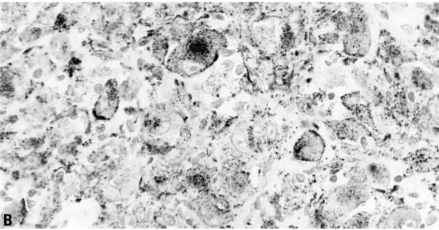

Fig. 3.107 Histiocytic sarcoma. **A** The neoplastic cells are large, and possess abundant eosinophilic cytoplasm. **B** The tumour cells show granular immunostaining for CD68 (PGM1).

(including over 50 cases) {405,774,949, 1140,1596}, there is only a single case with predominant involvement of the mediastinum {949}. There are reports on malignant histiocytosis or histiocytic sarcoma associated with mediastinal non-seminomatous germ cells tumours, but they lack vigorous documentation regarding the true histiocytic nature of the neoplasm {83,473,474,789,1460, 1461,2246}.

Histopathology
Histiocytic sarcoma is characterized by a diffuse infiltrate of large cells with voluminous eosinophilic, and sometimes finely vacuolated, cytoplasm. The nuclei are round, oval, indented, grooved or irregularly folded, often with vesicular chromatin and small nucleoli. Nuclear pleomorphism can be significant.
The diagnosis has to be confirmed by immunohistochemical staining: positive for CD68 and lysozyme; frequently posi-

tive for CD45, CD4, CD43, CD45RO and HLA-DR; occasionally positive for S100 protein; and negative for myeloid markers, dendritic cell markers (CD1a, CD21, CD35), T lineage-specific markers, B lineage-specific markers and CD30 {1596}.

Dendritic cell tumours

J.K.C. Chan
T. Grogan
S.A. Pileri
E.S. Jaffe

Follicular dendritic cell tumour / sarcoma

Definition
Follicular dendritic cell (FDC) tumour/sarcoma is a neoplastic proliferation of spindle to ovoid cells showing morphologic and phenotypic features of follicular dendritic cells. The terms tumour and sarcoma are both used because of the variable cytologic grade and indeterminate clinical behaviour of these neoplasms.

ICD-O code
Follicular dendritic cell tumour   9758/1
Follicular dendritic cell sarcoma 9758/3

Clinical features
These neoplasms are uncommon, with only a small number of cases having been reported to show primary involvement of the thymus or mediastinal lymph nodes {58,323,482, 560,1571,1596}. The patients are adults with a mean age of 46 years, being comparable to that of the same tumour occurring in other sites {323,1571}. However, they differ in showing marked male predominance, but this may be due to bias from the small number of cases. The patients are asymptomatic, or present with cough, haemoptysis or chest discomfort.

Etiology and precursor lesions
A proportion of cases of follicular dendritic tumour/sarcoma arise in the setting of hyaline-vascular Castleman disease, often through an intermediary phase of follicular dendritic cell proliferation outside the follicles {320,323,1186}. Both components of hyaline-vascular Castleman disease and follicular dendritic cell tumour/sarcoma may be identified in the same tumour mass in the mediastinum {482}.

Histopathology
Tumours are often large, with a broad. histologic spectrum. The growth pattern can be storiform, whorled, fascicular, nodular, diffuse or even trabecular. The individual tumour cells are spindle or

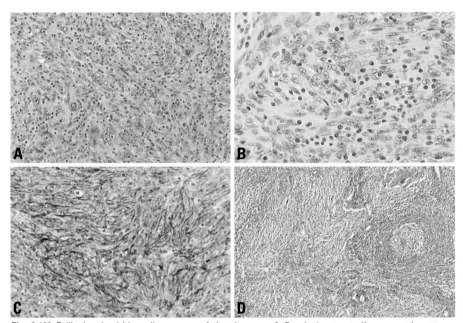

Fig. 3.108 Follicular dendritic cell sarcoma of the thymus. **A** Fascicular to storiform growth pattern. Characteristic irregular clustering of nuclei and sprinkling of small lymphocytes. **B** This tumour comprises spindle cells with indistinct cell borders, elongated pale nuclei and small distinct nucleoli. The nuclei appear irregularly clustered. Sprinkling of small lymphocytes. **C** Membrane immunostaining for CD21 in a meshwork pattern. **D** On the right a component resembling hyaline-vascular Castleman disease.

ovoid, and the lightly eosinophilic cytoplasm often exhibits indistinct cell borders. The nuclei are elongated or oval, with thin nuclear membrane, vesicular or granular chromatin, and small distinct nucleoli. There is often an irregular clustering of the nuclei, and occasional multinucleated tumour giant cells can be seen. Some cases can exhibit significant nuclear pleomorphism, mitotic activity and coagulative necrosis. The tumour is typically sprinkled with small lymphocytes, which can show clustering around blood vessels. A diagnosis of follicular dendritic cell sarcoma should be confirmed by immunohistochemical studies (positive for CD21 and CD35, and variably CD23), and preferably also by ultrastructural studies (numerous long slender cytoplasmic processes and mature desmosomes).

Differential diagnosis
Mediastinal follicular dendritic cell sarcoma can be mistaken for type A thymoma

because of the mediastinal location, spindle cell growth and lymphocytic infiltration. To add to the confusion, follicular dendritic cell sarcoma can exhibit jigsaw puzzle-like lobulation and perivascular spaces as commonly seen in thymomas {359}. In contrast to type A thymoma, there is no focal glandular differentiation, cytokeratin is negative, and follicular dendritic cell-associated markers are expressed.

Histogenesis
Follicular dendritic cells of the B-cell follicle.

Prognosis and predictive factors
Among 5 patients with mediastinal FDC tumour/sarcoma with follow-up information, two developed pulmonary metastases after two years, one developed local recurrence at 3 years, and two were alive without evidence of disease after surgery and radiochemotherapy.

Interdigitating dendritic cell tumour / sarcoma

Definition
Interdigitating dendritic cell sarcoma/ tumour is a neoplastic proliferation of spindle to ovoid cells with phenotypic features similar to those of interdigitating dendritic cells.

ICD-O code
Interdigitating dendritic cell tumour
9757/1
Interdigitating dendritic cell sarcoma
9757/3

Epidemiology, localization and clinical features
Interdigitating dendritic cell sarcomas are very rare, and mediastinal involvement is even rarer. The few reported cases have involved the mediastinal lymph nodes as a component of disseminated disease {569,1309,1635,1698, 2067}. There is a reported case of mediastinal tumour showing hybrid features of follicular dendritic cells and interdigitating dendritic cells {499}.

Histopathology
The tumour shows a fascicular, storiform, whorled or diffuse growth pattern, comprising spindle or plump cells with indistinct cell borders and abundant eosinophilic cytoplasm. The nuclei often exhibit finely dispersed chromatin and distinct nucleoli. Cytologic atypia is variable.

Differential diagnosis
The diagnosis should always be confirmed by immunohistochemical staining, with or without ultrastructural studies (complex interdigitating cell processes lacking well-formed macula adherens-type desmosomes and lacking Birbeck granules). The neoplastic cells strongly express S-100 protein, and often show variable weak staining for CD68, lysozyme, CD4 and CD45. They should be negative for CD1a, follicular dendritic cell markers (CD21, CD35), myeloperoxidase, T lineage specific markers, B-cell-specific markers and CD30.

Myeloid sarcoma and extramedullary acute myeloid leukaemia

A. Orazi

Definition

Myeloid sarcoma is a mass forming neoplastic proliferation of myeloblasts or immature myeloid cells occurring in an extramedullary site. It may occur *de novo* or simultaneously with acute myeloid leukaemia (AML), myeloproliferative disorders, or myelodysplastic syndromes, but may also be the first manifestation of leukaemic relapse in a previously treated patient {1518}. Interstitial infiltration of myeloid blasts without a nodular mass can be termed extramedullary AML.

ICD-O code   9930/3

Synonyms

Extramedullary myeloid tumour; granulocytic sarcoma; chloroma

Clinical features

Mediastinal myeloid sarcoma has been reported in association with a superior vena cava syndrome {1643}. Most mediastinal cases occur simultaneously with AML or are followed by AML shortly. Patients who presented with "primary" mediastinal granulocytic sarcoma without concurrent AML, all eventually relapsed as frank leukaemia {369}.

Histopathology

The most common type of myeloid sarcoma occurring in the mediastinum is known as granulocytic sarcoma {2193}, a tumour composed of myeloblasts and promyelocytes. The degree of maturation is variable in different cases. The blastic subtype is entirely composed of myeloblasts; in the more differentiated subtypes, promyelocytes are also present {919,2108}. Rare cases composed of monoblasts (termed monoblastic sarcoma), can also occur in this location. Cases associated with acute transformation of an underlying myeloproliferative disorder may show foci of trilineage extramedullary hematopoiesis associated with the blastic proliferation.

In patients with mediastinal germ cell tumours with mediastinal myeloid sarcoma or extramedullary myeloid leukaemia, the possibility of a "local" origin of the tumour should also be considered

Cytochemistry and immunophenotype
Cytochemical stains to detect myeloid differentiation in AML can be applied to imprints of biopsy material. Flow cytometry may demonstrate myeloid antigen expression. Myeloid associated markers which that can confirm the diagnosis include lysozyme, myeloperoxidase, CD43, CD117, CD68, and CD61. The lack of expression of lymphoid associated antigens helps in the differential diagnosis *versus* large cell lymphomas and lymphoblastic lymphoma. The histochemical stain for chloroacetate esterase may be helpful in identifying promyelocytes and more differentiated myeloid elements in differentiated myeloid sarcoma subtypes.

Differential diagnosis

The major differential diagnosis is with non-Hodgkin lymphomas, lymphoblastic lymphoma and diffuse large cell lymphoma; in children, the differential includes various metastatic small round cell tumours. Cases of myeloid sarcoma with prominent sclerosis may closely mimic sclerosing mediastinal (thymic) large B-cell lymphoma. In patients with mediastinal germ cell tumours, the possi-

bility of a "local" origin of the myeloid sarcoma from haematopoietic precursor cells occurring within the germ cell tumour should also be considered {1278}.

Somatic genetics

AML with t(8;21) has an increased frequency of granulocytc sarcomas, as do monocytic and monoblastic leukemias with 11q23 abnormalities.

The presence of genetic abnormalities in myeloid sarcoma, can be detected by reverse transcriptase-polymerase chain reaction, conventional cytogenetics, or fluorescence in-situ hybridization studies.

Prognosis and predictive factors

Mediastinal myeloid sarcoma is an aggressive disease. Patients who presented with a "primary" mediastinal MS and were treated by local irradiation only (prior to developing AML), eventually all relapsed as frank leukaemia and died soon afterwards {369}. In contrast, patients who were considered to have AML and given upfront systemic chemotherapy achieved better outcomes, their prognosis being that of the underlying leukaemia {369,919}.

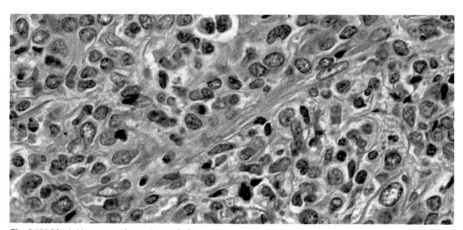

Fig. 3.109 Myeloid sarcoma (monoblastic). Sclerotic bands divide the neoplasm into irregular alveolar clusters and cords. Note the kidney shaped immature nuclei with vesicular or granular chromatin, multiple small nucleoli, and pale abundant cytoplasm.

Soft tissue tumours of the thymus and mediastinum

A. Marx
T.T. Kuo
Ph. Ströbel
P.J. Zhang
Y. Shimosato
J.K.C. Chan

A variety of mesenchymal and neurogenic tumours can arise in the mediastinum. For those that occur in the anterior mediastinum, it is often difficult to ascertain whether they are of thymic origin or derived from other mediastinal constituents {1529}. An exception is thymolipoma, since the intimate admixture of lipomatous tissue with thymic parenchyma strongly supports its thymic derivation. Some sarcomas arise in mediastinal germ cell tumours {1230, 1932}.

Principles of the classification

The classification of mesenchymal and neurogenic tumours of the thymus and mediastinum follows the WHO classifications of tumours of soft tissues and bone {590} and of tumours of the nervous system {1026}. Since thymolipoma is a unique thymic tumour with a predominant mesenchymal component, it is described and discussed here in more detail.

Epidemiology

Mesenchymal and neurogenic tumours of the thymus and mediastinum are all very rare, constituting less than 10% of all mediastinal neoplasms. Almost all neurogenic neoplasms of the mediastinum occur in the posterior mediastinum.

Clinical features

Mesenchymal and neurogenic tumours of the anterior mediastinum or thymus are frequently detected incidentally, but may present as cough, chest pain, pleural effusion, respiratory distress or the superior vena cava syndrome. Hypoglycaemia is a rare complication of solitary fibrous tumour {2164}. Tumours in the middle and posterior mediastinum, which are mostly neurogenic neoplasms, often produce symptoms due to compression of large vessels, heart, nerves or spinal cord.

Thymolipoma

Definitions

Thymolipoma is a well-circumscribed tumour consisting of mature adipose tissue with interspersed islands of non-neoplastic thymic tissue.

ICD-O code   8850/0

Synonym

Thymolipomatous hamartoma

Epidemiology

Thymolipomas are rare tumours (about 80-100 published cases) that may occur at any age, but are most commonly encountered in young adults (10-30 years, mean age 33 years) {1352,1683}. There is no sex predilection.

Localization

All documented cases arose in the anterior mediastinum.

Clinical features

Thymolipomas may remain asymptomatic for a long period. The majority of cases are incidental findings on routine chest radiographs and may simulate cardiomegaly {44,1818} or other mediastinal neoplasms. Thymolipomas may become symptomatic either due to the size of the lesion, or, less frequently, due to associated autoimmune phenomena. Among these, myasthenia gravis is the most frequent (about 7% of cases {1352}), but single cases with other manifestations such as aplastic anaemia {113} and Graves disease {147} have been reported.

Macroscopy

The size of thymolipoma ranges from 4 to over 30 cm {1352}. The tumours are yellow, soft, fairly well circumscribed with scattered white streaks or focal solid areas on the cut surface.

Histopathology

Histologically, they consist of abundant mature adipose tissue admixed with areas containing remnants of thymic tissue. The fat cells show no cytologic atypia or mitotic activity {1352}. The thymic tissue component may vary from strands of atrophic thymic epithelium to large

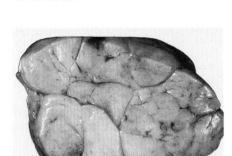

Fig. 3.110 Thinly encapsulated thymolipoma in a 6-year-old male child. The cut surface is yellow, bulging, and lobulated, resembling lipoma. From Y. Shimosato and K. Mukai {1808}.

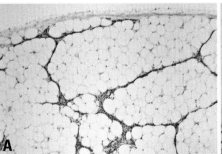
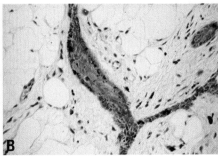

Fig. 3.111 Thymolipoma. **A** Thymolipoma showing a delicate but distinct fibrous capsule and thin septae of atrophic thymic tissue. **B** Strands of thymic epithelial cells within thymolipoma. The lymphocyte content is virtually absent in this case, possibly related to the age of the patient. The content of fibrous tissue may be extensive: 'Thymofibrolipoma' {1372}. Note single melanocytes scattered among thymic epithelial cells.

areas containing inconspicuous thymic parenchyma containing numerous, often calcified, Hassall's corpuscles {1352}. Myoid cells are present {907}. The thymic compartment may show single lymph follicles.

Differential diagnosis
Diagnosis of thymolipoma is usually not problematic. However, due to the large size of some lesions, careful sampling is necessary in order to rule out the possibility of atypical or malignant areas. In rare cases, thymomas may arise within thymolipomas {69}. Histologically, the main differential diagnoses include lipoma of the thymus (no thymic epithelial component) and mediastinal liposarcomas (scattered lipoblasts).

Histogenesis
The pathogenesis and biological nature of thymolipoma are controversial, but most authors favour a benign neoplasm {69, 763,1352}. An origin from specialized thymic stroma has been postulated {69, 763}.

Prognosis and predictive factors
There have been no reports on recurrences, metastasis or tumour-related deaths, and local excision is curative.

Thymoma in thymolipoma
There is a single case report about thymoma within a thymolipoma occurring in a 67 years old female patient without myasthenia gravis {69}. The thymoma was classified as "cortical" (type B2). There was no recurrence within 10 years after radical surgery. We observed an almost identical case.

Lipoma

ICD-O code   8850/0

Lipoma is the most common benign mesenchymal tumour of the mediastinum {1529,1932}. In contrast to thymolipoma it does not contain foci of thymic parenchyma. Other rare benign lipomatous tumours are lipoblastoma/lipoblastomatosis {517}, hibernoma {31}, and angiolipoma {1031}.

Liposarcoma

ICD-O code   8850/3

Liposarcoma is the most common sarcoma in the anterior mediastinum, and some cases may represent thymic stromal sarcomas {801,938}, i.e. malignant counterparts of thymolipoma (*thymoliposarcoma*) {1030}. Mediastinal liposarcoma usually occurs in adults (mean age 43 years), and is rare in children {357}. In some cases, there is synchronous

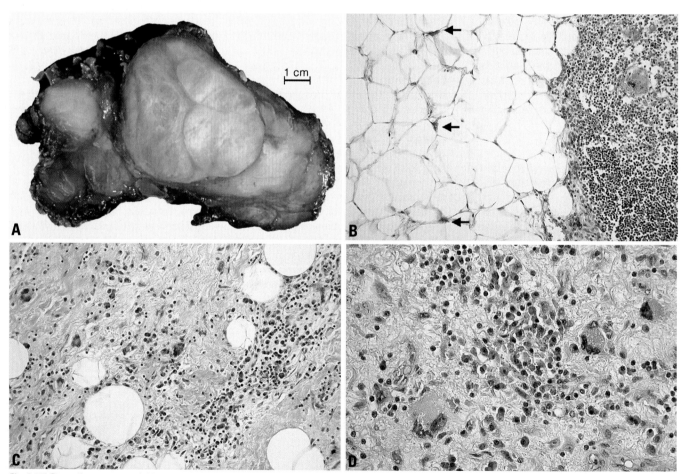

Fig. 3.112 Thymoliposarcoma. **A** Macroscopy of a recurrent tumour (2 years after first treatment): well circumscribed and partially encapsulated tumour from the anterior mediastinum. **B** Bland looking well differentiated (lipoma-like) liposarcoma adjacent to thymic remnant tissue with some lipoblasts (arrows). **C** Multinucleated neoplastic lipoblasts and a heavy inflammatory reaction in the more fibrotic stroma of the recurrent tumour. **D** Higher magnification demonstrating multinucleated tumour cells and the inflammatory reaction.

involvement of other sites such as the retroperitoneum.

Well-differentiated liposarcoma is the most frequent subtype (60% of cases), including lipoma-like, inflammatory {1030} spindle cell {1138,1835}, leiomyomatous and dedifferentiated variants {601}, followed by myxoid liposarcoma (28%), and other subtypes (12%) {1030}, such as the highly aggressive pleomorphic liposarcoma {513}. In some cases, the presence of heavy lymphoid infiltration may result in mimicry of lymphoma or an inflammatory process {1030}.

Like the same tumour occurring in other sites, mediastinal myxoid liposarcoma shows TLS/FUS-CHOP fusion transcripts {1762}.

The tumours are curable by surgical excision in some patients {47,256, 357,740}, but recurrences develop in up to 32% of cases after a mean interval of 36 months. Myxoid liposarcoma has a worse prognosis than well-differentiated liposarcoma {1030}.

Solitary fibrous tumour

Definition
Solitary fibrous tumour (SFT) is an uncommon, locally aggressive mesenchymal neoplasm with highly variegating morphologic appearance, characterized by two basic elements encountered in varying proportions: a solid spindle cell component and a diffuse sclerosing component.

ICD-O code   8815/0

Epidemiology
Mediastinal SFT is a rare tumour of adults (28-78 years of age) {999}. Mediastinal SFT on average account for 15% of all SFT, and about 25% of extrapleural SFT {772,791,999,1384}.

Localization
Some mediastinal SFT may represent extensions from pleural SFT, but others arise from the mediastinal (including thymic) stroma {1685}.

Macroscopy
Mediastinal SFT can reach a large size, of up to 16 cm {2164}.

Table 3.13
Comparison of immunophenotype of solitary fibrous tumour (SFT) with other spindle cell tumours of the thymus and mediastinum.

Diagnosis	CD34	Bcl-2	CD99	CK[1]	S100	Desmin
SFT	+++	+++	+++	-	-	-/+
Type A Thymoma	-	-	-[2]	+++	-	-
Spindle Cell Liposarcoma	+++	+	+/-	-	+	-
Synovial Sarcoma	-	+++	+/-	+/++	-	-
Fibromatosis	-	-	-	-	-	-
Leiomyoma	-	-	-/+[3]	-	-	+++[3]
Nerve Sheath Tumour	-[4]	+++ > -	-	-[5]	+++[6]	-

[1]CK, cytokeratin; [2]Immature T-cells may be +; [3]An identical phenotype is observed in some angiomatoid fibrous histiocytomas; [4]S100-negative "dendritic cells" may be positive {1000,2121}; [5]Rare glandular structures may be +; [6]Malignant peripheral nerve sheath tumours may be negative.

Histopathology
Solitary fibrous tumour (SFT) of the mediastinum is identical to SFT of the pleura in terms of morphology and immunophenotype [CD34+(>90%), CD99+ (>90%), bcl2+ (80-90%), cytokeratin-] {772,791,999,1384,2063}.

In contrast to the usually bland-looking pleural or thyroid SFT {1674,2164}, high mitotic activity (> 1-4/10HPF), cytologic atypia and coagulative necrosis occur in more than 50% of mediastinal SFT, suggesting a high propensity for sarcomatous transformation {637,772,2164}. In such cases there is sometimes an identifiable component of bland-looking SFT.

Differential diagnosis
The typical collagenous stroma around individual tumour cells and the charac-

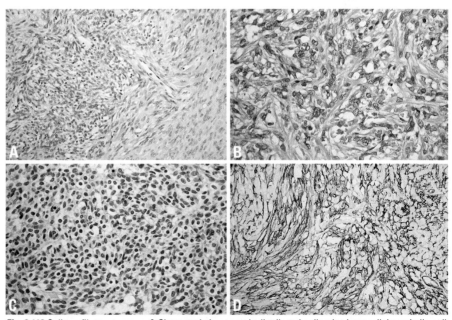

Fig. 3.113 Solitary fibrous tumour. **A** Characteristic unevenly distributed celluarity: hypocellular spindle cell area (on the right side), and a cellular area on the left. Note the inconspicuous vessels. **B** Patternless architecture composed of spindle cells in a haphazard arrangement. **C** Cellular area in the same tumour as shown B. Bland looking spindle cells with inconspicuous cell borders and oval nuclei. **D** Characteristic strong cell membrane CD34 expression in almost all tumour cells.

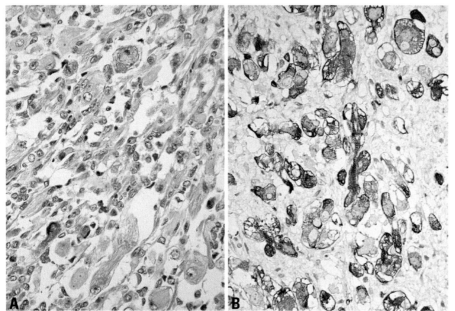

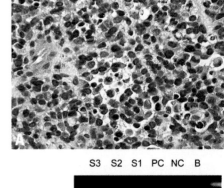

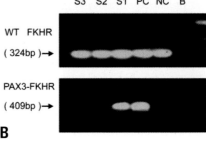

Fig. 3.114 Embryonal rhabdomyosarcoma. A Embryonal rhabdomyosarcoma of the mediastinum. B Desmin expression with occasional cells showing cross-striations.

Fig. 3.116 Alveolar rhabdomyosarcoma. A Solid variant in the anterior mediastinum in a 2 months-old girl. Primitive round cells are arranged in solid sheets, with focal alveolar pattern. Tumour cells have a high N:C ratio and dense chromatin, many apoptotic bodies and mitoses. B RT-PCR analysis of solid variant of alveolar rhabdomyosarcoma (RMS) in a 2 months old girl (same case as A). Note the 409 bp PAX3-FKHR fusion product in frozen tumour tissue (lower panel). Abbreviations: B, blank; NC, negative control (tonsil); PC, positive control [t(2;13) positive RMS]; S1, specimen 1, current case; S2-S3, two other RMS specimens negative for t(2;13); WT, wild type FKHR segment (324bp; upper panel). Molecular size markers (ladder) on the right side in the upper panel. For RT-PCR protocol see refs {114,658}.

teristic immunophenotype distinguish SFT from type A thymoma, synovial sarcoma, low-grade spindle cell liposarcoma, leiomyomatous tumours and neural tumours {1908}.

Somatic genetics
Genetic findings in mediastinal SFT have not been reported.

Prognosis and predictive factors
Primary mediastinal SFT are more aggressive than pleural or thyroid SFT {1674}. Local recurrences and tumour-related deaths occur in about 50% and 25% of cases, respectively {2164}. SFT may recur late (13 years after surgery) and can rarely develop intrathoracic metastases {2164}. High mitotic activity

(>1/10 HPF) and necrosis herald an aggressive course.

Rhabdomyosarcoma (RMS)

ICD-O code   8900/3

RMS most commonly arise in thymic germ cell tumour {1932}, or may occur as a component of sarcomatoid thymic carcinoma {1509}, but can also rarely arise de novo. Embryonal, pleomorphic and alveolar RMS of the thymus, one with unusual clear cell features, have been reported {135,1922,1932}. The tumours can occur in adults and children, and follow a very aggressive clinical course {135,1922}.
The t(2;13)(q35; q14) translocation resulting in a PAX3/FKHR fusion gene

has been observed in an example of mediastinal alveolar RMS of the solid variant {1742}. "Rhabdomyomatous thymomas" {1351,1730} with myoid cells, should not be mistaken for RMS.

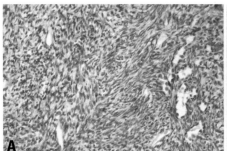

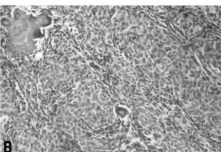

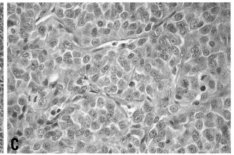

Fig. 3.115 Synovial sarcoma (SS). A Monophasic spindle cell SS focally with gaping vessels resembling haemangiopericytoma. B Spindle cell component calcifying SS (30% of all SS cases). Unusual biphasic type: solid epithelial cords and few spindle cells. C Round cell component. High power of the solid epithelial component (if single component: = "monophasic epithelial SS").

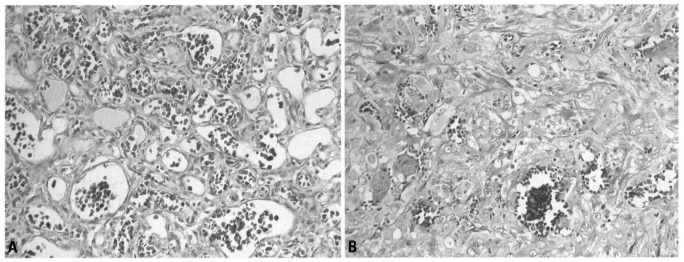

Fig. 3.117 A Capillary haemangioma of the anterior mediastinum. The tumour forms distinct lobules separated by a loose stroma. **B** Epithelioid haemangioendothelioma. Cords of tumour cells with abundant eosinophilic cytoplasm. Occasional tumour cells show vacuolation. Some primitive vascular channels contain blood. This case also shows interspersed osteoclastic giant cells.

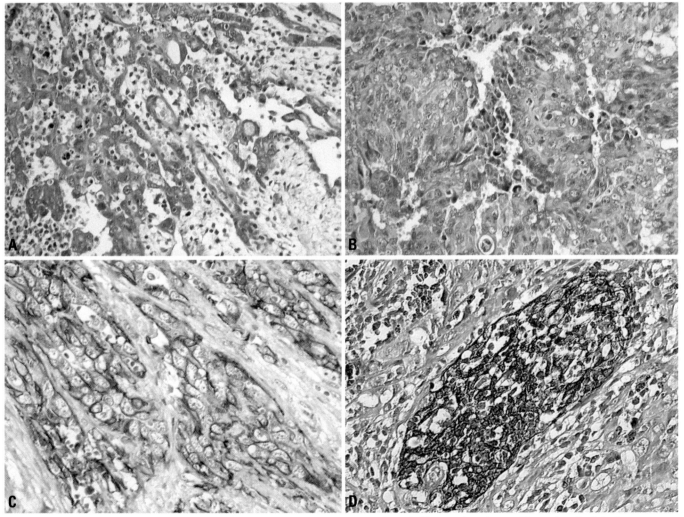

Fig. 3.118 Angiosarcoma. **A** The tumour forms anastomosing channels, and the lining cells show significant nuclear pleomorphism and atypia. **B** Angiosarcoma can show a solid growth, obscuring the vascular nature of this malignant tumour. **C** Typical immunostaining of tumour cell membranes for CD31. **D** Immunostaining of remnant thymic epithelial cell network for cytokeratin 19.

Synovial sarcoma (SS)

ICD-O code   9040/3

Several cases of SS have been reported {871,2033,2163}. The tumours usually occur in adults but rarely in children {871} and manifest by pain, dyspnoea or superior vena cava syndrome. Most cases followed an aggressive clinical course, with 3 of 5 patients dying of tumour on follow-up of 10 months to 4 years. Detection of SYT-SSX chimeric RNA transcripts, resulting from the t(X;18) translocation is often essential to distinguish SS from mesothelioma, sarcomatoid (thymic and other) carcinomas, malignant peripheral nerve sheath tumour with glandular differentiation, germ cell tumour-associated sarcomas or metastases {71,2033}.

Vascular tumours

Mediastinal lymphangioma is a common mediastinal tumour in children {1932}. Hemangiomas of the cavernous, and less frequently, capillary subtype have been reported and may be complicated by the Kasabach-Merritt syndrome {838,1353, 1932}. Hemangiopericytoma, epithelioid hemangioendothelioma and angiosarcoma (the latter usually arising from a thymic germ cell tumour {1230,1356})

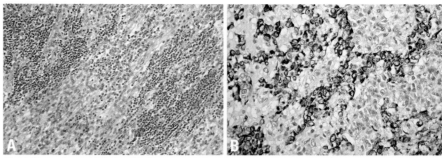

Fig. 3.120 Angiomatoid fibrous histiocytoma of the central mediastinum involving the ascending aorta and thymus. **A** The tumour typically comprises spindle cells that may raise the differential diagnosis of leiomyoma. In contrast to leiomyoma, AFH is typically accompanied in the tumour periphery by a dense inflammatory infiltrate composed of lymphocytes and plasma cells. **B** Desmin positivity in the neoplastic cells. Inflammatory cells are negative.

have also been described {962,1921, 1932}

Leiomyomatous tumours

Leiomyomas, probably derived from the aortic arch {1789}, and even rarer, leiomyosarcomas {96,1370} have been reported in the mediastinum, including its anterior compartment. They should be distinguished from liposarcomas with leiomyomatous differentiation {601}, and angiomatoid fibrous histiocytomas (AFH) of the mediastinum. AFH can exhibit spindle cell features, and half of the cases show desmin expression. However, it is often accompanied by an infiltrate of lymphocytes and plasma cells, particularly in the peripheral portion. Frequent coexpression of CD99, CD68 and EMA, and a characteristic t(12;16)(q13; p11) translocation generating FUS/ATF1 fusion transcripts distinguish AFH from leiomyoma and leiomyosarcoma {590}.

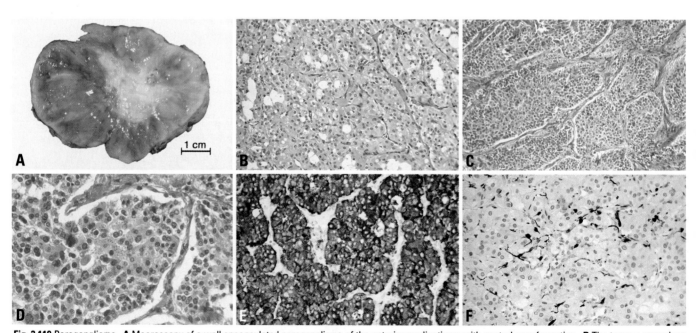

Fig. 3.119 Paraganglioma. **A** Macroscopy of a well encapsulated paraganglioma of the anterior mediastinum with central scar formation. **B** The tumour comprises packets of cells with abundant eosinophilic cytoplasm, traversed by a delicate vasculature. **C** Low power histology showing the "Zellballen-Pattern" of a mediastinal paraganglioma. **D** High power of the same case shows marked variability of cell and nuclear size. **E** Typical strong cytoplasmic granular immunostaining for synaptophysin. **F** Immunostaining for S100 protein reveals the delicate sustentacular cells that wrap around the tumour cell packets.

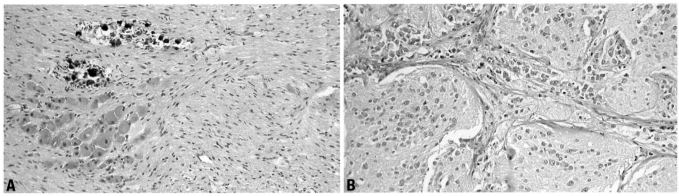

Fig. 3.121 A Ganglioneuroma of the posterior mediastinum. Clusters of ganglion cells merge into a spindle cell component that resembles neurofibroma or schwannoma. Calcification is common. By definition, there should not be identifiable neuroblasts. **B** Differentiating neuroblastoma of the posterior mediastinum with abundant neuropil. The latter should not be confused with the schwannian stroma required for a diagnosis of ganglioneuroblastoma.

Neurogenic tumours

Neurogenic tumours of the mediastinum occur almost exclusively in the middle and posterior compartments, where they constitute the most frequent neoplasms. However, benign *schwannomas* {1597}, and malignant peripheral nerve sheath tumours, including malignant Triton tumours {1525} have also been described in the anterior mediastinum, mainly in patients with neurofibromatosis {1726,1851}.

About 20% of mediastinal *paragangliomas* occur in the anterior compartment {1365} and they may be pigmented {1350}. They tend to occur in older individuals (mean age 46 years). The patients are asymptomatic, or present with compression symptoms, or rarely with Cushing syndrome {1548}. Posterior mediastinal paragangliomas tend to occur in younger patients (mean age 29 years), and about half of the cases have hypertension or other symptoms due to release of catecholamines by the tumours {1350}. They recur locally and metastasize in 55% and 26% of cases, respectively {1123}. Paragangliomas typ-

ically show a nesting pattern associated with a prominent vasculature. The tumour cells are immunoreactive for synaptophysin, and S100 protein positive sustentacular cells are often demonstrable around tumour cell nests. In contrast to neuroendocrine carcinomas, paragangliomas do not form ribbons or rosette-like structures, and cytokeratin is usually negative.

Tumours related to the sympathetic ganglia include *neuroblastoma, ganglioneuroblastoma and ganglioneuroma*. They occur almost exclusively in the posterior mediastinum, although neuroblastomas {70} and ganglioneuroblastomas have also been rarely described in the thymus {76,1964,2141}. In fact, neuroblastoma is the most common malignant tumour of the posterior mediastinum in young children. Ganglioneuroblastoma and ganglioneuroma occur mostly in adults.

Primary *ependymoma* of the posterior mediastinum in adults, is typically associated with a prolonged indolent course {503,2153}.

Other rare neoplasms

Other thymic/mediastinal soft tissue tumours include Ewing sarcoma which usually extends into the mediastinum from the thoracic wall {690}, malignant rhabdoid tumour {166,1160,1691}, inflammatory myofibroblastic tumour (inflammatory pseudotumour) {422,467}, calcifying fibrous tumour {1443}, giant cell angiofibroma {636}, elastofibrolipoma {455}, desmoid fibromatosis {1036}, benign mesenchymoma {2054}, rhabdomyoma {1315}, alveolar soft part sarcoma {593} and malignant fibrous histiocytoma {344,1932}.

Primary malignant melanoma {42,642, 1804,2088} probably arises from thymic nevus cell aggregates {642,1552}. Other rare tumours include meningioma {553, 2150}, osteosarcoma {454,739,888}, chondrosarcoma {1592}, giant cell tumour {622}, chordoma {32,1675,1910}, myelolipoma {1008,1706,1884}, and extramedullary haematopoietic tumours {449,834,1366,1400,1481,1788}.

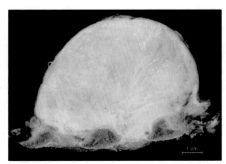

Fig. 3.122 Fibromatosis (desmoid tumour) of the thoracic wall and pleura.

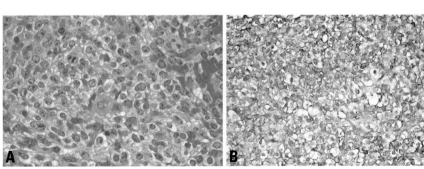

Fig. 3.123 A Ewing sarcoma of the mediastinum with **B** CD99 (MIC-2) expression.

Ectopic thyroid and parathyroid tumours

J.K.C. Chan

Ectopic thyroid tumour

Definition
Ectopic thyroid tumour is a thyroid neoplasm that occurs in sites other than the cervical thyroid gland proper.

Thyroid tumours occurring in the mediastinum are often of cervical thyroid gland origin with extension into the mediastinum. Ectopic thyroid tumours arising in the mediastinum without connection to the cervical thyroid gland are very rare. They are either discovered incidentally, or present with symptoms referable to a mediastinal mass. The nomenclature and diagnostic criteria of these thyroid tumours should follow those of the World Health Organization classification of tumours of endocrine organs {9}. Follicular adenoma and papillary carcinoma are the commonest, but other tumour types have also been described, such as follicular carcinoma, oncocytic (Hürthle cell) carcinoma and poorly differentiated insular carcinoma {507,966, 1191,1328,1527,1889,2133}. If there are uncertainties as to whether the tumour is of thyroid origin, positive immunostaining for thyroglobulin would provide a strong support for the diagnosis. Information on the behaviour of these tumours is limited, but it is likely that the outcome is similar to comparable stage tumours occurring in the cervical thyroid gland {2133}.

Histogenesis
Thyroid tissue that has aberrantly migrated to the mediastinum during embryologic development is the cell of origin for the ectopic thyroid tumours in the mediastinum.

Ectopic parathyroid tumour

Definition
Ectopic parathyroid tumour is a parathyroid cell neoplasm occurring in sites other than the usual locations of the parathyroid glands in the neck {1889}.

Epidemiology, clinical features
Approximately 10-20% of all parathyroid adenomas (including lipoadenomas) occur in the mediastinum, most commonly the anterosuperior mediastinum in the vicinity or within the thymus gland {376,399,1444,2103,2141}. The patients present with symptoms due to hyperparathyroidism. Ectopic parathyroid carcinomas of the mediastinum are very rare, and they may or may not be functional {990,1412,1627}.

Histopathology
The nomenclature and diagnostic criteria for ectopic parathyroid tumours should follow those of the World Health Organization Classification of endocrine tumours (see "World Health Organization Classification of Tumours: Pathology and Genetics of Tumours of Endocrine Organs"). Parathyroid adenomas are circumscribed or thinly encapsulated tumours comprising sheets, cords and acini of polygonal cells traversed by a delicate vasculature. There is often a mixture of tumour cells with clear, lightly eosinophilic and oxyphilic cytoplasm. Some tumours have abundant interspersed adipose cells (lipoadenomas) {1444,2167}. Mitotic figures are absent or rare, and focal nucleomegaly is acceptable. Parathyroid carcinomas often show capsular or vascular invasion, sclerotic bands, and mitotic figures. If there are uncertainties whether a neoplasm is of parathyroid origin, positive immunostaining for parathyroid hormone would provide a strong support for the diagnosis.

Histogenesis
Ectopic or supernumerary parathyroid gland in the anterosuperior mediastinum is the cell of origin for the ectopic parathyroid tumours. Such a localization for the parathyroid gland is not surprising since the inferior parathyroid glands share a common origin with the thymus from the third branchial pouch {2141}.

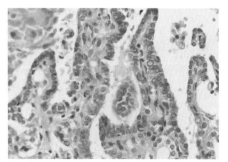

Fig. 3.124 Ectopic papillary thyroid carcinoma of the anterior mediastinum. The tumour comprises papillae lined by cells with overlapping and pale nuclei.

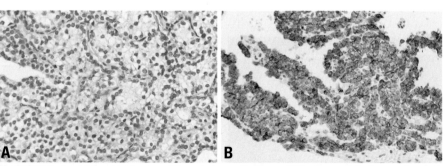

Fig. 3.125 Ectopic parathyroid adenoma of the anterior mediastinum. A The tumour cells form packets and acini, separated by a delicate vasculature. Many clear cells are evident. B Positive immunostaining for parathyroid hormone provides confirmation that the tumour is of parathyroid origin.

Metastases to thymus and anterior mediastinum

H.K. Müller-Hermelink
Ph. Ströbel
A. Zettl
A. Marx

Definition

Malignant tumours that metastasize to the thymus or anterior mediastinum from distant primary tumours. Neoplasms that extend directly from adjacent organs or tissues are also included in this category.

The most common primary tumours involving these sites are lung, thyroid, breast and prostatic carcinomas {948, 1188,1287,1288,1305}, while melanoma and various sarcomas (liposarcoma, osteosarcoma, rhabdomyosarcoma, Kaposi sarcoma and malignant fibrous histiocytoma) are rare primary tumours {33,702,843,1852,1865}.

The distinction between squamous and neuroendocrine carcinomas of the thymus and mediastinal metastases with this differentiation can be difficult. In about 50% of carcinomas, morphological and immunohistochemical features can clarify the thymic derivation, while clinical staging procedures are required to clarify the derivation of the other cases. The different genetic characteristics of carcinomas of the thymus {896,2238,2242} compared to those of lung and the head and neck region {188,1582,1585,1866} are of diagnostic value.

Clinical data is also necessary to distinguish primary thymic melanomas {42, 642,1804,2088} or sarcomas {256,1742, 1932} from metastasis with a respective differentiation.

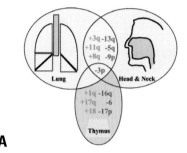

A

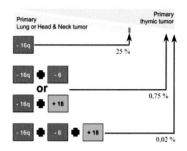

B

Fig. 3.126 Metastases to thymus and anterior mediastinum. **A** Summary of recurrent genetic gains and losses as determined by CGH discriminating between squamous cell carcinomas of the thymus, lung and head & neck region. There is considerable overlap between the carcinomas arising in the lung and head & neck. By contrast, the major genetic aberrations of thymic carcinomas are not shared with lung and head & neck carcinomas. **B** Diagnostic value of CGH-based genetic profiles for the distinction between squamous cell carcinomas of the thymus and mediastinal metastases of primary lung and head and neck tumours. Percentages indicate the probabilities for a primary lung or head and neck carcinoma in the presence of highly discriminating genetic alterations {188,1267,1866,2238}.

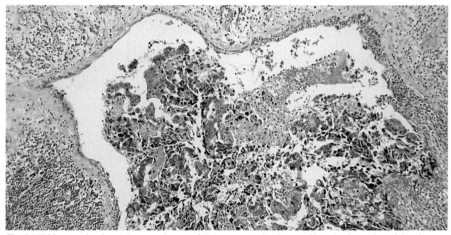

Fig. 3.127 Metastasis of an adenocarcinoma of the rectum to the thymus. Note the formation of thymic cyst adjacent to and infiltrated by the metastatic tumour.

Table 3.14

Morphological and immunohistochemical criteria for the differential diagnosis of features of primary thymic carcinomas from metastases to the anterior mediastinum arising from carcinomas of the lung and head and neck region.

Tumour	Primary of the thymus	Primary of lung or head and neck
Squamous cell, basaloid, lympho-epithelioma-like carcinoma	Lobular growth pattern 70% Perivascular spaces 50% CD5 expression 50% CD70 expression 50% CD117 expression 40-100%[1]	Lobular growth pattern rare Perivascular spaces very rare CD5 not expressed CD70 not expressed CD117 not expressed
Neuroendocrine carcinoma[2]	TTF-1 expression absent[3]	TTF-1 expression frequent

[1]Ströbel et al. in a series of 34 thymic carcinomas (unpublished) [2]Oliveira et al, 2001 {1513}; Pomplun et al. 2002 {1609}; [3]Muller-Hermelink et al. in a series of 15 neuroendocrine carconomas (unpublished).

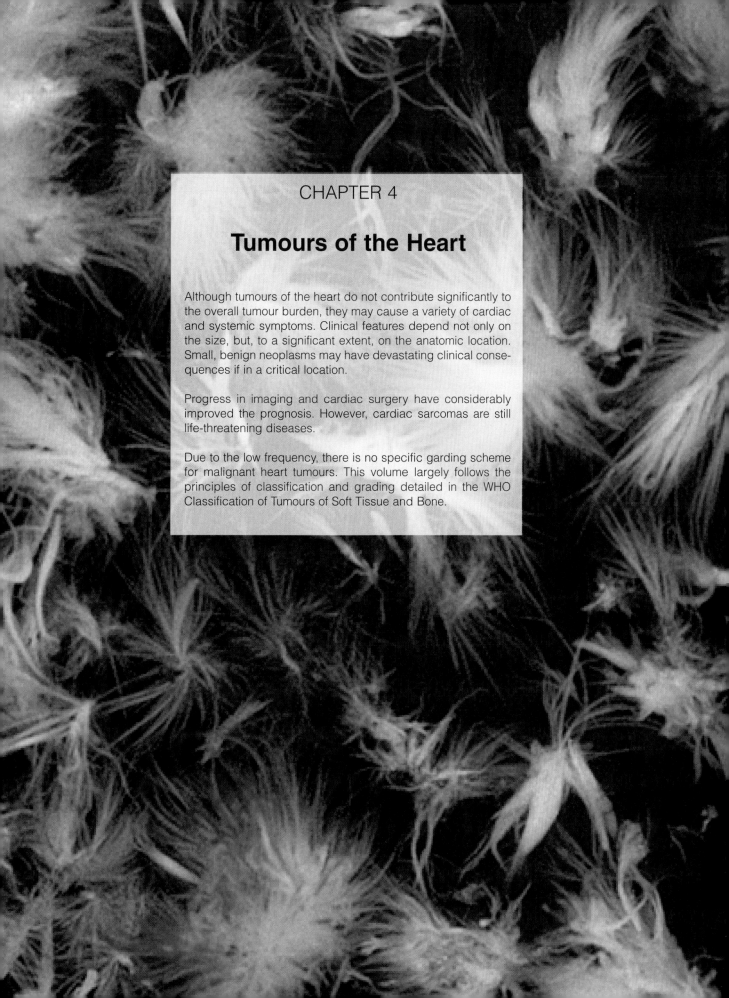

CHAPTER 4

Tumours of the Heart

Although tumours of the heart do not contribute significantly to the overall tumour burden, they may cause a variety of cardiac and systemic symptoms. Clinical features depend not only on the size, but, to a significant extent, on the anatomic location. Small, benign neoplasms may have devastating clinical consequences if in a critical location.

Progress in imaging and cardiac surgery have considerably improved the prognosis. However, cardiac sarcomas are still life-threatening diseases.

Due to the low frequency, there is no specific garding scheme for malignant heart tumours. This volume largely follows the principles of classification and grading detailed in the WHO Classification of Tumours of Soft Tissue and Bone.

WHO histological classification of tumours of the heart

Benign tumours and tumour-like lesions

Rhabdomyoma	8900/0
Histiocytoid cardiomyopathy	
Hamartoma of mature cardiac myocytes	
Adult Cellular Rhabdomyoma	8904/0
Cardiac myxoma	8840/0
Papillary fibroelastoma	
Haemangioma	9120/0
Cardiac fibroma	8810/0
Inflammatory myofibroblastic tumor	8825/1
Lipoma	8850/0
Cystic tumour of the atrioventricular node	

Malignant tumours

Angiosarcoma	9120/3
Epithelioid haemangioendothelioma	9133/3
Malignant pleomorphic fibrous histiocytoma	
(MFH)/Undifferenciated pleomorphic sarcoma	8830/3
Fibrosarcoma and myxoid fibrosarcoma	8840/3
Rhabdomyosarcoma	8900/3
Leiomyosarcoma	8890/3
Synovial sarcoma	9040/3
Liposarcoma	8854/3
Cardiac lymphomas	
Metastatic tumours	

Pericardial tumours

Solitary fibrous tumour	8815/1
Malignant mesothelioma	9050/3
Germ cell tumours	
Metastatic pericardial tumours	

[1] Morphology code of the International Classification of Diseases for Oncology (ICD-O) {6} and the Systematized Nomenclature of Medicine (http://snomed.org). Behaviour is coded /0 for benign tumours, /3 for malignant tumours, and /1 for borderline or uncertain behaviour.

Tumours of the heart: Introduction

A.P. Burke
J.P. Veinot
R. Loire
R. Virmani

H. Tazelaar
H. Kamiya
P.A. Araoz
G. Watanabe

Epidemiology

The estimated frequency of cardiac tumours ranges from 0.0017-0.33% {2165}. In a review of 22 autopsy-based series of primary cardiac tumours a frequency of 0.021% was identified among 731,309 patients {1656}. In one 20-year (1972-1991) review of 12,485 autopsy cases, there was a 0.056% incidence of primary tumours and a 1.23% incidence of secondary tumours {1116}. However, these data may have a high referral bias and may not reflect population-based incidence rates {2079}. At the Mayo Clinic, the autopsy incidence of primary cardiac tumours from 1915 to 1931 was 0.05%, but more than tripled to 0.17% between 1954 and 1970 {2165}; again, referral bias may have played a role in this change.

When most cardiac tumours were diagnosed at autopsy, myxomas and sarcomas were reported at a similar frequency. With the utilization of cardiopulmonary bypass and surgical excision, the reported frequency of myxomas as opposed to cardiac sarcomas has increased substantially {249,1568}. In a review of surgical series, cardiac myxomas constitute 77% of surgically excised tumours, and cardiac sarcomas, 10% {249}.

In children, cardiac tumours are not common and most are benign {249}. The most common pediatric tumours include rhabdomyomas, fibromas, myxomas, and teratomas {249,356}.

Secondary cardiac tumours, either metastatic or by direct invasion, outnumber primary cardiac neoplasms {1116}. A review of 3,314 autopsies found a 2.9% frequency of metastatic tumours involving the heart {12}. The most common primary sites are lung, breast, and cutaneous melanoma.

Clinical features

Cardiac neoplasms may cause a variety of signs and symptoms {1225,1791, 2079}. The clinical presentation depends on the size of the tumour and its anatomic location. Growth rate, friability, and invasiveness are also important factors

that determine clinical features {737}. Large tumours may be relatively silent, whereas small tumours in a critical location may give rise to devastating clinic consequences.

Left atrial tumours, especially those that are mobile or pedunculated, may lead to systemic embolism involving the coronary, cerebral and peripheral circulations {737,1568,2077}, resulting in myocardial infarction, stroke or ischemic viscera or limbs. Left atrial tumours may also interfere with mitral valve function resulting in mitral stenosis or regurgitation. Cardiac murmurs and a characteristic tumour "plop" may be auscultated. Valve dysfunction manifests as left-sided heart failure with shortness of breath, orthopnea, paroxysmal nocturnal dyspnoea, pulmonary edema, fatigue, cough, and chest pain {356}.

Intramural left ventricular tumours may be asymptomatic or present with a mass effect. With protrusion into the cavity, hemodynamic compromise may result {1225}. Local extension of the tumour may cause conduction or coronary artery compromise with chest pain, myocardial infarction, arrhythmia, heart block or sudden death {356,737,1225,1791}.

Right atrial or right ventricular tumours may result in right heart failure from atrioventricular or pulmonary outflow obstruction, resulting in peripheral edema, hepatomegaly, ascites, shortness of breath, syncope and sometimes, sudden death {737}. If the tumours interfere with valve function they may result in regurgitation or stenosis {1791}.

Right-sided cardiac tumours may embolize to the lungs and present as pulmonary emboli with chest pain, pulmonary infarction and haemoptysis {1634,1791}. Chronic embolization may also mimic chronic thromboembolic disease with signs and symptoms of pulmonary hypertension.

Pericardial tumours may cause chest pain typical of pericarditis {1225,1568}. The tumours may be haemorrhagic and cause pericardial effusion and tamponade {1634}. However, constrictive peri-

carditis may also result from tumour infiltration.

Rarely, tumours such as myxoma, cause *systemic symptoms,* including anorexia, weight loss, fatigue and malaise which may mimic a variety of systemic disorders {356,737,1774,2077}. Interestingly, they may also cause haematologic abnormalities, including anemia, polycythemia, leukocytosis, thrombocytosis and elevated sedimentation rate {1225}. Tumour production of mediators, including interleukins, has been reported {1774}.

Imaging

Primary tumours of the heart and pericardium may be detected as an abnormal finding on a chest radiogram or another imaging test obtained for an unrelated reason. Once detected cardiac imaging is needed to define (1) tumour location, extent and boundaries; (2) relationships with adjacent key cardiac structures such as valves and coronary arteries; (3) tumour type; and (4) presence and degree of functional impairment. The main non-invasive imaging modalities for evaluating primary cardiac tumours each have advantages and disadvantages. They are often used together in a complementary manner for diagnosis and surgical planning.

Echocardiography.
The primary advantage of echocardiography is that it has the best spatial and temporal resolution and provides excellent anatomic and functional information {492,705,1070,1162,2104,2215}. It is the optimal imaging modality for small masses (<1 cm) or masses arising from valves. A second major advantage of echocardiography is the ability to image velocities with Doppler, which allows for assessment of presence, degree, and location of obstructions to blood flow or valve regurgitation. Echocardiography is typically the modality used for the initial evaluation of cardiac tumours and may be the only diagnostic test required in some patients. Disadvantages include

suboptimal image quality in patients with poor acoustic windows, inability to image extent of disease outside of the mediastinum, and relatively low soft tissue contrast, which limits detection of tumour infiltration and characterization of tumour tissue. Also, intravenous contrast agents are not routinely used with echocardiography, which limits the ability to characterize tumour vascularity.

Magnetic Resonance Imaging (MRI)

The primary advantage of MRI is its excellent soft tissue contrast which makes it the most sensitive modality for detection of tumour infiltration. MRI has more manipulable imaging parameters than other imaging modalities. Because of this, MRI is the best modality for characterizing tumour tissue {1003,1768, 1831,2156}. For example, a T2-weighted standard or fast spin echo sequence distinguishes tumours with high water content, such as haemangioma, from tumours with low water content, such as fibroma. A third advantage of MRI is the ability to characterize tumour vascularity with intravenous contrast. Though not as flexible as echocardiography, MRI does allow assessment of wall motion and assessment of velocities through large vessels. This allows for characterization of ventricular function, inflow or outflow obstruction and valve regurgitation. The primary disadvantage of MRI is long examination times, which translates into the need for sedation in children, and the need for reliable ECG gating. MRI should be considered when the tissue type, exact location, or the relationships of the tumour with neighbouring structures are not completely defined by echocardiography or when surgical resection of the tumour is considered.

Computed Tomography (CT)

ECG gated CT scans with the latest generation of multidetector scanners or with electron beam scanners are also very useful for cardiac imaging {65,275}. In many ways, the advantages and disadvantages of CT are intermediate between those of echocardiography and MRI. Modern CT scanners have excellent spatial resolution, which is better than that of MRI, but not as high echocardiograpy. CT has better soft tissue contrast than echocardiography, and can be used to definitively characterize fatty content and calcifications; however, the overall soft

Fig. 4.01

Parameters of the grading system for sarcomas of the Féderation Nationale des Centres de Lutte Contre le Cancer (FNCLCC).

Tumour differentiation

Score 1: Sarcomas closely resembling normal adult mesenchymal tissue (e.g., low-grade leiomyosarcoma).

Score 2: Sarcomas for which histological typing is certain (e.g., Myxoid Fibrosarcoma)

Score 3: Undifferentiated, angiosarcoma

Mitotic count

Score 1: 0-9 mitoses per 10 HPF*

Score 2: 10-19 mitoses per 10 HPF

Score 3: ≥20 mitoses per 10 HPF

Tumour necrosis

Score 0: No necrosis

Score 1: <50% tumour necrosis

Score 2: ≥50% tumour necrosis

Histologic grade

Grade 1: Total score 2,3

Grade 2: Total score 4,5

Grade 3: Total score 6, 7, 8

Modified from Trojani et al {2031}.

*A high-power field (hpf) measures 0.1734mm^2

---

tissue contrast and ability to characterize tumour infiltration and tumour type is less than that of MRI. Intravenous contrast can provide information about tumour vascularity, an advantage CT shares with MRI. CT may be used as an adjunct to both echocardiography and MRI.

Cardiac Catheterization

This is seldom required for diagnosis of cardiac tumours, but may be performed in adults to exclude coronary artery disease. Angiography provides indirect and nonspecific imaging based on filling defects within the cardiac chambers and displacement of the coronary arteries {347,1840}. Two exceptions are worth noting. First, endomyocardial biopsy for tissue typing may be considered in selected patients. Second, selective coronary angiography is helpful when planning surgical resection of an intramyocardial tumour.

Tumour grading and staging

Given the low frequency of malignant cardiac tumours, there is no grading scheme specifically referring to malignant heart tumours. This volume uses the criteria published in the recent WHO

Classification of Tumours of Soft Tissue and Bone {590}. The concept of grading sarcomas was first introduced in 1977 {1712}. Several grading systems have since been proposed which have shown to correlate with prognosis {412,1247, 1418,2031,2070}. The two most important parameters in non-cardiac soft tissue seem to be the mitotic index and extent of tumour necrosis {1793,2031, 2070}. Most pathologists recognize three grades of malignancy: G1, low grade; G2, intermediate grade; and G3, high grade. Some use a 4-tiered system.

The two most widely used systems are those of the NCI (U.S. National Cancer Institute) {412,413} and the FNCLCC (Fédération Nationale des Centres de Lutte Contre le Cancer) {387-389,748, 2031}.

According to the methodology defined in 1984 {412} and refined in 1999 {413}, the NCI system uses a combination of histologic type, cellularity, pleomorphism and mitotic rate for attributing grade 1 or 3. All the other types of sarcomas are classified as either grade 2 or grade 3 depending on the amount of tumour necrosis, with 15% necrosis as the threshold for separation of grade 2 and grade 3 lesions.

The FNCLCC system is based on a score obtained by evaluating three features: tumour differentiation, mitotic rate and amount of tumour necrosis {2031}. A score is attributed independently to each parameter and the grade is obtained by adding the three attributed scores. Tumour differentiation is highly dependent on histologic type and subtype. The reproducibility of this system has been tested by 15 pathologists: the crude proportion of agreement was 75% for tumour grade, but only 61% for histologic type {748}.

Because of the limitations and pitfalls of grading, the following guidelines have been suggested to improve reliablility:

> Grading should be used only for untreated primary soft tissue sarcomas.

> Grading should be performed on representative and well-processed material.

> Grading is not a substitute for a histologic diagnosis and does not differentiate benign and malignant lesions. Before grading a soft tissue lesion, one must be sure that one is dealing with a true sarcoma and not a pseudosarcoma.

> Parameters of grading must be carefully evaluated, particularly the mitotic rate.

The WHO Classification of Tumuors of Soft Tissue and Bone {590} offers additional information on the grading of soft tissue sarcomas. There is no TNM classification for cardiac malignancies.

Treatment and prognosis

In general, surgical resection, when possible, is the treatment of choice for primary cardiac tumours in symptomatic patients. It is also highly desirable for patients whose tumours are identified incidentally because of the ever-present risk of sudden death, embolism, obstruction, or arrhythmia {307,952}. In patients with rhabdomyomas and so called histiocytoid cardiomyopathy, predominantly children, there are some who suggest that surgical intervention is only necessary in the face of life-threatening symptoms, as these tumours are benign and known to regress with age {1880}.

Surgical strategy varies by tumour type. Cardiac myxomas arise mainly from the left atrial septum, and the surgical strategy usually includes complete tumour resection with underlying stalk. Sometimes reconstruction using a prosthetic patch is necessary {952}. The prognosis of patients with cardiac myxomas is excellent. They may occasionally recur, especially in patients with Carney complex, an autosomal dominant syndrome characterized by associated skin lesions, endocrine abnormalities and other unusual tumours {1018}. It is difficult to suggest a regular surgical strategy for other cardiac tumours as they arise in various locations. The prognosis for other benign tumours is generally favourable with low recurrence, and it is quite good even if incompletely excised {307,952,1880}. Orthotopic heart transplantation is an option if tumour resection

and reconstruction would be expected to cause irreparable damage to essential cardiac structures {731}.

For malignant cardiac tumours, complete resection is often impossible because of local spread {2071}. The prognosis of patients with primary malignant cardiac tumours is very poor even if complete resection is attempted {952,2071}. Adjuvant chemotherapy and irradiation are usually also given, but these are not effective in most cases {2071}. Favourable results of heart transplantation for primary malignant cardiac tumours have been reported despite immunosuppression {731,733, 1962, 2071}.

Benign tumours with myocyte differentiation

A.P. Burke
H. Tazelaar
C.R. Patel
R. Virmani

T. Geva
G. Tornambene
D.J. Radford

Rhabdomyoma

Definition
A benign tumour of the cardiac myocyte, which can be solitary or multiple. The cells typically contain large glycogen filled vacuoles.

ICD-O code
8900/0

Epidemiology
Cardiac rhabdomyoma is commonly associated with tuberous sclerosis, an autosomal dominant disorder with a high mutation rate. It involves multiple organs including brain, kidney, pancreas, retina and skin. In autopsy series, patients with tuberous sclerosis have a 30% incidence of cardiac rhabdomyoma {571}. However, the actual incidence is likely higher since series that have evaluated patients with echocardiography have found an incidence between 40% and 86% {119,492,777}. The presence of multiple cardiac rhabdomyomas prenatally may be the earliest manifestation of tuberous sclerosis.

Localization
Rhabdomyomas are firm, white, well-circumscribed lobulated nodules that occur in any location in the heart, but are more common in the ventricles. In patients with tuberous sclerosis, tumours are usually multiple (> 90%) and can consist of numerous miliary nodules measuring less than 1 mm; in this instance, the term "rhabdomyomatosis" has been used. The most common locations are the left ventricle and ventricular septum, although 30% will have atrial wall or right ventricular involvement {1602}. In contrast to patients with tuberous sclerosis, approximately 50% of sporadic rhabdomyomas occur singley.

Clinical features
Signs and symptoms
Rhabdomyomas are the most common tumours in the pediatric age group. They are also the tumours most commonly diagnosed during the prenatal period by foetal echocardiography. Intrauterine as well as sudden death after birth has been attributed to these tumours.

Clinical and hemodynamic findings are related to the number, position, and size of the tumours. For instance large intramural or intracavitary tumours may obstruct valvular orifices, or occlude intracavitory spaces {1254}. Foetal dysrhythmias or non-immune hydrops may be identified as early as 21 weeks by ultrasound {863}. The tumours may cause infant respiratory distress, congestive heart failure, or low cardiac output. Right-sided tumours that cause obstruction may cause cyanosis, or features suggestive of tetralogy of Fallot or pulmonary stenosis {41,583}. Left-sided tumours may present as subaortic obstruction, or hypoplastic left heart syndrome {2068}. Rarely they can be associated with structural cardiac defects {2113}. Patients with "rhabdomyomatosis" or diffuse microscopic involvement of the myocardium may present as though they have a cardiomyopathy. Spontaneous regression is a common feature {1254,1840}.

Electrocardiographic abnormalities will vary depending on location, but evidence of ventricular hypertrophy and ST-T wave abnormalities consistent with ischemia and/or strain are common. The conduction abnormalities consist of bundle branch block, preexcitation, and first to third degree atrioventricular block.

Imaging
At echocardiography rhabdomyomas appear as homogeneous, well-circumscribed echogenic masses in the ventricular myocardium, possibly protruding into the ventricular cavity. Although uncommon, extensive rhabdomyomas can be associated with ventricular dysfunction. Given that the finding of multiple cardiac masses is diagnostic of rhabdomyoma, especially in patients with tuberous sclerosis, and that the tumours are not infiltrative, echocardiography usually provides adequate information for diagnosis and clinical management. If there is question of tumour type or of tumour invasion, MRI or CT may be used to further define the tumours. At MRI, rhabdomyomas appear as well-circumscribed masses with signal characteristics similar to that of normal myocardium {155,737,1003}. Compared with the signal from uninvolved myocardium, the masses are hypointense on postgadolinium imaging. At CT, rhabdomy-

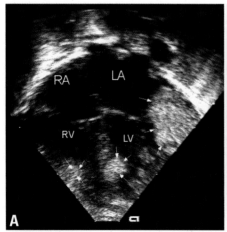
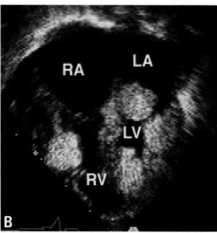

Fig. 4.01 Rhabdomyoma. **A** Echocardiogram of an infant who presented with supraventricular tachycardia. There are multiple rhabdomyomas. These eventually regressed and the arrhythmias resolved. **B** Echocardiographic imaging from the apical chamber view, showing multiple cardiac rhabdomyomas involving the left (LV) and right (RV) ventricles.

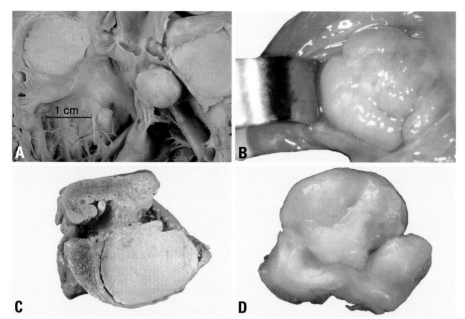

Fig. 4.02 Cardiac rhabdomyoma. **A** Multiple rhabdomyomas in an infant with tuberous sclerosis complex (courtesy of William D. Edwards, M.D.). **B** Intraoperative photograph. The tumour nearly fills the ventricular cavity, and is glistening and polypoid. **C** Stillborn child with a ventricular rhabdomyoma. **D** Subaortic rhabdomyoma in an 5 months old child.

omas also appear as multiple nodules, which may be hyper or hypoattenuating compared to normal myocardium. With MRI or CT, the rest of the body can be imaged for signs of tuberous sclerosis. However, because rhabdomyoma has many imaging features similar to normal myocardium, echocardiography, MRI, and CT may be complementary as rhabdomyomas that are not visible by one modality may be visible on another {737}.

Macroscopy

Single or multiple, they are well-circumscribed, non-capsulated white or grey white nodules which may vary in size from millimeters to several centimeters. Tumours can become quite large, espe-cially in sporadic cases. In one series of 14 cases, the range was 0.3-9.0 cm, with a mean of 3.4 cm {248}. They most often occur in the ventricle, but can be found in the atria, at the cavoatrial junction and on the epicardial surface. Large tumours may obliterate and distort a ventricular cavity.

Histopathology

Cardiac rhabdomyomas are well-demar-cated nodules of enlarged cardiac myocytes with cleared cytoplasm. In some cells, strands of eosinophilic cyto-plasm stretch from a central nucleus to the cell membrane giving rise to cells that resemble a spider ("spider cells"). The majority of cells show vacuolization

with sparse myofilaments. There is a strong reaction with periodic acid-Schiff reagent, reflecting the presence of abundant intracellular glycogen.

Immunoprofile

Immunohistochemical studies document the striated muscle characteristics of rhabdomyoma cells, which express myoglobin, desmin, actin, and vimentin. Tumour cells do not express cell prolifer-ation markers such as Ki-67 and PCNA, indicating that the lesions are more likely hamartomas as opposed to neoplasms {248}.

Electron microscopy

By electron microscopy, the cells resem-ble altered myocytes. They possess abundant glycogen, small and sparse mitochondria, and cellular junctions resembling intercalated disks surround the cell periphery. In contrast, the inter-calated disks of differentiated myocytes are located exclusively at the poles of the cell. Intercalated discs and myofibrils or collections of Z band material are pres-ent. Rarely one may observe there primi-tive T-tubules. Leptomeric fibers close to the sarcolemma may also be identified.

Differential diagnosis

The diagnosis of cardiac rhabdomyoma in infants and young children is straight-forward. In patients with multiple non-cal-cifying masses, especially with other manifestations of tuberous sclerosis complex, a tissue diagnosis is unneces-sary. However, because the tumours have been shown to regress with age and multiple biopsies do not allow for evaluation of the morphologic changes that characterize this process, the rela-tionship between persistent rhabdomy-omas and so-called adult rhabdomy-

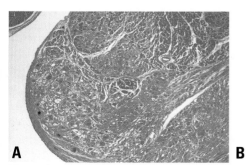

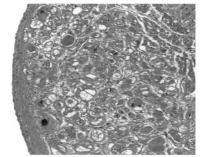

Fig. 4.03 Rhabdomyoma. **A** The subendocardium shows a poorly demarcated area of cellular vacuolization. **B** A higher magnification note "spider" cells, several vacuolated tumor cells, and cells with abundant eosinophilic cytoplasm , which is more typical for rhabdomyomas in older children.

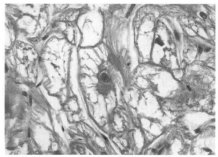

Fig. 4.04 Cardiac rhabdomyoma with classic spider cell.

omas and hamartomas is not clear. In the rare examples of rhabdomyomas in older children, there is often a paucity of spider cells, resulting in a tumour with some characteristics of adult rhabdomyomas, but without the proliferative activity. Hamartoma of mature cardiac myocytes, which, like rhabdomyoma, is a non-proliferative hamartomatous lesion, occurs in adults. These tumours lack circumscription and spider cells.

Genetic alterations
The familial form of tuberous sclerosis, which is present in up to 50% of patients with cardiac rhabdomyoma, exhibits autosomal dominant inheritance. Two disease genes have been identified: TSC-1 at chromosome 9q34, and TSC-2 at chromosome 16p13 {1613}. The TSC-1 gene encodes hamartin, and TSC-2 tuberin, proteins involved in tumour suppression. Loss of heterozygosity is often found at these loci in tumours from patients with tuberous sclerosis. The precise roles of TSC-1 and TSC-2 in the development of cardiac tumours and regulation of embryonic and neonatal cardiomyocyte growth remain to be elucidated.

Treatment and Prognosis
Rhabdomyomas have a natural history of spontaneous regression {204,556,1840}. However, serious symptoms may precipitate the need for surgical resection. When arrhythmias are the presenting symptom, treatment with anti-arrhythmic drugs is commenced. If control is achieved by that means, then drugs can

be continued until the arrhythmias or tumours regress. If drugs fail to control arrhythmias, surgical resection is indicated. When a tumour is causing intracardiac obstruction, surgery is necessary {180,525,538,1289}.

Histiocytoid cardiomyopathy

Definition
Histiocytoid cardiomyopathy is a rare, but distinctive arrhythmogenic disorder caused by a neoplastic or hamartomatous proliferation of cardiac cells with some Purkinje cell characteristics.

Synonyms
Purkinje cell hamartoma, arachnocytosis of the myocardium, infantile cardiomyopathy, infantile xanthomatous cardiomyopathy, oncocytic cardiomyopathy, focal lipid cardiomyopathy, isolated cardiac lipidosis, infantile cardiomyopathy with histiocytoid changes, myocardial or conduction system hamartoma, foamy myocardial transformation, and congenital cardiomyopathy.

Epidemiology
Histiocytoid cardiomyopathy occurs predominantly in the first two years of life; 20% of cases are diagnosed in the first month, 60% in the first year, and less than 3% after two years of life. The prevalence of this disease may be higher than the reported cases would suggest, since some cases are undoubtedly diagnosed as Sudden Infant Death Syndrome (SIDS).

The female preponderance is 3:1. In approximately 5% of cases there seems to be a familial tendency.

Clinical features
Histiocytoid cardiomyopathy is an arrhythmogenic disorder; 70% of published cases the patients present with a spectrum of arrhythmias and electrical disturbances including: paroxysmal atrial tachycardia, atrial fibrillation, ventricular fibrillation, ventricular tachycardia, premature atrial contractions, premature ventricular contractions, Wolff-Parkinson-White syndrome, and right or left bundle branch block.

Approximately 20% of patients present as sudden death and often such cases have been misclassified as Sudden Infant Death Syndrome (SIDS). Other infants experience flu-like symptoms preceding or accompanying the cardiac manifestations. The majority of patients (95%) display cardiomegaly, but may also have a number of associated anomalies, including cardiac malformation (16%): ventricular and atrial septal defects, hypoplastic left heart syndrome; and endocardial fibroelastosis. Extracardiac anomalies occur in 17% of patients including corneal opacities, microcephaly, cataract, aphakia, hydrocephalus, agenesis of the corpus callosum, cleft palate, laryngeal web, and linear skin defect. Combined cardiac and extracardiac anomalies occur in 4%, and 7% show extracardiac histiocytoid cells in exocrine and endocrine glands {1794}.

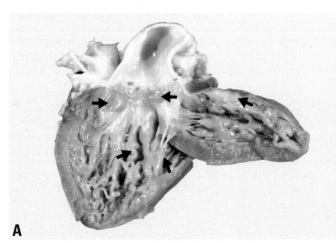 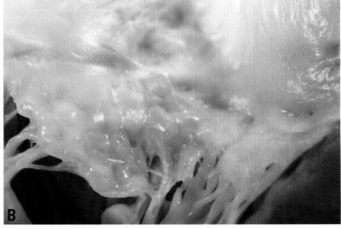

Fig .4.05 Histiocytoid cardiomyopathy. **A** Gross picture of the heart, showing multiple histiocytoid nodules in the aortic valve leaflets, endocardium, and papillary muscles (arrows). **B** Macroscopic photograph of a heart demonstrating the left ventricle and portion of the mitral valve. Note pale tan endocardial nodules at the level of the annulus.

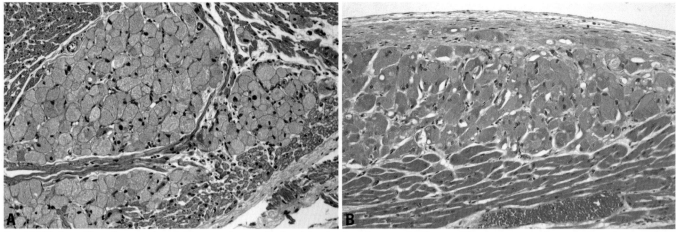

Fig. 4.06 Histiocytoid cardiomyopathy. **A** Discrete, circumscribed nodule of pale cells, superficially resembling foamy macrophages in the subendocardium. **B** Subendocardial histiocytoid nodule. Note the ill-defined border with adjacent myocardial fibers.

Etiology

Many theories of the etiopathogenesis have been proposed, including viral infection, myocardial ischemia, toxic exposure, and metabolic disorders such as glycogen storage disease, cardiac lipidosis, and various mitochondrial myopathies. However, the clinical, gross, microscopic, and ultrastructural findings show clear differences between the above-mentioned disorders and histiocytoid cardiomyopathy. The clinical presentation (arrhythmia), the distribution of histiocytoid cells, and their ultrastructural and immunohistochemical characteristics, all point to the cardiac conduction system as playing a key role. The primitive Purkinje cells of the developing heart show a striking resemblance to histiocytoid cells. Both types of cells show strong positivity for cholinesterase by frozen section histochemistry and for neutral lipids with the Sudan Black stain. Cholinesterase is present only in the conduction tissue of the heart; it is not present in contractile myocytes {1794}.

Macroscopy

Single or multiple subendocardial yellow-tan nodules or plaques ranging from 1-15 mm may be seen in both ventricles, the septum, and on all four cardiac valves. Although these nodules are mainly seen beneath the endocardium following the distribution of the bundle branches of the conduction system, they can also be seen in the inner myocardium and subepicardial areas. Lesions may be grossly inapparent as nodules, but multiple cross sections of the myocardium may show a mottled appearance with irregular ill-defined yellowish-tan areas.

Histopathology

Histiocytoid cardiomyopathy lesions appear as multifocal, ill-defined islands of large polygonal cells with granular eosinophilic cytoplasm, small round to oval shaped nuclei containing occasional nucleoli. The cytoplasmic appearance is due to extensive accumulation of mitochondria. The cells are distributed along the bundle branches of the conduction system. The sinoatrial and atrioventricular nodes are involved in 28% of cases; however, these areas are not sampled routinely {1794}.

Immunoprofile

Histiocytoid cardiomyopathy cells react with anribodies to desmin, myoglobin, myosin, and muscle specific actin. There is no expression of macrophage or histiocyte antigens (CD68, CD69, MAC 387, LN3, HAM-56). The cells also fail to react with antibodies to vimentin and cytokeratin (CAM-5.2), whereas S-100 protein reactivity is variable. Cell proliferation markers (Ki-67 and MIB-1) are usually negative {682,1713}.

Electron microscopy

Ultrastructurally, the cells of histiocytoid cardiomyopathy show poorly developed intercellular junctions. Their cytoplasm contains a superabundance of swollen mitochondria with disorganized cristae and dense membrane bounded granules, which push the diminished myofibrils to the periphery of the cell. The cytoplasm also contains lipid droplets of vari-

able size, scattered desmosomes, intercalated discs, and leptometric fibers.

Differential diagnosis

The disease has been confused with mitochondrial cardiomyopathy. However, there are major gross, light microscopic, and ultrastructural differences between the two diseases. Mitochondrial cardiomyopathy shows no discrete nodules as present in histiocytoid cardiomyopathy. Additionally, in mitochondrial cardiomyopathy, all myocytes are affected, but to a variable degree, whereas in histiocytoid cardiomyopathy, only focal areas of the heart are involved, but the affected cells are affected totally. The ultrastructural changes in histiocytoid cardiomyopathy cells consist of increased numbers of mitochondria with and without structural changes and reduced myofibrils. In mitochondrial cardiomyopathy, the mitochondria are consistently abnormal in a varitey of ways. They are enlarged, show variation in size and shape, contain occasional glycogen particles, and have cristae which are increased in number and on cross section, are arranged in a concentric circular fashion (like growth rings of a tree) surrounding occasional dense bodies.

Genetic susceptibility

Familial recurrence of histiocytoid cardiomyopathy in 5% of cases has led to several proposals of a genetic mechanism. The female preponderance of cases suggests an X-linked mutation causing prenatal lethality in the homozygous male {168,234,1898}. A female infant with "oncocytic cardiomyopathy" and microphthalmia with linear skin defects showed monosomy for Xp22 {1543}. Biochemical {1543} and molecular (mitochondrial DNA) {57} evidence suggest a defect of complex III (reduced coenzyme Q-cytochrome c reductase) of the respiratory chain in cardiac mitochondria. Such a mechanism could be responsible for the mitochondrial changes observed by light and electron microscopy, and the systemic involvement in some patients. It has been suggested that the disease is due to a mutation in Sox6 gene (p[100H]), which is associated with widespread myopathies {385}. From reported cases with known ethnic background, histiocytoid cardiomyopathy appears to be more common in Caucasian (80%) followed by African-American (15%), and Latin-American infants (3%); it is rare in Asian infants {1794}.

Prognosis and predictive factors
Histiocytoid cardiomyopahty causes incessant ventricular tachycardia in small children and can result in sudden death. Surgical excision or direct-vision cryoablation of the multiple small nodular tumours is required for long-term cure {665}. Surgical intervention, electrophysiologic mapping, and ablation of the arrhythmogenic foci result in a survival rate of approximately 80%. Some authors have found that aggressive anti-arrhythmic treatment may allow the tumours to regress without subjectiing patients to surgery. A few patients with extensive disease have undergone cardiac transplant {664,678,984,1286}.

Hamartoma of mature cardiac myocytes

Definition
The term "hamartoma" has been loosely applied to several cardiac tumours, most commonly histiocytoid cardiomyopathy ("Purkinje cell hamartoma"). The term has also been applied to lesions or malformations composed of a variety of cardiac elements, and other tumours composed primarily of a single cell type (e.g., rhabdomyoma). The term hamartoma of mature cardiac myocytes is used for a distinct tumour in adults, composed of cardiac myocytes. This lesion may be single or multiple.

Etiology

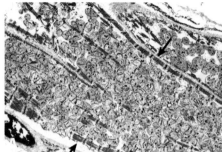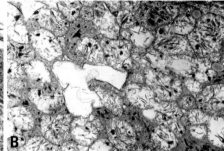

Fig. 4.07 Histiocytoid cardiomyopathy. **A** Electron microscopic illustration showing histiocytoid cells packed with mitochondria. The diminished myofibrils are displaced to the periphery of the cell (arrows). **B** Higher magnification showing abundant swollen mitochondria with disorganized cristae and dense membrane bounded granules.

The etiology of cardiac hamartoma is unknown. Some have suggested that these tumours may represent maturing congenital rhabdomyomas. However, there has been no association of hamartoma of mature cardiac myocytes with other syndromes including the tuberous sclerosis complex, making this unlikely.

Localization
Hamartomas of mature cardiac myocytes may occur in the ventricles or atria, and may be single or multiple {243}. Unusual examples of diffuse multiple tumourlets similar to so-called rhabdomyomatosis, have also been described.

Clinical features
As is the case with most cardiac tumours, the clinical features depend on the location. Tumours in the atria may result in supraventricular arrhythmias and Wolf Parkinson White syndrome, and those in the ventricles sudden death, or no symptoms at all.

Macroscopy
They are usually poorly demarcated firm white masses and range in size from 2 mm to 5 cm in greatest dimension. They resemble normal myocardium, but the bundles of muscle may appear disorganized and associated with bands of connective tissue.

Histopathology
They are composed of enlarged myocytes with obvious cross striations, and contain enlarged, irregular nuclei. They are poorly demarcated and may interdigitate with normal myocytes at the edges of the tumour. The interstitium demonstrates increased collagen.

Interspersed fat cells may be present in small numbers.

Immunoprofile
The tumours are similar to normal cardiac myocytes, and express actin and myosin. Abnormal accumulations of these intermediate filaments may be appreciated, particularly of actin. There is no evidence of proliferation by immunohistochemical stains for Ki-67 or PCNA.

Electron microscopy
The cells show features of myocytes, but abnormal accumulations of actin and myosin may be identified.

Differential diagnosis
The disorganized hypertrophied muscle fibers of a hamartoma are also reminiscent of the disarray characteristic of hypertrophic cardiomyopathy, but with rare exception (apical variant), hypertrophic cardiomyopathy is not associated with a focal mass lesion.

Prognosis and predictive factors
These tumours are benign neoplasms and can be excised, resulting in cure. However, arrhythmias and sudden death may be the initial presentation.

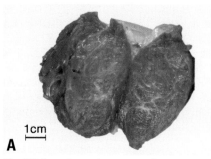

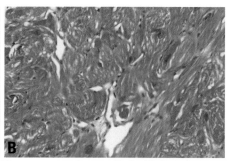

Fig. 4.08 Hamartoma of mature cardiac myocytes. **A** The tumour was circumscribed, with the appearance of muscle. **B** The tumour cells are hypertrophic, forming disorganized bundles with interstitial fibrosis.

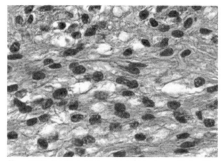

Fig. 4.09 Adult cellular rhabdomyoma. Note the monomorphic, bland spindled cells; their myogenic nature is not clearly evident on routine stains.

Adult cellular rhabdomyoma

Definition
Adult cellular rhabdomyoma is a benign neoplasm of striated myocytes. A similar tumour frequently occurs in the head and neck region (extracardiac rhabdomyoma).

ICD-O code   8904/0

Epidemiology
The adult form of extracardiac rhabdomyoma occurs primarily in the head and neck region of men and women over 40 years. Four cases of "extracardiac" rhabdomyomas have been described in the heart {241,2226}.

Clinical features and localization
Three of the four reported cases of adult cellular rhabdomyoma have occurred in the atria, and all have occurred in adults from 35-55 years of age. Common to any heart tumour, the mode of presentation is often electrical disturbance such as supraventricular tachycardia or nonsustained ventricular tachycardia. The masses may be identified incidentally.

Macroscopy
They range in size from 2–5 cm. The tumours are soft, bulging, tan to brown and have a pseudocapsule. These fea-

tures distinguish these tumours from other cardiac tumours with muscle differentiation.

Histopathology
These tumours are histologically distinct from cardiac rhabdomyomas, and are composed of tightly packed, round to polygonal cells with eosinophilic, finely granular cytoplasm, occasional vacuoles and occasional spider cells. Conversely, cardiac rhabdomyomas are composed of large cells with clear cytoplasm containing abundant glycogen and many spider cells.

Differential diagnosis
In contrast to congenital rhabdomyomas, adult cellular rhabdomyomas occur in adults, demonstrate evidence of cellular proliferation e.g. by expression of Ki-67 antigen, and contain relatively few vacuolated or spider cells. Unlike hamartoma of mature cardiac myocytes, the tumours are well circumscribed, and although not as frequent as in congenital rhabdomyoma, some vacuolated cells are usually present. Furthermore, the disorganized masses of myofilaments characteristic of hamartoma of mature cardiac myocytes are not seen. Rhabdomyosarcoma shares some features with adult cellular rhabdomyoma. Despite the evidence of cell proliferation in the latter

tumours, the absence of tumour necrosis, mitotic figures, myogenin expression, and the presence of a well-defined pseudocapsule help to distinguish it from rhabdomyosarcoma.

Histogenesis
The lesion is believed to be a true neoplasm of striated muscle origin.

Somatic genetics
Due to the rarity of these lesions, molecular and genetic characterization has not been undertaken. In extracardiac rhabdomyoma, a reciprocal translocation between chromosomes 15 and 17 and abnormalities of the long arm of chromosome 10 have been described {680}.

Prognosis and predictive factors
The prognosis of adult cellular rhabdomyoma is unknown, but presumed to be benign, based on the biologic behaviour of extracardiac rhabdomyomas in adults. Late recurrences have been described in extracardiac rhabdomyoma {680}.

Benign tumours of pluripotent mesenchyme

A.P. Burke
H. Tazelaar
J.J. Gomez-
Roman
R. Loire
P. Chopra
M. Tomsova
J.P. Veinot
T. Dijkhuizen

C.T. Basson
R. Rami-Porta
E. Maiers
A.E. Edwards
P. Walter
J.R. Galvin
S. Tsukamoto
D. Grandmougin
P.A. Araoz

Cardiac myxoma

Definition
Myxoma is a neoplasm composed of stellate to plump cytologically bland mesenchymal cells set in a myxoid stroma.

ICD-O code   8840/0

Epidemiology
Cardiac myxoma represents one of the most common benign cardiac tumours {2013,2165}. In most surgical series, they account for almost 80% of cases {249,1986}. In large registries and repositories with significant referral bias myxomas represent between 20 and 40% of primary cardiac tumours {249,1338}. Patient age ranges from 2-97 years. Mean age at presentation is 50 years {1133}. About 90% of individuals are between the ages of 30 and 60 years {2165}. A recent analysis of 1,195 individuals with myxomas revealed that 67% were female and 33% were male {2212}. Patients with the myxoma (Carney) complex are generally younger and more often male than patients with sporadic myxomas.

Clinical features
Clinical presentation is diverse and dependent upon tumour location and to a lesser extent morphology {175,643, 1598,1616}. About 20% of cardiac myxomas are asymptomatic; they are usually smaller than 40 mm {722,736}.

Cardiac symptoms
In over 50% of patients left atrial myxomas cause symptoms of mitral valve stenosis or obstruction (dyspnoea and orthopnoea from pulmonary oedema or heart failure). Right atrial myxomas may obstruct the tricuspid valve and cause symptoms of right-sided heart failure.
The majority of patients have an abnormal physical examination, most characteristically a diastolic or systolic murmur. A "tumour plop" may be occasionally heard in early diastole {722,1598,1616}. Abnormal, but nonspecific electrocardiographic changes may be identified in 20-40% of patients and include atrial fibrillation or flutter and left and right bundle branch block {643,1616}. Chest roentgenograms also show only nonspecific findings, including cardiomegaly, chamber enlargement, and pulmonary oedema {1616}.

Embolism
Embolic phenomena are the second most common manifestation (30-40% of patients). Frequent sites of embolization include the central nervous system, kidney, spleen and extremities. Coronary embolism may result in myocardial infarction {524,1542}. There is some evidence that fibrous lesions are more likely to produce valvular obstruction while polypoid and myxoid ones are more likely to embolize {722,736}.

Systemic symptoms
These are possibly related to IL-6 production by tumour cells. They are seen in approximately 20% of patients and include myalgia, muscle weakness, arthralgia, fever, fatigue and weight loss. Although infection of a myxoma is rare, when present the initial manifestations mimic those of infective endocarditis, and can include fever, chills, petechiae, subconjunctival haemorrhages, Osler nodes and positive blood culture.
Anaemia, leukocytosis and elevated erythrocyte sedimentation rate are the most common laboratory findings {175,1616}. Most myxomas are sporadic, although syndromic and familial cases (Carney or myxoma complex) are well recognised. In familial cases, the patients present at a younger age, they occur in unusual locations and have a higher recurrence rate than in non-familial cases {296,2114}.

Imaging
At echocardiography carciac myxomas typically appear as a mobile mass attached to the endocardial surface by a stalk, usually arising from the fossa ovalis. Myxomas with this appearance can be confidently diaganosed by echocardiography and further imaging is not necessary {1298}. In fact, because the tumours are usually small and mobile, myxomas are typically better defined by echocardiography than by either MRI or CT, because echocardiog-

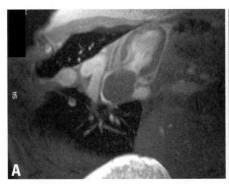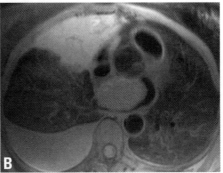

Fig. 4.10 Cardiac myxoma. **A** Long axis MRI view of the left ventricle demonstrating a well-circumscribed myxoma (T) centered in the left atrium. The inferior portion of the mass abuts the tricuspid valve. **B** The mass seen in the previous figure (T) originates from the atrial septum and is best demonstrated on the axial view. The right-sided effusion and consolidation (E) are unrelated to the myxoma (the patient had metastatic malignant melanoma, with an incidental cardiac myxoma).

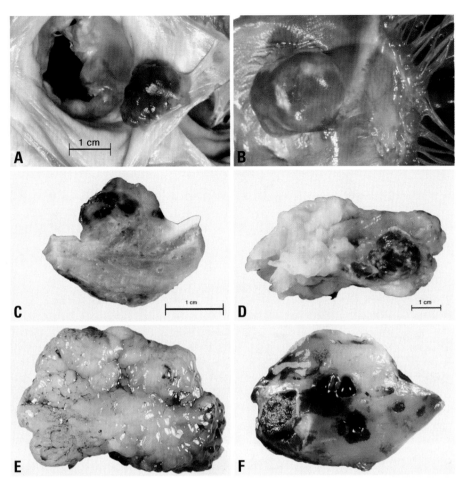

Myxomas are ovoid, globular, lobulated or polypoid. They may be smooth and glistening or have multiple papillary, villous, finger-like projections. They may be grey white and fibrous, gelatinous and myxoid, or a combination of both. The papillary structures may be quite friable increasing the risk of embolisation. Superficial thrombi also embolize. Marked variation in colour is characteristic. Pale grey, pearly white or yellow brown areas are frequently admixed with haemorrhagic dark brown or red areas. Tumour consistency depends on the quantity and distribution of fibrous tissue, and calcification. Rarely, the bulk of the tumour becomes calcified {120,1180}.

Histopathology

The myxoma cells may be arranged singly, in cords, or in vasoformative ring structures {245,361,1625}. The cells can be elongated, fusiform or stellate. They contain modest amounts of eosinophilic cytoplasm. Nuclei are oval, round, or elongated and mitoses are very rare. Myxoma cells have a tendency to form primitive or differentiated vessels, reflected in expression of endothelial markers. Less myxoid stroma often forms a halo around the vascular formations.

The stroma contains variable amounts of proteoglycans, collagen and elastin. It shows strong reactivity with alcian blue, resistant to predigestion by hyaluronidase. The vessels within the tumour are thin-walled and lack pericytes. Occasionally, cavernous vascular spaces containing blood or proteinaceous material are encountered. Thick walled blood vessels with prominent muscular walls are present predominantly at the base of tumour and in the stalk. Extravasated red cells, foci of recent and organizing haemorrhage and hemosiderin deposition are frequent. Hemosiderin is seen free within the stroma, within histiocytes and myxoma cells. Variable numbers of lymphocytes, plasma cells, macrophages, dendritic cells, and mast cells may be present.

Gamna-Gandy bodies as seen in chronic venous congestion of the spleen may be encountered infrequently. Calcification and metaplastic bone formation may also occur. The latter are more frequent in right atrial myxomas. The surface is usually composed of a single layer of flattened cells, but multilayering and tufting may occur.

Fig. 4.11 Cardiac myxoma. **A** This incidental finding at autopsy is a sessile smooth surfaced mass attached to the endocardium of the let atrium at the level of the oval fossa. Note the relationship to the mitral valve, which may often become partly obstructed in patients with left atrial myxoma, resulting in pulmonary hypertension. **B** Myxoma of the left atrium, with typical localization at the fossa ovalis. **C** Cut surface of a papillary myxoma of the left atrium. **D** Papillary myxoma with necrosis, left atrium. **E** Left atrial myxoma after resection. **F** Left atrial myxoma with an old and recent haemorrhages.

raphy has the best spatial and temporal resolution. If the narrow stalk is not visible, the diagnosis cannot be made by echocardiography and further imaging, usually MRI, is necessary to show the tumour's margins and to exclude tumour infiltration. At MRI and CT myxoma appears as an intracavitary heterogeneous, lobular mass. As with echocardiography, if the narrow stalk is visible, myxoma can be diagnosed by MRI or CT {66}.

Macroscopy

Cardiac myxomas are intracavitary masses that occur most often in the left atrium {361}. They arise from the endocardium of the atrial septum near the fossa ovalis in 85-90% of cases. Most of the remainder are located in the right atrium. Rarely, they arise in the ventricles.

Multiple tumours occurring at sites other than fossa ovalis and ventricles are generally found in the inherited form of cardiac myxoma. Very rarely, cardiac myxomas have also been documented to occur on valves and chordae tendineae.

The external appearance, consistency, size and weight are extremely variable. They may be as small as a few millimeters and as large as 14 cm in diameter. The weight ranges from 2-250 gm. Tiny cardiac myxomas may be totally asymptomatic and discovered incidentally at surgery for another purpose or autopsy. Larger ones are either sessile or pedunculated, but the site of attachment is always discrete and usually in the region of the fossa ovalis. Occasionally, the stalk may be long, resulting in free mobility of the tumour within the atrial cavity.

Heterologous components

Well-defined columnar epithelium, occasionally forming glands occurs in about 2% of myxomas. The epithelium may show moderate cytologic atypia, mitotic activity and express cytokeratin. Age and sex distribution of patients, signs and symptoms, frequency of syndromic association and sites of occurrence are similar for cardiac myxoma with or without glands. Recognition of the glands as a component of a myxoma is important since these structures may be confused with metastatic adenocarcinoma. The glandular cells are positive for PAS-diastase, alcian blue and mucicarmine; they stain for cytokeratin (diffuse cytoplasmic staining with antibodies to cytokeratin 7, AE1/AE3, 4betaE12 and Cam 5.2; and focal staining for cytokeratin 20), EMA (diffuse cytoplasmic), and CEA (apical cell border). Reactivity for CA19.9 has also been observed on the apical epithelial membrane of the glandular component of a myxoma from a patient with elevated serum CA19 {1190}. Foci of extramedullary haematopoiesis may be seen in 7% of myxomas {245}. Thymic rests have also been observed {245}.

Immunoprofile

The cells are cytokeratin negative, variably S-100 positive, and variably positive for smooth muscle and endothelial markers e.g. CD 34 and CD31 {362,1269, 1625,2013}. Calretinin is expressed in about 75% of cardiac myxomas {16}.

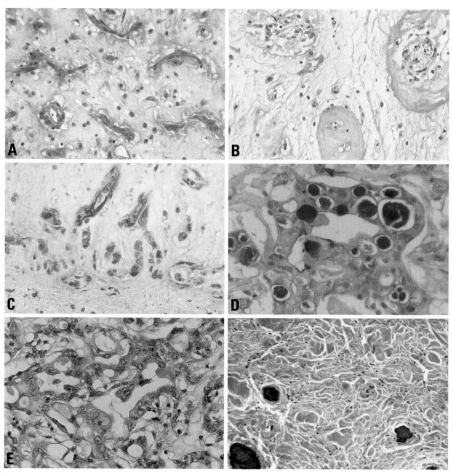

Fig. 4.12 Cardiac myxoma. **A** Numerous rudimentary vessels. **B** Three stages of rudimentary vessels. **C** A primitive endothelial marker, CD34 is often present within the central areas of the vascular structures formed by cardiac myxoma. **D** Cardiac myxoma glands with PAS-positive-diastase resistant material consistent with mucus. **E** Cardiac myxoma with complex glands whose cells show moderate cytologic atypia. **F** Cytokeratin 7 staining of a cardiac myxoma with heterologous components.

Histogenesis

Some years ago myxomas were considered nothing more than organised thrombi. Their neoplastic nature is supported by the presence of chromosomal abnormalities {489}, abnormal DNA content {1226} and the presence of microsatellite instability {1853}. The presence of heterologous elements, however, still suggest to some that they may be reactive or hamartomatous {1925}. The origin of myxoma cells is unclear. They are thought to arise from subendothelial vasoformative reserve cells or primitive cells which reside in the fossa ovalis and surrounding endocardium. The minute endocardial structures described by Prichard {1618} do not seem to correspond to the hypothetical subendothelial pluripotential vasoformative reserve cells from which the myxomas would arise, because they do not share the immuno-

histochemical properties of myxoma cells {15,16}. On the other hand, cardiomyocyte-specific transcription factor mRNAs have been recently found in RNA extracted from myxoma lysates, suggesting cardiomyogenic differentiation in myxoma cells and a possible origin in cardiomyocyte progenitor cells {1037}.

Genetic susceptibility

Although most myxomas are sporadic, some have been associated with the myxoma complex {295,483}. This autosomal dominat syndrome has been reported under the acronyms NAME (nevi, atrial myxoma, myxoid neurofibroma, ephelides), LAMB (lentigines, atrial myxoma, mucocutaneous myxomas, blue nevi), and more recently as Carney syndrome {295,299,530}. This syndrome includes cardiac myxomas and extracar-

diac manifestations: abnormal skin pigmentation (lentigines and blue nevi), calcifying Sertoli-Leydig testicular tumours, cutaneous myxomas, myxoid breast fibroadenomas, pigmented adrenal cortical hyperplasia, pituitary hyperactivity, psammomatous melanotic schwannoma and thyroid tumours {295}. Familial myxomas are estimated to account for 7% of atrial myxomas {299}, are more often multiple, recurrent and right sided, as compared to sporadic myxomas. The affected patients are also younger, most presenting at 20-30 years of age {530,1133,1544}.

Somatic genetics

The chromosomal patterns of sporadic cardiac myxoma are characterised by extensive intratumour heterogeneity. In the seventeen cases published to date, multiple unspecific chromosome aberrations have been reported, including dicentric chromosomes and, in particular, telomeric associations {489,497,498, 502}. Intratumour heterogeneity, as found in a variety of tumour types and grades {688}, is considered a sign of genetic instability presumably resulting from disruption of genes that control genomic integrity. Studies of cardiac myxomas suggest that the chromosomal regions 12p1 and 17p1 may play a specific role in the development of these neoplasms since they are frequently rearranged {497}.

Cytogenetic analyses of three cases of cardiac myxoma derived from patients with the myxoma syndrome reveal chromosome patterns similar to those observed in sporadic cases {489,1658, 1882}. Whether there is a common genetic mechanism underlying sporadic and familial cardiac myxomas is unclear. Based on linkage analysis, 2 loci have been proposed for genes causally related to the myxoma syndrome: 2p16 {1882} and 17q2 {299}. Recently, a gene located at 17q24 was cloned that showed mutations in myxoma patients {122,598,1018}. This gene, *PRKAR1A*, represents a putative tumour suppressor gene, coding for the type 1 alpha regulatory subunit of protein kinase A (CNC1, OMIM #160980). No causal gene has been identified at the 2p16 locus, and some families that were initially thought to have disease related to this locus actually have chromosome 17q24 *PRKAR1A* mutations {122}. At least one further locus remains to be identified. As yet, neither mutations of *PRKAR1A* nor loss of heterozygosity of markers at 17q2 and 2p16 have been found in sporadic cardiac myxomas {598}.

Flow cytometry shows abnormally high tetraploid DNA patterns in all cases of syndromic myxomas, whereas in sporadic myxomas it is present only in about 20%.

Prognosis and predictive factors

There is a remarkably different prognosis between patients with sporadic and familial myxomas. Patients with sporadic tumours have a good prognosis, with 1-3% recurrence rate {1275,296,2227}. However, about 10% of patients with familial myxomas either have recurrent tumours or develop another tumour in a different location {1276,1598}. The recur-

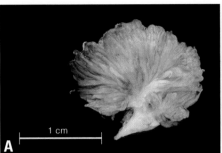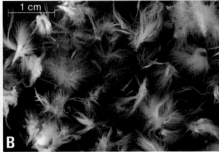

Fig. 4.13 Papillary fibroelastoma. **A** Papillary fibroelastoma from aortic valve. Note multiple translucent papillary fronds. **B** Multiple papillary fibroelastomas (greater than 40) developing 17 years following open heart surgery. From A.N. Kurup et al. {1105}.

rence interval in one series was 47.8 months {296}. The probability of recurrence has been related to DNA chromosomal pattern {296,1276}. Patients with a familial tumour need to followed long term.

Embolization is the major complication of myxoma and may result in ischemic symptoms in a variety of arterial beds. Intracranial aneurysm due to embolization is also a rare, but potentially morbid, complication. The etiology of these aneurysms is unclear but histologic verification of myxoma cells in arterial walls has been reported {1758}.

Treatment

Immediate surgical resection is advised when the diagnosis of cardiac myxoma is suspected {1454}, because of the risk of embolism {2001}. The tumour is removed under cardiac arrest with cardiopulmonary bypass. Minimal manipulation and gentle management of the heart is recommended so as not to precipitate embolism. After the tumour is resected, the cardiac chamber should be irrigated with saline solution to wash out residual tumour fragments.

The approach to a left atrial myxoma is usually through a vertical incision. When the tumour is not large, a transseptal approach useful, whereas a transseptal biatriotomy {516} is recommended for a large tumour. As the majority of left atrial myxomas arise from the interatrial septum, the tumours can be removed en bloc with a 5 mm margin of normal tissue. The fossa ovalis, where the pretumour cells of myxomas are thought likely to exist {2102}, should also be excised if possible. For a right atrial myxoma, direct caval cannulation avoids tumour fragmentation. When direct cannulation to the inferior vena cava is

impractical, a cannula should be inserted from the femoral vein for the inferior vena cava. Tumour resection with the full thickness of the septum and patch repair is required for tumours with a broad based attachment. However, when the tumour originates from the atrial wall, resection of the attachment, and 5 mm of normal tissue including endocardium and underlying myocardium are recommended.

Papillary fibroelastoma

Definition

An endocardial based papilloma lined by endothelial cells with proteoglycan rich avascualar stroma, usually rich in elastin.

Synonyms

Giant Lambl excrescence, fibroelastic papilloma

Epidemiology

Papillary fibroelastoma is a rare and benign tumour representing less than 10% of primary cardiac tumours {121,247}. The true incidence is difficult to determine, as the tumour may be overlooked and there is morphologic overlap with Lambl excresences, a reactive age-related valvular lesion {249,2080} In recent series of surgically excised cardiac tumours papillary fibroelastoma represents the second most frequent benign lesion.

Papillary fibroelastoma is the most common primary tumour of cardiac valves. In two recent series of primary valve tumours, papillary fibroelastoma constituted 73% and 89% of cases {531,1714}. Mean age of the patients is 60 years (range, newborn to 83 years) and there is an equal gender predilection {1714, 1903}.

Etiology

The histogenesis continues to be a source of controversy. Various gross, microscopic, and molecular characteristics of papillary fibroelastoma have led to the lesions' being described as neoplasms, hamartomas, organized thrombi, and unusual endocardial responses to trauma. The histochemical presence of fibrin, hyaluronic acid, and laminated elastic fibers within the fronds supports the hypothesis that papillary fibroelastomas may be related to organizing thrombi. Evidence favouring the hamartoma hypothesis includes a histologic appearance that suggests the proliferation of miniature tendinous cords and apparent congenital papillary fibroelastomas associated with other congenital cardiac anomalies. Due to the presence of dendritic cells and cytomegalovirus in the intermediate layers of some papillary fibroelastomas, a recent study proposed that papillary fibroelastomas may be related to a chronic form of viral endocarditis {734}.

Repetitive hemodynamic trauma may contribute to their development as they have been reported in association with diseases resulting in abnormal flow of blood in the heart including rheumatic heart disease, hypertrophic cardiomyopathy, mitral valve prolapse and atrial septal defect, among other diseases. However, the mechanisms by which such hemodynamic abnormalities contribute to papillary fibroelastoma growth are unclear. There is increasing evidence that at least a subset (18%) of these tumours develop as a result of iatrogenic factors, including thoracic irradiation and open-heart surgery (subaortic septal myectomy, valve repair, valve replacement and repair of congenital defects {1105}. In contrast to sporadic cases, which are most common on cardiac valves, iatrogenic papillary fibroelastomas tend to occur in a variety of non-valvular endocardial surfaces, usually in close proximity to the predisposing iatrogenic factor, e.g. in the chamber most closely associated with the site of surgery.

Localization

Ninety percent of papillary fibroelastomas occur on heart valves, including aortic, posterior and anterior mitral leaflets {531,597,842,1397,1819,2015}, mitral chordae and papillary muscles {313,659}. Unusual locations include the

Table 4.02

Immunohistochemical profile of cardiac papillary fibroelastomas. From D. Grandmougin et al. {734}

Marker	Central fibrous core	Intermediate layer	Endothelial border
Vimentin	(+)	(+)	(+)
S 100 Protein	(-)	(+)	(-)
CD 31	(-)	(-)	(+)
CD 34	(-)	(-)	(+)
Factor VIII	(-)	(-)	(+)*
CMV-LMP-1		(+)	
EBV-LMP-1		(-)	

*Staining intensity decreased in comparison to the adjacent normal endocardial endothelium with an immunoreactivity ratio of 0.4

tricuspid and pulmonary valves, right and left atrial and ventricular endocardial walls, Chiari's network, and coronary ostia {43,202,254,913,977,1179,1770, 2249}. Autopsy series show an equal right and left heart distribution {205, 531,1274}. However, surgical series have a high prevalence (81%) of left sided papillary fibroelastomas because left-sided lesions are much more frequently symptomatic.

Tumours are found most commonly (69.5%) on diseased valves - 37.8% post-rheumatic valves and 62.2% valves with fibrosis and calcification {1903}.

Papillary fibroelastomas have been likened to Lambl excrescence, but unlike Lambl excrescences, which occur at the line of closure of semilunar valves, papillary fibroelastomas occur anywhere on the valve surface.

Clinical features

The clinical diagnosis of papillary fibroelastoma can be difficult because embolic complications can mimic a variety of underlying diseases {1714}. Integrity of the superficial endothelial layer of the fronds has been demonstrated to be the main element leading to occurrence of embolic events {734}. Embolism is related to the aggregation of platelets and fibrin {567,734,742}. Lesions adjacent to coronary ostia may prolapse resulting in angina, syncope or sudden death {205,262}. The majority of

surgically excised cases occur in patients with symptoms related to cerebral ischemia. The diagnosis is made by multiplanar transthoracic and transesophageal echocardiography {713, 1151,1770,2015}. High-resolution echocardiography shows an echolucent centre.

Macroscopy

Papillary fibroelastomas range in size from 2-50 mm in greatest dimension, although the majority are less than 10 mm. They are generally opalescent white, but this colour may be obscured by thrombus. They are usually attached to the endocardial surface by a short single stalk, but those with more than one attachment to the endocardium have been observed. Papillary fibroelastomas have multiple papillary fronds and, particularly when immersed in water, they resemble a pom-pom or sea anemone. Papillary fibroelastomas most often occur singly (80-90%), but among patients with iatrogenic tumours, multiple tumours (2 to greater than 40) occur with great frequency (67%). Such tumours are less likely to occur on the valves and have been reported in a wide variety of locations (on papillary muscles, tendinous cords, and atrial and ventricular septal and free walls).

Histopathology

Papillary fibroelastomas have a superficial endothelial layer, an intermediate

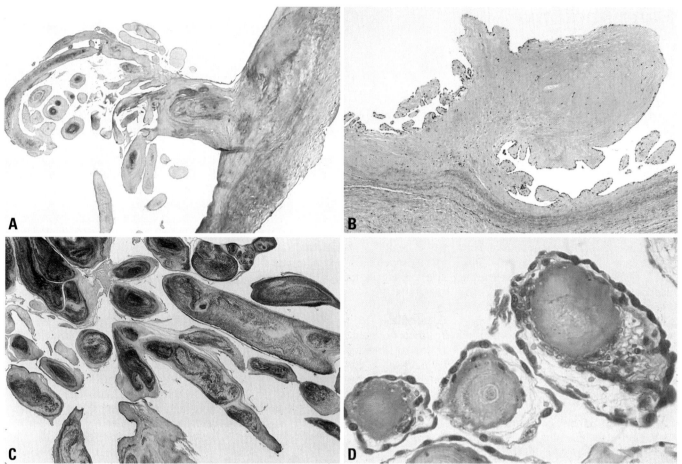

Fig. 4.14 Papillary fibroelastoma. **A** Location at the aortic valve. **B** Movat pentachrome stain demonstrating an incidental papillary fibroelastoma on the surface of the valve. In this example, there is little elastic tissue within the papillae. **C** Papillary fibroelastoma showing multiple fronds with prominent elastic tissue cores (elastic van Gieson). **D** Fibroelastic papilloma with young vegetations.

layer rich in proteoglycans and a central avascular core. The inner layers contain fibroblasts and occasional inflammatory cells including macrophages and dendritic cells {742,1703}. Elastic fibres are most prominent in the core but may be sparse or absent in the distal parts of the papillae. Acute and organizing thrombi may be seen on the surface and obscure the papillary surfaces.

Immunohistochemistry
Immunohistologic studies demonstrate a disparity between surface and deeper layers. Surface endothelial cells express vimentin and CD34 with some loss of intensity for CD31 and factor VIII related antigen in comparison to normal endocardial endothelium. It has been proposed that the decreased expression of endothelial markers indicates endothelial

trauma or dysfunction {734,1200,1703}. Spindle cells in deeper layers may focally express S100 protein. The S100 cells likely represent competent antigen presenting dendritic cells. The presence of T cells has not been investigated in these regions.

Haemangioma

H. Tazelaar
A.P. Burke
G. Watanabe
C.T. Basson

Definition

Haemangiomas (angiomas) are benign tumours composed predominantly of blood vessels. The histologic classification includes those composed of multiple dilated thin-walled vessels (cavernous type), smaller vessels resembling capillaries (capillary type), and dysplastic malformed arteries and veins (arterio-venous haemangioma, cirsoid aneurysm). Cardiac haemangiomas often have combined features of cavernous, capillary and arteriovenous haemangiomas, and many contain fibrous tissue and fat. These features are reminiscent of intramuscular haemangiomas of skeletal muscle.

ICD-O code   9120/0

Clinical features

Most cardiac haemangiomas are discovered incidentally but patients may present with dyspnoea on exertion, arrhythmias, right-sided heart failure, pericarditis, pericardial effusion, and failure to thrive. Patients may have associated vascular syndomes e.g. Kasabach-Merritt {675}.

Imaging

At echocardiography, haemangiomas are usually hyperechoic, circumscribed, and intracavitary solitary masss. At MRI, hemaniogmas may be intermediate to high on T1 weighted images, often are very intense on T2 weighted images, and also enhnance brightly with contrast administration. {1003}. At CT the tumors are usually circumscribed, low attenuation, heterogeneous and also enhance brightly with contrast administration. {737}. The circumscribed, non-infiltrative appearance of haemangioma, particularly on MRI which is most sensitive to tissue infiltration, can be used to suggest that the neoplasm is benign, but a specific diagnosis cannot be made with imaging.

Localization

The most frequent locations are the lateral wall of the left ventricle (21%), the anterior wall of the right ventricle (21%), the interventricular septum (17%) and occasionally, the right ventricular outflow tract {226}.

Macroscopy

The tumours are often large and gross appearance depends on the size of the vascular spaces in the tumour. The capillary type is frequently slightly raised from the endocardial sruface and appears red to purple. Intramuscular types will appear infiltrative. Cavernous haemangiomas are usually large and are also poorly circumscribed.

Histopathology

Capillary haemangiomas are composed of nodules of small capillary-size vessels, each of which is subserved by a "feeder" vessel. This lobular or grouped arrangement of vessels is helpful for distinguishing these benign from malignant vascular proliferations. Mast cells and factor XIII-positive interstitial cells are a consistent feature.

Intramuscular cardiac haemangioma has superficial resemblance to arteriovenous malformation, with the presence of heterogeneous vessel types, including muscularized arteries, veins, and capillaries. In contrast to capillary haemangioma, they are infiltrative lesions and occur within the myocardium. They are histologically identical to intramuscular haemangiomas within skeletal muscle, and may possess, in addition to the vessels, fat and fibrous tissue. Because of the latter features, some intramuscular cardiac haemangiomas are misclassified as lipomas or fibrolipomas.

Cavernous haemangiomas are composed of large dilated vascular spaces. They tend to infiltrate the myocardium. The lining cells are bland and flattened and mitotically inactive.

Genetic susceptibility

Genetic susceptibility to cardiac haemangiomas has not been identified. Extracardiac haemangiomas occur in a variety of contexts. They may be single sporadic lesions or multiple lesions that are components of complex genetic syndromes. Capillary haemangiomas occur in up to 10% of live births and are the most frequent tumour in newborns {1409}. When these tumours occur in the absence of associated syndromes, they may represent manifestations of an autosomal dominant mendelian trait (OMIM #602089) {7}. Linkage analyses {224, 2101} of multiplex kindreds affected by hereditary capillary haemangiomas have identified loci on chromosome 5 (q31-q33 and q13-q22) that appear to contain as yet unidentified causal disease genes.

A wide array of complex syndromes, such as von Hippel Lindau syndrome (OMIM #193300) and SC phocomelia/ Roberts syndrome (OMIM #269000), that

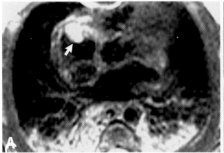
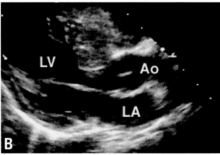

Fig. 4.15 Cardiac haemangioma. **A** MRI of right atrial haemangioma in a newborn who underwent partial surgical resection of the tumor. ECG-triggered breath-hold T2-weighted fast spin echo sequence shows a markedly hyperintense signal from the tumor (arrow). **B** Echocardiographic imaging of cardiac haemangioma involving the interventricular septum in a 7-year-old boy.

can be transmitted in a mendelian fashion include haemangiomas as components of their clinical presentations. The Klippel-Trenaunay-Weber syndrome, in which cutaneous haemangiomas occur in the setting of osseous hypertrophy, shows familial clustering, but a clear mode of inheritance has not been established. Autosomal paradominant and dominant modes of inheritance have been proposed {306,775}. Translocations {2105 2130} have been identified in 2 Klippel-Trenaunay-Weber patients, t(5;11) (q13.3;p15.1) and t(8;14)(q22.3; q13), but specific gene defects remain to be identified.

Somatic genetics

Specific genes have been associated with two disorders involving arteriovenous malformations. Mutations in the gene on chromosome 9p21 encoding the endothelial cell-specific receptor tyrosine kinase TIE2 cause the autosomal dominant Bean or "Blue rubber-bleb nevus" syndrome (OMIM #112200) and familial multiple cutaneous and mucosal venous malformations (OMIM#600195) {2084}. At least some cases of hereditary cerebral cavernous malformations (OMIM #116860) are caused by mutations in the chromosome 7q21-q22 Krev interaction trapped-1, *KRIT-1*, gene {1110}. KRIT1 normal binds to RAP1A, a Ras GTPase, and the disease causing mutations appear to disrupt these interactions. Other genetic loci for this disorder have been identified at chromosomes 17p15-p13 and 3q25.2-q27 and remain to be studied. The genetic and clinical relationship of this disorder to hereditary neuro-cutaneous angioma (OMIM #106070) is unclear.

Syndromic associations

The majority of cardiac haemangiomas are sporadic, without evidence of extracardiac vascular lesions. Rarely, there may be extracardiac haemangiomas of the gastrointestinal tract and port-wine stain of the face. Giant cardiac haemangiomas can result in thrombosis and coagulopathies (Kasabach-Merritt syndrome) {239,675}.

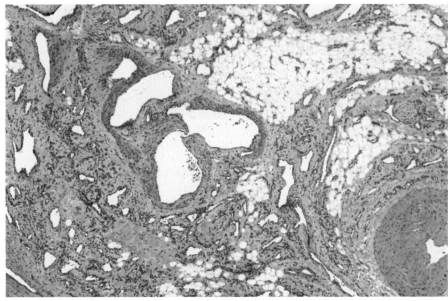

Fig. 4.16 Haemangioma. This lesion has some features of arteriovenous malformation, with a non-uniform collection of thick walled arteries, dilated veins and capillaries. In addition, there is fat and fibrous tissue, as ooccasionally seen in an intramuscular haemangioma.

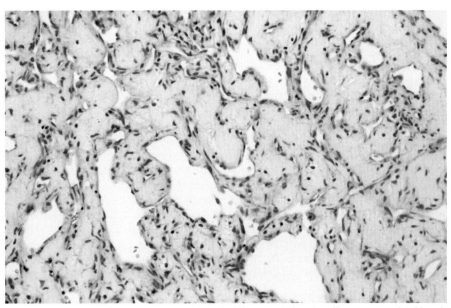

Fig. 4.17 Haemangioma. This tumor shows a relatively uniform population of capillary type vessels with variable degrees of dilatation. The myxoid background may suggest myxoma, but other features of myxoma are absent, and the vessels are mature.

Benign tumours with myofibroblastic differentiation

E. Dulmet
A.P. Burke
T. Geva
H. Kamiya
H. Tazelaar

V. T. de Montpréville
C.T. Basson
G. Watanabe
P.A. Araoz

Cardiac fibroma

Definition
Fibroma is a rare primary heart tumour composed of fibroblasts or myofibroblasts with a matrix containing collagen. It almost exclusively occurs within the myocardium of the ventricles or ventricular septum. It is not clear whether it is a hamartoma or a true neoplasm. Because most cases occur in infants and children it is likely congenital.

ICD-O code   8810/0

Synonyms
Fibroelastic hamartoma, fibrous hamartoma.

Epidemiology
Most cardiac fibromas are discovered in children and often before one year of age {737,1944}. Prenatal diagnosis with sonography is possible {121,134,538}. However, cases are also reported in adults {307} and even as an incidental finding in the elderly {2093}. There is no sex predominance. The incidence is very low with only about 200 cases reported to date.

Localization
The most common site of cardiac fibroma is the ventricular septum, but the free walls of the left and right ventricle are other common locations. Atrial fibromas are quite rare.

Clinical features
One-third of cardiac fibromas cause symptoms because of their mass effect, either through obstruction of blood flow or interference with valvular function and patients present with cardiac failure or cyanosis. In another third of the cases, cardiac fibromas, whatever their location, cause significant arrhythmias, syncope or sudden death. The remaining patients are asymptomatic and tumours are discovered because of heart murmur or a radiographic abnormality. Embolic phenomena are not a feature of cardiac fibromas {121,134,538,737,1944}.

Imaging At echocardiography fibromas typically appear as a large, well-circumscribed, solitary mass in the septum or ventricular free wall {1010,1242} and in some cases may be confused with hypertrophic cardiomyopathy {66}. The tumors are frequently very large and may cause obstruction, which can be assessed by colour Doppler. MRI likewise shows a large, solitary, homogeneous myocardial mass centered in the ventricles {1003, 1215,1660}. Because of the fibrous nature of the tumour, the signal intensity is often less than that of adjacent uninvolved myocardium, and contrast-enhanced imaging usually

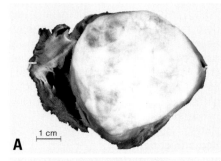

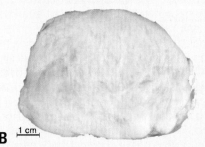

Fig. 4.19 Cardiac fibroma. **A** The tumour fills the left ventricular cavity, which is obliterated. The right ventricle and tricuspid valve are on the left. **B** Cardiac fibroma with prominent whorled surface.

demonstrates a hypoperfused tumour core. CT also shows a large, solitary, ventricular mass, which is usually low attenuation on CT. Unlike other imaging modalities CT may detect calcification which is a helpful feature in making a confident diagnosis. {66}. Overall, the imaging finding of a solitary, very large,

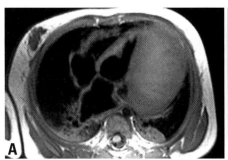

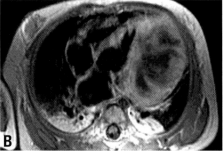

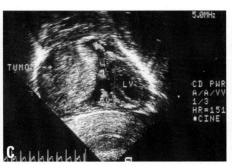

Fig. 4.18 Cardiac fibroma. **A** Left ventricular fibroma in a 6-month-old infant. A. ECG-triggered breath-hold proton-density fast spin echo MRI with double inversion recovery sequence in the axial plane showing a large inhomogeneous mass involving the left ventricular free wall. **B** MRI of left ventricular fibroma in a 6-months-old infant. Post-gadolinium imaging shows enhancement of the uninvolved myocardium and the tumour's periphery. Note the hypoperfused tumor core. **C** Echocardiogram of an infant with a large right ventricular fibroma causing right ventricular outflow tract obstruction.

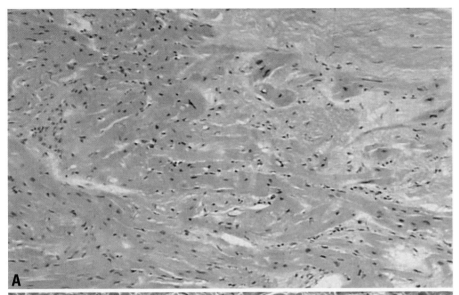

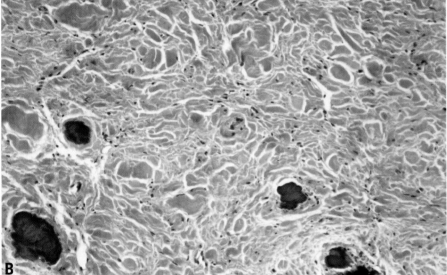

Fig. 4.20 Cardiac fibroma. **A** Fibroma infiltration into adjacent myocardium. **B** Calcifications in a fibrous lesion from a 19-year-old patient.

hypovascular mass in a child is suggestive of a cardiac fibroma.

Macroscopy
They are typically rounded masses that are fibrous, white and whorled, reminiscent of uterine leimyomas. The margin may be either circumscribed or infiltrative. In some cases, fibromas are massive and can obliterate ventricular cavities. They are nearly always mural, although polypoid endocardial based lesions have been reported. Most occur singly. The mean diameter is 5 cm.

Histopathology
Fibromas are composed of bland-looking spindle cells forming loose intersecting bundles. They are not encapsulated and extend into the surrounding myocardium. Even in grossly circumscribed cases, entrapped myocytes can often be seen deep within the tumours, far from the gross margins {244,451}. The fibroma cells have oval or tapered nuclei without nucleoli. Their cytoplasm is pale. These cells are associated with abundant collagenous stroma, which increases with the age of the patient. Cellular lesions are observed in infants during their first months of life, while fibromas in older patients contain large amounts of collagen. Mitoses and foci of extramedullary haematopoiesis may be present in cellular tumours {451}. Calcification is observed in lesions from patients of all

ages, but is somewhat more common in older individuals. Wavy elastic fibers are frequent and may be prominent. Focal myxoid change in the stroma and chronic inflammation may also be present {244}.

Immunoprofile
Tumour cells express vimentin and smooth muscle actin, both in cellular and fibrous lesions. They do not express desmin, CD34 or S-100 protein. Reacitivity for markers of proliferation, are much more frequent in cellular tumours than in the fibrous ones {451}.

Somatic genetics
A clonal translocation has been described in cell cultures of a subepicardial fibroma resected from an infant. Cytogenetic analysis in this tumor showed a clonal reciprocal translocation, 46,XY,t(1;9)(q32;q22),inv(9)(p11q12)c {572}.

Genetic susceptibility
Approximately 3% of patients with Gorlin syndrome have cardiac fibromas {418, 547,716}. Gorlin syndrome (or nevoid basal cell carcinoma syndrome) is an autosomal dominant disorder characterized by generalized body overgrowth, jaw keratocysts, developmental abnormalities of the skeleton, and a predisposition to neoplasms, specifically cardiac fibroma. Gorlin syndrome results from germline mutations in the PTC gene, which maps to chromosome 9q22.3 and is homologous to the Drosophila patched (*ptc*) gene {756}. The *ptc* gene encodes a transmembrane protein in Drosophila that represses the Hedgehog signaling pathway to control cell fate, growth, and development {756,893}. These data suggest that the *PTC* gene not only functions as a tumour suppressor gene, but also plays a critical role in development. However, the precise role of the *PTC* gene in myocardial cell growth and differentiation and its role in the development of cardiac fibroma remains to be defined {2077}.
Associated hydrocephalus, cleft lip and palate, and Sotos syndrome (megalencephaly with gigantism) have been reported {446,1242}.

Prognosis and predictive factors
The cardiac fibroma is benign, but its nature of slow but continuous growth

may cause conduction defects and arrhythmias. Extension into the ventricular free walls may result in atrioventricular valve inflow or arterial outflow obstruction. Spontaneous regression as can occur with congenital rhabdomyoma has not been observed.

Treatment
Operative intervention is usually required {451,615,2071}. When the tumour proves unresectable, heart transplantation is an option {731,2071}. However, favourable late results even after incomplete excision have been reported {132,307,1880}.

Inflammatory myofibroblastic tumour

Definition
Inflammatory myofibroblastic tumour is composed of myofibroblasts accompanied by a variable number of inflammatory cells including lymphocytes, macrophages, plasma cells and eosinophils.

ICD-O code   8825/1

Synonyms
Plasma cell granuloma, inflammatory pseudotumour and possibly inflammatory fibrosarcoma

Epidemiology
These tumours are very rare in the heart, and only small series and case reports appear in the literature.

Localization
Although there is a predilection for the ventricles, especially the right ventricular outflow tract, any site in the heart may be involved {1177}.

Clinical features
Signs and symptoms
There are no specific signs or symptoms related to cardiac inflammatory myofibroblastic tumour, as these are related to location within the heart. One cardiac

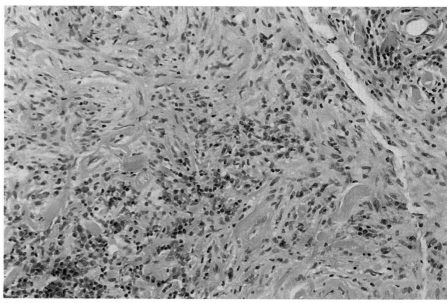

Fig. 4.21 Inflammatory myofibroblastic tumour of the left ventricle. Plump spindle cells are arranged in a haphazard fashion and focally surround myocytes. A modest chronic inflammatory cell infiltrate including plasma cells is also present.

inflammatory myofibroblastic tumour has been reported in a patient with systemic vasculitis and another tumour regressed spontaneously.

Macroscopy
Inflammatory myofibroblastic tumours of the heart are large lesions, measuring up to 8 cm {451}. Grossly, they tend to have relatively narrow attachments to the endocardium and project into the ventricular lumen.

Histopathology
Inflammatory myofibroblastic tumor is composed of spindled myofibroblasts, fibroblasts, chronic inflammatory cells and sometimes eosinophils. Various combinations of these cell types make these tumours quite variable from one case to another Occasional mitoses and foci of necrosis may be present.

Immunoprofile
The tumour cells strongly express actin and vimentin, but not desmin, CD34, S-

100 protein and p53. It is unknown if ALK-1 expression is diagnostically useful in cardiac inflammatory myofibroblastic tumours as is the case with extracardiac tumours.

Differential diagnosis
In contrast to fibromas, inflammatory myofibroblastic tumours are endocardial lesions, and there is often organizing fibrin thrombus on the surface. In addition the tumours are more histologically variable, the spindle cells are larger than in fibromas and the cells often have nucleoli.

Prognosis and predictive factors
The biologic behavior of inflammatory myofibroblastic tumour is that of a low-grade lesion with the propensity for recurrence, but overt malignancy is rare. No case of metastases arising from cardiac inflammatory myofibroblastic tumour has been reported.

Cardiac lipoma

A.P. Burke
P.A. Araoz

Definition
Benign tumour composed of mature, white adipocytes.

ICD-O code   8850/0

Epidemiology
Cardiac lipoma is rare and found in fewer than 1 in 10,000 autopsies {1116}. Lipomas generally account for only 0.5-3% of excised heart tumours {121,573, 952,1257,1672}. Higher estimates of up to 10% of heart tumours are likely because lipomatous hypertrophy, a separate entity, has been included {1257,1628}. Lipomas occur in children, but account for less than 2% of heart tumours similar to the relative incidence in adults {134}.

Localization
Cardiac lipomas may occur anywhere in the heart. There is a predilection for the pericardium and epicardial surfaces {540,1125,1628,2060}, where they may attain enormous sizes. Other sites include the ventricular septum {1869}, and cardiac valves. When they involve

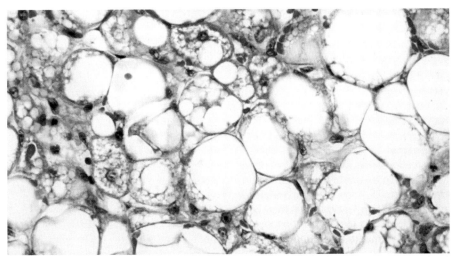

Fig. 4.23 Lipomatous hypertrophy. Lipomatous hypertrophy of atrial septum. Note the multivacuolated adipocytes which can mimic liposarcoma.

the latter site, the designation "fibrolipoma" has been used {149,280,1562}.

Clinical features
As is the case with other heart tumours, the presentation is varied, and depends on location. Many cardiac lipomas are incidental findings, or cause a variety of arrhythmias, syncope and electrocardiographic abnormalities {342,638,1383, 1562,1735}. Rarely, outflow tract obstruction may occur {1869}. Computed tomography and magnetic resonance imaging may establish the fatty nature of the tumour {1383}. Recurrences are rare {2146}.

Imaging
The echocardiographic appearance of cardiac lipomas varies with their location. Lipomas in the pericardial space have variable echogenecity but are often hypoechogenic, while intracavitary lipomas are typically echogenic {66}. The reason for this difference is unknown. At echocardiography, intracavitary lipomas are usually circumscribed but cannot be differentiated from other circumscribed cardiac masses. However, MRI and CT both allow for very specific identification of fat and therefore can be used to definitively diagnose lipomas {66}.

Histopathology
Similar to extracardiac lipomas, cardiac lipomas are circumscribed masses of mature adipocytes. Unusual histologic variants of lipoma have not been described in the heart, with the exception of pediatric cardiac lipoblastoma in a child, which possessed immature and mature adipocytes, with focal vascular myxoid areas containing lipoblasts {500}.

Differential diagnosis
The main differential is lipomatous hypertrophy, a non-encapsulated lesion composed of mature fat and adipocytes resembling brown fat cells intermixed with enlarged cardiac myocytes occurring solely in the interatrial septum. Lipomatous hypertrophy is most often an incidental finding at autopsy, but may uncommonly be the cause of unexplained atrial arrhythmias, congestive heart failure, or superior vena cava obstruction {242,365}.
The differential diagnosis also includes the intramuscular variant of haemangioma, which may contain variable numbers of adipocytes.

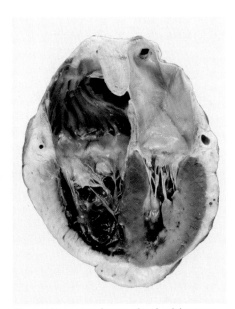

Fig. 4.22 Lipomatous hypertophy of atrial septum.

Cystic tumour of atrioventricular node

A.P. Burke
P.A. Araoz

Definition
Congenital multicystic tumour or rest located at the base of the atrial septum in the region of the atrioventricular node. Lining cells may be derived from primitive endoderm.

ICD-O code   8454/0

Synonyms
Mesothelioma of atrioventricular node, lymphangioma, endothelioma, inclusion cyst, Tawarian node, benign mesothelioma of Mahaim, endodermal rest, congenital polycystic tumour of atrioventricular node, intracardiac endodermal heterotopia.

Epidemiology
The mean age at presentation is 38 years (range birth- 78 years) and women are more frequently affected than men (approximately 3:1). One patient with long standing heart block survived to age 95, at which time the diagnosis was made at autopsy {64}.

Etiology
Because most patients have a history of congenital heart block, they likely are congenital rests. In 10% of patients the tumours occur in association with other midline defects {240,1189,1617,1719, 2021}. The precise intrauterine migration defect is unknown. The cell of origin is foregut endoderm, not mesothelium as previously believed. Because diagnosis in advanced years occurs, the congenital nature is not proved in all. Evidence that limited cell proliferation occurs in some cases may explain presentation later in life, and patients may live for decades with complete heart block {64}.

Localization
By definition they occur adjacent to the atrioventricular node. Similar lesions have not been described elsewhere in the body.

Clinical features
Two-thirds of patients present with complete heart block, 15% with lesser degress of atrioventricular block, and 10% with sudden death without documented history of heart block {240}. The remainder are incidental findings in newborns and infants with structural heart defects. Only rarely are atrioventricular nodal tumours detected in patients with normal sinus rhythm. Most tumours have first been diagnosed at autopsy but *in vivo* diagnosis has been reported {102}.

Macroscopy
They range in size from 2-20 mm and are multicystic, the cysts often barely perceptible.

Histopathology
They arise in the inferior interatrial septum and generally respect the boundaries of the central fibrous body, and do not involve ventricular myocardium or the valves. Tumour cells occur in nests or line the variably sized cystic spaces. Cells can interdigitate with myocytes within the inferior septum, resulting in degenerative changes within the myocytes. Cells may be cuboidal, transitional, squamoid or show sebaceous differentiation. Multilayering may occur along the cyst walls {240,1157,1189}.

Immunohistochemistry
The cells strongly express cytokeratin, epithelial membrane antigen, carcinoembryonic antigen and B72.3. Cells may also express calcitonin and serotonin. {465,523,1173,1345}.

Electron microscopy
Two cells types are characteristic. Within the solid nests, cells have well formed basement membrane, cytoplasmic tonofilaments and desmosomes. Cells lining the spaces are also connected by desmosomes, have short microvilli and may contain electron dense material {240}.

Prognosis
The tumours are benign neoplasms but may result in significant arrythmias or sudden death. Surgical excision has been reported in a few patients {951,1541}.

Cardiac sarcomas

A.P. Burke
H. Tazelaar
J.W. Butany
D. El-Demellawy
R. Loire
T. Geva
F. Bonilla
J.R. Galvin

J.P. Veinot
R. Virmani
H. Kamiya
G. Watanabe
D. Grandmougin
M. Horimoto
H. Hiraga

Angiosarcoma

Definition
Angiosarcoma is a malignant tumour whose cells display endothelial differentiation.

ICD-O code   9120/3

Synonyms
Haemangioendothelioma, malignant haemangioendothelioma, haemangiosarcoma, haemangioendothelial sarcoma, malignant haemangioma and malignant angioendothelioma {1179}.

Epidemiology
Angiosarcomas are the most common malignant differentiated cardiac neoplasms {259,691}. They occur over a wide age range (36 months to 80 years) {259,1693} with a peak incidence in the fourth decade. It occurs with equal frequency in men and women.

Localization
It most often arises in the right atrium near the atrioventricular groove (80%), but has been reported in the other three chambers as well as in the pericardium {921,1654}. Left atrial involvement is unusual though it has been reported {203,478,799}. In one series the right atrium was involved in 55.6% and showed co-involvement of the right ventricle (6.5%), pericardium (6.5%), and the left atrium (0.9%) {1653}.

Clinical features
Signs and symptoms
Clinical features reflect location, size and the extent of regional involvement, and the presence or absence of metastases {259}. Most are initially silent. Because of frequent pericardial involvement {1653}, dyspnoea is not an early symptom as is the case with other cardiac sarcomas. The most common presenting symptom is chest pain (46%) {259}. Right-sided heart failure, often associated with hemopericardium and supraventricular arrhythmias are also frequent {1128A, 1398A}. A significant number of patients present with or have co-existent haemorrhagic episodes, coagulopathy, anaemia, persistent haematomas or easy bruisability {25}. Sometimes, early pericardial involvement may lead to pericardial biopsy during emergency surgical cardiac decompression for tamponade. Cardiac rupture may occur, but is rare. Presentation with lung metastases is not uncommon {23,186,2216}. In 10% of cases, fever, weight loss, and fatigue remain unexplained for several months, resulting in delayed diagnosis, large tumour size, and advanced stage when surgery is performed.

The predominant right-sided location allows for diagnosis by endomyocardial biopsy, generally out of reach of other sarcoma types (which have a predilection for the left atrium). Sometimes the neoplasm remains undiagnosed in life due to the absence of specific symptoms.

Imaging
At echocardiography angiosarcomas typically appear as an echogenic, nodular or lobulated mass in the right atrium. Pericardial effusion or direct pericardial extension/invasion are frequently seen {66}. At MRI angiosarcoma also usually appears as a heterogeneous, nodular mass in the right atrium. MRI imaging sequences sensitive for hemorrhage (T1 weighted images) may show areas of hemorrhage which may be diffuse or nodular {65}. After administration of intravenous contrast (gadolinium-DTPA) enhancement along vascular lakes may be seen which has been described as a "sunray" appearance {527}. Like echocardiography, MRI may also show pericardial effusion or direct pericardial invasion, though MRI is more sensitive than echocardiography for distinguishing between pericardial fluid and pericardial tumour. CT findings are similar to the MRI findings. CT usually shows a heterogeneous, nodular mass in the right atrium

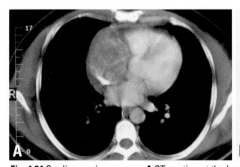
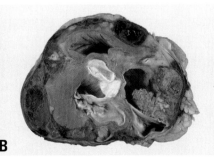
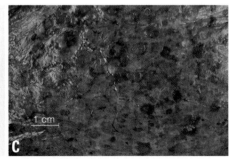

Fig. 4.24 Cardiac angiosarcoma. **A** CT section at the level of the aortic valve demonstrates a soft tissue mass completely filling the right atrium. **B** Cardiac angiosarcoma arising in right atrioventricular groove, forming a papillary right atrial mass. Note the extensive pericardial involvement. **C** Metastatic angiosarcoma to the lung, forming multiple haemorrhagic subpleural nodules (courtesy of Dr. William D. Edwards).

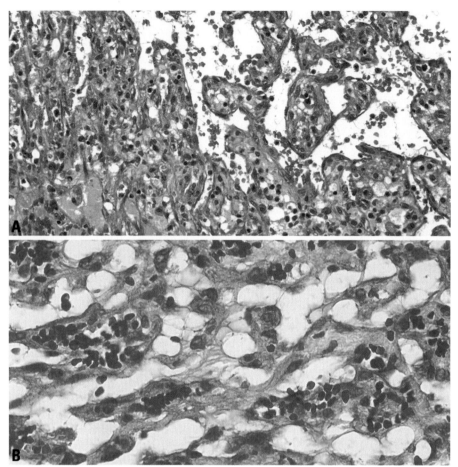

Fig. 4.25 Cardiac angiosarcoma. **A** Cardiac angiosarcoma with papillary features. Serpiginous and gaping vascular spaces lined by plump hyperchromatic endothelial cells. **B** Cardiac angiosarcoma with irregular vascular spaces lined by atypical hyperchromatic, somewhat epithelioid endothelial cells.

Histopathology

Over two-thirds of cardiac angiosarcomas are well to moderately differentiated showing well-formed vascular channels and papillary structures. The vascular channels are irregular, anastomosing, and sinusoidal. The lining cells are usually pleomorphic and atypical. They may form cord-like structures in which lumina are difficult to demonstrate. Mitoses are usually present {249,259,590}. The remaining third are poorly differentiated and composed predominantly of anaplastic spindle cells. In angiosarcoma with a focal or dominant spindle cell pattern, poorly formed vascular channels and extravascular red blood cells can usually be identified focally. Generous sampling may be necessary in order to identify diagnostic areas in such cases {249}. Often, metastatic as opposed to primary lesions, show areas of better differentiation. Angiosarcoma with a solid pattern of growth and individual cells having epithelioid features have been reported {2059}. In these cases the neoplastic cells have eosinophilic cytoplasm with occasional cytoplasmic vacuoles. The nuclei in this variety are usually large, hyperchromatic and have prominent eosinophilic nucleoli. The stroma can be abundant and hyalinized.

Immunoprofile

Immunohistochemical staining is important for the definitive diagnosis of vascular lesions, especially those with poorly differentiated patterns in which vascular channels are difficult to identify. Most angiosarcomas express, to variable degrees, usual endothelial cell antigens including factor VIII (von Willebrand factor), CD31 and CD34. Of these, CD31 gives the most consistent results, has good specificity and excellent sensitivity (approximately 90%) {462,2119}. Vascular channels may be highlighted by the use of laminin and type IV collagen. Cytokeratin and epithelial membrane antigen may be focally positive in conventional angiosarcoma and may be diffusely positive in epithelioid angiosarcomas {2247}.

Electron microscopy

With the wide availability of immunohistochemistry, ultrastructural study is less critical for diagnosis. The classic ultrastructural feature of endothelial cells, the Weibel-Palade body, is not demonstrable

with possible pericardial effusion or invasion. At CT angiosarcomas are usually low attenuation due to necrosis but may have focal high areas of attenuation due to hemorrhage. CT may show a similar pattern of contrast enhancement as MRI. With MRI or CT, the presence of a hemorrhagic, irregular right atrial mass is very suggestive of angiosarcoma, especially if accompanied by a pericardial effusion {66}.

Macroscopy

Angiosarcomas usually form lobulated variegated masses in the right atrial wall, protruding into the chamber. They range from 2.0 cm to several centimeters. The masses are classically dark, grey-brown to black in colour and may resemble a melanoma {249}, but tumours with less well-developed vascular spaces may appear firm, yellow-white in colour, lacking the classic hemorrhagic appearance. The pericardium is frequently involved

and hence a hemorrhagic pericardial effusion is a frequent accompaniment. While involvement of the tricuspid valve and extension or invasion of the vena cavae is reported, involvement of the pulmonary artery and interatrial septum are unusual. In rare instances, the pericardium is the sole site of involvement.

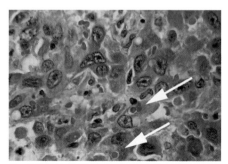

Fig. 4.26 Epithelioid angiosarcoma. Note the prominent eosinophilic cytoplasm (arrows).

in most neoplastic cells. However, pinocytotic vesicles, abundant intermediate filaments, and a moderate amount of rough endoplasmic reticulum and Golgi apparatus may be identified. Pericytes may be demonstrated adjacent to tumour cells {1291}.

Differential diagnosis
In cases with a dominant spindle cell pattern distinction from an unclassified spindle cell sarcoma, fibrosarcoma or malignant fibrous histiocytoma may be difficult. The detection of endothelial vacuoles or papillary structures are helpful. Immunohistochemical stains for laminin, type IV collagen and even reticulin stains may help highlight the vascular lumina {545}. The increasing incidence of Kaposi sarcoma makes differentiation from the spindle cell areas of angiosarcoma essential, though cardiac Kaposi sarcoma is usually metastatic.

Pericardial angiosarcomas can be mistaken for mesotheliomas {1277} and clumps of reactive mesothelial cells may be trapped in areas of an angiosarcoma. Stains for cytokeratin, calretinin, cytokeratin 5/6 and CD31 can help to differentiate the two populations of cells.

Genetics
Genetics studies involving cardiac angiosarcomas are rare and they only analyze isolated patients with heart primary tumours. Cytogenetic analyses of cardiac angiosarcoma show no consistent chromosomal abnormality {590}. A case of right atrial angiosarcoma demonstrated hyperdiploid clonal populations with changes in chromosome number, as follows: 55, XY, +der (1;17) (q10:q10), +2,+7, +8, +19, +20, +21, +22, as well as polysomy of chromosome 8 {2247}. Other chromosomal changes reported are gains of 5pter-p11, 8p12-qter, 20pter-q12 and losses of 4p, 7p15-pter-y and abnormalities involving 22q {310,590}. Molecular analyses on tumour tissues have focused on genetic alterations of TP53 and K-ras. The few reports available show that TP53 is more frequently altered than K-ras. Mutations of the TP53 tumour suppressor gene have been revealed by PCR-SSCP and sequencing studies and by immunohistochemical staining in up to 50% of tumours studied {662,1428,2247}. A K-ras mutation has also been documented in heart angiosarcoma {662}: a G-to-A

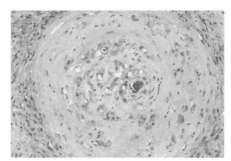

Fig. 4.27 Epithelioid haemangioendothelioma. There are cords of tumor cells arranged circumferentially within a vessel wall. The cells show focal vacuolization, representing intracytoplasmic vascular lumina.

transition at the first base of codon 13, which resulted in one amino acid substitution (Gly-13-Ser), in 2 relatively young patients (31 and 36 years old).

Prognosis and predictive factors
Cardiac angiosarcomas have an especially poor prognosis because they typically present in the face of advanced disease {249}. In one study, 80% of patients had metastatic disease at the time of diagnosis and 90% survived less than nine months {921}. A mean survival of ten months after surgical excision, with or without adjuvant therapy, has been reported in another study {823}. In soft tissue angiosarcomas, morphologic features that have statistically correlated with poor outcome include age, large size and high proliferative (Ki-67) index {478,590}. Metastases occur most frequently to the lung (70%), then liver. No significant correlation has been reported between DNA ploidy patterns and clinical outcome {590}.

Treatment
There are no randomized treatment trials, but patients are generally treated by a combination of surgery and radiation with or without sarcoma-type chemotherapy. Surgical resection is necessary, but complete excision cannot be achieved in most cases, because lack of a dissection plane and myocardial encroachment of tumoural tissue. However, even partial resection (with possible valve repair) may provide some months of symptom-free survival. However, local recurrence is the rule, even when resection was thought to be complete. Heart transplantation has been used to treat cardiac angiosarcoma, but without long-term survival {1654, 2043}.

Epithelioid haemangioendothelioma

Definition
Epithelioid haemangioendothelioma is a vascular tumour composed of epithelioid cells arranged in short strands or solid nests. The constituent endothelial cells are round or oval, contain small intracellular lumina, and frequently infiltrate muscular walls of vessels.

ICD-O code   9133/3

Epidemiology
Fewer than five have been reported in the heart {26,249,1241}. Epithelioid haemangioendothelioma has been reported in association with myelodysplastic syndrome {26}.

Histopathology
The intracellular lumens of epithelioid haemangioendothelioma may mimic the vacuoles of adenocarcinoma, which may be initially considered in the microscopic differential diagnosis. Immuno-histochemical stains for factor VIII-related antigen, CD31, or CD34 identify the cells as endothelial. The differential diagnosis also includes epithelioid haemangioma, a tumour even rarer as a cardiac primary {453}.

Prognosis
Approximately 10% of extracardiac haemangioendotheliomas develop metastases, and up to one third recur. The biologic behaviour of epithelioid haemangioendotheliomas of the heart is unknown. They should be considered low-grade malignant, based on available data on histologically similar extracardiac tumours, and a case report of a tumour that developed distant metastases {1241}.

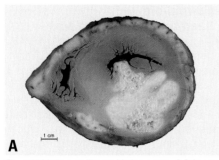
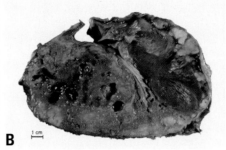
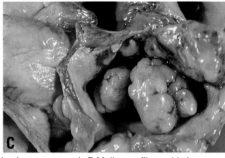

Fig. 4.28 Malignant fibrous histiocytoma. **A** Primary malignant fibrous histiocytoma with ossesous differentiation (osteosarcoma). **B** Malignant fibrous histiocytoma with osseous differentiation (osteosarcoma). **C** Large nodules in the right atrium.

Pleomorphic malignant fibrous histiocytoma (MFH) / Undifferentiated pleomorphic sarcoma

Definition

Malignant fibrous histiocytoma or undifferentiated plemorphic sarcoma is high-grade malignancy showing fibroblastic or myobroblastic differentiation and areas of marked cellular pleomorphism. Malignant fibrous histiocytomas and fibrosarcomas represent a broad spectrum of mesenchymal tumours and the degree of cellular pleomorphism is the major distinguishing feature.

ICD-O code

Malignant fibrous
histiocytoma   8830/3

Synonym

Malignant fibrous histiocytoma is now regarded as synonymous with undifferentiated pleomorphic sarcoma, as many tumours formerly classified as MFH have been found to have evidence of myogenic or other more specific differentiation.

Epidemiology

Malignant fibrous histiocytoma, as historically defined, is the second most common malignant cardiac sarcoma in adults and, if considered with all undifferentiated sarcomas represents the most common sarcoma. There is no gender predilection and the mean age is around 45 years (range, 20-80 years). Rare cases have been reported in infants.

Localization

Malignant fibrous histiocytoma tends to be located in the left atrium of the heart, most commonly the posterior wall and / or interatrial septum {1056,1142,1526}.

In a recent review, 81% of 47 cases were left atrial {1508}. The other reported locations included the pericardial space (3 cases), right ventricle/ pulmonary valve (3 cases), right atrium (1 case), and left ventricle (1 case) {1508}. Although the majority occur in the left atrium, where they most often present like cardiac myxomas, they more commonly arise along the posterior wall in comparison to the septum {1056,1142,1526}.

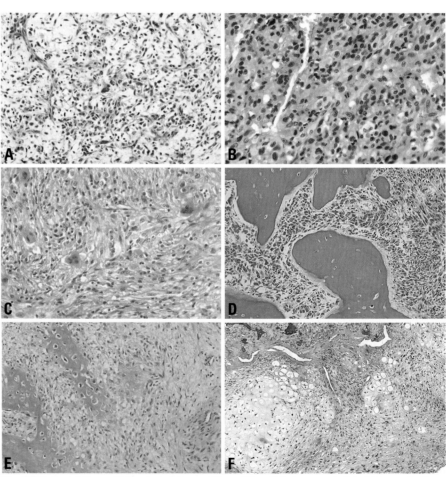

Fig. 4.29 Malignant fibrous histiocytoma (pleomorphic undifferentiated sarcoma). **A** In this example, there is a myxoid background and a prominent vascular pattern reminiscent of myxoid malignant fibrous histiocytoma found in soft tissue. **B** Malignant fibrous histiocytoma arising in left atrium where it initially mimicked a cardiac myxoma. Note mitotic activity. **C** Note pleomorphic growth pattern. **D** Malignant fibrous histiocytoma with osseous differentiation (osteosarcoma). Note formation of the mature bone trabeculae. **E** Osteoid formation. **F** Cartilagenous differentiation.

Clinical features

Most occur on the left side of the heart and cause signs and symptoms related to pulmonary congestion, mitral stenosis and pulmonary vein obstruction. Tumours may also present with metastases and the lungs, lymph nodes, kidney and skin are common sites.

Constitutional signs and symptoms may precede symptoms referable to the heart. Diagnosis of cardiac sarcoma rests on echocardiography; MRI is helpful preoperatively to determine precise tumour size, location, and adjacent tissues invasion, and post-operatively for assessment of excision and recurrence.

Macroscopy

Malignant fibrous histiocytoma typically presents as a soft or firm polypoid endocardial based tumour. It may be sessile or pedunculated, simulating myxoma, but unlike myxoma, may form multiple masses not obviously part of the same tumour {1142}. The mass may distend the atrium and impinge upon the mitral valve. Extension into the pulmonary veins and lung parenchyma may be present {1056} They may be uniform tan-white or variegated due to haemorrhage and necrosis. Calcification is uncommon.

Histopathology

Malignant fibrous histiocytoma or undifferentiated pleomorphic sarcoma is a diagnosis of exclusion, and immunohistochemical studies are important in ruling out metastatic myogenic, melanocytic and neurogenic tumours as well as sarcomatoid carcinomas. Of the subtypes of malignant fibrous histiocytoma described in the soft tissue, the pleomorphic (greater than 90%) and giant cell subtypes have been recognized in the heart. The tumours are heterogeneous in appearance and are variably cellular. The constituent cells may be spindled or epithelioid and sometimes have abundant eosinophilic cytoplasm. Intermixed giant cells are common. A storiform arrangement of tumour cells is common and they usually have marked pleomorphism. Mitotic activity is easy to find.

Osteosarcoma

Undifferentiated pleomorphic sarcomas demonstrate areas of osseous differentiation in 15% of cases. There is debate as to whether these tumours should be classified as extra skeletal osteosarcomas or

undifferentiated pleomorphic sarcomas with osteosarcomatous differentiation. Virtually all osteosarcomas of the heart reported thus far have occurred in the left atrium. Like skeletal osteosarcoma, areas of malignant giant cell tumour (giant cell malignant fibrous histiocytoma), chondroid differentiation, and osseous differentiation have been found to coexist in variable amounts in a single lesion.

Genetics

Genetic studies of cardiac sarcomas are limited. In studies of extra cardiac malignant fibrous histiocytoma, the common signature of genetic alterations includes recurring low-level copy number increases at new sites on chromosome 7, and losses of chromosome 2 sequences {1546}. Genomic imbalance at chromosome 13 has also been observed, with high gains for Xp and bands 1q21-22, 1p31, 3q27 and 9q3. The losses at chromosome 13 were observed in a large proportion at regions 13q12-14 and 13q21-22 {1131,1224}. Specific losses in regions that harbour tumour suppressor genes like INK4a (9p21) and RB1 (13q14) have been revealed by Southern blot and comparative genomic hybridization {1828}. RB1 gene is probably implicated in tumourigenesis of malignant fibrous histiocytoma due to the high correlation between absence of RB1 protein expression and chromosome 13 losses and mutations found in this gene {353}. Mutations localized to the core domain of TP53 have been found by immunohistochemical and sequencing procedures {1982}, as have other abnormalities like protein accumulation {1647}. TP53 mutations and accumulation of p53 protein have been detected in tumours with MDM2 gene amplification {1647}.

Treatment

Complete resection of malignant primary cardiac tumours can rarely be achieved, but palliative surgery is usually undertaken because many patients present with mechanical obstruction {731}. Adjunctive chemotherapy, radiation therapy or both are sometimes used {731}, however, the optimal protocol and efficacy are unclear {731,1508,1962,2043}. Patients with unresectable primary malignant cardiac tumours who are free of metastases may be considered for heart transplantation {731,1962,2043}.

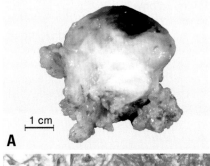

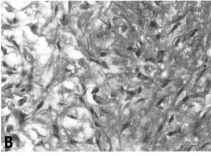

Fig. 4.30 A Myxosarcoma from the left atrium. Cut surface showing variable solid, soft and haemorrhagic regions. **B** Fibromyxosarcoma. A portion of the tumor near the endocardial surface shows an undifferentiated spindle cell sarcoma without prominent vascularity or pleomorphism and an abundant proteoglycan matrix.

Prognosis and predictive factors

For malignant fibrous histiocytoma and fibrosarcoma there is some evidence that grading is useful in predicting survival, but the majority of patients with these tumours die of either local or metastatic disease {731,952,1508}. The mean postoperative survival is 5-18 months. The cause of death may be related to metastatic disease, bulky intracardiac recurrences, or general debilitation.

Fibrosarcoma and myxosarcoma

Definition

Fibrosarcoma is a malignant tumour composed of fibroblasts with variable amounts of intercellular collagen and a classic herringbone architecture. Some fibrosarcomas with abundant myxoid stroma have been called myxosarcomas but are not considered malignant variants of cardiac myxoma. Tumours with marked pleomorphism, or a prominent vascular or storiform pattern are better classified as malignant fibrous histiocytoma.

ICD-O code

Fibrosarcoma   8810/3

Epidemiology

Fibrosarcoma represents 5-10% of all cardiac sarcomas depending on the criteria used for diagnosis. Fibrosarcomas are less frequent, and occur over a broader age range than malignant fibrous histiocytoma, some having been reported in children.

Localization

Fibrosarcomas are most common in the left atrium, but have been reported to arise in all chambers. Fibrosarcomas may also infiltrate the pericardial space, thus mimicking mesothelioma {1034}.

Clinical features

The clinical features of fibrosarcomas have not been well-delineated from related cardiac sarcomas such as malignant fibrous histiocytoma (undifferentiated pleomorphic sarcoma) as the classification of these lesions has not been standardized in large series. As with other sarcomas, signs and symptoms vary depending on the location of the tumour. Because most occur on the left side of the heart, signs and symptoms related to pulmonary congestion, mitral stenosis and pulmonary vein obstruction are most frequent. Rarely, cardiac fibrosarcoma may present with metastases in the lungs, lymph nodes, skin, and kidney.

Macroscopy

Fibrosarcoma typically presents as a soft polypoid tumour projecting into the chamber from whose walls they arise. They have a gross appearance similar to MFH {329}, but haemorrhage, necrosis, and variegation are less common.

Histopathology

Fibrosarcoma of adult type is composed of spindle shaped cells arranged in sweeping fascicles that are often arranged at angles to one another resulting in a "herringbone" pattern. The nuclei are usually elongate with tapered ends and darkly staining. Mitotic activity is variable. In the myxoid variant tumour cells spindling is less pronounced and cells may take on a stellate or ovoid configuration. However in all types pleomorphism is minimal and prominent vascularity is absent.

Differential diagnosis

The differential diagnosis for the typical variant of fibrosarcoma includes mono-

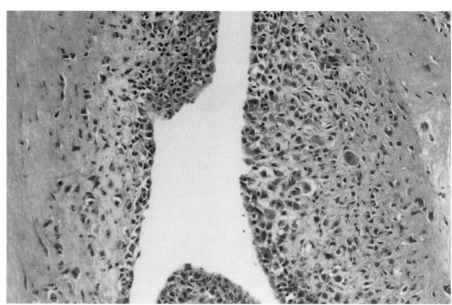

Fig. 4.31 Embryonal rhabdomyosarcoma predenting as small cell undifferentiated tumor with cellular areas concentrated towards the surface.

phasic synovial sarcoma, inflammatory myofibroblastic tumours and localized fibrous tumours, and for the myxoid variant, other myxoid sarcomas (MFH, leiomyosarcoma, etc.) and cardiac myxoma. The latter is generally distinguished by the presence of myxoma cells, abundant organizing hemorrhage, and absence of mitotic figures and high cellularity. Fibromas are easily distinguished from typical fibrosarcoma by lack of cellularity and abundant collagen.

Prognosis and predictive factors

See discussion on treatment of maligant fibrous histiocytoma. There is no proven difference in prognosis between cardiac fibrosarcoma and malignant fibrous histiocytoma as demonstrated in a meta-analysis using actuarial methods {249}.

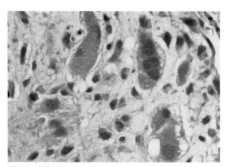

Fig. 4.32 Embryonal rhabdomyosarcoma with rhabdomyoblasts containing abundant eosinophilic cytoplasm.

Rhabdomyosarcoma

Definition

Rhabdomyosarcoma is a malignant tumour with striated muscle differentiation.

ICD-O code   8900/3

Epidemiology

Rhabdomyosarcoma is a very rare subtype of cardiac sarcoma. In the past, before immunohistochemical documentation of tumour histogenesis was routine, it was stated that a large proportion of cardiac sarcomas were rhabdomyosarcomas. However, in more recent series, the proportion is less than 5% {250}, and in one recent series of cardiac sarcomas with rigorous immunohistochemical documentation, none of 24 was classified as rhabdomyosarcoma {509}.

Localization

Rhabdomyosarcomas occur anywhere in the heart. Approximately 50% occur in the atria, and 50% in the ventricles. The frequency of ventricular involvement is greater than other cardiac sarcomas. Contrary to sarcomas with fibro- or myofibroblastic differentiation, they are not usually intracavitary tumours, but are more often mural.

Clinical features

Cardiac rhabdomyosarcomas are usually of the embryonal variant and, there-

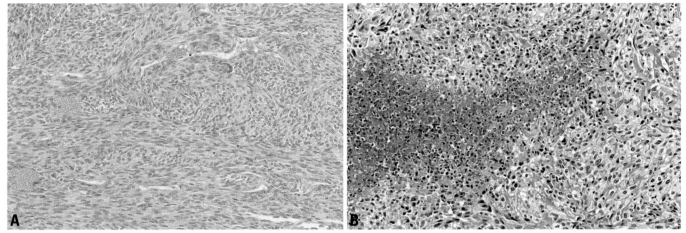

Fig. 4.33 Leiomyosarcoma. **A** The tumour is cellular, composed of fascicles of relatively uniform cells. **B** Note tumour cellularity and focal necrosis.

fore, occur most frequently in children and young adults; it is the most common primary cardiac malignancy in children. The mean age at presentation is approximately 20 years, compared to 40-50 years of age for other subtypes of cardiac sarcoma. Rhabdomyosarcoma is more likely than other primary cardiac sarcomas to involve the valves. The clinical presentation, as with other cardiac tumours, depends on the cardiac location.

Macroscopy
Cardiac rhabdomyosarcomas are bulky, invasive tumours that may be grossly mucoid or gelatinous, similar to cardiac myxoma, or soft and necrotic, with variegation and heterogeneity. They usually arise within the myocardium and are less likely than sarcomas with myofibroblastic or fibroblastic differentiation to be endocardial based, luminal tumours.

Tumour spread and staging
Sites of metastatic spread are, in order of descending frequency: lungs, regional lymph nodes, central nervous system, gastrointestinal tract, kidney, adrenals, thyroid, ovary, bone and pancreas.

Histopathology
Cardiac rhabdomyosarcomas are almost exclusively embryonal. Embryonal rhabdomyosarcoma is small cell neoplasm with variable numbers of PAS-positive rhabdomyoblasts (tadpole or strap cells). Well-differentiated embryonal rhabdomyosarcoma has numerous tadpole-shaped rhabdomyoblasts. Nuclear staining with antibodies against myo-

genin greatly facilitates the diagnosis {1630}. Desmin is also useful in documenting muscular differentiation. Alveolar rhabdomyosarcoma, characterized by a collagenous stroma and a paucity of rhabdomyoblasts, has been described in the heart generally as a metastatic lesion. Sarcoma botryoides, with characteristic grape-like structures and a so-called cambium layer, a form of embryonal rhabdomyosarcoma, has also been described in the heart {760}.

Differential diagnosis
The differential diagnosis includes other cardiac sarcomas, especially undifferentiated lesions and metastatic small round cell tumours in children and young adults. Immunohistochemical stains are vital in identifying rhabdomyoblasts. Adult cellular rhabdomyomas, in contrast to rhabdomyosarcoma, lack significant mitotic activity, necrosis, and do not express myogenin.

Electron microscopy
The diagnostic features are thick and thin filaments reminiscent of normal striated muscle. Internal A and I banding may or may not be present, but Z-bands are frequently well formed. Plentiful glycogen granules and abundant mitochondria are also present. Tumour nuclei are lobulated, containing variable amounts of condensed chromatin. Occasionally, several grids must be examined before rhabdomyoblasts are identified.

Somatic genetics
At exon 1 of K-ras, a mutation at the first base of codon 13 (G to A transition) has

been detected in cardiac rhabdomyosarcoma {662}.

Treatment
Surgery
Surgical resection of the tumour is usually indicated even if it is considered as palliative to relieve obstruction to cardiac blood flow and to clarify the diagnosis {301,470,952}. Total orthotopic heart transplantation may offer relatively long-term survival {67,701,733} if there are no distant metastases.

Chemotherapy
Although the outcome of chemotherapy on cardiac rhabdomyosarcoma has not been fully studied, due to the rarity of the tumour, there have been advances in the treatment of soft tissue rhabdomyosarcoma {423,529, 1194,1749} with a three-year progression-free survival of approximately 65%. Neoadjuvant chemotherapy may optimize a surgical approach {1749}.

Radiotherapy
Adjuvant radiotherapy is commonly mandatory to preclude local relapse or to optimize the results of a surgical approach. However radiotherapy may be used preoperatively to decrease tumor size and allow surgical resection.

Prognosis and predictive factors
Specific prognostic microscopic features have not been devised for cardiac rhabdomyosarcomas. However, grading is similar for other subtypes of cardiac sarcomas, and includes an assessment of mitotic activity and necrosis {509}. The

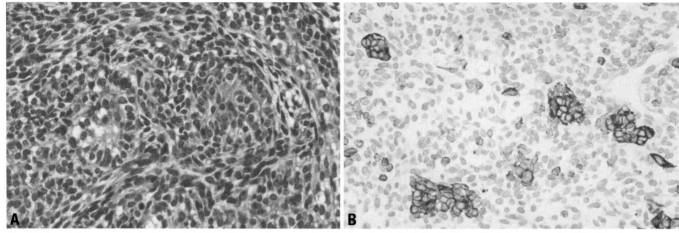

Fig. 4.34 Synovial sarcoma. **A** The tumour is highly cellular and composed predominantly of spindled cells. The epithelial areas may be difficult to discern on routine stains. **B** Immunohistochemical stain demonstrating expression of pancytokeratin in islands of epithelial cells.

prognosis is poor, with recurrence and eventual metastasis with death of the patient within months the rule {1944}. The mean survival rarely exceeds 12 months.

Leiomyosarcoma

Definition
A malignant tumour composed of cells with distinct smooth muscle features.

ICD-O code 8890/3

Epidemiology
Cardiac leiomyosarcoma is uncommon, representing less 10% of cardiac sarcomas. There is no sex predilection, and most occur in patients between 40 and 50 years of age.

Clinical features
Dyspnoea is the main clinical feature. Sometimes patients present with chest pain, cough, atrial arrythmias, or haemoptysis.

Macroscopy
Most of them are located in the left atrium (posterior wall) and invade pulmonary veins or mitral valve. But, tumours can arise elsewhere, including the right atrium and ventricle, or pulmonary valve or trunk. The tumours tend to be firm, fleshy, grey and sessile. They may present as multiple intra-cavitary nodules.

Histopathology
Leiomyosarcoma is composed of compact bundles of spindle cells that possess blunt-ended nuclei and are often oriented at sharp angle or 90° to one another. Inconstant characteristic features include the presence of cytoplasmic glycogen and perinuclear vacuoles. Pleomorphic and giant cells may be present. Zones of necrosis and mitotic figures are generally plentiful. Usual immunohistochemical markers of neoplastic cells are smooth muscle alpha actin and desmin. Alpha actin also shows numerous normal little vessels in the tumour tissue. There may occasionally be aberrant expression of cytokeratin and epithelial membrane antigen. Demonstration of smooth muscle cell derivation virtually confirms malignancy, as leiomyomas remain undescribed in this location.

Treatment and prognosis
Treatment consists of surgical excision, almost always incomplete. This may allow some patients several months of symptom free survival, typically less than one year. Chemotherapy and radiation therapy may provide palliation.

Synovial sarcoma

Definition
Synovial sarcoma is a biphasic tumour composed of spindled and epithelioid areas, characterized by X;18 chromosomal translocations.

ICD-O code 9040/3

Epidemiology
Synovial sarcomas account for approximately 5% of cardiac sarcomas {173, 300,400,1466}. The true incidence has probably been underestimated, as molecular studies can now confirm the diagnosis in the monophasic variant, which is the most common form in the heart. An association between cardiac synovial sarcoma and asbestos exposure has been reported {1144}.

Localization
There is a predilection for the atria and pericardial surfaces.

Clinical features
Clinical symptoms may arise from obstruction, embolism, and tamponade.

Macroscopy
Synovial sarcomas are bulky, infiltrative tumours that are typically firm and white. Necrosis or hemorrhage may be present.

Histopathology
The classic lesion is biphasic, but the monomorphic variant is especially common in the heart. The spindle component resembles a fibrosarcoma, but alternating cellular and oedematous areas are typical. The spindle cells are small, compact, and often infiltrated by sparse mononuclear lymphoid cells. The epithelioid cells form clusters and nests, and occasionally larger gland–like spaces which may show branching. Immunohistochemically, cytokeratin and epithelial membrane antigen are strongly expressed in the epithelioid cells. Staining for these markers in the spindle cells may be very focal. Spindle cells express vimentin and occasionally smooth muscle actin. The cells do not express CD34.

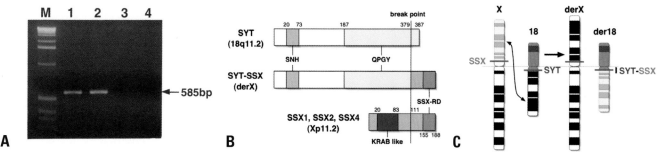

Fig. 4.35 Synovial sarcoma. **A** An example of detection of fusion SS18/SSX transcripts by RT-PCR. M; 1kb ladder, lane 1; a biphasic synovial sarcoma of soft tissue, lane 2; a synovial sarcoma of peritoneum, lane 3; a malignant mesothelioma, lane 4; an adenocarcinoma of the lung. **B** Schematic diagram of domain structure of the SS18, SSX, and SS18/SSX proteins. SNH (SS18 amino terminal domain) might act as a inhibitor of the QPGY domain, which is a C-Terminal domain rich in glutamine, proline, glycine and tyrosine and might function as a transcription activation domain. KRAB (kruppel-associated box) is a transcription repression domain. However, the KRAB-like domain of SSX appears to be an inefficient or even inactive repressor domain. SSX-RD is a novel repressor domain, which is highly conserved in the SSX family. **C** Schematic representation of the translocation t(X;18)(p11.2;q11.2).

Differential diagnosis

Distinction of synovial sarcoma from mesothelioma, another biphasic tumour, can usually be made on the basis of tumour location (mesotheliomas do not occur within the atria) and growth pattern (synovial sarcoma is usually a circumscribed solitary lesion while mesothelioma tends to grow diffusely over the pericardium. Additionally, the spindle cell areas of synovial sarcoma tend to be relatively monomophic. The X;18 translocation may be confirmed on formalin fixed, paraffin embedded tissues and has a high degree of sensitivity and specificity {1506}. Reactivity for calretinin has been described in both mesothelioma and synovial sarcoma, and is not helpful in the differential diagnosis. Unlike mesothelioma, solitary fibrous tumour is generally lower-grade, usually expresses CD34 antigen, is less cellular and tends to have alternating hyper- and hypocellular areas.

Somatic genetics

Cytogenetically the reciprocal translocation t(X;18)(p11.2;q11.2) is seen in more than 90% of soft tissue synovial sarcomas {1330}. This is considered to be the primary cytogenetic abnormality and specific for synovial sarcomas.

The breakpoints of the t(X;18) have been cloned, and it has been shown that this translocation results in fusion of *SS18* gene (previously described as SYT or SSXT) at the chromosome 18q11.2 to either of two genes, *SSX1* or *SSX2*, at Xp11.2. This rearrangement of genes produces a chimeric *SS18 /SSX* transcript, which could be implicated in tumourigenesis {375}. The *SS18/SSX* transcripts can be specific markers of synovial sarcoma that can be detected by the reverse transcriptase-polymerase chain reaction (RT-PCR). The transcripts can be identified in almost all synovial sarcomas when there is adequate tumour RNA {837}. This molecular diagnostic method also can be applied to paraffin-embedded tissue {747}.

Cardiac lymphomas

G. Rolla
F. Calligaris-Cappio
A.P. Burke

Definition

Primary cardiac lymphoma (PCL) is an extra-nodal lymphoma involving only the heart and/or the pericardium. A less restrictive definition includes small secondary lesions elsewhere, with the vast bulk of the tumour arising in the heart. It is clinically defined as a lymphoma presenting as cardiac disease with the bulk of the tumour being intra-pericardial. Cardiac involvement by disseminated non-Hodgkin lymphoma should be excluded.

Epidemiology

PCL is an uncommon malignancy, accounting for 1.3% of primary cardiac tumours and 0.5% of extranodal lymphomas {249,273,1679}. The published series account for about 80 cases, while cardiac involvement in disseminated lymphoma has been documented in nearly 20% of autopsy cases {1280}. The appearance of PCL in patients with AIDS {1736} and in a kidney recipient {1667} suggests that immunodeficiency may be a predisposing factor. However, the heart is an uncommon site for immunodeficiency-related lymphoma. Most PCL arise in immunocompetent patients. The median age of the reported cases is 62 years (range, 5-90 years) with a male-to-female ratio of 3:1.

The clinical course is generally short, with a mean survival of 7 months (range, 0-48 months).

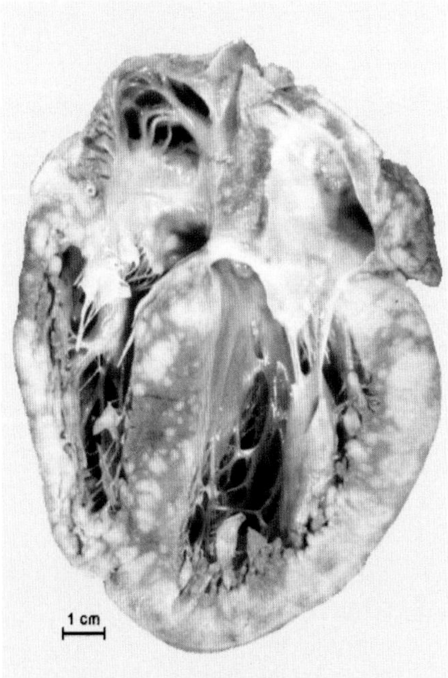

Clinical features

Signs and symptoms

The clinical course is generally acute in onset. There is no pathognomonic clinical presentation and patients are generally investigated because of chest pain, pericardial effusion, refractory heart failure, arrhythmia, or lightheadness and syncope due to a myxoma-like intracavitary mass {308}. Superior vena cava obstruction {363}, multiple pulmonary emboli and infarction {1832} and hypertrophic cardiomyopathy {266} have also been reported as initial diagnosis in patients with PCL. Complete atrio-ventricular block may be the major clinical presentation {1416}.

Imaging

Because the gross pathologic features of primary cardiac lymphoma are variable, the imaging findings are variable. Cardiac lymphomas most commonly manifest as circumscribed, nodular masses in the myocardium, often with an associated pericardial effusion. These findings are usually well seen at echocardiography, MRI, and CT. Lymphoma may also manifest as an ill-defined, infiltrative mass, in which case, they are typically best depicted with MRI because of its superior soft tissue contrast {66}. Internal imaging features and contrast enhancement patterns are very variable with cardiac lymphomas. Lymphomas may have high or low signal on MRI, may have similar attenuation as muscle or lower attenuation than muscle on CT, and may show increased, or decreased contrast enhancement. In some cases, pericardial effusion or pericardial thickening may be the only findings. In additon to echocardiography, MRI, and CT, nuclear medicine techniques may be useful procedures for the non-invasive assessment of cardiac lymphomas. Gallium-67 uptake is non-specific, though a marked accumulation in the heart without extracardiac uptake can suggest the diagnosis of PCL {1680}.

Diagnostic approach

When pericardial effusion is present its drainage may have both palliative and diagnostic purposes. Lymphoma cells may be detected in serous fluid in up to 88% of cases {308}.

When cytology is not available, the diagnosis of PCL is usually assessed by explorative thoracotomy with cardiac mass biopsy. Recently, less invasive procedures have been performed, such as transoesophageal echocardiography (TEE) guided percutaneous intracardiac biopsy {46,947}.

Macroscopy

PCL may arise in either atrium or ventricle. Usually the tumour is large, infiltrating myocardium and extending into the right atrium and ventricle in the form of multiple intracavitary polypoid nodules, which may eventually obliterate the cavities. The right atrium is involved in more than 2/3 of patients. The pericardium is usually thickened by white-greyish tumour infiltration. Pericardial effusion, which is generally massive, may be isolated (12.5% of cases) or associated with a heart mass (near half of cases) {737}.

Cytology

A diagnostic cytologic sample sample is obtained in less than 20% of primary cardiac lymphomas (PCL) {1680}. It may be difficult to differentiate PCL from benign reactive lymphocytosis by cytology alone. Immunocytochemical staining {1724}, cytogenetic studies {1} and polymerase chain reaction {964} have been performed successfully to confirm the lymphoid lineage and detect the presence of a monoclonal population.

Fig. 4.36 Cardiac lymphoma. Mulitofocal masses involving both atria and ventricular walls.

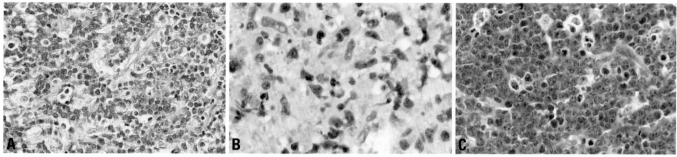

Fig. 4.37 Cardiac lymphomas. **A** Mass limited to the myocardium in a 40-year old man. Tumour cells are moderately sized with high mitotic rate; immunophenotype was consistent with diffuse large B-cell lymphoma. **B** In this example of a localized left ventricular tumour, the lymphoma cells are large and irregular. Immunophenotypically, the tumour typed as a diffuse large B-cell lymphoma. **C** Occasionally, cardiac lymphomas are of the high-grade small cell type (lymphoblastic lymphoma). In this lesion, the immunophenotype confirmed B-cell Burkitt subtype.

Histopathology
Diffuse large B-cell lymphoma is the subtype most frequently observed (80% of published cases). Non-cleaved small cell lymphoma has been reported in a few cases; the histopathology was unspecified in the other cases. Recently two cases of diffuse large B-cell lymphoma with CD5 expression have been reported {317}. This is a recently identified subgroup of diffuse large B-cell lymphomas, which differs for clinical characteristics (elderly, female and extranodal involvement) and aggressive clinical course {2181}. One case of Burkitt lymphoma in an immunocompetent patient has been described {317}.

Somatic genetics
A complex abnormal karyotype containing t(8;14) (q24;q32) has been reported in a case of diffuse large B-cell lymphoma mainly involving the heart with cells which were CD5+ and CD20+ with a c-myc rearrangement {1948}. In situ hybridization for EBER-1 was negative.

Prognosis and predictive factors
Late diagnosis appears to be a major factor in the poor outcome in PCL patients. Irrespective of the treatment applied, 60% of the patients died of their tumour 1.8 months after diagnosis {317}. Prompt anthracycline-based chemotherapy results in near 60% of complete response (mean follow-up 17 months; range 3-40 months). PCL should be treated like other aggressive lymphomas arising in other primary sites.

Metastatic tumours to the heart

G. Rolla
F. Calligaris-Cappio

Definition

Malignant cardiac neoplasm with a non-pericardial or myocardial primary site. Metastatic tumors that infiltrate myocardium are frequently accompanied by pericardial metastases, especially in the cases of carcinomas, which additionally involve mediastinal lymph nodes.

Epidemiology

In a series of 133 surgically resected cardiac tumors, 14% were metastatic {1411}. In a recent review, cardiac metastases were present in 12% of autopsies performed for widespread malignancy {12}. Primary tumors in decreasing order of frequency include carcinomas of the lung, lymphomas, carcinomas of the breast, leukemia, carcinomas of the stomach, malignant melanoma, hepatocellular carcinoma and carcinomas of the colon. The following tumors have an especially high rate of cardiac metastasis if the incidence of the primary tumor is considered: leukemia, melanoma, thyroid carcinoma, extracardiac sarcomas, lymphomas, renal cell carcinomas, carcinomas of the lung and carcinomas of the breast. These tumors all had a greater than 15% rate of cardiac metastasis in a large autopsy study {1398}.

The rate of cardiac involvement by metastatic disease has not appeared to change over a 14-year period, indicating that current treatment modalities may not have a significant effect on the rate of metastatic malignancy to the heart.

Clinical features

The cardiac location of the tumor greatly affects the signs and symptoms. These can include symptoms related pericardial effusions, arrhythmias, or congestive heart failure. Obstruction of the mitral or aortic valve may cause syncope. Involvement of the right heart and tricuspid valves may give rise to right-sided failure.

Localization

Malignancies spread to the heart by direct extension, usually from mediastinal tumor; haematogenously; via lymphatics; and rarely by intracavitary extension from the inferior vena cava or pulmonary veins. Lymphatic spread is generally accompanied by involvement and enlargement of pulmonary hilar or mediastinal lymph nodes. Haematogenous spread is characterized by myocardial involvement.

Epithelial malignancies typically spread to the heart by lymphatics. Melanoma, sarcomas, leukemia and renal cell carcinoma metastasize to the heart by a haematogenous route. Melanomas, renal tumours, including Wilms' tumour and renal cell carcinoma, adrenal tumours, liver tumours, and uterine tumours are the most frequent intracavitary tumours.

Metastatic cardiac tumours affect the right side of the heart in 20-30% of cases, the left side in 10-33% of cases, and show bilateral or diffuse involvement in approximately 30-35% of cases. The endocardium or chamber cavities are involved in 5% of cases {1398}. The most common epithelial malignancies to metastasize to the heart are carcinomas of the breast and lung. In most cases there is pericardial involvement with superficial myocardial infiltration. The valves and endocardium are usually spared. Generally, the heart is not the only organ involved, and metastatic deposits are usually present in extracardiac sites.

The myocardium is involved in virtually 100% of cases of metastatic melanoma,

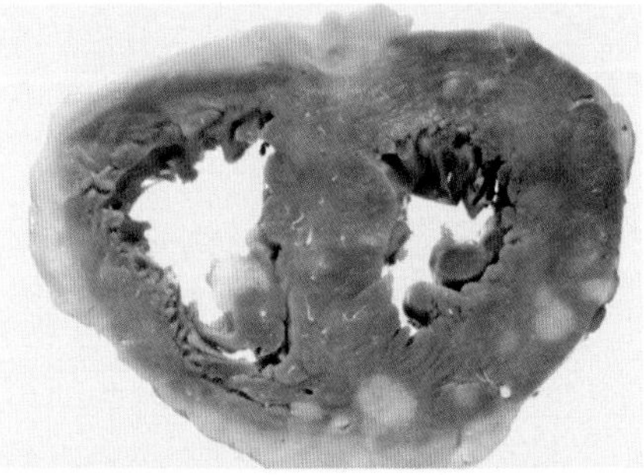

Fig. 4.38 Metastases of a large cell carcinoma of the lung in the heart.

and there is less frequent infiltration of epi- and endocardium.

Leukemic and lymphomatous infiltrates are typically widespread, involving the epicardium (61%), and myocardium diffusely. The left ventricle is involved in 55%, and right atrium in 54% of cases. Sarcomatous deposits are found within the myocardium (50%), pericardium (33%), or both myocardium and pericardium (17% of cases). Valvular metastases are uncommon {764}. Osteosarcoma, liposarcoma, leiomyosarcoma, unclassifiable sarcomas, rhabdomyosarcoma, neurofibrosarcoma, synovial sarcoma, and maligant fibrous histiocytoma have been reported to involve the heart secondarily.

Pathologic findings

Metastatic deposits may be diffuse, multinodular, or consist of a single dominant mass. Especially with carcinomas, there may be diffuse studding and thickening of the pericardial surfaces. This pattern can grossly be confused with mesothelioma, or benign fibrosing pericarditis. The tumour burden in the heart is the highest with melanoma, as compared to any other malignancy.

Carcinomatous spread in the myocardium is frequently most prominent in subepicardial lymphatics, whereas melanomas, sarcomas, renal cell carcinomas and lymphoid neoplasms form intramyocardial interstitial tumours. The histopathologic distinction between primary and metastatic sarcoma may be impossible upon surgical resection of a cardiac tumour. Most sarcomas metastatic to the heart cause symptoms at their primary site before cardiac symptoms are evident, however {764}. Although primary sarcomas of the heart are uncommon, extracardiac sarcomas presenting as cardiac metastases are even rarer.

Pericardial tumours

A. Burke
R. Loire
R. Virmani

Solitary fibrous tumour

Definition
An uncommon, spindle-cell, fibroblastic tumour which often shows a prominent haemangiopericytoma-like vascular pattern.

ICD-O code
Solitary fibrous tumour 8815/1

Synonyms
Benign mesothelioma, fibrous mesothelioma, submesothelial fibroma

Localization
The most common locations, outside the pleura, include the head and neck, especially orbit, soft tissue, especially abdomen, extremities, and meninges {233,1384,1473}. As with any lesion common to the pleura, there have been examples of solitary fibrous tumour reported in the pericardium and rarely within the heart.

Clinical features
Clinical features are related to pericardial mass effect.

Macroscopy
Solitary fibrous tumours tend to be well-circumscribed, firm, fleshy or white although diffuse mesothelial surface involvement has been described.

Histopathology
Histologic variability is the rule and multiple growth patterns have been described. Most tumours will have a predominant monomorphic spindle cell pattern resembling low-grade fibrosarcoma although broad tumour cell fascicles are rare. Areas of hypercellularity typically alternate with those that are less cellular. The less cellular areas can by myxoid or contain abundant collagen {459}. Typically the nuclei of tumour cells are closely apposed to collagen bundles. A haemangiopericytoma-like vascular pattern may be conspicuous, present in a small portion of the lesion, or absent. The differential diagnosis includes other monomorphic spindle cell tumours, including neurogenic tumours, spindle cell mesotheliomas, monophasic synovial sarcoma, and fibrosarcoma {1311}. Recently, desmoid tumour of the pleura has been added in the list of differential diagnostic considerations {2151}. See pleural section for additional information.

Immunoprofile
Solitary fibrous tumours are CD34 and bcl-2 positive. They are consistently negative for epithelial markers, muscle spe-

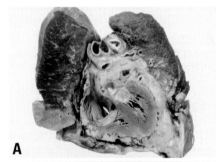
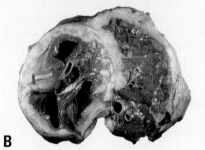

Fig. 4.39 Mesothelioma of pericardium. **A** Note the extensive tumour encasing the pericardium. **B** In many cases, the pericardial mass is in continuity with pleural mesothelioma.

cific actin, desmin, CD31, CD117 (c-kit), S-100 protein calretinin, and inhibin {596,772,1473,2127}.

Differential diagnosis
Sarcomatous mesotheliomas of the pericardium are distinguished from solitary fibrous tumours by their diffuse growth pattern, and keratin and calretinin reactivity. On the other hand, solitary fibrous tumour may closely mimic monophasic synovial sarcoma and low- grade fibrosarcoma. Fibrosarcoma tends to be more architecturally monomorphic and negative for CD34. Monophasic synovial sarcoma has higher grade cytology, plumper nuclei and shows focal keratin reactivity. Endometrial stromal sarcoma, and metastatic granulosa cell tumour may be excluded by negative reactivity for cytokeratin, estrogen and progesterone receptors, and inhibin.

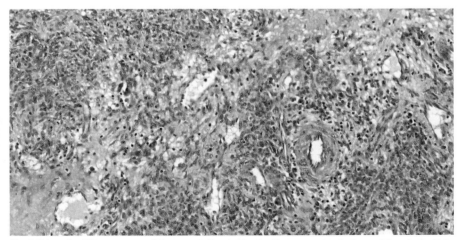

Fig. 4.40 Localized fibrous tumor of the mesothelium is identical in appearance to those of the pleura. Note the spindle cell growth with prominent vascularity and variable cellularity.

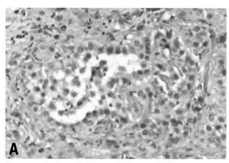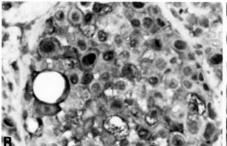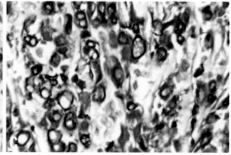

Fig. 4.41 Pericardial mesothelioma. **A** The majority of pericardial mesotheliomas are epithelioid. **B** Strong expression of calretinin. **C** Strong expression of cytokeratin 7.

Prognosis and predictive factors
The prognosis is generally good, although recurrences and local spread have been reported. Criteria for malignancy of pleural tumours include necrosis and a mitotic count of greater than 4 per 10 high powered fields, but the applicability of these criteria to tumours in the heart and pericardium is unknown.

Malignant mesothelioma

Definition
Malignant mesothelioma arises from mesothelial cells or demonstrates mesothelial differentiation. The definition of primary pericardial mesothelioma stipulates that there is no tumour present outside the pericardium, with the exception of lymph node metastases.

ICD-O code   9050/3

Epidemiology
Mesothelioma of the pericardium represents approximately 0.7% of malignant mesotheliomas {831}. As with mesotheliomas in other sites, the incidence may be increasing, due to the latency between asbestos exposure and tumour development {1074}.

Etiology
Like pleural mesotheliomas, a large proportion of mesotheliomas of the pericardium are induced by asbestos {1074}. Iatrogenically induced pericardial mesotheliomas have been reported decades after exposure to pericardial dusting with asbestos and fibreglass as a treatment for angina pectoris. Therapeutic radiation for breast cancer and mediastinal lymphoma has also been implicated in rare patients. However, there remains a subset of patients with mesothelioma who have no known exposure history.

Clinical features
Signs and symptoms
The mean age of patients with pericardial mesothelioma is about 45 years, with a wide age range, including elderly, older children and young adults. The initial course is usually related to pericardial effusions. Tamponade may eventually occur {1202}.

Imaging
Echocardiography usually shows pericardial effusions and may show pericardial thickening. However, because pericardium is at the periphery of the field of view obtainable with echocardiography, MRI or CT are usually necessary. MRI and CT usually demonstrate pericardial fluid as well as pericardial thickening and/or pericardial masses {737}.

Macroscopy
Malignant mesotheliomas of the pericardium can form bulky nodules that fill the pericardial cavity. The tumour can also spread diffusely over the pericardial surface and completely encase the heart. They can further encircle the great vessels and may obstruct the venae cavae.

Histopathology
Malignant mesotheliomas of the pericardium resemble pleural mesotheliomas. Although the majority are of the epithelioid type, forming tubules, papillary structures, and cords of infiltrating cells that can incite a desmoplastic response, the sarcomatous variant is also common. Variants similar to those described in the pleura may also be seen in the pericardium e.g. microcystic, adenomatoid, deciduoid {1649,1802}.

Immunoprofile
The immunohistochemical profile of pericardial mesothelioma is similar to that of pleural mesothelioma. Expression of mesothelial antigens, such as calretinin, and cytokeratins 5/6 are helpful in the diagnosis, as are negative reactions for adenocarcinoma markers, such as carcinoembryonic antigen.

Electron microscopy
Ultrastructurally, mesothelioma cells from epithelioid areas contain branched, bushy microvilli. Cytoplasmic tonofibrils are present in approximately 50% of tumours. Asbestos bodies may be identified within pericardial mesothelioma, but are of no diagnostic utility.

Differential diagnosis
The distinction between mesothelioma and pleural-based lung adenocarcinoma can be quite difficult, and is generally based on immunohistochemical findings. Distinction from reactive mesothelial cell proliferations may also be difficult; in comparison to reactive pleural mesothelial proliferations, reactive pericardial mesothelial cells may be more deeply "invasive". Reactive stromal cells may also often attain bizarre and pleomorphic shapes, confusing the histopathologic picture. Other malignancies that may be confused with mesothelioma include pericardial-based angiosarcoma, which may elicit a prominent mesothelial response, malignant solitary fibrous tumour and synovial sarcoma. Immunohistochemistry is invaluable in such circumstances. Mesothelioma lacks the X;18 translocation of synovial sarcoma.

Prognosis and predictive factors
The prognosis of pericardial mesothelioma is poor. Fifty per cent of patients

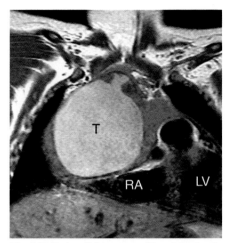

Fig. 4.42 Pericardial teratoma. T1-weighted spin echo MR image in the coronal plane showing large pericardial teratoma (T). The right atrium (RA) is compressed by the tumour.

survive 6 months, and an exceptional patient may live as long as 48 months {248}.

Germ cell tumours

Definition
A neoplasm of germ cell origin classified by histologic type into seminoma (dysgerminoma), embryonal carcinoma, yolk sac tumour (endodermal sinus tumour), choriocarcinoma, and teratoma.

Epidemiology
Approximately 100 cases of intrapericardial germ cell tumours have been report-

ed, over 90% within the pericardium, and the remainder in the myocardium. The majority are pericardial teratomas {248}, and the remainder are yolk sac tumours {411,1178}. Reports of intrapericardial teratoma describing the presence of only one or two germ cell layers may represent misclassified bronchogenic cysts.

Clinical features
Patient age ranges from intrauterine life to 66 years {411}. Teratomas generally occur in infants while adults tend to have malignant germ cell tumours. Over 75% of cardiac teratomas occur in children under age 15. There is a slight female predominance. Symptoms include respiratory distress, pericardial tamponade, and cyanosis. Occasionally mediastinal teratomas in adults may secondarily involve the pericardium.

Due to the routine use of fetal echocardiography, an increasing number of pericardial teratomas are being diagnosed in second and third trimester fetuses {1615, 1786,2005}. Neonates may die at birth from cardiac tamponade and cardiac compression. Prenatal resection and intrauterine pericardiocentesis have been successfully accomplished {1615, 1935}.

Intramyocardial teratomas have occurred in the newborn period or in the first 6 years of life {1615}. Most patients are symptomatic and present with congestive heart failure; rarely, a patient may be asymptomatic, or sudden death may

be the first symptom, due to acute arrhythmia caused from the tumour's interventricular location.

Macroscopy
Cardiac teratomas may be massive, measuring up to 15 cm. They have a smooth surface and are lobulated. The tumours are multicystic with intervening solid areas. The tumours usually displace the heart and rotate it along its longitudinal axis. Intrapericardial teratomas are usually located on the right side of the heart, displacing the organs to the left and posteriorly; those located on the left side will produce the opposite effect. Teratomas are usually attached by a pedicle to one of the great vessels with arterial supply directly from the aorta.

Histopathology
Teratomas of the heart are similar to extracardiac teratomas. A minority of germ cell tumours of the pericardium are yolk sac tumours {248,411,1792}.

Histogenesis
The cell of origin of extragonadal teratoma, including pericardial teratoma, is the primordial germ cell. Although normal germ cells migrate from the yolk sac to the gonad, they may lodge early in embryogenesis in midline structures such as the mediastinum.

Treatment
Surgical excision is the only effective treatment for cardiac teratoma. Since the blood supply is usually from the root of the ascending aorta, the surgeon must perform a careful dissection and ligation of these vessels to prevent massive hemorrhage. Intracardiac teratomas, because of their location in the interventricular septum, are more difficult to remove than pericardial teratomas. Malignant germ cell tumours require standard chemotherapy.

Metastatic pericardial tumours

A high percentage of pericardial biopsies occur in patients in whom the diagnosis of malignancy has not yet been made, either for life-threatening tamponade or to establish the cause of pericarditis {1201,1499}. In about two-thirds of patients with positive pericardial biopsy, the clinical diagnosis is pericarditis,

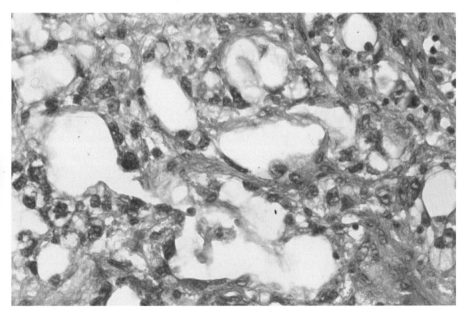

Fig. 4.43 Yolk sac tumour. The patient was a young woman with a pericardial mass, detected incidentally.

Table 4.03

Table 4.03
Malignant tumours diagnosed at pericardial biopsy {1201}.

Tumour type	Number	Fraction
Carcinoma	54	68%
Adenocarcinoma	32	40%
Squamous cell	14	18%
Large cell	7	9%
Small cell	1	1%
Lymphoma	12	15%
Sarcoma	7	9%
MFH	3	3%
Angiosarcoma	2	2%
Leiomyosarcoma	1	1%
Neurofibrosarcoma		
Thymoma	5	6%
Melanoma	2	2%
Total	**80**	**100%**

the lung or an undetermined primary site. Breast carcinoma, unlike lung carcinoma, usually manifests as pericardial disease only after the primary site is known. Other tumours found in pericardial biopsies include lymphoma, melanoma, multiple myeloma, thymoma, metastatic seminoma {121,249,1398}. The sites of origin of tumours discovered initially at pericardial biopsy are shown in Table 4.03.

The distinction between reactive mesothelial hyperplasia and metastatic carcinoma can be difficult, and is assisted by immunohistochemistry. The presence of carcinoembryonic antigen, berEP4, B72.3 antigen, and Leu M1 favour carcinoma over mesothelial hyperplasia. Calretinin and cytokeratin 5/6 reactivity favour the diagnosis of a mesothelial process.

The treatment of malignant pericardial disease includes establishing a pericardial window, sclerosis with tetracycline or other agents, and radiation therapy {1069}. Malignant pericardial effusions are generally a sign of rapidly progressive disease, necessitating emergency treatment. Patients with metastatic pericardial disease have a mean survival of 4.3 months {1201}. In contrast, patients

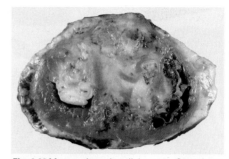

Fig. 4.44 Metastatic pericardial tumors. Gross large metastatic nodules in cardiac chambers and myocardium (renal cell carcinoma).

with pericardial malignant lymphoma or with involvement by thymoma often fare significantly better.

and in the remainder, tamponade. False negative biopsies may occur due to sampling, and it is not uncommon to have a positive cytology and a negative biopsy. Most adenocarcinomas presenting as pericardial metastases originate either in

Contributors

Dr. Seena AISNER
Department of Pathology, UMDNJ
New Jersey Medical School E-155
University Hospital
185 South Orange Avenue
Newark, NJ 07103 USA
Tel. +1 973 972 5726 / 5723
Fax. +1 973 972 5724
aisnersc@umdnj.edu

Dr. Philip A. ARAOZ
Department of Radiology
Mayo Clinic
200 First Street SW
Rochester MN 55905
USA
Tel. +1 507 255 8454 / 3853
Fax. +1 507 255 4068
araoz.philip@mayo.edu

Dr. Hisao ASAMURA
Division of Thoracic Surgery
National Cancer Center Hospital
5-1-1, Tsukiji, Chuo-ku
Tokyo, 104-0045
JAPAN
Tel. +81 3 3542 2511
Fax. +81 3 3542 3815
hasamura@ncc.go.jp

Dr. Marie-Christine AUBRY
Department of Pathology
Mayo Clinic
200 First Street
Rochester, MN 55905
USA
Tel. +1 507 284 1190
Fax. +1 507 284 1599
aubry.mariechristine@mayo.edu

Dr. P.M. BANKS
Department of Pathology & Lab. Medicine
Carolinas Medical Center
1000 Blythe blvd.
28203 Charlotte, NC
USA
Tel. +1 704 355 2251
Fax. +1 704 355 2156
peter.banks@carolinas.org

Dr. Mattia BARBARESCHI
Unità Operativa di Anatomia Patologica
Ospedale S. Chiara
Largo Medaglie d'Oro 9
38100 Trento
ITALY
Tel. +39 0461 903092
Fax. +39 0461 903389
barbareschi@tn.apss.tn.it

---

* The asterisk indicates participation
in the Working Group Meeting on the
WHO Classification of Tumours of the
Lung, Pleura, Thymus and Heart that
was held in Lyon, France, March 12-
16, 2003.

Dr. Helmut BARTSCH
Toxicology and Cancer Risk Factors
German Cancer Research Center (DKFZ)
Im Neuenheimer Feld 280
D-69120 Heidelberg
GERMANY
Tel. +49 6221 423 300
Fax. +49 6221 423 359
h.bartsch@dkfz-heidelberg.de

Dr. Craig T. BASSON
Greenberg Division of Cardiology,
Department of Medicine
Weill Medical College of Cornell University
525 E.68th Street
New York, NY 10021, USA
Tel. +1 212 746 2201
Fax. +1 212 746 2222
ctbasson@med.cornell.edu

Dr. Audrey S. BAUR
Institut Universitaire de Pathologie
25 Rue de Bugnon
CH-1011 Lausanne
SWITZERLAND
Tel. +41 21 314 7111
Fax. +41 21 314 7115
audrey.baur@hospvd.ch

Dr. Mary Beth BEASLEY
Dept. of Pathology
Providence Portland Medical Center
4805 N.E. Glisan St.
Portland, OR 97213
USA
Tel. +1 503 215 5778
Fax. +1 503 215 6855
marybeth.beasley@providence.org

Dr. Paolo BOFFETTA
Unit of Environmental Cancer Epidemiology
International Agency for
Research on Cancer (IARC)
150 cours Albert-Thomas
F-69008 Lyon, FRANCE
Tel. +33 4 72 73 84 41
Fax. +33 4 72 73 83 20
boffetta@iarc.fr

Dr. Carsten BOKEMEYER
Medizinische Universitätsklinik,
Universitätklinikum Tübingen
Otfried-Mueller-Str. 10
D-72076 Tübingen, GERMANY
Tel. +49 7071 29 82711
Fax. +49 7071 29 5332
carsten.bokemeyer@med.uni-
tuebingen.de

Dr. Félix BONILLA
Department of Medical Oncology
Hospital Universitario Puerta de Hierro
C/ San Martin de Porres, 4
28035 Madrid, SPAIN
Tel. +34 91 386 65 27
Fax. +34 91 373 76 67
felixbv@stnet.es

Dr. Michael BOROWITZ
Department of Pathology
Johns Hopkins Medical Institutions
Weinberg 2335
401 N Broadway
21232 Baltimore, MD, USA
Tel. +1 410 614 2889
Fax. +1 410 502 1493
mborowit@jhmi.edu

Dr. Christian BRAMBILLA
Service de Pneumologie
Centre Hospitalier Universitaire de
Grenoble
B.P. 217
38043 Grenoble, FRANCE
Tel. +33 4 76 76 55 91
Fax. +33 4 76 76 53 64
cbrambilla@chu-grenoble.fr

Dr. Elizabeth BRAMBILLA*
Département d'Anatomie et de
Cytologie Pathologique
Centre Hospitalier Universitaire, B.P. 217
F-38043 Grenoble Cedex 09
FRANCE
Tel. +33 4 76 76 54 86
Fax. +33 4 76 76 59 49
ebrambilla@chu-grenoble.fr

Dr. Allen BURKE*
Department of Pathology
Shady Grove Adventist Hospital
9901 Medical Center Dr.
20850 Rockville, MD, USA
Tel. +1 301 279 6097
Fax. +1 202 782 9021/
+1 301 217 5209
aburke1029@mac.com

Dr. Louise M. BURKE
Department of Histopathology
Cork University Hospital
Cork
IRELAND
Tel. +353 21 4922127 / 4922514
Fax. +353 21 4922774
burkel@shb.ie

Dr. Jagdish W. BUTANY
Department of Laboratory Medicine and
Pathobiology, E4-316
Toronto General Hospital
200 Elizabeth Street
M5G 2C4 Toronto, Ontario, CANADA
Tel. +1 416 340 3003
Fax. +1 416 586 9901
jagdish.butany@uhn.on.ca

Dr. Philip T. CAGLE*
Center for Pulmonary Pathology
Department of Pathology
Baylor College of Medicine
1 Baylor Plaza
Houston, TX 77030, USA
Tel. +1 713 394 6478
Fax. +1 713 798 3779
pcagle@bcm.tmc.edu

Dr. Federico CALIGARIS-CAPPIO
Dipartimento di Oncologia
Instituto Scientifico San Raffaele
Via Olgettina, 60
20132 Milano Mi
ITALY
Tel. +39 2 26432390
Fax. +39 2 26410154
caligaris.federico@hsr.it

Dr. Vera Luiza CAPELOZZI
Department of Surgical Pathology
Hospital Das Clinicas
University of Sao Paolo School of Medicine
Av. Dr. Arnaldo 455
01246-903 Sao Paolo SP, BRAZIL
Tel. +55 11 3064 2744
Fax. +55 11 5096 0761
vcapelozzi@lim05.fm.usp.br

Dr. Neil CAPORASO
National Cancer Institute EPS 7116
National Institutes of Health
6120 Executive Blvd
Bethesda, MD 20892 , USA
Tel. +1 301 496 4377
Fax. +1 301 402 4489
caporaso@nih.gov

Dr. Frédérique CAPRON
Service d'Anatomie et de Cytologie
Pathologiques, Hôpital de la Pitié
83, Boulevard de l'hôpital
75651 Paris Cedex 13, FRANCE
Tel. +33 1 42 17 77 74
Fax. +33 1 42 17 77 77
frederique.capron@psl.ap-hop-paris.fr

Dr. J.A. CARNEY
Department of Laboratory Medicine and
Pathology
Mayo Clinic
200 First Street SW
Rochester, MN USA 55905, USA
Tel. +1 507 284 2691
Fax. +1 507 284 5036
carney.aidan@mayo.edu

Dr. Lina CARVALHO
Anatomia Patologica
Hospitais da Universidade de Coimbra
Av. Bissaya Barreto
3000 Coimbra, PORTUGAL
Tel. +351 239 400 524
Fax. +351 239 835 451
lcarvalho@huc.min-saude.pt /
sap@huc.min-saude.pt

Dr. Alexander C.L. CHAN
Department of Pathology
Queen Elyzabeth Hospital
Wylie Road, Kowloon
Hong Kong,
SAR CHINA
Fax. +852 238 524 55
chancl@ha.org.hk

Dr. John K.C. CHAN
Department of Pathology
Queen Elizabeth Hospital
Wylie Road, Kowloon
Hong Kong
SAR CHINA
Tel. +852 2 958 6830
Fax. +852 2 385 2455
jkcchan@ha.org.hk

Dr. Yih-Leong CHANG
Department of Pathology
National Taïwan University Hospital
6F-1, 99, Section 3, Roosevelt Road
Taipei, 106
TAIWAN / CHINA
Tel. +886 2 2312 3456 (ext. 5460)
Fax. +886 2 2362 5176
damu@ha.mc.ntu.edu.tw

Dr. Gang CHEN
Department of Pathology
Shanghai Chest Hospital
241 Huai Hai Road West
200030 Shanghai
CHINA
Tel. +86 021 628 219 90 9616
Fax. +86 021 628 011 09
chengang888@online.sh.cn

Dr. Roberto CHIARLE
Department of Pathology
Hospital S. Giovanni Battista
Università di Torino
Via Santena 7,
I-10126 Torino, ITALY
Tel. +39 011 633 6860
Fax. +39 011 633 6500
roberto.chiarle@unito.it

Dr. Prem CHOPRA
Department of Pathology
All India Institute of Medical
Sciences (A.I.M.S.)
Ansari Nagar
110 029 New Delhi, INDIA
Tel.+91 11 6190067/6853600
Fax. + 91 11 2686 2663
premchopra@hotmail.com

Dr. Andrew CHURG*
Department of Pathology
University of British Columbia
2211 Wesbrook Mall
V6T2B5 Vancouver, BC
CANADA
Tel. +1 604 822 7775
Fax. +1 604 822 7635
achurg@interchange.ubc.ca

Dr. Thomas V. COLBY*
Department of Pathology
Mayo Clinic Scottsdale
13400 E. Shae Blvd
Scottsdale, AZ 85259, USA
Tel. +1 480 301 8021 /
+1 480 342 2456
Fax. +1 480 301 8372
colby.thomas@mayo.edu

Dr. Bryan CORRIN*
Imperial College School of Medicine
Royal Brompton Hospital
London, SW3 6NP
UNITED KINGDOM
Tel. +44 20 7351 8420
Fax. +44 20 7351 8293
b.corrin@imperial.ac.uk

Dr. David H. DAIL*
Department of Pathology
Virginia Mason Clinic C6 Path
1100 Ninth Ave.
Seattle, WA 98101
USA
Tel. +1 206 223 6861
Fax. +1 206 341 0525
david.dail@vmmc.org

Dr. Daphne DE JONG
Department of Pathology
The Netherlands Cancer Institute
Plesmanslaan 121
NL-1066 CX Amsterdam
THE NETHERLANDS
Tel. +31 20 512 2752
Fax. +31 20 512 2759
d.d.jong@nki.nl

Dr. Vincent T. DE MONTPREVILLE
Département de Pathologie
Centre Chirurgical Marie Lannelongue
133 Avenue de la Résistance
F-92350 Le Plessis Robinson
FRANCE
Tel. +33 1 40 94 28 07
Fax. +33 1 40 94 28 05
de-montpreville@ccml.com

Dr. Louis P. DEHNER
Department of Anatomic Pathology
Washington University School of Medicine
660 S.Euclid Ave.
Campus Box 8118
St Louis, MO 63110, USA
Tel. +1 314 362 0150
Fax. +1 314 362 0327
dehner@path.wustl.edu

**Dr. Mojgan DEVOUASSOUX-
SHISHEBORAN***
Département de Pathologie
Hôpital de la Croix Rousse
93 Grande Rue de la Croix Rousse
F-69317 Lyon, FRANCE
Tel. +33 4 72 07 18 75, Fax. +33 4 72 07 18 79
mojgan.devouassoux-shisheboran@chu-lyon.fr

Dr. T. DIJKHUIZEN
Department of Medical Genetics
University of Groningen
Antonius Deusinglaan 4
9713 AW Groningen
THE NETHERLANDS
Tel. +31 50 363 2925
Fax. +31 50 363 2947
t.dijkhuizen@medgen.azg.nl

Dr. Elizabeth DULMET
Département de Pathologie
Centre Chirurgical Marie Lannelongue
133 avenue de la Résistance
92350 Le Plessis-Robinson
FRANCE
Tel. +33 1 40 94 28 08
Fax. +33 1 40 94 28 05
dulmet@ccml.com

Dr. Alberto EDWARDS
Cardiovascular Center
University of Chili
Av. Santos Dumont 999, p.3-E
Santiago
CHILI
Tel. +56 2 737 1414
Fax. +56 2 737 1414
aedwards@ns.hospital.uchile.cl

Dr. Tadaaki EIMOTO
Department of Pathology
Nagoya City University Medical School
1 Kawasumi, Mizuho-ku
Nagoya 467 8601
JAPAN
Tel. +81 52 853 8161
Fax. +81 52 851 4166
teimoto@med.nagoya-cu.ac.jp

Dr. Dina EL-DEMELLAWY
Department of Laboratory Medicine and
Pathobiology, E4-316
Toronto General Hospital
200 Elizabeth Street
M5G 2C4 Toronto, Ontario, CANADA
Tel. +1 416 340 3003
Fax. +1 416 586 9901
din9@mail.com

Dr. Peter ENGEL
Department of Pathology
Roskilde County Hospital
Kogevej 7-13
DK-4000 Roskilde
DENMARK
Tel. +45 46 30 29 59
Fax. +45 46 35 29 83
rspen@ra.dk

Dr. Emilio Alvarez FERNANDEZ
Departamento de Anatomía Patológica
Hospital General "Gregorio Marañón"
c/ Dr. Esquerdo, 46
E-28007 Madrid
SPAIN
Tel. +34 91 586 81 63
Fax. +34 91 586 80 18
ealvarez.hgugm@salud.madrid.org

Dr. Sydney D. FINKELSTEIN
Redpath Integrated Pathology
816 Middle Street
Pittsburgh, PA 15212
USA
Tel. +1 412 231 3600
Fax. +1 412 231 2207
sdf@redpathip.com

Dr. Jonathan A. FLETCHER
Department of Pathology
Thorn 528
Brigham and Women's Hospital
75, Francis Street,
Boston, MA 02115, USA
Tel. +1 617 732 7883
Fax. +1 617 278 6921
jfletcher@partners.org

Dr. Douglas B. FLIEDER*
Department of Pathology and
Laboratory Medicine
New York-Presbyterian Hospital-Weill
Cornell Medical Center
525 East 68th Street
New York, NY 10021, USA
Tel. +1 212 746 2741, Fax. +1 212 746 8624
dbf2001@med.cornell.edu

Dr. Armando E. FRAIRE
Department of Pathology
University of Massachussets Medical
Center
55 Lake Avenue, North
Worcester, MA 01655, USA
Tel. +1 508 334 1395
Fax. +1 508 334 5775
fraireA@ummhc.org.

Dr. Wilbur A. FRANKLIN*
Department of Pathology
University of Colorado Health Sciences
Center, Campus Box B216
4200 East Nine Avenue
Denver, CO 80262, USA
Tel. +1 303 315 1807 / 7183
Fax. +1 303 315 1835
wilbur.franklin@uchsc.edu

Dr. Teri J. FRANKS
Department of Pulmonary and
Mediastinal Pathology
Armed Forces Institute of Pathology
6825 16th Street, NW
Washington, DC 20306-6000, USA
Tel. +1 202 782 1782
Fax. +1 202 782 5017
frankst@afip.osd.mil

Dr. Christopher A. FRENCH
Brigham and Women's Hospital
Depart. of pathology
75 Francis Street,
Boston, MA 02115
USA
Tel. +1 617 732 7483
Fax. +1 617 278 6996
cfrench@partners.org

Dr. Takeshi FUJII
Department of Pathology
International Medical Center of Japan
1-21-1 Toyama, Shinjuku
Tokyo 162-8655
JAPAN
Tel. +81 3 3202 7181 (ext. 5441)
Fax. +81 3 3207 1038
tafujii@imcj.hosp.go.jp

Dr. Masashi FUKAYAMA
Department of Pathology
University of Tokyo
7-3-1 Hongo, Bunkyo-ku
113-0033 Tokyo, JAPAN
Tel. +81 3 5841 3344
Fax. +81 3 5800 8785
mfukayama-tky@umin.ac.jp

Dr. Anthony GAL
Department of Pathology, Room H-171
Emory University Hospital
1364 Clifton Road, NE
Atlanta, GA 30322,
USA
Tel. +1 404 712 7320
Fax. +1 404 712 4754
E-mail agal@emory.edu

Dr. Françoise GALATEAU-SALLE*
Departement de Pathologie
Centre Hospitalier Regional et
Universitaire de Caen
Groupe Mesopath. PNSM-INVS
Côte de Nacre
F-14033 Caen, FRANCE
Tel. +33 2 31 06 44 07, Fax. +33 2 31 06 50 63
E-mail galateausalle-f@chu-caen.fr

Dr. Jeffrey GALVIN
Department of Radiologic Pathology
Armed Forces Institute of Pathology
6825, NW 16th Street,
Washington, DC 20306-6000
U.S.A.
Tel. +1 202 782 2155 / 2167
Fax. +1 202 782 0768
E-mail galvin@afip.osd.mil

Dr. Philippe GAULARD
Département de Pathologie
Hôpital Henri Mondor
51 Av du Maréchal de Lattre de Tassigny
F-94010 Créteil Cedex, FRANCE
Tel. + 33 1 49 81 27 43
Fax. +33 1 49 81 27 33
E-mail philippe.gaulard@hmn.ap-hop-
paris.fr

Dr. Adi F. GAZDAR*
Department of Pathology
Hamon Ctr. Ther. Onc. Res.
University of Texas Southwestern
Medical Center, Rm NB8-206
5323 Harry Hines Boulevard
Dallas, TX 75390-8593, USA
Tel. +1 214 648 4900, Fax. +1 214 648 4940
adi.gazdar@utsouthwestern.edu

Dr. Kim GEISINGER*
Department of Pathology
Wake Forest University School of Medicine
Medical Center Boulevard
Winston-Salem, NC 27157
USA
Tel. +1 336 716 2608
Fax. +1 336 716 7595
kgeis@wfubmc.edu

Dr. Tal GEVA
Department of Cardiology
Children's Hospital
Harvard Medical School
300 Longwood Avenue
02115 Boston, Masssachussets, USA
Tel. +1 617 355 6000/7655
Fax. +1 617 739 3784
tal.geva@chboston.org

Dr. Allen R. GIBBS*
Department of Histopathology
Llandough Hospital
Penlan Road South Glamorgan
Penarth, CF64 2XX
WALES UNITED KINGDOM
Tel. +44 29 207 15283
Fax. +44 29 207 12979
allen.gibbs@cardiffandvale.wales.nhs.uk

Dr. Ulrich GÖBEL
Clinic of Pediatric Oncology,
Hematology, and Immunology
Heinrich-Heine-Universität
Moorenstr. 5
D-40225 Düsseldorf, GERMANY
Tel. +49 211 81 17680
Fax. +49 211 81 16206
dominik.schneider@uni-duesseldorf.de

Dr. José Javier GOMEZ-ROMAN
Dpto Anatomia Patologica
Hospital Universitario Marqués de
Valdecilla
Avd. de Valdecilla s/n
E-39008 Santander, SPAIN
Tel. +34 942 20 33 90 / 25 20
Fax. +34 942 20 26 55 / 34 92
apagrj@humv.es

Dr. John R. GOSNEY
Department of Pathology
Duncan Building, 5th Floor
Royal Liverpool University Hospital
Daulby Street
Liverpool, L69 3GA, UNITED KINGDOM
Tel. +44 1 51 706 4490
Fax. +44 1 51 706 5859
john.gosney@rlbuht.nhs.uk

Dr. Daniel GRANDMOUGIN
Service de Chirurgie Cardio-Vasculaire
Hôpital Nord CHU
F-42055 St Etienne Cedex 2
FRANCE
Tel. +33 4 77 82 83 35
Fax. +33 4 77 82 84 53
daniel.grandmougin@chu-st-etienne.fr

Dr. Thomas GROGAN
Department of Pathology, rm 5212
Arizona Health Sciences Center
1501 N. Campbell Avenue
Tucson, AZ 85724
USA
Tel. +1 520 626 2212
Fax. +1 520 626 6081
tmgrogan@email.arizona.edu

Dr. DONALD G. GUINEE
Department of Pathology
Virginia Mason Clinic
1100 Ninth Avenue
Seattle, WA 98111
USA
Tel. +1 206 223 6861
Fax. +1 206 341 0525
donald.guinee@vmmc.org

Dr. Pierre HAINAUT
Unit oF Molecular Carcinogenesis
International Agency for
Research on Cancer (IARC)
150 cours Albert-Thomas
69372 Lyon, FRANCE
Tel. +33 4 72 73 85 32
Fax. +33 4 72 73 83 22
hainaut@iarc.fr

Dr. Samuel P. HAMMAR
Department of Pathology
Diagnostic Specialties Laboratory
700 Lebo boulevard
Bremerton, WA 98310, USA
Tel. +1 360 479 7707
Fax. +1 360 479 7886
shammar@hmh.westsound.net
shammar@comcast.net

Dr. Samir M. HANASH
Department of Pediatrics
University of Michigan Medical Center
A520 MSRB1
Ann Arbor, MI 48109-0718
USA
Tel. +1 734 763 9311
Fax. +1 734 647 8148
shanash@umich.edu

Dr. Curtis C. HARRIS
Laboratory of Human Carcinogenesis
National Cancer Institute
Center for Cancer Research
National Institutes of Health
Building 37, Room 3068
Bethesda, MD 20892-4255, USA
Tel. +1 301 496 2048, Fax. +1 301 496 0497
curtis_harris@nih.gov

Dr. Nancy Lee HARRIS*
Department of Pathology
Massachussets General Hospital
55 Fruit Street, WRN 219
Boston, MA 02114-2699
USA
Tel. +1 617 726 5155
Fax. +1 617 726 9353
nlharris@partners.org

Dr. J.T. HARTMANN
Department of Hematology / Oncology
Eberhard-Karls-University Tuebingen
Otfried-Mueller-Strasse 10
72076 Tuebingen
GERMANY
Tel. +49 7071 29 82127
Fax. +49 7071 29 5689
joerg.hartmann@med.uni-tuebingen.de

Dr. Philip S. HASLETON*
Pulmonary Pathology
Wythenshawe Hospital, University of
Manchester School of Medicine
Southmoor Road
Manchester, M23 9 LT, UNITED KINGDOM
Tel. +44 161 291 2144 / 2122
Fax. +44 161 291 2125
philip.hasleton@man.ac.uk

Dr. Aage HAUGEN
Department of Toxicology
National Institute of Occupational Health
P.O. Box 8149 Dep
N-0033 Oslo
NORVEGE
Tel. +47 23 19 52 70
Fax. +47 23 19 52 03
age.haugen@stami.no

Dr. Douglas W. HENDERSON
Anatomical Pathology Department
Flinders University School of Medicine
Flinders Medical Center
Bedford Park 5042
AUSTRALIA
Tel. +618 8204 5135 / 4414
Fax. +618 8374 1437
douglas.henderson@flinders.edu.au

Dr. Kristin HENRY
Department of Histopathology
Imperial College London
Charing Cross Hospital
Fulham Palace Road
London, W6 8 RF, UNITED KINGDOM
Tel. +44 208 846 7133
Fax. +44 208 846 1364
k.henry@imperial.ac.uk

Dr. Claudia I. HENSCHKE
Department of Radiology
Weill Medical College of Cornell University
525 East 68th Street, J-030
New York, NY 10021
USA
Tel. +1 212 746 2529
Fax. +1 212 746 2811
chensch@med.cornell.edu

Dr. Elizabeth P. HENSKE
Department of Medical Oncology
Fox Chase Cancer Center
7701 Burholme Avenue
Philadelphia, Pa 19111
USA
Tel. +1 215 728 2428
Fax. +1 215 214 1623
elizabeth.henske@fccc.edu

Dr. Hiroaki HIRAGA
Dep. of Clinical Research
Division of Orthopedics
Hokkaido Cancer Center
Kikusui 4-2, Shiroishi-Ward
003-0804 Sapporo, JAPAN
Tel. +81 11 811 9111
Fax. +81 11 811 9159
hhiraga@sap-cc.go.jp

Dr. Fred R. HIRSCH*
Department of Pathology
University of Colorado
Health Sciences Center
4200 East Ninth Avenu
Denver, CO 80262, USA
Tel. +1 303 315 1814
Fax. +1 303 315 1835 / 3304
fred.hirsch@uchsc.edu

Dr. Tsunekazu HISHIMA
Department of Pathology
Tokyo Metropolitan Komagome Hospital
3-18-22 Honkomagome
113-8677 Bunkyo-ku, Tokyo
JAPAN
Tel. +81 3 3823 2101 ext 4410
Fax. +81 3 4463 7561
hishima@cick.jp

Dr. Masashi HORIMOTO
Division of Cardiovascular Disease
Chitose City Hospital
Hokko 2-1-1
Chitose City, 066-8550
JAPAN
Tel. +81 123 24 3000
Fax. +81 123 24 3005
masashi.horimoto@city.chitose.hokkaido.jp

Dr. Hiroshi INAGAKI
Department of Pathology
Nagoya City University School of Medicine
1 Kawasumi, Mizuho-ku
Nagoya, 467-8601
JAPAN
Tel. +81 52 853 8161
Fax. +81 52 851 4166
hinagaki@med.nagoya-cu.ac.jp

Dr. Kouki INAI
Department of Pathology
Hiroshima University School of Medicine
1-2-3 Kasumi Minami Ku
734-8551 Hiroshima
JAPAN
Tel. +81 82 257 5150
Fax. +81 82 257 5154
koinai@hiroshima-u.ac.jp

Dr. Masayoshi INOUE
Department of General Thoracic
Surgery (E1)
Osaka University Graduate School of
Medicine
2-2 Yamadaoka, Suita
Osaka 565-0871, JAPAN
Tel. +81 6 6879 3152, Fax. +81 6 6879 3164
masa@surg1.med.osaka-u.ac.jp

Dr. Elaine S. JAFFE
Laboratory of Pathology
Hematopathology Section
National Cancer Institute, NIH
10 Center Drive, MSC 1500
Bethesda, MD 20892-1500, USA
Tel. +1 301 496 0183
Fax. +1 301 402 2415
elainejaffe@nih.gov

Dr. Nirmala A. JAMBHEKAR
Department of Pathology 8th Floor
Tata Memorial Hospital Annexe Building
Dr. Ernest Borges Road, Parel
400 012 Mumbai / Bombay
INDIA
Tel. +91 22 2414 6750
Fax. +91 22 2414 6937
najambhekar@rediffmail.com

Dr. Jin JEN
Laboratory of Population Genetics
Center for Cancer Research
National Cancer Institute
41 Library Drive, Rm D702
Bethesda, MD 20892, USA
Tel. +1 301 435 8958
Fax. +1 301 435 8963
jenj@mail.nih.gov

Dr. S.X. JIANG
Department of Pathology
Kitasato University School of Medicine
1-15-1 Kitasato, Sagamihara
Kanagawa, 228-8555
JAPAN
Tel. +81 42 778 9020
Fax. +81 42 778 9123
sxjiang@med.kitasato-u.ac.jp

Dr. Hiroyuki KAMIYA
Department of General and
Cardiothoracic Surgery
Kanazawa University Hospital
Takaramachi 13-1
Kanazawa 920-8641, JAPAN
Tel. +81 76 265 2355
Fax. +81 76 222 6833
h.kamiya88@yahoo.co.jp

Dr. Toshiaki KAWAI
Department of Pathology
National Defense Medical College
3 Tokorozawa, 359 Saitama
JAPAN
Tel. +81 42 995 1505
Fax. +81 42 996 5192
tkawai@cc.ndmc.ac.jp

Dr. Keith M. KERR*
Department of Pathology
Aberdeen University Medical School
Aberdeen Royal Infirmary, Foresterhill
Aberdeen, AB25 2ZD
UNITED KINGDOM
Tel. +44 1 224 552 414
Fax. +44 1 224 663 002
k.kerr@abdn.ac.uk

Dr. Andras KHOOR
Department of Pathology
Mayo Clinic
4500 San Pablo Road
Jacksonville, FL 32224
USA
Tel. +1 904 296 3745
Fax. +1 904 296 5904
khoor.andras@mayo.edu

Dr. Hitoshi KITAMURA
Department of Pathology
Yokohama City University
Graduate School of Medicine
3-9 Fukuura, Kanazawa-ku
Yokohama, 236-0004 , JAPAN
Tel. +81 45 787 2581 / 2583
Fax. +81 45 789 0588
pathola@med.yokohama-cu.ac.jp

Dr. Paul KLEIHUES
Department of Pathology
University Hospital
Schmelzbergstr. 12
CH-8091 Zurich
SWITZERLAND
Tel. +41 1 255 3516
Fax. +41 1 255 2525
paul.kleihues@usz.ch

Dr. Michael N. KOSS
Department of Pathology
Keck School of Medicine
University of Southern California
Hoffman Building Rm 209
2011 Zonal Avenue
Los Angeles, CA 90033, USA
Tel. +1 323 226 6507, Fax. +1 323 226 7069
mnkoss@earthlink.net

Dr. Tseng-tong KUO*
Department of Pathology
Chang Gung Memorial Hospital
199 Tun Hwa Road
Taipei, 105
TAIWAN / CHINA
Tel. +886 3 328 1200 (Ext. 2727)
Fax. +886 3 328 0147
ttkuo@cgmh.org.tw

Dr. Michael O. KURRER
Department of Pathology
University Hospital Zurich
Schmelzbergstr. 12
CH-8091 Zürich
SWITZERLAND
Tel. +41 1 255 3922
Fax. +41 1 255 4416
michael.kurrer@usz.ch

Dr. R. Hubert LAENG
Department of Pathology
Kantonsspital Aarau
Buchserstrasse
CH-5001 Aarau
SWITZERLAND
Tel. +41 62 838 6105
Fax. +41 62 838 5299
laeng@ksa.ch

Dr. Stephen LAM
Department of Respiratory Medicine
British Columbia Cancer Agency and the
University of British Columbia
601 West, 10th Avenue
V5Z 4E6 Vancouver BC, CANADA
Tel. +1 604 877 6098 (ext.2080)
Fax. +1 604 875 5799
sclam@interchange.ubc.ca

Dr. Sylvie LANTUEJOUL
Département d'Anatomie et Cytologie
Pathologique
Centre Hospitalier Universitaire, B.P. 217
F-38043 Grenoble Cedex 09
FRANCE
Tel. +33 4 76 76 54 86
Fax. +33 4 76 76 59 49
slantuejoul@chu-grenoble.fr

Dr. Kevin LESLIE
Department of Laboratory Medicine
and Pathology
Mayo Clinic Scottsdale
13400 E. Shae Boulevard
Scottsdale, AZ 85259, USA
Tel. +1 480 301 8021
Fax. +1 480 301 8372
leslie.kevin@mayo.edu

Dr. Robert LOIRE*
17, rue du Clos Bergier
F-69660 Collonges au Mont d'Or
FRANCE
Tel. +33 4 78 22 59 07

Dr. Emilio MAIERS
Cardiovascular Center
University of Chili
Av Santos Dumont 999, p. 3-E
Santiago
CHILE
Tel. +56 2 271 6241
Fax. +56 2 271 6241
maiers@vtr.net

Dr. Toshiaki MANABE
Laboratory of Anatomic Pathology
Kyoto University Hospital
54, Shogoin Kawahara-cho, Sakyo-ku
606-8507 Kyoto
JAPAN
Tel. +81 75 751 3488 / 3520
Fax. +81 75 751 4948
manabet@kuhp.kyoto-u.ac.jp

Dr. Alberto M. MARCHEVSKY
Department of Pathology and
Laboratory Medicine
Cedars-Sinai Medical Center
8700 Beverly Boulevard
Los Angeles, CA 90048-1869, USA
Tel. +1 310 423 6629 / 6621
Fax. +1 310 423 0122
marchevsky@cshs.org

Dr. Mirella MARINO
Department of Pathology
Regina Elena Cancer Institute
Via E. Chianesi, 53
I-00144 Roma
ITALY
Tel. +39 06 5266 5581
Fax. +39 06 5266 6102/5523
mirellamarino@inwind.it

Dr. Alexander MARX*
Department of Pathology
University of Wuerzburg
Josef-Schneider-Strasse 2
97080 Wuerzburg
GERMANY
Tel. +49 931 201 47 421 / 420
Fax. +49 931 201 47 505
alex.marx@mail.uni-wuerzburg.de

Dr. Akira MASAOKA
Second Department of Surgery
Nagoya City University
Nagoya, 467-8602
JAPAN
Tel. +81 52 853 8231
Fax. +81 52 853 6440

Dr. Yoshihiro MATSUNO
Cytopathology Section
National Cancer Center Hospital
1-1 Tsukiji 5-chome, Chuo-ku
104-0045 Tokyo
JAPAN
Tel. +81 3 3542 2511 (ext 7096}
Fax. +81 3 3248 2463
ymatsuno@ncc.go.jp

Dr. Frank MAYER
Abteilung für Onkologie,
Medizinische Klinik
Universität Tübingen
Otfried-Mueller-Str. 10
D-72076 Tübingen, GERMANY
Tel. +49 7071 298 2711,
Fax. +49 7071 29 5332
frank.mayer@med.uni-tuebingen.de

Dr. Fabio MENESTRINA*
Inst. di Anatomia Patologica
Università degli Studi di Verona
Policlinico G.B. Rossi
P.le L.A. Scuro n.10
I-37134 Verona, ITALY
Tel. +39 045 8027135 / 8074323
Fax. +39 045 8027136
f.menestrina@univr.it

Dr. Matthew MEYERSON
Department of Adult Oncology
Dana-Farber Cancer Institute
Harvard Medical School
44 Binney Street
Boston, MA 02115, USA
Tel. +1 617 632 4768
Fax. +1 617 582 7880
matthew_meyerson@dfci.harvard.edu

Dr. Markku MIETTINEN
Department of Soft Tissue Pathology
Armed Forces Institute of Pathology
6825, 16th Street, N.W.
Washington, DC 20306-6000
USA
Tel. +1 202 782 2793
Fax. +1 202 782 9182
miettinen@afip.osd.mil

Dr. Thierry J. MOLINA
Service Central d'Anatomie et de
Cytologie Pathologiques
Hotel Dieu
1 Place du Parvis Notre Dame
F-75181 Paris cedex 04, FRANCE
Tel. +33 1 42 34 82 82
Fax. +33 1 42 34 86 41
thierry.molina@htd.ap-hop-paris.fr

Dr. Peter MÖLLER*
Institute of Pathology
University Hospital
University of Ulm
Albert-Einstein-Allee 11
D-89081 Ulm, GERMANY
Tel. +49 731 50023320
Fax. +49 731 50023884
peter.moeller@medizin.uni-ulm.de

Dr. Cesar MORAN
Department of Pathology
MD Anderson Cancer Center
1515 Holcombe Boulevard
Houston, TX 77030, USA
Tel. +1 713 792 8134
Fax. +1 713 792 4094 /
+1 713 745 3740
cesarmoran@mdanderson.org

Dr. Kiyoshi MUKAI
Department of Diagnostic Pathology
Tokyo Medical University
Nishi-Shinjuku 6-7-1, Shinjuku-ku
160-0023 Tokyo
JAPAN
Tel. +81 3 3342 6111 (Ext.5933)
Fax. +81 3 3342 7717
kmukai@tokyo-med.ac.jp

Dr. Klaus-Michael MÜLLER
Bergmannsheil University Hospital
Institute of Pathology
Bürkle-de-la-Camp-Platz 1
D-44789 Bochum
GERMANY
Tel. +49 234 302 6600
Fax. +49 234 302 6671
patho-bhl@ruhr-uni-bochum.de

Dr. H. Konrad MÜLLER-HERMELINK*
Department of Pathology
University of Würzburg
Josef-Schneider-Strasse 2
D-97080 Würzburg
GERMANY
Tel. + 49 931 201 47776/47777
Fax. + 49 931 201 47440
path062@mail.uni-wuerzburg.de

Dr. Shigeo NAKAMURA
Department of Pathology
Aichi Cancer Center
1-1 Kanokoden, Chikusa-ku
464-8681 Nagoya
JAPAN
Tel. +81 52 762 6111.
Fax. +81 52 763 5233
snakamur@aichi-cc.jp

Dr. Yukio NAKATANI
Department of Basic Pathology
Chiba University Graduate
School of Medicine
1-8-1 Inohana, Chuo-ku
Chiba, 260-8670, JAPAN
Tel. +81 43 222 7171
Fax. +81 43 226 2013
nakatani@ma.kcom.ne.jp

Dr. Oscar NAPPI
U.O.C. di Anatomia Patologica
Azienda Ospedaliera A. Cardarelli
Via A. Cardarelli 9
I-80131 Napoli NA
ITALY
Tel. +39 081 747 3550 / 3541 / 3542
Fax. +39 081 747 3550
oscarnappi@tin.it

Dr. Andrew G. NICHOLSON*
Department of Histopathology
Royal Brompton Hospital
Sydney Street
London SW3 6NP
UNITED KINGDOM
Tel. +44 20 7351 8425
Fax. +44 20 7351 8293
a.nicholson@rbh.nthames.nhs.uk

Dr. Siobhan NICHOLSON
Department of Histopathology
Central Pathology Laboratory
St James's Hospital
James's Street
Dublin 8, IRELAND
Tel. +353 1 416 2903 / 2992
Fax. +353 1 410 3514
snicholson@stjames.ie

Dr. Seiji NIHO
Division of Thoracic Oncology
National Cancer Center Hospital East
6-5-1, Kashiwanoha, Kashiwa
277-8577 Chiba
JAPAN
Tel. +81 4 7133 1111
Fax. +81 4 7131 4724
siniho@east.ncc.go.jp

Dr. Masayuki NOGUCHI*
Department of Pathology
Institute of Basic Medical Sciences
University of Tsukuba
1-1-1 Tennodai, Tsukuba-shi
305-8575 Ibaraki, JAPAN
Tel. +81 29 853 3750
Fax. +81 29 853 3150
nmasayuk@md.tsukuba.ac.jp

Dr. N. Paul OHORI
Department of Pathology
University of Pittsburgh Medical
Center Presbyterian, A610
200 Lothrop Street
Pittsburgh, PA 15213-2582, USA
Tel. +1 412 647 9843 / 3478
Fax. +1 412 647 3455
ohorinp@msx.upmc.edu

Dr. Attilio ORAZI
Department of Pathology
Division of Hematopathology, Room 0969
Indiana University Medical Center
Riley Hospital
702 Barrhill Drive
Indianapolis, IN 46202-5200, USA
Tel. +1 317 274 7250, Fax. +1 317 274 0149
aorazi@iupui.edu

Dr. Nelson G. ORDONEZ
Department of Pathology
MD Anderson Cancer Center
1515 Holcombe Boulevard
Houston, TX 77030
USA
Tel. +1 713 792 3167
Fax. +1 713 792 3696 / +1-713 745 3501
nordonez@mdanderson.org

Dr. Giorgio PALESTRO
Dipartimento di Scienze Biomediche e
Oncologia Umana
Università di Torino
Via Santena 7
I-10126 Torino, ITALY
Tel. +39 11 670 65 17
Fax. +39 11 633 65 00
giorgio.palestro@unito.it

Dr. D. Maxwell PARKIN
Unit of Descriptive Epidemiology
International Agency for
Research on Cancer (IARC)
150, cours Albert Thomas
69372 Lyon Cedex 08, FRANCE
Tel. +33 4 72 73 84 82
Fax. +33 4 72 73 86 96
parkin@iarc.fr

Dr. Chandrakant R. PATEL
Heart Center
Children's Hospital Medical
Center of Akron
1 Perkins Square
Akron, OH 44308, USA
Tel. +1 330 543 8030
Fax. +1 330 543 8311
cpatel@chmca.org

Dr. Elizabeth J. PERLMAN
Department of Pathology
Children's Memorial Hospital
2300, Children's Plaza, Box 17
IL 60614 Chicago
USA
Tel. +1 773 880 4306
Fax. +1 773 880 3858
eperlman@childrensmemorial.org

Dr. Iver PETERSEN
Institute of Pathology
University Hospital Charité
Humboldt-University
Schumannstrasse 20-21
D-10098 Berlin, GERMANY
Tel. +49 30 450 536 050,
Fax. +49 30 450 536 902
iver.petersen@charite.de

Dr. Nicolai PETROVITCHEV
Department of Pathology
Cancer Research Center
Kashirskoye Street 24
Moscow, 115478
RUSSIA
Tel. +7 095 324 96 44
Fax. +7 095 323 57 10
n_petrovichev@mtu-net.ru

Dr. Stefano A. PILERI
Pathology and Haematopathology
Institute of Haematology and
Clinical Oncology "Seragnoli"
Bologna University
Via Massarenti 9
I-40138 Bologna, ITALY
Tel. +39 051 6363044, Fax. +39 051 6363606
pileri@med.unibo.it

Dr. Helmut POPPER
Institute of Pathology
University of Graz School of Medicine
Auenbruggerplatz 25
A-8036 Graz
AUSTRIA
Tel. +43 316 380 4405
Fax. +43 316 384 329
helmut.popper@meduni-graz.at

Dr. Marlene PRAET
Department of Pathology, Blok A 503
University Hospital
De Pintelaan, 185
9000 Ghent
B-BELGIUM
Tel. +32 92 40 36 64
Fax. +32 92 40 49 65
marleen.praet@ugent.be

Dr. Robert PUGATCH
Department of Diagnostic Radiology
University of Maryland Medical System
22 South Greene Street
Baltimore, MD 21201-1595
USA
Tel. +1 410 328 3938
Fax. +1 410 328 0641
rpugatch@umm.edu

Dr. D.J. RADFORD
The Prince Charles Hospital
Queensland Centre for
Congenital Heart Disease
The Prince Charles Hospital
Rode Road
Chermside, QLD 4032, AUSTRALIA
Tel. +61 7 3350 8111, Fax. +61 7 3350 8715
dorothy_radford@health.qld.gov.au

Dr. Ramón RAMI-PORTA
Thoracic Surgery Service
Hospital Mutua de Terrassa
Plaça Dr. Robert 5
08221 Barcelona (Terrassa)
SPAIN
Tel. +34 93 736 5050
Fax. +34 93 736 5059
rramip@teleline.es

Dr. Angela RISCH
Toxicology and Cancer Risk Factors
DKFZ - Deutsches Krebsforschungszentrum
Im Neuenheimer Feld 280
69120 Heidelberg, GERMANY
Tel. +49 6221 42 43 22
Fax. +49 6221 42 43 23
a.risch@dkfz-heidelberg.de

Dr. Victor ROGGLI*
Department of Pathology (113) Rm F3196
Durham VA and
Duke University Medical Center
508 Fulton
Durham, N.C. 27705, USA
Tel. +1 919 286 0411 X6615
Fax. +1 919 286 6818
roggl002@mc.duke.edu

Dr. Giovanni ROLLA
Department of Human Oncology
University of Torino
Ospedale Mauriziano Umberto I
Largo Turati 62
10128 Torino, ITALY
Tel. +39 011 5082 083
Fax. +39 011 5682 588
giovanni.rolla@unito.it

Dr. Juan ROSAI
Dipartimento di Patologia
Istituto Nazionale Tumori
Via Venezian,1
I-20133 Milano
ITALY
Tel. +39 02 2390 2876
Fax. +39 02 2390 2877
juan.rosai@istitutotumori.mi.it

Dr. Andreas Rosenwald
Institute of Pathology
University of Würzburg
Josef-Schneider-Strasse 2
D-97080 Würzburg
GERMANY
Tel. +49 931 201 47 424
Fax. +49 931 201 47 440
rosenwald@mail.uni-wuerzburg.de

Dr. Giulio ROSSI
Dipartimento di Scienze Morfologiche
Sezione di Anatomia Patologica
University of Modena and Reggio Emilia
Via del Pozzo, 71
I-41100 Modena, ITALY
Tel. +39 059 422 38 90
Fax. +39 059 422 48 20
rossi.giulio@unimo.it

Dr. Thomas RÜDIGER
Department of Pathology,
University of Würzburg
Josef-Schneider-Str. 2
97080 Würzburg
GERMANY
Tel. +49 931 201 47783
Fax. +49 931 888 7518
thomas.ruediger@mail.uni-wuerzburg.de

Dr. Valerie RUSCH
Thoracic Service
Memorial Sloan-Kettering Cancer Center
1275 York Avenue
New York, N.Y. 10021
USA
Tel. +1 212 639 8695
Fax. +1 212 717 3682
ruschv@mskcc.org

Dr. Jonathan M. SAMET
Department of Epidemiology
Bloomberg School of Public Health
The John Hopkins University
615 N. Wolfe Street, Ste W6041
Baltimore, MD 21205-2179, USA
Tel. +1 410 955 3286
Fax. +1 410 614 0467
jsamet@jhsph.edu

Dr. Rodolfo SARACCI
International Agency for Research on
Cancer (IARC)
150 cours Albert-Thomas
F-69008 Lyon, FRANCE
Tel. +33 4 72 73 84 08
Fax. +33 4 72 73 83 61
saracci@iarc.fr

Dr. Dominik T. SCHNEIDER
Clinic of Pediatric Oncology,
Hematology, and Immunology
Heinrich-Heine-University
Moorenstr. 5,
D-40225 Duesseldorf, GERMANY
Tel. +49 211 81 16491
Fax. +49 211 81 16206
dominik.schneider@uni-duesseldorf.de

Dr. Mary N. SHEPPARD
Department of Histopathology
Royal Brompton National Heart
and Lung Hospital
Sydney Street
London SW3 6NP, UNITED KINGDOM
Tel. +44 207 351 8424 / 8423 / 8420
Fax. +44 207 351 8293 / 8435
m.sheppard@rbh.nthames.nhs.uk

Dr. Peter G. SHIELDS
Cancer Genetics and Epidemiology
Lombardi Cancer Center
Georgetown University Medical Center
3800 Reservoir Rd., NW. Rm. 150,
Washington, DC 20057-1465, USA
Tel. +1 202 687 0003
Fax. +1 202 687 0004
pgs2@georgetown.edu

Dr. Yukio SHIMOSATO*
4-26-1-603 Minamiogikubo Suginamiku
167-0052 Tokyo
JAPAN
Tel. +81 3 3331 0603
Fax. +81 3 3331 0603
uhi55656@nifty.com

Dr. Ivy SNG
Singapore General Hospital
Department of Pathology
Outram Road
Singapore 169608
SINGAPORE
Tel. +65 6321 4926
Fax. +65 6222 6826
gptsng@sgh.com.sg

Dr. Leslie H. SOBIN*
Department of Hepatic and
Gastrointestinal Pathology
Armed Forces Institute of Pathology
14th Street and Alaska Avenue
Washington, DC 20306, USA
Tel. +1 202 782 2880
Fax. +1 202 782 9020
sobin@afip.osd.mil

Dr. Gabriella SOZZI
Molecular Cytogenetics Unit
Department of Experimental Oncology
Istituto Nazionale Tumori
Via Venezian 1
20133 Milano, ITALY
Tel. +39 02 23902232 / 2643
Fax. +39 02 23902764
gabriella.sozzi@istitutotumori.mi.it

Dr. Philipp STRÖBEL
Department of Pathology
University of Würzburg
Josef-Schneider-Strasse 2
D-97080 Würzburg
GERMANY
Tel. +49 931 201 47878
Fax. +49 931 201 47440
philipp.stroebel@mail.uni-wuerzburg.de

Dr. Saul SUSTER
Department of Pathology E 409 Doan Hall
The Ohio State University Medical Center
410 W. Tenth Avenue
Colombus (Ohio), 43210-1228
USA
Tel. +1 614 293 7625
Fax. +1 614 293 7626
suster.3@osu.edu

Dr. Takashi TAKAHASHI
Division of Molecular Oncology
Aichi Cancer Center Research Institute
1-1 Kanokoden, Chikusa-Ku
Nagoya 464-8681
JAPAN
Tel. +81 52 764 2983/2993
Fax. +81 52 764 2983
tak@aichi-cc.jp

Dr. Hisashi TATEYAMA
Department of Pathology
Nagoya City University Medical School
1 Kawasumi, Mizuho-ku
Nagoya 467-8601
JAPAN
Tel. +81 52 853 8161
Fax. +81 52 851 4166
htate@med.nagoya-cu.ac.jp

Dr. Henry TAZELAAR*
Department of Pathology
Mayo Clinic
200 First St., SW
Rochester, MN 55905, USA
Tel. +1 507 284 1192 /
+1 507 284 6348 direct
Fax. +1 507 284 1875 /1599
tazelaar.henry@mayo.edu

Dr. Joseph R. TESTA
Human Genetics Program
Fox Chase Cancer Center
333 Cottman Avenue
Philadelphia, PA 19111, USA
Tel. +1 215 728 2610
Fax. +1 215 214 1623
jr_testa@fccc.edu

Dr. Françoise THIVOLET-BEJUI*
Service d' Anatomie et Cytologie
Pathologiques
Hôpital Louis Pradel
28, Avenue Doyen Jean Lepine
69677 Bron Cedex, FRANCE
Tel. +33 4 72 11 80 74
Fax. +33 4 72 35 73 47
francoise.thivolet-bejui@chu-lyon.fr

Dr. F.B. THUNNISSEN
Department of Pathology C66
Canisius Wilhelmina Ziekenhuis
PO BOX 9015
6500 GS Nijmegen
THE NETHERLANDS
Tel. +31 24 365 8510
Fax. +31 24 365 8844
e.thunnissen@cwz.nl

Dr. Joseph F. TOMASHEFSKI, JR.
Department of Pathology
MetroHealth Medical Center
2500 MetroHealth Drive
Cleveland, OH 44109
USA
Tel. +1 216 778 5181
Fax. +1 216 778 7112
jtomashefski@metrohealth.org

Dr. Marketa TOMSOVA
The Fingerland Department of Pathology
Charles University Faculty of Medicine and
Faculty Hospital
CZ-500 05 Hradec Králové
CZECH REPUBLIC
Tel. +42 049 583 3187
Fax. +42 049 583 2004
tomsovam@lfhk.cuni.cz

Dr. G. TORNAMBENE
Cattedra di Neonatologia Pediatrica E
U.O. Cardiologia Pediatrica
Università di Catania
Via S. Sofia 78
I-95125 Catania, ITALY
Tel. +39 095 580578 / 580448
Fax. +39 095 223068
giacomotornambene@tin.it

Dr. WILLIAM D. TRAVIS*
Dept. of Pulmonary &
Mediastinal Pathology, Bld 54, Rm 2071
Armed Forces Institute of Pathology
6825 NW 16th St.
Washington, DC 20306-6000
USA
Tel. +1 202 782 1781, Fax. +1 202 782 5016
travis@afip.osd.mil

Dr. S. TSUKAMOTO
Second Department of Surgery
Nihon UniversIty School of Medicine
30-1 Oyaguchi-Kamimachi, Itabashi-Ku
173-8610 Tokyo
JAPAN
Tel. +81 03 3972 8111
Fax. +81 3 3955 9818
tsuka@tdmc.hosp.go.jp

Dr. Jerzy E. TYCZYNSKI
Cancer Prevention Institute
41000 S. Kettering Blvd
Dayton, OH 45439
USA
Tel. +1 937 293 8508
Fax. +1 937 293 7652
tyczynski@hotmail.com

Dr. James W. VARDIMAN
Department of Pathology
University of Chicago Medical Center
5841 South Maryland Ave., MC0008 Rm
TW-055
Chicago IL 60637-1470, USA
Tel. +1 773 702 6196
Fax. +1 773 702 1200
jvardima@uchospitals.edu

Dr. Madeline F. VAZQUEZ
Department of Cytopathology
New York Presbyterian Hospital
Weill Medical College of Cornell University
525 East 68th Street
New York, NY 10021, USA
Tel. +1 212 746 2766
Fax. +1 212 746 8359
mfv2001@mail.med.cornell.edu

Dr. John P. VEINOT
Department of Laboratory Medicine, Rm 123
Ottawa Heart Institute
Ottawa Hospital, Civic Campus
1053 Carling Avenue
Ottawa, Ontario K1Y 4E9, CANADA
Tel. +1 613 761 4344
Fax. +1 613 761 4846
jpveinot@ottawahospital.on.ca

Dr. Jean-Michel VIGNAUD
Laboratoire d'Anatomie Pathologique
Centre Hospitalier Universitaire de Nancy
Hôpital Central
29, Av. du Maréchal de Lattre de Tassigny
F-54035 Nancy, FRANCE
Tel. +33 3 83 85 13 51
Fax. +33 3 83 85 13 31
jm.vignaud@chu-nancy.fr

Dr. Paolo VINEIS
Dipartimento di Scienze Biomediche e
Oncologia Umana
Università di Torino e CPO-Piemonte
Via Santena 7
I-10126 Torino, ITALY
Tel. +39-011 6706525 / 6702526
Fax. +39-011 6706692
paolo.vineis@unito.it

Dr. Renu VIRMANI
Department of Cardiovascular Pathology
Armed Forces Institute of Pathology (AFIP)
6825 16th Street, NW
Washington, DC 20306-6000
USA
Tel. +1 202 782 2844
Fax. +1 202 782 9021
virmani@afip.osd.mil

Dr. Peter VOGT
Department of Pathology
University Hospital
Schmelzbergstrasse 12
CH-8091 Zürich
SWITZERLAND
Tel. +41 1 255 25 24
Fax. +41 1 255 45 51
peter.vogt@usz.ch

Dr. Paul WALTER
Service d'Anatomie Pathologique
Hôpital Hautepierre
Avenue Moliere
67098 Strasbourg Cedex
FRANCE
Tel. +33 3 88 12 70 49
Fax. +33 3 88 12 70 52
paul.walter@chru-strasbourg.fr

Dr. R.A. WARNKE
Department of Pathology
Stanford University Medical Center
300 Pasteur Dr., Rm. L235
94305-5324 Stanford, California
Tel. +1 650 725 5167
Fax. +1 650 725 6902
rwarnke@stanford.edu

Dr. Go WATANABE
Department of General and
Cardiothoracic Surgery
Kanazawa University School of Medicine
13-1 Takara-machi
920-8641 Kanazawa, JAPAN
Tel. +81 76 265 2354
Fax. +81 76 222 6833
go@med.kanazawa-u.ac.jp

Dr. Hans WEILL
10 Falcon Drive
Mandeville, LA 70471
USA
Tel. +1 985 624 5458 /
+1 970 927 9321
Fax. +1 206 238 6383
hweill@earthlink.net

Dr. William H. WESTRA
Department of Pathology
Johns Hopkins Medical Institutions
401 N. Broadway, Weinberg 2242
Baltimore, MD 21231 USA
Tel. +1 410 955 2163
Fax. +1 410 955 0115
wwestra@jhmi.edu

Dr. Mark R. WICK
Department of Pathology
University of Virginia Health System
Occupational Health. Room 3882 OMS,
Campus Box 800214
2200 Jefferson Park Avenue
Charlottesville, VA 22908-0214, USA
Tel. +1 434 243 4818, Fax. +1 434 924 0217
mrw9c@virginia.edu

Dr. Ignacio I. WISTUBA
Department of Anatomic Pathology
Pontificia Universidad Catolica de Chile
Marcoleta 367, P.O. Box 114-D
Santiago
CHILE
Tel. +56 2 354 3209
Fax. +56 2 639 5101
iwistuba@med.puc.cl

Dr. Eunhee S. YI
Department of Pathology
University of California San Diego
Medical Center
200 West Arbor Drive
San Diego CA 92103-8720, USA
Tel. +1 619 543 5288
Fax. +1 619 543 5249
jeyi@ucsd.edu

Dr. Tomoyuki YOKOSE
Pathology Division, Ibaraki Prefectural
Central Hospital and Cancer Center
Koibuchi 6528
Tomobemachi, Nishiibaraki-gun
309-1793 Ibaraki, JAPAN
Tel. +81 296 77 1121 (Ext.2284)
Fax. +81 296 77 2886
t-yokose@chubyoin.pref.ibaraki.jp

Dr. Satoshi YONEDA
Division of General Thoracic Surgery
Imakiire General Hospital
4-16, Shimotatsuo-chou
892-8502 Kagoshima City
JAPAN
Tel. +81 99 226 2211
Fax. +81 99 222 7906
binyoneda@imakiire.or.jp

Dr. Samuel A. YOUSEM
Department of Pathology A610
University of Pittsburgh Medical Center
Presbyterian Campus
200 Lothrop Street
Pittsburgh, PA 15213-2582, USA
Tel. +1 412 647 6193
Fax. +1 412 647 3399
yousemsa@msx.upmc.edu

Dr. Andreas ZETTL
Department of Pathology
University of Würzburg
Josef-Schneider-Strasse 2
D-97080 Würzburg
GERMANY
Tel. +49 931 201 47796
Fax. +49 931 201 47440
andreas.zettl@mail.uni-wuerzburg.de

Dr. Paul J. ZHANG
Department of Pathology and
Laboratory Medicine
6 Founders Pavilion
3400 Spruce Street
Philadelphia, PA 10147, USA
Tel. +1 215 662 6503
Fax. +1 215 349 5910
pjz@mail.med.upenn.edu

Source of charts and photographs

1.

1.1	Dr. D.M. Parkin
1.2 A,B	Dr. R. Peto
1.3A	Dr. P. Boffetta
1.3B	World Cancer Report {2250}
1.4	Dr. R. Peto
1.5	Dr. J. Yokota
1.6 - 1.007	Dr. P. Hainaut
1.8A-C	Dr. F. Thivolet-Bejui
1.9A	Dr. E.A. Fernandez
1.9B	Dr. P. Vogt
1.9C	Dr. E.A. Fernandez
1.9D-1.10B	Dr. K.M. Kerr
1.11A-1.12B	Dr. W.D. Travis
1.11C*	Dr. W.D. Travis
1.13A	Dr. I. Petersen
1.13B*	Dr. W.D. Travis
1.14A-B	Dr. P. Vogt
1.15	Dr. F. Thivolet-Bejui
1.16A-1.017B	Dr. W.D. Travis
1.18A-B	Dr. I. Petersen
1.19A	Dr. C.I. Henschke
1.19B,C	Dr. K.M. Kerr
1.20A-C	Dr. C.I Henschke
1.21A-C	Dr. F. Thivolet-Bejui
1.22A-C	Dr. K. Geisinger
1.23	Dr. P. Ohori
1.24A#,B	Dr. T.V. Colby
1.25*	Dr. T.V .Colby
1.26A*	Dr. W.D. Travis
1.26B-1.028	Dr. T.V. Colby
1.29	Dr. M. Noguchi
1.30A*	Dr. T.V .Colby
1.30B	Dr. M. Noguchi
1.31-1.32C	Dr. T.V .Colby
1.33A,B*	Dr. T.V. Colby
1.34A	Dr. K.M. Kerr
1.34B-D*	Dr. T.V. Colby
1.35-1.036	Dr. I. Petersen
1.37A	Dr. K.M. Kerr
1.37B*	Dr. W.D. Travis
1.38	Dr. K. Geisinger
1.39A	Dr. E. Brambilla
1.39B*	Dr. W.D. Travis
1.39C	Dr. E. Brambilla
1.39D*	Dr. W.D. Travis

The copyright remains with the authors. Requests for permission to reproduce figures or charts should be directed to the respective contributor. For addresses see Contributors List.

*Reproduced from W.D. Travis et al. (eds.). World Health Organization (WHO) Histological Typing of Lung and Pleural Tumours (1999) with kind permission from Springer Verlag, Heidelberg. Ref. {2024}

#Reproduced from T.V. Colby et al. (eds.). Tumors of the Lower Respiratory Tract. (1995) with kind permission from Armed Forces Institute of Pathology, Washington, DC. Ref. {391}

1.40A-1.041C	Dr. E. Brambilla
1.42*	Dr. W.D. Travis
1.43A,B	Dr. E. Brambilla
1.44	Dr. E. Brambilla
1.45A*	Dr. W.D. Travis
1.45B,C	Dr. E. Brambilla
1.046A*	Dr. W.D. Travis
1.46B	Dr. Y.L. Chang
1.47A*	Dr. W.D. Travis
1.47B	Dr. E. Brambilla
1.48	Dr. I. Petersen
1.49*	Dr. T.V. Colby
1.50	Dr. E. Brambilla
1.51A,B	Dr. K. Geisinger
1.52A-C	Dr. G. Rossi
1.52D*	Dr. T.V. Colby
1.53A,B	Dr. G. Rossi
1.54*	Dr. W.D. Travis
1.55-1.56	Dr. G. Rossi
1.57	Dr. M.N. Koss
1.58*	Dr. W.D. Travis
1.059A,B	Dr. M.N. Koss
1.59C,D*	Dr. W.D. Travis
1.60	Dr. W.D. Travis
1.61A	Dr. F. Thivolet-Bejui
1.61B	Dr. K. Geisinger
1.62A,B	Dr. P.S. Hasleton
1.62C	Dr. P. Vogt
1.63A-D*	Dr. W.D. Travis
1.64A-1.65B*	Dr. W.D. Travis
1.66	Dr. D.B. Flieder
1.67A-D	Dr. S.A. Yousem
1.68	Dr. P. Vogt
1.69-1.70B	Dr. S.A. Yousem
1.70C, D	Dr. F. Thivolet-Bejui
1.71A	Dr. W.D. Travis
1.71B-D	Dr. E. Brambilla
1.72	Dr. K.M. Muller
1.73A-F	Dr. S .Lam
1.74	Dr. W.A. Franklin
1.75	Dr. I.I. Wistuba
1.76A,B	Dr. K.M. Kerr
1.77*	Dr. W.D. Travis
1.78A,B	Dr. K.M. Kerr
1.78C	Dr. W.D. Travis
1.78D	Dr. K.M. Kerr
1.79A-C	Dr. H. Kitamura
1.80A,B*	Dr. W.D. Travis
1.81-1.82B	Dr. D.B. Flieder
1.82C-1.85A*	Dr. W.D. Travis
1.85B	Dr. L.M. Burke
1.86A	Dr. D.B. Flieder
1.86B-1.087*	Dr. W.D. Travis
1.088A-C	Dr. D.B. Flieder
1.88D*	Dr. W.D. Travis
1.89	Dr. D.B. Flieder
1.90A,B*	Dr. W.D. Travis
1.91	Dr. A. Nicholson
1.92A	Dr. F. Thivolet-Bejui
1.92B*	Dr. T.V. Colby
1.092C,D	Dr. A. Nicholson
1.93*	Dr. T.V. Colby
1.94-1.97B	Dr. M.N. Koss
1.97C	Dr. D. Guinee
1.98*	Dr. W.D. Travis
1.99A	Dr. T.V. Colby

1.99B*	Dr. W.D .Travis
1.100	Dr. T.V. Colby
1.101A,B*-1.102	Dr. W.D. Travis
1.103	Dr. H. Tazelaar
1.104A	Dr. L.P. Dehner
1.104B	Dr. H. Tazelaar
1.104C,D	Dr. L.P. Dehner
1.105-1.106B	Dr. H. Tazelaar
1.107A-1.108	Dr. L.P. Dehner
1.109A-1.110B*	Dr. T.V. Colby
1.111	Dr. S.A. Yousem
1.112A-D*	Dr. W.D. Travis
1.113	Dr. H. Tazelaar
1.114*	Dr. W.D. Travis
1.115	Dr. H. Tazelaar
1.116A-1.117D	Dr. E.S. Yi
1.118A,B	Dr. H. Tazelaar
1.119A	Dr. A. Nicholson
1.119B-1.120B	Dr. J. Tomashefski
1.120C,D*	Dr. W.D. Travis
1.121A-C	Dr.M.N.Devouassoux-Shisheboran
1.122A*	Dr. W.D. Travis
1.122B,C	Dr.M.N.Devouassoux-Shisheboran
1.123-1.126C*	Dr. W.D. Travis
1.127A,B*#	Dr. T.V. Colby
1.128A,B*	Dr. W.D. Travis
1.129A,B*#	Dr. T.V. Colby
1.130	Dr. K. Geisinger
1.131A,B*	Dr. D.H. Dail
1.132A-D	Dr. D.H. Dail
1.133	Dr. W.D. Travis

2.

2.3A,B	Dr. P. Vogt
2.4A-C	Dr. P.T. Cagle
2.4D	Dr. P. Vogt
2.6A	Dr. A. Churg
2.6B,2.7	Dr. P. Vogt
2.8A-2.9A*	Dr. W.D. Travis
2.9B	Dr. V. Roggli
2.10A-2.12*	Dr. W.D. Travis
2.13A	Dr. F. Galateau-Salle
2.13B	Dr. F. Galateau-Salle
2.14	Dr. Kutsal Turhan, Dr. Recep Savas and Dr. Ali Veral, Turkey
2.15*	Dr. W.D. Travis
2.16	Dr. P. Vogt
2.17	Dr. W.D. Travis
2.18A-D	Dr. P. Gaulard
2.19	Dr. P. Vogt
2.20	Dr. H. Tazelaar
2.21A-C	Dr. N.G. Ordonez
2.22*	Dr. W.D. Travis
2.23A*	Dr. W.D. Travis
2.23B,C	Dr. M. Miettinen

3.

3.1A-F	Dr. A. Marx
3.2A-C	Dr. H.K. Muller-Hermelink
3.3A,B	Dr. P. Ströbel
3.4A-C	Dr. G. Chen
3.5-3.9C	Dr. T.T. Kuo
3.10	Dr. A. Zettl
3.11A-3.14B	Dr. T.T. Kuo
3.14C-3.16D	Dr. A. Marx
3.17A-3.18A	Dr. H.K. Muller-Hermelink
3.18B	Dr. A. Marx
3.18C	Dr. H.K. Muller-Hermelink
3.18D	Dr. A. Marx
3.19A	Dr. H.K. Muller-Hermelink
3.19B-3.020D	Dr. A. Marx
3.21	Dr. P.J. Zhang
3.22	Dr. B. Schalke Dept. of Neurology, Univ. of Regensburg, D-93053 Regensburg Germany
3.23	Dr. R.H. Laeng
3.24	Dr. T. Kirchner Inst. of Pathology, University of Erlangen-Nuremberg, D-91054 Erlangen, Germany
3.25A	Dr. H.K. Muller-Hermelink
3.25B	Dr. A. Marx
3.25C,D	Dr. H.K. Muller-Hermelink
3.26A	Dr. A. Marx
3.26B-E	Dr. H.K. Muller-Hermelink
3.26F-3.27C	Dr. A. Marx
3.28A,B	Dr. A. Zettl
3.29	Dr. T.T. Kuo
3.30–3.31B	Dr. A. Marx
3.31C	Dr. R.H. Laeng
3.31D	Dr. A. Marx
3.32A-3.34C	Dr. J.K.C. Chan
3.35A,B	Dr. T.T. Kuo
3.36	Dr. A. Marx
3.37A	Dr. T.T. Kuo
3.37B	Dr. A. Marx
3.38A-3.40	Dr. M. Fukayama
3.41A,B	Dr. A. Zettl
3.42A	Dr. A. Marx
3.42B	Dr. M. Fukayama
3.43A	Dr. A.S. Baur
3.43B	Dr. A. Marx
3.44A	Dr. J. Rosai
3.44B	Dr. M.R. Wick
3.45-3.47D	Dr. T.T. Kuo
3.47E	Dr. A. Marx
3.47F	Dr. T.T. Kuo
3.48A-3.50D	Dr. J.K.C. Chan
3.52,3.53	Dr. J. Rosai
3.54	Dr. M.O. Kurrer
3.55A,B	Dr. A. Marx
3.56A-3.58B	Dr. C.A. French
3.59A,B	Dr. A. Marx

3.60A,B	Dr. J.K.C. Chan	3.106B	Dr. A. Marx
3.61	Dr. T.T. Kuo	3.107A-3.108D	Dr. J.K.C. Chan
3.62	Dr. J.K.C. Chan	3.109	Dr. A. Orazi
3.63A	Dr. T.T. Kuo	3.110	Dr. Y. Shimosato
3.63B,C	Dr. J.K.C. Chan	3.111A	Dr. A. Marx
3.63D	Dr. T.T. Kuo	3.111B	Dr. H.K. Muller-Hermelink
3.64A,B	Dr. J.K.C. Chan	3.112A-D	Dr. Wei-Jen Chen, Dept. of Pathology, Chang Gung Memorial Hospital, Kaohsiung, Taiwan / China
3.64C,D	Dr. T.T. Kuo		
3.65A,B	Dr. J.K.C. Chan		
3.65C,D	Dr. J. Rosai		
3.66, 3.67	Dr. T.T. Kuo		
3.68A	Dr. A. Marx		
3.68B	Dr. M.R. Wick	3.113A-3.114A	Dr. A. Marx
3.69A	Dr. J.K.C. Chan	3.114B	Dr. A. Marx
3.69B	Dr. M.R. Wick	3.115A-C	Dr. R. Chiarle
3.69C	Dr. J.K.C. Chan	3.116A,B	Dr. P.J. Zhang
3.69D	Dr. M.R. Wick	3.117A-3.118B	Dr. J.K.C. Chan
3.70A	Dr. A. Marx	3.118C,D	Dr. A. Marx
3.70B	Dr. J.K.C. Chan	3.119A	Dr. T.T. Kuo
3.70C	Dr. A. Marx	3.119B	Dr. J.K.C. Chan
3.70D	Dr. J. Rosai	3.119C,D	Dr. T.T. Kuo
3.71A	Dr. T.T. Kuo	3.119E,F	Dr. J.K.C. Chan
3.71B	Dr. J.K.C. Chan	3.120A,B	Dr. A. Marx
3.72A	Dr. T.T. Kuo	3.121A,B	Dr. J.K.C. Chan
3.72B,C	Dr. E.J. Perlman	3.122	Dr. P. Vogt
3.72D	Dr. M.R. Wick	3.123A	Dr. R. Chiarle
3.73-3.74A	Dr. J.K.C. Chan	3.123B	Dr. A. Marx
3.74B	Dr. A. Marx	3.124-3.125B	Dr. J.K.C. Chan
3.75A	Dr. E.J. Perlman	3.126A,B	Dr. P. Strobel
3.075B	Dr. T.T. Kuo	3.127	Dr. T.T. Kuo
3.76-3.77B	Dr. J.K.C. Chan		
3.77C-E	Dr. E.J. Perlman		
3.77F-3.78A	Dr. J.K.C. Chan	**4.**	
3.78B	Dr. E.J. Perlman		
3.79	Dr. T.T. Kuo	4.1A	Dr. D.J. Radford
3.80	Dr. E.J. Perlman	4.1B	Dr. T. Geva
3.081A,B	Dr. J.K.C. Chan	4.2A	Dr. W.D. Edwards, Division of Anatomic Pathology, Mayo Clinic, Rochester, MN 55905, USA
3.82A	Dr. E.J. Perlman		
3.82B-3.86D	Dr. J.K.C. Chan		
3.86a A-D	Dr. H.K. Muller-Hermelink		
3.87, 3.88	Dr. F. Menestrina		
3.089	Dr. P. Moller	4.2B	Dr. A. Burke
3.90A	Dr. H.K. Müller-Hermelink	4.2C	Dr. R. Loire
		4.2D	Dr. P. Vogt
3.90B	Dr. F. Menestrina	4.3A,B	Dr. A. Burke
3.90C	Dr. T. Rüdiger	4.4	Dr. H. Tazelaar
3.90D	Dr. F. Menestrina	4.5A	Dr. B.M. Shehata Dept. of Pathology, Egleston Children's Hospital, Emory University, Atlanta, Ga, USA
3.90E,F	Dr. T. Rüdiger		
3.91	Dr. F. Menestrina		
3.92-3.94D	Dr. J.K.C. Chan		
3.95	Dr. H.K. Müller-Hermelink		
3.96A-3.97D	Dr. N.L. Harris	4.5B,4.6A	Dr. A. Burke
3.98A,B	Dr. H.K. Muller-Hermelink	4.6B-4.7B	Dr. B.M. Shehata
		4.8A-4.9	Dr. A. Burke
3.099	Dr. S. Nakamura	4.10A,B	Dr. J. Galvin
3.100	Dr. N.L. Harris	4.11A	Dr. A. Burke
3.101	Dr. H.K. Muller-Hermelink	4.11B-D	Dr. P. Vogt
		4.11E-4.12B	Dr. R. Loire
3.102A,B	Dr. N.L. Harris.	4.12C	Dr. A. Burke
3.103A-C	Dr. A. Marx	4.12D,E	Dr. H. Tazelaar
3.104	Dr. A. Rosenwald	4.12F	Dr. P. Walter
3.105A-3.105D	Dr. H.K. Muller-Hermelink	4.13A,B	Dr. H. Tazelaar
		4.14A	Dr. R. Loire
3.106A	Dr. J.K.C. Chan	4.14B	Dr. A. Burke

4.14C	Dr. H. Tazelaar
4.14D	Dr. R. Loire
4.15A,B	Dr. T. Geva
4.16,4.17	Dr. A. Burke
4.18 A,B	Dr. T. Geva
4.18C	Dr. C.R. Patel
4.19A	Dr. A. Burke
4.19B,4.20A	Dr. H. Tazelaar
4.20B	Dr. V.T. De Montpreville
4.21-4.23	Dr. H. Tazelaar
4.24A	Dr. J. Galvin
4.24B	Dr. H. Tazelaar
4.24C	Dr. W.D. Edwards
4.25A	Dr. H. Tazelaar
4.25B	Dr. H. Tazelaar
4.26,4.27	Dr. A. Burke
4.28A,B	Dr. H. Tazelaar
4.28C	Dr. R. Loire
4.29A	Dr. A. Burke
4.29B	Dr. H. Tazelaar
4.29C	Dr. R. Loire
4.29D-4.29F	Dr. H. Tazelaar
4.30A	Dr. J.P. Veinot
4.30B-4.33A	Dr. A. Burke
4.33B	Dr. H. Tazelaar
4.34A,B	Dr. A. Burke
4.35A,B	Dr. H. Hiraga
4.36-4.37C	Dr. A. Burke
4.38,4.39A	Dr. P. Vogt
4.39B	Dr. R. Loire
4.40-4.41C	Dr. A. Burke
4.42	Dr. T. Geva
4.43	Dr. A. Burke
4.44	Dr. R. Loire

References

1. Anon. (1987). Case records of the Massachusetts General Hospital. Weekly clinicopathological exercises. Case 22-1987. A 58-year-old woman with progressive pericardial disease. N Engl J Med 316: 1394-1404.

2. Anon. (1993). A predictive model for aggressive non-Hodgkin's lymphoma. The International Non-Hodgkin's Lymphoma Prognostic Factors Project. N Engl J Med 329: 987-994.

3. Anon. (1997). A clinical evaluation of the International Lymphoma Study Group classification of non-Hodgkin's lymphoma. The Non-Hodgkin's Lymphoma Classification Project. Blood 89: 3909-3918.

4. Anon. (1997). International Germ Cell Consensus Classification: a prognostic factor-based staging system for metastatic germ cell cancers. International Germ Cell Cancer Collaborative Group. J Clin Oncol 15: 594-603.

5. Anon. (1997). Pretreatment evaluation of non-small-cell lung cancer. The American Thoracic Society and The European Respiratory Society. Am J Respir Crit Care Med 156: 320-332.

6. Anon. (2000). International Classification of Diseases for Oncology. Third ed. World Health Organization (WHO): Geneva.

7. Anon. (2003). Online Mendelian Inheritance in Man, OMIM (TM). McKusick-Nathans Institute for Genetic Medicine, Johns Hopkins University (Baltimore, MD) and NationalCenter for Biotechnology Information, National Library of Medicine (Bethesda, MD), 2000 http://www.ncbi.nlm.nih.gov/omim/ .

8. Anon. (2003). Surveillance, Epidemiology and End Results (SEER), Cancer Statistics Review 1973-1999. http://seer cancer gov/csr/1973_1999/overview/overview21 pdf

9. DeLellis RA, Heitz PhU, Lloyd RV, , Eng C (Eds.) World Health Organization Classification of Tumours. Pathology and Genetics of Tumours of Endocrine Organs. IARC Press: Lyon 2004

10. Abbondanzo SL, Rush W, Bijwaard KE, Koss MN (2000). Nodular lymphoid hyperplasia of the lung: a clinicopathologic study of 14 cases. Am J Surg Pathol 24: 587-597.

11. Ablin AR, Krailo MD, Ramsay NK, Malogolowkin MH, Isaacs H, Raney RB, Adkins J, Hays DM, Benjamin DR, Grosfeld JL (1991). Results of treatment of malignant germ cell tumors in 93 children: a report from the Childrens Cancer Study Group. J Clin Oncol 9: 1782-1792.

12. Abraham KP, Reddy V, Gattuso P (1990). Neoplasms metastatic to the heart: review of 3314 consecutive autopsies. Am J Cardiovasc Pathol 3: 195-198.

13. Abrams HL, Spiro R, Goldstein N (1950). Metastases in carcinoma - analysis of 1000 autopsied cases. Cancer 3: 74-85.

14. Abutaily AS, Addis BJ, Roche WR (2002). Immunohistochemistry in the distinction between malignant mesothelioma and pulmonary adenocarcinoma: a critical evaluation of new antibodies. J Clin Pathol 55: 662-668.

15. Acebo E, Val-Bernal JF, Gomez-Roman JJ (2001). Prichard's structures of the fossa ovalis are not histogenetically related to cardiac myxoma. Histopathology 39: 529-535.

16. Acebo E, Val-Bernal JF, Gomez-Roman JJ (2001). Thrombomodulin, calretinin and c-kit (CD117) expression in cardiac myxoma. Histol Histopathol 16: 1031-1036.

17. Adachi Y, Okamura M, Yasumizu R, Nagata N, Inaba M, Sugihara A, Kumamoto T, Umemoto M, Saito Y, Genba H (1995). [An autopsy case of immature teratoma with choriocarcinoma in the mediastinum]. Kyobu Geka 48: 829-832.

18. Adams VI, Unni KK, Muhm JR, Jett JR, Ilstrup DM, Bernatz PE (1986). Diffuse malignant mesothelioma of pleura. Diagnosis and survival in 92 cases. Cancer 58: 1540-1551.

19. Addis BJ, Corrin B (1985). Pulmonary blastoma, carcinosarcoma and spindle-cell carcinoma: an immunohistochemical study of keratin intermediate filaments. J Pathol 147: 291-301.

20. Addis BJ, Dewar A, Thurlow NP (1988). Giant cell carcinoma of the lung—immuno-histochemical and ultrastructural evidence of dedifferentiation. J Pathol 155: 231-240.

21. Addis BJ, Hyjek E, Isaacson PG (1988). Primary pulmonary lymphoma: a re-appraisal of its histogenesis and its relationship to pseudolymphoma and lymphoid interstitial pneumonia. Histopathology 13: 1-17.

22. Addis BJ, Isaacson PG (1986). Large cell lymphoma of the mediastinum: a B-cell tumour of probable thymic origin. Histopathology 10: 379-390.

23. Adem C, Aubry MC, Tazelaar HD, Myers JL (2001). Metastatic angiosarcoma masquerading as diffuse pulmonary hemorrhage: clinicopathologic analysis of 7 new patients. Arch Pathol Lab Med 125: 1562-1565.

24. Afifi HY, Bosl GJ, Burt ME (1997). Mediastinal growing teratoma syndrome. Ann Thorac Surg 64: 359-362.

25. Afzal MN, Alguacil-Garcia A (1997). Primary cardiac angiosarcoma: clinical and pathological diagnostic problems. Can J Cardiol 13: 293-296.

26. Agaimy A, Kaiser A, Wunsch PH (2002). [Epithelioid hemangioendothelioma of the heart in association with myelodysplastic syndrome.] Z Kardiol 91: 352-356.

27. Agoff SN, Lamps LW, Philip AT, Amin MB, Schmidt RA, True LD, Folpe AL (2000). Thyroid transcription factor-1 is expressed in extrapulmonary small cell carcinomas but not in other extrapulmonary neuroendocrine tumors. Mod Pathol 13: 238-242.

28. Aguayo SM, King TEJr, Waldron JAJr, Sherritt KM, Kane MA, Miller YE (1990). Increased pulmonary neuroendocrine cells with bombesin-like immunoreactivity in adult patients with eosinophilic granuloma. J Clin Invest 86: 838-844.

29. Aguayo SM, Miller YE, Waldron JAJr, Bogin RM, Sunday ME, Staton GWJr, Beam WR, King TEJr (1992). Brief report: idiopathic diffuse hyperplasia of pulmonary neuroendocrine cells and airways disease. N Engl J Med 327: 1285-1288.

30. Ahmed T, Bosl GJ, Hajdu SI (1985). Teratoma with malignant transformation in germ cell tumors in men. Cancer 56: 860-863.

31. Ahn C, Harvey JC (1990). Mediastinal hibernoma, a rare tumor. Ann Thorac Surg 50: 828-830.

32. Ahrendt MN, Wesselhoeft CW (1992). Chordoma presenting as a posterior mediastinal mass in a pediatric patient. J Pediatr Surg 27: 1515-1518.

33. Akman ES, Ertem U, Tankal V, Pamir A, Tuncer AM, Uluoglu O (1989). Aggressive Kaposi's sarcoma in children: a case report. Turk J Pediatr 31: 297-303.

34. Akyuz C, Koseoglu V, Gogus S, Balci S, Buyukpamukcu M (1997). Germ cell tumours in a brother and sister. Acta Paediatr 86: 668-669.

35. al Kaisi N, Abdul-Karim FW, Mendelsohn G, Jacobs G (1988). Bronchial carcinoid tumor with amyloid stroma. Arch Pathol Lab Med 112: 211-214.

36. al Saati T, Delecluze HJ, Chittal S, Brousset P, Magaud JP, Dastugue N, Cohen-Knafo E, Laurent G, Rubin B, Delsol G (1992). A novel human lymphoma cell line (Deglis) with dual B/T phenotype and gene rearrangements and containing Epstein-Barr virus genomes. Blood 80: 209-216.

37. Alexandrov K, Cascorbi I, Rojas M, Bouvier G, Kriek E, Bartsch H (2002). CYP1A1 and GSTM1 genotypes affect benzo[a]pyrene DNA adducts in smokers' lung: comparison with aromatic/hydrophobic adduct formation. Carcinogenesis 23: 1969-1977.

38. Alexiou C, Obuszko Z, Beggs D, Morgan WE (1998). Inflammatory pseudotumors of the lung. Ann Thorac Surg 66: 948-950.

39. Alguacil-Garcia A, Halliday WC (1987). Thymic carcinoma with focal neuroblastoma differentiation. Am J Surg Pathol 11: 474-479.

40. Aliotta PJ, Castillo J, Englander LS, Nseyo UO, Huben RP (1988). Primary mediastinal germ cell tumors. Histologic patterns of treatment failures at autopsy. Cancer 62: 982-984.

41. Allen HD, Blieden LC, Stone FM, Bessinger FBJr, Lucas RVJr (1974). Echocardiographic demonstration of a right ventricular tumor in a neonate. J Pediatr 84: 854-856.

42. Alli PM, Crain BJ, Heitmiller R, Argani P (2000). Malignant melanoma presenting as an intrathymic tumor: a primary thymic melanoma? Arch Pathol Lab Med 124: 130-134.

43. Almagro UA, Perry LS, Choi H, Pintar K (1982). Papillary fibroelastoma of the heart. Report of six cases. Arch Pathol Lab Med 106: 318-321.

44. Almog C, Weissberg D, Herczeg E, Pajewski M (1977). Thymolipoma simulating cardiomegaly: a clinicopathological rarity. Thorax 32: 116-120.

45. Alobeid B, Beneck D, Sreekantaiah C, Abbi RK, Slim MS (1997). Congenital pulmonary myofibroblastic tumor: a case report with cytogenetic analysis and review of the literature. Am J Surg Pathol 21: 610-614.

46. Alter P, Grimm W, Tontsch D, Maisch B (2001). Diagnosis of primary cardiac lymphoma by endomyocardial biopsy. Am J Med 110: 593-594.

47. Alvarez-Sala R, Casadevall J, Caballero P, Prados C, Ortega B (1995). Long-term survival in a surgically treated non-encapsulated mediastinal primary liposarcoma. Diagnostic utility of core-needle biopsy for mediastinal tumors. J Cardiovasc Surg (Torino) 36: 199-200.

48. Amo-Takyi BK, Gunther K, Peters I, Mittermayer C, Eblenkamp M, Tietze L (2001). Benign solitary fibrous pleural tumour. Evidence of primitive features and complex genomic imbalances, including loss of 20q. APMIS 109: 601-606.

49. Anagnostaki L, Krag Jacobsen G, Horn T, Sengelov L, Braendstrup O (1992). Melanotic neuroectodermal tumour as a predominant component of an immature testicular teratoma. Case report with immunohistochemical investigations. APMIS 100: 809-816.

50. Anagnostopoulos I, Hansmann ML, Franssila K, Harris M, Harris NL, Jaffe ES, Han J, van Krieken JM, Poppema S, Marafioti T, Franklin J, Sextro M, Diehl V, Stein H (2000). European Task Force on Lymphoma project on lymphocyte predominance Hodgkin disease: histologic and immunohistologic analysis of submitted cases reveals 2 types of Hodgkin disease with a nodular growth pattern and abundant lymphocytes. Blood 96: 1889-1899.

51. Anami Y, Matsuno Y, Yamada T, Takeuchi T, Nakayama H, Hirohashi S, Noguchi M (1998). A case of double primary adenocarcinoma of the lung with multiple atypical adenomatous hyperplasia. Pathol Int 48: 634-640.

52. Anbazhagan R, Tihan T, Bornman DM, Johnston JC, Saltz JH, Weigering A, Piantadosi S, Gabrielson E (1999). Classification of small cell lung cancer and pulmonary carcinoid by gene expression profiles. Cancer Res 59: 5119-5122.

53. Anderson C, Ludwig ME, O'Donnell M, Garcia N (1990). Fine needle aspiration cytology of pulmonary carcinoid tumors. Acta Cytol 34: 505-510.

54. Anderson M, Sladon S, Michels R, Davidson L, Conwell K, Lechner J, Franklin W, Saccomanno G, Wiest J (1996). Examination of p53 alterations and cytokeratin expression in sputa collected from patients prior to histological diagnosis of squamous cell carcinoma. J Cell Biochem Suppl 25: 185-190.

55. Anderson MB, Kriett JM, Kapelanski DP, Tarazi R, Jamieson SW (1995). Primary pulmonary artery sarcoma: a report of six cases. Ann Thorac Surg 59: 1487-1490.

56. Andre F, Fizazi K, Culine S, Droz J, Taupin P, Lhomme C, Terrier-Lacombe M,

Theodore C (2000). The growing teratoma syndrome: results of therapy and long-term follow-up of 33 patients. Eur J Cancer 36: 1389-1394.
57. Andreu AL, Checcarelli N, Iwata S, Shanske S, Dimauro S (2000). A missense mutation in the mitochondrial cytochrome b gene in a revisited case with histiocytoid cardiomyopathy. Pediatr Res 48: 311-314.
58. Andriko JW, Kaldjian EP, Tsokos M, Abbondanzo SL, Jaffe ES (1998). Reticulum cell neoplasms of lymph nodes: a clinicopathologic study of 11 cases with recognition of a new subtype derived from fibroblastic reticular cells. Am J Surg Pathol 22: 1048-1058.
59. Andrion A, Mazzucco G, Gugliotta P, Monga G (1985). Benign clear cell (sugar) tumor of the lung. A light microscopic, histochemical, and ultrastructural study with a review of the literature. Cancer 56: 2657-2663.
60. Ansari MQ, Dawson DB, Nador R, Rutherford C, Schneider NR, Latimer MJ, Picker L, Knowles DM, McKenna RW (1996). Primary body cavity-based AIDS-related lymphomas. Am J Clin Pathol 105: 221-229.
61. Anton RC, Schwartz MR, Kessler ML, Cagle PT (1998). Metastatic carcinoma of the prostate mimicking primary carcinoid tumor of the lung and mediastinum. Pathol Res Pract 194: 753-758.
62. Aoki Y, Yarchoan R, Braun J, Iwamoto A, Tosato G (2000). Viral and cellular cytokines in AIDS-related malignant lymphomatous effusions. Blood 96: 1599-1601.
63. Aozasa K, Ohsawa M, Iuchi K, Tajima K, Komatsu H, Shimoyama M (1993). Artificial pneumothorax as a risk factor for development of pleural lymphoma. Jpn J Cancer Res 84: 55-57.
64. Arai T, Kurashima C, Wada S, Chida K, Ohkawa S (1998). Histological evidence for cell proliferation activity in cystic tumor (endodermal heterotopia) of the atrioventricular node. Pathol Int 48: 917-923.
65. Araoz PA, Eklund HE, Welch TJ, Breen JF (1999). CT and MR imaging of primary cardiac malignancies. Radiographics 19: 1421-1434.
66. Araoz PA, Mulvagh SL, Tazelaar HD, Julsrud PR, Breen JF (2000). CT and MR imaging of benign primary cardiac neoplasms with echocardiographic correlation. Radiographics 20: 1303-1319.
67. Aravot DJ, Banner NR, Madden B, Aranki S, Khaghani A, Fitzgerald M, Radley-Smith R, Yacoub MH (1989). Primary cardiac tumours—is there a place for cardiac transplantation? Eur J Cardiothorac Surg 3: 521-524.
68. Argani P, Askin FB, Colombani P, Perlman EJ (2000). Occult pulmonary synovial sarcoma confirmed by molecular techniques. Pediatr Dev Pathol 3: 87-90.
69. Argani P, de Chiocca IC, Rosai J (1998). Thymoma arising with a thymolipoma. Histopathology 32: 573-574.
70. Argani P, Erlandson RA, Rosai J (1997). Thymic neuroblastoma in adults: report of three cases with special emphasis on its association with the syndrome of inappropriate secretion of antidiuretic hormone. Am J Clin Pathol 108: 537-543.
71. Argani P, Zakowski MF, Klimstra DS, Rosai J, Ladanyi M (1998). Detection of the SYT-SSX chimeric RNA of synovial sarcoma in paraffin-embedded tissue and its application in problematic cases. Mod Pathol 11: 65-71.
72. Arguello M, Sgarbanti M, Hernandez E, Mamane Y, Sharma S, Servant M, Lin R, Hiscott J (2003). Disruption of the B-cell specific transcriptional program in HHV-8 associated primary effusion lymphoma cell lines. Oncogene 22: 964-973.
73. Ariyoshi N, Miyamoto M, Umetsu Y, Kunitoh H, Dosaka-Akita H, Sawamura Y, Yokota J, Nemoto N, Sato K, Kamataki T (2002). Genetic polymorphism of CYP2A6 gene and tobacco-induced lung cancer risk in male smokers. Cancer Epidemiol Biomarkers Prev 11: 890-894.
74. Armas OA, White DA, Erlandson RA, Rosai J (1995). Diffuse idiopathic pulmonary neuroendocrine cell proliferation presenting as interstitial lung disease. Am J Surg Pathol 19: 963-970.
75. Arrigoni MG, Woolner LB, Bernatz PE (1972). Atypical carcinoid tumors of the lung. J Thorac Cardiovasc Surg 64: 413-421.
76. Asada Y, Marutsuka K, Mitsukawa T, Kuribayashi T, Taniguchi S, Sumiyoshi A (1996). Ganglioneuroblastoma of the thymus: an adult case with the syndrome of inappropriate secretion of antidiuretic hormone. Hum Pathol 27: 506-509.
77. Asamura H, Nakayama H, Kondo H, Tsuchiya R, Shimosato Y, Naruke T (1996). Lymph node involvement, recurrence, and prognosis in resected small, peripheral, non-small-cell lung carcinomas: are these carcinomas candidates for video-assisted lobectomy? J Thorac Cardiovasc Surg 111: 1125-1134.
78. Asano S, Hoshikawa Y, Yamane Y, Ikeda M, Wakasa H (2000). An intrapulmonary teratoma associated with bronchiectasia containing various kinds of primordium: a case report and review of the literature. Virchows Arch 436: 384-388.
79. Ascani S, Piccioli M, Poggi S, Briskomatis A, Bolis GB, Liberati F, Frongillo R, Caramatti C, Fraternali-Orcioni G, Gamberi B, Zinzani PL, Lazzi S, Leoncini L, O'Leary J, Piccaluga PP, Pileri SA (1997). Pyothorax-associated lymphoma: description of the first two cases detected in Italy. Ann Oncol 8: 1133-1138.
80. Ascoli V, Mecucci C, Knuutila S (2001). Genetic susceptibility and familial malignant mesothelioma. Lancet 357: 1804.
81. Ascoli V, Scalzo CC, Bruno C, Facciolo F, Lopergolo M, Granone P, Nardi F (1998). Familial pleural malignant mesothelioma: clustering in three sisters and one cousin. Cancer Lett 130: 203-207.
82. Ascoli V, Signoretti S, Onetti-Muda A, Pescarmona E, Della-Rocca C, Nardi F, Mastroianni CM, Gastaldi R, Pistilli A, Gaidano G, Carbone A, Lo-Coco F (2001). Primary effusion lymphoma in HIV-infected patients with multicentric Castleman's disease. J Pathol 193: 200-209.
83. Ashby MA, Williams CJ, Buchanan RB, Bleehen NM, Arno J (1986). Mediastinal germ cell tumour associated with malignant histiocytosis and high rubella titres. Hematol Oncol 4: 183-194.
84. Ashley DJ, Davies HD (1967). Mixed glandular and squamous-cell carcinoma of the bronchus. Thorax 22: 431-436.
85. Ashmore PG (1954). Papilloma of the bronchus - case report. J Thorac Surg 27: 293-294.
86. Astrinidis A, Khare L, Carsillo T, Smolarek T, Au KS, Northrup H, Henske EP (2000). Mutational analysis of the tuberous sclerosis gene TSC2 in patients with pulmonary lymphangioleiomyomatosis. J Med Genet 37: 55-57.
87. Attanoos RL, Dojcinov SD, Webb R, Gibbs AR (2000). Anti-mesothelial markers in sarcomatoid mesothelioma and other spindle cell neoplasms. Histopathology 37: 224-231.
88. Attanoos RL, Papagiannis A, Suttinont P, Goddard H, Papotti M, Gibbs AR (1998). Pulmonary giant cell carcinoma: pathological entity or morphological phenotype? Histopathology 32: 225-231.
89. Aubry MC, Bridge JA, Wickert R, Tazelaar HD (2001). Primary monophasic synovial sarcoma of the pleura: five cases confirmed by the presence of SYT-SSX fusion transcript. Am J Surg Pathol 25: 776-781.
90. Aubry MC, Myers JL, Colby TV, Leslie KO, Tazelaar HD (2002). Endometrial stromal sarcoma metastatic to the lung: a detailed analysis of 16 patients. Am J Surg Pathol 26: 440-449.
91. Aubry MC, Myers JL, Douglas WW, Tazelaar HD, Washington Stephens TL, Hartman TE, Deschamps C, Pankratz VS (2002). Primary pulmonary carcinoma in patients with idiopathic pulmonary fibrosis. Mayo Clin Proc 77: 763-770.
92. Aubry MC, Myers JL, Ryu JH, Henske EP, Logginidou H, Jalal SM, Tazelaar HD (2000). Pulmonary lymphangioleiomyomatosis in a man. Am J Respir Crit Care Med 162: 749-752.
93. Auerbach O, Gere JB, Forman JB, Petrick TG, Smolin HJ, Muehsam GE, Kassouny DY, Stout AP (1957). Changes in the bronchial epithelium in relation to smoking and cancer of the lung. N Engl J Med 256: 97-104.
94. Auerbach O, Hammond EC, Garfinkel L (1979). Changes in bronchial epithelium in relation to cigarette smoking, 1955-1960 vs. 1970-1977. N Engl J Med 300: 381-385.
95. Auerbach O, Stout AP, Hammond EC, Garfinkel L (1961). Changes in bronchial epithelium in relation to cigarette smoking and in relation to lung cancer. N Engl J Med 265: 253-267.
96. Auliac JB, Cuvelier A, Peillon C, Louvel JP, Metayer J, Muir JF (1999). [Mediastinal leiomyosarcoma]. Rev Mal Respir 16: 210-213.
97. Avila NA, Kelly JA, Chu SC, Dwyer AJ, Moss J (2000). Lymphangioleiomyomatosis: abdominopelvic CT and US findings. Radiology 216: 147-153.
98. Babu MK, Nirmala V (1994). Thymic carcinoma with glandular differentiation arising in a congenital thymic cyst. J Surg Oncol 57: 277-279.
99. Baez-Giangreco A, Afzal M, Hamdy MG, Antonious J (1997). Pleuropulmonary blastoma of the lung presenting as posterior mediastinal mass: a case report. Pediatr Hematol Oncol 14: 475-481.
100. Bajorin DF, Motzer RJ, Rodriguez E, Murphy B, Bosl GJ (1993). Acute nonlymphocytic leukemia in germ cell tumor patients treated with etoposide-containing chemotherapy. J Natl Cancer Inst 85: 60-62.
101. Baker PB, Goodwin RA (1985). Pulmonary artery sarcomas. A review and report of a case. Arch Pathol Lab Med 109: 35-39.
102. Balasundaram S, Halees SA, Duran C (1992). Mesothelioma of the atrioventricular node: first successful follow-up after excision. Eur Heart J 13: 718-719.
103. Balsara BR, Bell DW, Sonoda G, De Rienzo A, du Manoir S, Jhanwar SC, Testa JR (1999). Comparative genomic hybridization and loss of heterozygosity analyses identify a common region of deletion at 15q11.1-15 in human malignant mesothelioma. Cancer Res 59: 450-454.
104. Balsara BR, Testa JR (2002). Chromosomal imbalances in human lung cancer. Oncogene 21: 6877-6883.
105. Baranzelli MC, Kramar A, Bouffet E, Quintana E, Rubie H, Edan C, Patte C (1999). Prognostic factors in children with localized malignant nonseminomatous germ cell tumors. J Clin Oncol 17: 1212.
106. Barbanti-Brodano G, Sabbioni S, Martini F, Negrini M, Corallini A, Tognon M (2004). Simian virus 40 infection in humans and association with human diseases: results and hypotheses. Virology 318: 1-9.
107. Barbareschi M, Ferrero S, Aldovini D, Leonardi E, Colombetti V, Carboni N, Mariscotti C (1990). Inflammatory pseudotumour of the lung. Immunohistochemical analysis on four new cases. Histol Histopathol 5: 205-211.
108. Barbareschi M, Ferrero S, Frigo B, Mariscotti C, Mosca L (1988). Bronchial carcinoid with S-100 positive sustentacular cells. Tumori 74: 705-711.
109. Barbareschi M, Frigo B, Mosca L, Carboni N, Arrigoni GP, Leonardi E, Wilander E, Siegal GP, Shiro BC (1990). Bronchial carcinoids with S-100 positive sustentacular cells. A comparative study with gastrointestinal carcinoids, pheochromocytomas and paragangliomas. Pathol Res Pract 186: 212-222.
110. Barbareschi M, Murer B, Colby TV, Chilosi M, Macri E, Loda M, Doglioni C (2003). CDX-2 homeobox gene expression is a reliable marker of colorectal adenocarcinoma metastases to the lungs. Am J Surg Pathol 27: 141-149.
111. Barnard M, Bayani J, Grant R, Teshima I, Thorner P, Squire J (2000). Use of multicolor spectral karyotyping in genetic analysis of pleuropulmonary blastoma. Pediatr Dev Pathol 3: 479-486.
112. Barnes LD, Garrison PN, Siprashvili Z, Guranowski A, Robinson AK, Ingram SW, Croce CM, Ohta M, Huebner K (1996). Fhit, a putative tumor suppressor in humans, is a dinucleoside 5',5"'-P1,P3-triphosphate hydrolase. Biochemistry 35: 11529-11535.
113. Barnes RDS, Ogorman P (1962). Two cases of anaplastic anaemia associated with tumours of thymus. J Clin Pathol 15: 264.
114. Barr FG, Chatten J, D'Cruz CM, Wilson AE, Nauta LE, Nycum LM, Biegel JA, Womer RB (1995). Molecular assays for chromosomal translocations in the diagnosis of pediatric soft tissue sarcomas. JAMA 273: 553-557.
115. Barth TF, Martin-Subero JI, Joos S, Menz CK, Hasel C, Mechtersheimer G, Parwaresch RM, Lichter P, Siebert R, Moeller P (2003). Gains of 2p involving the REL locus correlate with nuclear c-Rel protein accumulation in neoplastic cells of classical Hodgkin's lymphoma. Blood 101: 3681-6.
116. Barton AD (1997). T-cell lymphocytosis associated with lymphocyte-rich thymoma. Cancer 80: 1409-1417.
117. Bartsch H, Nair U, Risch A, Rojas M, Wikman H, Alexandrov K (2000). Genetic polymorphism of CYP genes, alone or in combination, as a risk modifier of tobacco-related cancers. Cancer Epidemiol Biomarkers Prev 9: 3-28.
118. Basheda S, Gephardt GN, Stoller JK (1991). Columnar papilloma of the bronchus. Case report and literature review. Am Rev Respir Dis 144: 1400-1402.
119. Bass JL, Breningstall GN, Swaiman KF (1985). Echocardiographic incidence of cardiac rhabdomyoma in tuberous sclero-

sis. Am J Cardiol 55: 1379-1382.
120. Basso C, Valente M, Casarotto D, Thiene G (1997). Cardiac lithomyxoma. Am J Cardiol 80: 1249-1251.
121. Basso C, Valente M, Poletti A, Casarotto D, Thiene G (1997). Surgical pathology of primary cardiac and pericardial tumors. Eur J Cardiothorac Surg 12: 730-737.
122. Basson CT, Aretz HT (2002). Case records of the Massachusetts General Hospital. Weekly clinicopathological exercises. Case 11-2002. A 27-year-old woman with two intracardiac masses and a history of endocrinopathy. N Engl J Med 346: 1152-1158.
123. Bath LE, Walayat M, Mankad P, Godman MJ, Wallace WH (1997). Stage IV malignant intrapericardial germ cell tumor: a case report. Pediatr Hematol Oncol 14: 451-455.
124. Battifora H (1976). Spindle cell carcinoma: ultrastructural evidence of squamous origin and collagen production by the tumor cells. Cancer 37: 2275-2282.
125. Baudis M (2003). Progenetix CGH online database. Bioinformatics http://www.progenetix.net.
126. Baumgartner WA, Mark JB (1980). Metastatic malignancies from distant sites to the tracheobronchial tree. J Thorac Cardiovasc Surg 79: 499-503.
127. Beasley MB, Lantuejoul S, Abbondanzo S, Chu WD, Hasleton PS, Travis WD, Brambilla E (2003). The p16/cyclin D1/Rb pathway in neuroendocrine tumors of the lung. Hum Pathol 34: 136-142.
128. Beasley MB, Thunnissen FB, Brambilla E, Hasleton P, Steele R, Hammar SP, Colby TV, Sheppard M, Shimosato Y, Koss MN, Falk R, Travis WD (2000). Pulmonary atypical carcinoid: predictors of survival in 106 cases. Hum Pathol 31: 1255-1265.
129. Beasley SW, Tiedemann K, Howat A, Werther G, Auldist AW, Tuohy P (1987). Precocious puberty associated with malignant thoracic teratoma and malignant histiocytosis in a child with Klinefelter's syndrome. Med Pediatr Oncol 15: 277-280.
130. Beaty MW, Kumar S, Sorbara L, Miller K, Raffeld M, Jaffe ES (1999). A biphenotypic human herpesvirus 8—associated primary bowel lymphoma. Am J Surg Pathol 23: 992-994.
131. Beaty MW, Toro J, Sorbara L, Stern JB, Pittaluga S, Raffeld M, Wilson WH, Jaffe ES (2001). Cutaneous lymphomatoid granulomatosis: correlation of clinical and biologic features. Am J Surg Pathol 25: 1111-1120.
132. Becker AE (2000). Primary heart tumors in the pediatric age group: a review of salient pathologic features relevant for clinicians. Pediatr Cardiol 21: 317-323.
133. Beer DG, Kardia SL, Huang CC, Giordano TJ, Levin AM, Misek DE, Lin L, Chen G, Gharib TG, Thomas DG, Lizyness ML, Kuick R, Hayasaka S, Taylor JM, Iannettoni MD, Orringer MB, Hanash S (2002). Gene-expression profiles predict survival of patients with lung adenocarcinoma. Nat Med 8: 816-824.
134. Beghetti M, Gow RM, Haney I, Mawson J, Williams WG, Freedom RM (1997). Pediatric primary benign cardiac tumors: a 15-year review. Am Heart J 134: 1107-1114.
135. Begin LR, Schurch W, Lacoste J, Hiscott J, Melnychuk DA (1994). Glycogen-rich clear cell rhabdomyosarcoma of the mediastinum. Potential diagnostic pitfall. Am J Surg Pathol 18: 302-308.
136. Begley CG, Green AR (1999). The SCL gene: from case report to critical hematopoietic regulator. Blood 93: 2760-2770.
137. Begueret H, Vergier B, Parrens M, Lehours P, Laurent F, Vernejoux JM, Dubus P, Velly JF, Megraud F, Taytard A, Merlio JP, de Mascarel A (2002). Primary lung small B-cell lymphoma versus lymphoid hyperplasia: evaluation of diagnostic criteria in 26 cases. Am J Surg Pathol 26: 76-81.
138. Bejarano PA, Baughman RP, Biddinger PW, Miller MA, Fenoglio-Preiser C, al Kafaji B, Di Lauro R, Whitsett JA (1996). Surfactant proteins and thyroid transcription factor-1 in pulmonary and breast carcinomas. Mod Pathol 9: 445-452.
139. Bejui-Thivolet F, Liagre N, Chignol MC, Chardonnet Y, Patricot LM (1990). Detection of human papillomavirus DNA in squamous bronchial metaplasia and squamous cell carcinomas of the lung by in situ hybridization using biotinylated probes in paraffin-embedded specimens. Hum Pathol 21: 111-116.
140. Belinsky SA, Nikula KJ, Palmisano WA, Michels R, Saccomanno G, Gabrielson E, Baylin SB, Herman JG (1998). Aberrant methylation of p16(INK4a) is an early event in lung cancer and a potential biomarker for early diagnosis. Proc Natl Acad Sci U S A 95: 11891-11896.
141. Belinsky SA, Palmisano WA, Gilliland FD, Crooks LA, Divine KK, Winters SA, Grimes MJ, Harms HJ, Tellez CS, Smith TM, Moots PP, Lechner JF, Stidley CA, Crowell RE (2002). Aberrant promoter methylation in bronchial epithelium and sputum from current and former smokers. Cancer Res 62: 2370-2377.
142. Bell DW, Jhanwar SC, Testa JR (1997). Multiple regions of allelic loss from chromosome arm 6q in malignant mesothelioma. Cancer Res 57: 4057-4062.
143. Ben Ezra J, Bailey A, Azumi N, Delsol G, Stroup R, Sheibani K, Rappaport H (1991). Malignant histiocytosis X. A distinct clinicopathologic entity. Cancer 68: 1050-1060.
144. Benhamou S, Lee WJ, Alexandrie AK, Boffetta P, Bouchardy C, Butkiewicz D, Brockmoller J, Clapper ML, Daly A, Dolzan V, Ford J, Gaspari L, Haugen A, Hirvonen A, Husgafvel-Pursiainen K, Ingelman-Sundberg M, Kalina I, Kihara M, Kremers P, Le Marchand L, London SJ, Nazar-Stewart V, Onon-Kihara M, Rannug A, Romkes M, Ryberg D, Seidegard J, Shields P, Strange RC, Stucker I, To-Figueras J, Brennan P, Taioli E (2002). Meta- and pooled analyses of the effects of glutathione S-transferase M1 polymorphisms and smoking on lung cancer risk. Carcinogenesis 23: 1343-1350.
145. Bennett WP, Colby TV, Travis WD, Borkowski A, Jones RT, Lane DP, Metcalf RA, Samet JM, Takeshima Y, Gu JR, Vahakangas KH, Soini Y, Paakko P, Welsh JA, Trump BF, Harris CC (1993). p53 protein accumulates frequently in early bronchial neoplasia. Cancer Res 53: 4817-4822.
146. Bennett WP, el Deiry WS, Rush WL, Guinee DGJr, Freedman AN, Caporaso NE, Welsh JA, Jones RT, Borkowski A, Travis WD, Fleming MV, Trastek V, Pairolero PC, Tazelaar HD, Midthun D, Jett JR, Liotta LA, Harris CC (1998). p21waf1/cip1 and transforming growth factor beta 1 protein expression correlate with survival in non-small cell lung cancer. Clin Cancer Res 4: 1499-1506.
147. Benton C, Gerard P (1966). Thymolipoma in a patient with Graves' disease. Case report and review of the literature. J Thorac Cardiovasc Surg 51: 428-433.
148. Bentz M, Barth TF, Bruderlein S, Bock D, Schwerer MJ, Baudis M, Joos S, Viardot A, Feller AC, Muller-Hermelink HK, Lichter P, Dohner H, Moller P (2001). Gain of chromosome arm 9p is characteristic of primary mediastinal B-cell lymphoma (MBL): comprehensive molecular cytogenetic analysis and presentation of a novel MBL cell line. Genes Chromosomes Cancer 30: 393-401.
149. Benvenuti LA, Mansur AJ, Lopes DO, Campos RV (1996). Primary lipomatous tumors of the cardiac valves. South Med J 89: 1018-1020.
150. Beresford L, Fernandez CV, Cummings E, Sanderson S, Ming-Yu W, Giacomantonio M (2003). Mediastinal polyembryoma associated with Klinefelter syndrome. J Pediatr Hematol Oncol 25: 321-323.
151. Berezowski K, Grimes MM, Gal A, Kornstein MJ (1996). CD5 immunoreactivity of epithelial cells in thymic carcinoma and CASTLE using paraffin-embedded tissue. Am J Clin Pathol 106: 483-486.
152. Berger MS, Gullick WJ, Greenfield C, Evans S, Addis BJ, Waterfield MD (1987). Epidermal growth factor receptors in lung tumours. J Pathol 152: 297-307.
153. Berger U, Khaghani A, Pomerance A, Yacoub MH, Coombes RC (1990). Pulmonary lymphangioleiomyomatosis and steroid receptors. An immunocytochemical study. Am J Clin Pathol 93: 609-614.
154. Bergmann M, Ackerman LV, Kemler RL (1951). Carcinoma of the lung - review of the literature and report of two cases treated by pneumonectomy. Cancer 4: 919-929.
155. Berkenblit R, Spindola-Franco H, Frater RW, Fish BB, Glickstein JS (1997). MRI in the evaluation and management of a newborn infant with cardiac rhabdomyoma. Ann Thorac Surg 63: 1475-1477.
156. Berkow RL, Kelly DR (1995). Isolated CNS metastasis as the first site of recurrence in a child with germ cell tumor of the mediastinum. Med Pediatr Oncol 24: 36-39.
157. Bernard A, Boumsell L, Reinherz EL, Nadler LM, Ritz J, Coppin H, Richard Y, Valensi F, Dausset J, Flandrin G, Lemerle J, Schlossman SF (1981). Cell surface characterization of malignant T cells from lymphoblastic lymphoma using monoclonal antibodies: evidence for phenotypic differences between malignant T cells from patients with acute lymphoblastic leukemia and lymphoblastic lymphoma. Blood 57: 1105-1110.
158. Bernatz PE, Clagett OT, Harrison EG (1961). Thymoma - A clinicopathologic study. J Thorac Cardiovasc Surg 42: 424-444.
159. Berruti A, Paze E, Fara E, Gorzegno G, Dogliotti L (1995). Acute myeloblastic leukemia associated with mediastinal non-seminomatous germ cell tumors. Report on two cases. Tumori 81: 299-301.
160. Berwick M, Matullo G, Vineis P (2002). Studies of DNA repair and human cancer: an update. In: Biomarkers of Environmentally Associated Disease, Wilson SH, Suk WA, eds., Lewis Publishers: Boca Raton .
161. Berwick M, Vineis P (2000). Markers of DNA repair and susceptibility to cancer in humans: an epidemiologic review. J Natl Cancer Inst 92: 874-897.
162. Beuschlein F, Hammer GD (2002). Ectopic pro-opiomelanocortin syndrome. Endocrinol Metab Clin North Am 31: 191-234.
163. Bhattacharjee A, Richards WG, Staunton J, Li C, Monti S, Vasa P, Ladd C, Beheshti J, Bueno R, Gillette M, Loda M, Weber G, Mark EJ, Lander ES, Wong W, Johnson BE, Golub TR, Sugarbaker DJ, Meyerson M (2001). Classification of human lung carcinomas by mRNA expression profiling reveals distinct adenocarcinoma subclasses. Proc Natl Acad Sci U S A 98: 13790-13795.
164. Bian Y, Jordan AG, Rupp M, Cohn H, McLaughlin CJ, Miettinen M (1993). Effusion cytology of desmoplastic small round cell tumor of the pleura. A case report. Acta Cytol 37: 77-82.
165. Bianchi AB, Mitsunaga SI, Cheng JQ, Klein WM, Jhanwar SC, Seizinger B, Kley N, Klein-Szanto AJ, Testa JR (1995). High frequency of inactivating mutations in the neurofibromatosis type 2 gene (NF2) in primary malignant mesotheliomas. Proc Natl Acad Sci U S A 92: 10854-10858.
166. Biggs PJ, Garen PD, Powers JM, Garvin AJ (1987). Malignant rhabdoid tumor of the central nervous system. Hum Pathol 18: 332-337.
167. Billmire D, Vinocur C, Rescorla F, Colombani P, Cushing B, Hawkins E, London WB, Giller R, Lauer S (2001). Malignant mediastinal germ cell tumors: an intergroup study. J Pediatr Surg 36: 18-24.
168. Bird LM, Krous HF, Eichenfield LF, Swalwell CI, Jones MC (1994). Female infant with oncocytic cardiomyopathy and microphthalmia with linear skin defects (MLS): a clue to the pathogenesis of oncocytic cardiomyopathy? Am J Med Genet 53: 141-148.
169. Biros E, Kalina I, Kohut A, Stubna J, Salagovic J (2001). Germ line polymorphisms of the tumor suppressor gene p53 and lung cancer. Lung Cancer 31: 157-162.
170. Biselli R, Ferlini C, Fattorossi A, Boldrini R, Bosman C (1996). Inflammatory myofibroblastic tumor (inflammatory pseudotumor): DNA flow cytometric analysis of nine pediatric cases. Cancer 77: 778-784.
171. Bishop PC, Wilson WH, Pearson D, Janik J, Jaffe ES, Elwood PC (1999). CNS involvement in primary mediastinal large B-cell lymphoma. J Clin Oncol 17: 2479-2485.
172. Bitar FF, el Zein C, Tawil A, Gharzuddine W, Obeid M (1998). Intrapericardial teratoma in an adult: a rare presentation. Med Pediatr Oncol 30: 249-251.
173. Bittira B, Tsang J, Huynh T, Morin JF, Huttner I (2000). Primary right atrial synovial sarcoma manifesting as transient ischemic attacks. Ann Thorac Surg 69: 1949-1951.
174. Bittmann I, Dose TB, Muller C, Dienemann H, Vogelmeier C, Lohrs U (1997). Lymphangioleiomyomatosis: recurrence after single lung transplantation. Hum Pathol 28: 1420-1423.
175. Bjessmo S, Ivert T (1997). Cardiac myxoma: 40 years' experience in 63 patients. Ann Thorac Surg 63: 697-700.
176. Bjorkqvist AM, Husgafvel-Pursiainen K, Anttila S, Karjalainen A, Tammilehto L, Mattson K, Vainio H, Knuutila S (1998). DNA gains in 3q occur frequently in squamous cell carcinoma of the lung, but not in adenocarcinoma. Genes Chromosomes Cancer 22: 79-82.
177. Bjorkqvist AM, Tammilehto L, Anttila S, Mattson K, Knuutila S (1997). Recurrent DNA copy number changes in 1q, 4q, 6q,

9p, 13q, 14q and 22q detected by comparative genomic hybridization in malignant mesothelioma. Br J Cancer 75: 523-527.

178. Bjorkqvist AM, Tammilehto L, Nordling S, Nurminen M, Anttila S, Mattson K, Knuutila S (1998). Comparison of DNA copy number changes in malignant mesothelioma, adenocarcinoma and large-cell anaplastic carcinoma of the lung. Br J Cancer 77: 260-269.

179. Bjorkqvist AM, Wolf M, Nordling S, Tammilehto L, Knuuttila A, Kere J, Mattson K, Knuutila S (1999). Deletions at 14q in malignant mesothelioma detected by microsatellite marker analysis. Br J Cancer 81: 1111-1115.

180. Black MD, Kadletz M, Smallhorn JF, Freedom RM (1998). Cardiac rhabdomyomas and obstructive left heart disease: histologically but not functionally benign. Ann Thorac Surg 65: 1388-1390.

181. Blackburn CC, Manley NR, Palmer DB, Boyd RL, Anderson G, Ritter MA (2002). One for all and all for one: thymic epithelial stem cells and regeneration. Trends Immunol 23: 391-395.

182. Bleisch VR, Kraus FT (1980). Polypoid sarcoma of the pulmonary trunk: analysis of the literature and report of a case with leptomeric organelles and ultrastructural features of rhabdomyosarcoma. Cancer 46: 314-324.

183. Blumberg D, Port JL, Weksler B, Delgado R, Rosai J, Bains MS, Ginsberg RJ, Martini N, McCormack PM, Rusch V (1995). Thymoma: a multivariate analysis of factors predicting survival. Ann Thorac Surg 60: 908-913.

184. Blumenfeld W, Turi GK, Harrison G, Latuszynski D, Zhang C (1999). Utility of cytokeratin 7 and 20 subset analysis as an aid in the identification of primary site of origin of malignancy in cytologic specimens. Diagn Cytopathol 20: 63-66.

185. Bocchetta M, Miele L, Pass HI, Carbone M (2003). Notch-1 induction, a novel activity of SV40 required for growth of SV40-transformed human mesothelial cells. Oncogene 22: 81-89.

186. Bocklage T, Leslie K, Yousem S, Colby T (2001). Extracutaneous angiosarcomas metastatic to the lungs: clinical and pathologic features of twenty-one cases. Mod Pathol 14: 1216-1225.

187. Bocklage TJ, Dail D, Colby TV (1998). Primary lung tumors infiltrated by osteoclast-like giant cells. Ann Diagn Pathol 2: 229-240.

188. Bockmuhl U, Wolf G, Schmidt S, Schwendel A, Jahnke V, Dietel M, Petersen I (1998). Genomic alterations associated with malignancy in head and neck cancer. Head Neck 20: 145-151.

189. Bodner SM, Koss MN (1996). Mutations in the p53 gene in pulmonary blastomas: immunohistochemical and molecular studies. Hum Pathol 27: 1117-1123.

190. Boffetta P, Agudo A, Ahrens W, Benhamou E, Benhamou S, Darby SC, Ferro G, Fortes C, Gonzalez CA, Jockel KH, Krauss M, Kreienbrock L, Kreuzer M, Mendes A, Merletti F, Nyberg F, Pershagen G, Pohlabeln H, Riboli E, Schmid G, Simonato L, Tredaniel J, Whitley E, Wichmann HE, Winck C, Zambon P, Saracci R (1998). Multicenter case-control study of exposure to environmental tobacco smoke and lung cancer in Europe. J Natl Cancer Inst 90: 1440-1450.

191. Boffetta P, Pershagen G, Jockel KH, Forastiere F, Gaborieau V, Heinrich J, Jahn I, Kreuzer M, Merletti F, Nyberg F, Rosch F, Simonato L (1999). Cigar and pipe smoking and lung cancer risk: a multicenter study from Europe. J Natl Cancer Inst 91: 697-701.

192. Boffetta P, Trichopoulos D (2002). Cancer of the lung, larynx, and pleura. In: Textbook of Cancer Epidemiology, Adami HO, Hunter D, Trichopoulos D, eds., Oxford University Press: Oxford , pp. 248-280.

193. Bohle A, Studer UE, Sonntag RW, Scheidegger JR (1986). Primary or secondary extragonadal germ cell tumors? J Urol 135: 939-943.

194. Bohm J, Fellbaum C, Bautz W, Prauer HW, Hofler H (1997). Pulmonary nodule caused by an alveolar adenoma of the lung. Virchows Arch 430: 181-184.

195. Boiselle PM, Patz EFJr, Vining DJ, Weissleder R, Shepard JA, McLoud TC (1998). Imaging of mediastinal lymph nodes: CT, MR, and FDG PET. Radiographics 18: 1061-1069.

196. Boix E, Pico A, Pinedo R, Aranda I, Kovacs K (2002). Ectopic growth hormone-releasing hormone secretion by thymic carcinoid tumour. Clin Endocrinol (Oxf) 57: 131-134.

197. Bokemeyer C, Droz JP, Horwich A, Gerl A, Fossa SD, Beyer J, Pont J, Schmoll HJ, Kanz L, Einhorn L, Nichols CR, Hartmann JT (2001). Extragonadal seminoma: an international multicenter analysis of prognostic factors and long term treatment outcome. Cancer 91: 1394-1401.

198. Bokemeyer C, Hartmann JT, Fossa SD, Droz JP, Schmol HJ, Horwich A, Gerl A, Beyer J, Pont J, Kanz L, Nichols CR, Einhorn L (2003). Extragonadal germ cell tumors: relation to testicular neoplasia and management options. APMIS 111: 49-59.

199. Bokemeyer C, Nichols CR, Droz JP, Schmoll HJ, Horwich A, Gerl A, Fossa SD, Beyer J , Pont J, Kanz L, Einhorn L, Hartmann JT (2002). Extragonadal germ cell tumors of the mediastinum and retroperitoneum: results from an international analysis. J Clin Oncol 20: 1864-1873.

200. Bonetti F, Chiodera PL, Pea M, Martignoni G, Bosi F, Zamboni G, Mariuzzi GM (1993). Transbronchial biopsy in lymphangiomyomatosis of the lung. HMB45 for diagnosis. Am J Surg Pathol 17: 1092-1102.

201. Bonetti F, Pea M, Martignoni G, Doglioni C, Zamboni G, Capelli P, Rimondi P, Andrion A (1994). Clear cell ("sugar") tumor of the lung is a lesion strictly related to angiomyolipoma—the concept of a family of lesions characterized by the presence of the perivascular epithelioid cells (PEC). Pathology 26: 230-236.

202. Boone S, Higginson LA, Walley VM (1992). Endothelial papillary fibroelastomas arising in and around the aortic sinus, filling the ostium of the right coronary artery. Arch Pathol Lab Med 116: 135-137.

203. Booth AM, LeGallo RD, Stoler MH, Waldron PE, Cerilli LA (2001). Pediatric angiosarcoma of the heart: a unique presentation and metastatic pattern. Pediatr Dev Pathol 4: 490-495.

204. Bosi G, Lintermans JP, Pellegrino PA, Svaluto-Moreolo G, Vliers A (1996). The natural history of cardiac rhabdomyoma with and without tuberous sclerosis. Acta Paediatr 85: 928-931.

205. Bossert T, Diegeler A, Spyrantis N, Mohr FW (2000). Papillary fibroelastoma of the aortic valve with temporary occlusion of the left coronary ostium. J Heart Valve Dis 9: 842-843.

206. Boucheix C, David B, Sebban C, Racadot E, Bene MC, Bernard A, Campos L, Jouault H, Sigaux F, Lepage E, Herve P, Fiere D (1994). Immunophenotype of adult acute lymphoblastic leukemia, clinical parameters, and outcome: an analysis of a prospective trial including 562 tested patients (LALA87). French Group on Therapy for Adult Acute Lymphoblastic Leukemia. Blood 84: 1603-1612.

207. Boucher LD, Yoneda K (1995). The expression of trophoblastic cell markers by lung carcinomas. Hum Pathol 26: 1201-1206.

208. Boudousquie AC, Lawce HJ, Sherman R, Olson S, Magenis RE, Corless CL (1996). Complex translocation [7;22] identified in an epithelioid hemangioendothelioma. Cancer Genet Cytogenet 92: 116-121.

209. Boulanger E, Agbalika F, Maarek O, Daniel MT, Grollet L, Molina JM, Sigaux F, Oksenhendler E (2001). A clinical, molecular and cytogenetic study of 12 cases of human herpesvirus 8 associated primary effusion lymphoma in HIV-infected patients. Hematol J 2: 172-179.

210. Bove KE, Hurtubise P, Wong KY (1985). Thymus in untreated systemic histiocytosis X. Pediatr Pathol 4: 99-115.

211. Brambilla E, Gazzeri S, Lantuejoul S, Coll JL, Moro D, Negoescu A, Brambilla C (1998). p53 mutant immunophenotype and deregulation of p53 transcription pathway (Bcl2, Bax, and Waf1) in precursor bronchial lesions of lung cancer. Clin Cancer Res 4: 1609-1618.

212. Brambilla E, Gazzeri S, Moro D, Caron de Fromentel C, Gouyer V, Jacrot M, Brambilla C (1993). Immunohistochemical study of p53 in human lung carcinomas. Am J Pathol 143: 199-210.

213. Brambilla E, Gazzeri S, Moro D, Lantuejoul S, Veyrenc S, Brambilla C (1999). Alterations of Rb pathway (Rb-p16INK4-cyclin D1) in preinvasive bronchial lesions. Clin Cancer Res 5: 243-250.

214. Brambilla E, Lantuejoul S, Sturm N (2000). Divergent differentiation in neuroendocrine lung tumors. Semin Diagn Pathol 17: 138-148.

215. Brambilla E, Moro D, Gazzeri S, Brambilla C (1999). Alterations of expression of Rb, p16(INK4A) and cyclin D1 in non-small cell lung carcinoma and their clinical significance. J Pathol 188: 351-360.

216. Brambilla E, Moro D, Veale D, Brichon PY, Stoebner P, Paramelle B, Brambilla C (1992). Basal cell (basaloid) carcinoma of the lung: a new morphologic and phenotypic entity with separate prognostic significance. Hum Pathol 23: 993-1003.

217. Brambilla E, Negoescu A, Gazzeri S, Lantuejoul S, Moro D, Brambilla C, Coll JL (1996). Apoptosis-related factors p53, Bcl2, and Bax in neuroendocrine lung tumors. Am J Pathol 149: 1941-1952.

218. Brambilla E, Travis WD, Colby TV, Corrin B, Shimosato Y (2001). The new World Health Organization classification of lung tumours. Eur Respir J 18: 1059-1068.

219. Bramwell NH, Burns BF (1986). Histiocytosis X of the thymus in association with myasthenia gravis. Am J Clin Pathol 86: 224-227.

220. Brauch H, Johnson B, Hovis J, Yano T, Gazdar A, Pettengill OS, Graziano S, Sorenson GD, Poiesz BJ, Minna J, Linehan M, Zbar B (1987). Molecular analysis of the short arm of chromosome 3 in small-cell and non-small-cell carcinoma of the lung. N Engl J Med 317: 1109-1113.

221. Bray F, Tyczynski JE, Parkin DM (2003). Going up or coming down? The changing phases of the lung cancer epidemic in the 15 European Union countries 1967-1999. Eur J Cancer .

222. Breeze RG, Wheeldon EB (1977). The cells of the pulmonary airways. Am Rev Respir Dis 116: 705-777.

223. Brennan P, Bray I (2002). Recent trends and future directions for lung cancer mortality in Europe. Br J Cancer 87: 43-48.

224. Breugem CC, Alders M, Salieb-Beugelaar GB, Mannens MM, Van der Horst CM, Hennekam RC (2002). A locus for hereditary capillary malformations mapped on chromosome 5q. Hum Genet 110: 343-347.

225. Briens E, Caulet-Maugendre S, Desrues B, Quinquenel ML, Lena H, Turlin B, Delaval P (1997). Alveolar haemorrhage revealing epithelioid haemangioendothelioma. Respir Med 91: 111-114.

226. Brizard C, Latremouille C, Jebara VA, Acar C, Fabiani JN, Deloche A, Carpentier AF (1993). Cardiac hemangiomas. Ann Thorac Surg 56: 390-394.

227. Brocheriou I, Carnot F, Briere J (1995). Immunohistochemical detection of bcl-2 protein in thymoma. Histopathology 27: 251-255.

228. Brown CC, Kessler LG (1988). Projections of lung cancer mortality in the United States: 1985-2025. J Natl Cancer Inst 80: 43-51.

229. Brown K, Collins JD, Batra P, Steckel RJ, Kagan AR (1989). Mediastinal germ cell tumor in a young woman. Med Pediatr Oncol 17: 164-167.

230. Brown MD, Reidbord HE (1967). Congenital pulmonary lymphangiectasis. Am J Dis Child 114: 654-657.

231. Brugieres L, Deley MC, Pacquement H, Meguerian-Bedoyan Z, Terrier-Lacombe MJ, Robert A, Pondarre C, Leverger G, Devalck C, Rodary C, Delsol G, Hartmann O (1998). CD30(+) anaplastic large-cell lymphoma in children: analysis of 82 patients enrolled in two consecutive studies of the French Society of Pediatric Oncology. Blood 92: 3591-3598.

232. Brundage MD, Davies D, Mackillop WJ (2002). Prognostic factors in non-small cell lung cancer: a decade of progress. Chest 122: 1037-1057.

233. Brunnemann RB, Ro JY, Ordonez NG, Mooney J, el Naggar AK, Ayala AG (1999). Extrapleural solitary fibrous tumor: a clinicopathologic study of 24 cases. Mod Pathol 12: 1034-1042.

234. Bruton D, Herdson PB, Becroft DM (1977). Histiocytoid cardiomyopathy of infancy: an unexplained myofibre degeneration. Pathology 9: 115-122.

235. Buckley C, Douek D, Newsom-Davis J, Vincent A, Willcox N (2001). Mature, long-lived CD4+ and CD8+ T cells are generated by the thymoma in myasthenia gravis. Ann Neurol 50: 64-72.

236. Bukowski RM (1993). Management of advanced and extragonadal germ-cell tumors. Urol Clin North Am 20: 153-160.

237. Bukowski RM, Wolf M, Kulander BG, Montie J, Crawford ED, Blumenstein B (1993). Alternating combination chemotherapy in patients with extragonadal germ cell tumors. A Southwest Oncology Group study. Cancer 71: 2631-2638.

238. Burbee DG, Forgacs E, Zochbauer-Muller S, Shivakumar L, Fong K, Gao B, Randle D, Kondo M, Virmani A, Bader S, Sekido Y, Latif F, Milchgrub S, Toyooka S, Gazdar AF, Lerman MI, Zabarovsky E, White M, Minna JD (2001). Epigenetic inac-

tivation of RASSF1A in lung and breast cancers and malignant phenotype suppression. J Natl Cancer Inst 93: 691-699.
239. Burke A, Johns JP, Virmani R (1990). Hemangiomas of the heart. A clinicopathologic study of ten cases. Am J Cardiovasc Pathol 3: 283-290.
240. Burke AP, Anderson PG, Virmani R, James TN, Herrera GA, Ceballos R (1990). Tumor of the atrioventricular nodal region. A clinical and immunohistochemical study. Arch Pathol Lab Med 114: 1057-1062.
241. Burke AP, Gatto-Weis C, Griego JE, Ellington KS, Virmani R (2002). Adult cellular rhabdomyoma of the heart: a report of 3 cases. Hum Pathol 33: 1092-1097.
242. Burke AP, Litovsky S, Virmani R (1996). Lipomatous hypertrophy of the atrial septum presenting as a right atrial mass. Am J Surg Pathol 20: 678-685.
243. Burke AP, Ribe JK, Bajaj AK, Edwards WD, Farb A, Virmani R (1998). Hamartoma of mature cardiac myocytes. Hum Pathol 29: 904-909.
244. Burke AP, Rosado-de-Christenson M, Templeton PA, Virmani R (1994). Cardiac fibroma: clinicopathologic correlates and surgical treatment. J Thorac Cardiovasc Surg 108: 862-870.
245. Burke AP, Virmani R (1993). Cardiac myxoma. A clinicopathologic study. Am J Clin Pathol 100: 671-680.
246. Burke AP, Virmani R (1993). Sarcomas of the great vessels. A clinicopathologic study. Cancer 71: 1761-1773.
247. Burke AP, Virmani R (1995). Atlas of Tumor Pathology. 3rd ed. Armed Forces Institute of Pathology: Washington, DC.
248. Burke AP, Virmani R (1996). Tumors of the Cardiovascular System. Armed Forces Institute of Pathology: Washington, DC.
249. Burke AP, Virmani R (1996). Tumors of the Heart and Great Vessels. 3rd ed. Armed Forces Institute of Pathology: Washington, DC.
250. Burke AP, Virmani R (2003). The cardiovascular system. In: Principles and Practice of Surgical Pathology and Cytopathology, Silverberg S, ed., Churchill Livingstone: New York .
251. Burke L, Khan MA, Freedman AN, Gemma A, Rusin M, Guinee DG, Bennett WP, Caporaso NE, Fleming MV, Travis WD, Colby TV, Trastek V, Pairolero PC, Tazelaar HD, Midthun DE, Liotta LA, Harris CC (1998). Allelic deletion analysis of the FHIT gene predicts poor survival in non-small cell lung cancer. Cancer Res 58: 2533-2536.
252. Burke LM, Rush WI, Khoor A, Mackay B, Oliveira P, Whitsett JA, Singh G, Turnicky R, Fleming MV, Koss MN, Travis WD (1999). Alveolar adenoma: a histochemical, immunohistochemical, and ultrastructural analysis of 17 cases. Hum Pathol 30: 158-167.
253. Burmeister B, Schwerdtle T, Poser I, Hoffmann E, Hartwig A, Muller WU, Rettenmeier AW, Seemayer NH, Dopp E (2004). Effects of asbestos on initiation of DNA damage, induction of DNA-strand breaks, P53-expression and apoptosis in primary, SV40-transformed and malignant human mesothelial cells. Mutat Res 558: 81-92.
254. Burn CG, Bishop MB, Davies JN (1969). A stalked papillary tumor of the mural endocardium. Am J Clin Pathol 51: 344-346.
255. Burns TR, Underwood RD, Greenberg SD, Teasdale TA, Cartwright JJr (1989). Cytomorphometry of large cell carcinoma of the lung. Anal Quant Cytol Histol 11: 48-52.
256. Burt M, Ihde JK, Hajdu SI, Smith JW, Bains MS, Downey R, Martini N, Rusch VW, Ginsberg RJ (1998). Primary sarcomas of the mediastinum: results of therapy. J Thorac Cardiovasc Surg 115: 671-680.
257. Bussey KJ, Lawce HJ, Himoe E, Shu XO, Heerema NA, Perlman EJ, Olson SB, Magenis RE (2001). SNRPN methylation patterns in germ cell tumors as a reflection of primordial germ cell development. Genes Chromosomes Cancer 32: 342-352.
258. Bussey KJ, Lawce HJ, Olson SB, Arthur DC, Kalousek DK, Krailo M, Giller R, Heifetz S, Womer R, Magenis RE (1999). Chromosome abnormalities of eighty-one pediatric germ cell tumors: sex-, age-, site-, and histopathology-related differences—a Children's Cancer Group study. Genes Chromosomes Cancer 25: 134-146.
259. Butany J, Yu W (2000). Cardiac angiosarcoma: two cases and a review of the literature. Can J Cardiol 16: 197-205.
260. Butkiewicz D, Cole KJ, Phillips DH, Harris CC, Chorazy M (1999). GSTM1, GSTP1, CYP1A1 and CYP2D6 polymorphisms in lung cancer patients from an environmentally polluted region of Poland: correlation with lung DNA adduct levels. Eur J Cancer Prev 8: 315-323.
261. Butnor KJ, Sporn TA, Hammar SP, Roggli VL (2001). Well-differentiated papillary mesothelioma. Am J Surg Pathol 25: 1304-1309.
262. Butterworth JS, Poindexter CA (1973). Papilloma of cusp of the aortic valve. Report of a patient with sudden death. Circulation 48: 213-215.
263. Byrd RB, Carr DT, Miller WE, Payne WS, Woolner LB (1969). Radiographic abnormalities in carcinoma of the lung as related to histological cell type. Thorax 24: 573-575.
264. Byrd RB, Miller WE, Carr DT, Payne WS, Woolner LB (1968). The roentgenographic appearance of squamous cell carcinoma of the bronchus. Mayo Clin Proc 43: 327-332.
265. Cabarcos A, Gomez Dorronsoro M, Lobo Beristain JL (1985). Pulmonary carcinosarcoma: a case study and review of the literature. Br J Dis Chest 79: 83-94.
266. Cabin HS, Costello RM, Vasudevan G, Maron BJ, Roberts WC (1981). Cardiac lymphoma mimicking hypertrophic cardiomyopathy. Am Heart J 102: 466-468.
267. Cacciotti P, Libener R, Betta P, Martini F, Porta C, Procopio A, Strizzi L, Penengo L, Tognon M, Mutti L, Gaudino G (2001). SV40 replication in human mesothelial cells induces HGF/Met receptor activation: a model for viral-related carcinogenesis of human malignant mesothelioma. Proc Natl Acad Sci U S A 98: 12032-12037.
268. Cagini L, Nicholson AG, Horwich A, Goldstraw P, Pastorino U (1998). Thoracic metastasectomy for germ cell tumours: long term survival and prognostic factors. Ann Oncol 9: 1185-1191.
269. Cagle PT, el Naggar AK, Xu HJ, Hu SX, Benedict WF (1997). Differential retinoblastoma protein expression in neuroendocrine tumors of the lung. Potential diagnostic implications. Am J Pathol 150: 393-400.
270. Cagle PT, Taylor LD, Schwartz MR, Ramzy I, Elder FF (1989). Cytogenetic abnormalities common to adenocarcinoma metastatic to the pleura. Cancer Genet Cytogenet 39: 219-225.
271. Cagle PT, Truong LD, Roggli VL, Greenberg SD (1989). Immunohistochemical differentiation of sarcomatoid mesotheliomas from other spindle cell neoplasms. Am J Clin Pathol 92: 566-571.
272. Cai YC, Banner B, Glickman J, Odze RD (2001). Cytokeratin 7 and 20 and thyroid transcription factor 1 can help distinguish pulmonary from gastrointestinal carcinoid and pancreatic endocrine tumors. Hum Pathol 32: 1087-1093.
273. Cairns P, Butany J, Fulop J, Rakowski H, Hassaram S (1987). Cardiac presentation of non-Hodgkin's lymphoma. Arch Pathol Lab Med 111: 80-83.
274. Cajal S, Suster S (1991). Primary thymic epithelial neoplasms in children. Am J Surg Pathol 15: 466-474.
275. Cane ME, Berrizbeitia LD, Yang SS, Mahapatro D, McGrath LB (1996). Paraganglioma of the interatrial septum. Ann Thorac Surg 61: 1845-1847.
276. Cangemi V, Volpino P, D'Andrea N, Puopolo M, Fabrizi S, Lonardo MT, Piat G (1995). Local and/or distant recurrences in T1-2/N0-1 non-small cell lung cancer. Eur J Cardiothorac Surg 9: 473-478.
277. Canty TG, Siemens R (1978). Malignant mediastinal teratoma in a 15-year-old girl. Cancer 41: 1623-1626.
278. Capello D, Gaidano G, Gallicchio M, Gloghini A, Medico E, Vivenza D, Buonaiuto D, Fassone L, Avanzi GC, Saglio G, Prat M, Carbone A (2000). The tyrosine kinase receptor met and its ligand HGF are co-expressed and functionally active in HHV-8 positive primary effusion lymphoma. Leukemia 14: 285-291.
279. Caputi M, Groeger AM, Esposito V, De Luca A, Masciullo V, Mancini A, Baldi F, Wolner E, Giordano A (2002). Loss of pRb2/p130 expression is associated with unfavorable clinical outcome in lung cancer. Clin Cancer Res 8: 3850-3856.
280. Caralps JM, Marti V, Ferres P, Ruyra X, Subirana MT (1998). Mitral valve repair after excision of a fibrolipoma. Ann Thorac Surg 66: 1808-1809.
281. Carbone A, Gloghini A, Cozzi MR, Capello D, Steffan A, Monini P, De Marco L, Gaidano G (2000). Expression of MUM1/IRF4 selectively clusters with primary effusion lymphoma among lymphomatous effusions: implications for disease histogenesis and pathogenesis. Br J Haematol 111: 247-257.
282. Carbone A, Gloghini A, Vaccher E, Zagonel V, Pastore C, Dalla Palma P, Branz F, Saglio G, Volpe R, Tirelli U, Gaidano G (1996). Kaposi's sarcoma-associated herpesvirus DNA sequences in AIDS-related and AIDS-unrelated lymphomatous effusions. Br J Haematol 94: 533-543.
283. Carbone M, Pass HI, Rizzo P, Marinetti M, Di Muzio M, Mew DJ, Levine AS, Procopio A (1994). Simian virus 40-like DNA sequences in human pleural mesothelioma. Oncogene 9: 1781-1790.
284. Carbone M, Rizzo P, Grimley PM, Procopio A, Mew DJ, Shridhar V, de Bartolomeis A, Esposito V, Giuliano MT, Steinberg SM, Levine AS, Giordano A, Pass HI (1997). Simian virus-40 large-T antigen binds p53 in human mesotheliomas. Nat Med 3: 908-912.
285. Carbone M, Rizzo P, Grimley PM, Procopio A, Mew DJ, Shridhar V, de Bartolomeis A, Esposito V, Giuliano MT, Steinberg SM, Levine AS, Giordano A, Pass HI (1997). Simian virus-40 large-T antigen binds p53 in human mesotheliomas. Nat Med 3: 908-912.
286. Carella R, Deleonardi G, D'Errico A, Salerno A, Egarter-Vigl E, Seebacher C, Donazzan G, Grigioni WF (2001). Immunohistochemical panels for differentiating epithelial malignant mesothelioma from lung adenocarcinoma: a study with logistic regression analysis. Am J Surg Pathol 25: 43-50.
287. Carey FA (1998). Pulmonary adenocarcinoma: classification and molecular biology. J Pathol 184: 229-230.
288. Carey FA, Wallace WA, Fergusson RJ, Kerr KM, Lamb D (1992). Alveolar atypical hyperplasia in association with primary pulmonary adenocarcinoma: a clinicopathological study of 10 cases. Thorax 47: 1041-1043.
289. Carles J, Rosell R, Ariza A, Pellicer I, Sanchez JJ, Fernandez-Vasalo G, Abad A, Barnadas A (1993). Neuroendocrine differentiation as a prognostic factor in non-small cell lung cancer. Lung Cancer 10: 209-219.
290. Carlin BW, Harrell JH, Olson LK, Moser KM (1989). Endobronchial metastases due to colorectal carcinoma. Chest 96: 1110-1114.
291. Carmelli D, Swan GE, Robinette D, Fabsitz R (1992). Genetic influence on smoking—a study of male twins. N Engl J Med 327: 829-833.
292. Carney JA (1979). The triad of gastric epithelioid leiomyosarcoma, functioning extra-adrenal paraganglioma, and pulmonary chondroma. Cancer 43: 374-382.
293. Carney JA (1985). Differences between nonfamilial and familial cardiac myxoma. Am J Surg Pathol 9: 53-55.
294. Carney JA (1999). Gastric stromal sarcoma, pulmonary chondroma, and extra-adrenal paraganglioma (Carney Triad): natural history, adrenocortical component, and possible familial occurrence. Mayo Clin Proc 74: 543-552.
295. Carney JA, Gordon H, Carpenter PC, Shenoy BV, Go VL (1985). The complex of myxomas, spotty pigmentation, and endocrine overactivity. Medicine (Baltimore) 64: 270-283.
296. Carney JA, Swee RG (2002). Carney complex. Am J Surg Pathol 26: 393.
297. Carsillo T, Astrinidis A, Henske EP (2000). Mutations in the tuberous sclerosis complex gene TSC2 are a cause of sporadic pulmonary lymphangioleiomyomatosis. Proc Natl Acad Sci U S A 97: 6085-6090.
298. Carter EJ, Bradburne RM, Jhung JW, Ettensohn DB (1990). Alveolar hemorrhage with epithelioid hemangioendothelioma. A previously unreported manifestation of a rare tumor. Am Rev Respir Dis 142: 700-701.
299. Casey M, Mah C, Merliss AD, Kirschner LS, Taymans SE, Denio AE, Korf B, Irvine AD, Hughes A, Carney JA, Stratakis CA, Basson CT (1998). Identification of a novel genetic locus for familial cardiac myxomas and Carney complex. Circulation 98: 2560-2566.
300. Casselman FP, Gillinov AM, Kasirajan V, Ratliff NB, Cosgrove DMI (1999). Primary synovial sarcoma of the left heart. Ann Thorac Surg 68: 2329-2331.
301. Castorino F, Masiello P, Quattrocchi E, Di Benedetto G (2000). Primary cardiac rhabdomyosarcoma of the left atrium: an unusual presentation. Tex Heart Inst J 27: 206-208.
302. Castro CY, Ostrowski ML, Barrios R, Green LK, Popper HH, Powell S, Cagle PT, Ro JY (2001). Relationship between Epstein-Barr virus and lymphoepithelioma-like carcinoma of the lung: a clinicopathologic study of 6 cases and review of the literature. Hum Pathol 32: 863-872.
303. Castro M, Shepherd CW, Gomez MR,

Lie JT, Ryu JH (1995). Pulmonary tuberous sclerosis. Chest 107: 189-195.
304. Cavazza A, Colby TV, Tsokos M, Rush W, Travis WD (1996). Lung tumors with a rhabdoid phenotype. Am J Clin Pathol 105: 182-188.
305. Cazals-Hatem D, Lepage E, Brice P, Ferrant A, d'Agay MF, Baumelou E, Briere J, Blanc M, Gaulard P, Biron P, Schlaifer D, Diebold J, Audouin J (1996). Primary mediastinal large B-cell lymphoma. A clinicopathologic study of 141 cases compared with 916 nonmediastinal large B-cell lymphomas, a GELA ("Groupe d'Etude des Lymphomes de l'Adulte") study. Am J Surg Pathol 20: 877-888.
306. Ceballos-Quintal JM, Pinto-Escalante D, Castillo-Zapata I (1996). A new case of Klippel-Trenaunay-Weber (KTW) syndrome: evidence of autosomal dominant inheritance. Am J Med Genet 63: 426-427.
307. Centofanti P, Di Rosa E, Deorsola L, Dato GM, Patane F, La Torre M, Barbato L, Verzini A, Fortunato G, di Summa M (1999). Primary cardiac tumors: early and late results of surgical treatment in 91 patients. Ann Thorac Surg 68: 1236-1241.
308. Ceresoli GL, Ferreri AJ, Bucci E, Ripa C, Ponzoni M, Villa E (1997). Primary cardiac lymphoma in immunocompetent patients: diagnostic and therapeutic management. Cancer 80: 1497-1506.
309. Cerfolio RJ, Allen MS, Nascimento AG, Deschamps C, Trastek VF, Miller DL, Pairolero PC (1999). Inflammatory pseudotumors of the lung. Ann Thorac Surg 67: 933-936.
310. Cerilli LA, Huffman HT, Anand A (1998). Primary renal angiosarcoma: a case report with immunohistochemical, ultrastructural, and cytogenetic features and review of the literature. Arch Pathol Lab Med 10: 929-935.
311. Cesarman E, Chang Y, Moore PS, Said JW, Knowles DM (1995). Kaposi's sarcoma-associated herpesvirus-like DNA sequences in AIDS-related body-cavity-based lymphomas. N Engl J Med 332: 1186-1191.
312. Cessna MH, Zhou H, Sanger WG, Perkins SL, Tripp S, Pickering D, Daines C, Coffin CM (2002). Expression of ALK1 and p80 in inflammatory myofibroblastic tumor and its mesenchymal mimics: a study of 135 cases. Mod Pathol 15: 931-938.
313. Cha SD, Incarvito J, Fernandez J, Chang KS, Maranhao V, Gooch AS (1981). Giant Lambl's excrescences of papillary muscle and aortic valve: echocardiographic, angiographic, and pathologic findings. Clin Cardiol 4: 51-54.
314. Chaganti RS, Houldsworth J (2000). Genetics and biology of adult human male germ cell tumors. Cancer Res 60: 1475-1482.
315. Chaganti RS, Ladanyi M, Samaniego F, Offit K, Reuter VE, Jhanwar SC, Bosl GJ (1989). Leukemic differentiation of a mediastinal germ cell tumor. Genes Chromosomes Cancer 1: 83-87.
316. Chaganti RS, Rodriguez E, Mathew S (1994). Origin of adult male mediastinal germ-cell tumours. Lancet 343: 1130-1132.
317. Chalabreysse L, Berger F, Loire R, Devouassoux G, Cordier JF, Thivolet-Bejui F (2002). Primary cardiac lymphoma in immunocompetent patients: a report of three cases and review of the literature. Virchows Arch 441: 456-461.
318. Chalabreysse L, Roy P, Cordier JF, Loire R, Gamondes JP, Thivolet-Bejui F (2002). Correlation of the WHO schema for the classification of thymic epithelial neoplasms with prognosis: a retrospective study of 90 tumors. Am J Surg Pathol 26: 1605-1611.
319. Chambers AF, Groom AC, MacDonald IC (2002). Dissemination and growth of cancer cells in metastatic sites. Nat Rev Cancer 2: 563-572.
320. Chan AC, Chan KW, Chan JK, Au WY, Ho WK, Ng WM (2001). Development of follicular dendritic cell sarcoma in hyaline-vascular Castleman's disease of the nasopharynx: tracing its evolution by sequential biopsies. Histopathology 38: 510-518.
321. Chan JK (2000). Images in Pathology. Int J Surg Pathol 8: 240.
322. Chan JK, Cheuk W, Shimizu M (2001). Anaplastic lymphoma kinase expression in inflammatory pseudotumors. Am J Surg Pathol 25: 761-768.
323. Chan JK, Fletcher CD, Nayler SJ, Cooper K (1997). Follicular dendritic cell sarcoma. Clinicopathologic analysis of 17 cases suggesting a malignant potential higher than currently recognized. Cancer 79: 294-313.
324. Chan JK, Hui PK, Tsang WY, Law CK, Ma CC, Yip TT, Poon YF (1995). Primary lymphoepithelioma-like carcinoma of the lung. A clinicopathologic study of 11 cases. Cancer 76: 413-422.
325. Chan JK, Sin VC, Wong KF, Ng CS, Tsang WY, Chan CH, Cheung MM, Lau WH (1997). Nonnasal lymphoma expressing the natural killer cell marker CD56: a clinicopathologic study of 49 cases of an uncommon aggressive neoplasm. Blood 89: 4501-4513.
326. Chan JK, Suster S, Wenig BM, Tsang WY, Chan JB, Lau AL (1997). Cytokeratin 20 immunoreactivity distinguishes Merkel cell (primary cutaneous neuroendocrine) carcinomas and salivary gland small cell carcinomas from small cell carcinomas of various sites. Am J Surg Pathol 21: 226-234.
327. Chan JK, Tsang WY, Seneviratne S, Pau MY (1995). The MIC2 antibody 013. Practical application for the study of thymic epithelial tumors. Am J Surg Pathol 19: 1115-1123.
328. Chan JKC, Yip TTC, Tsang WYW, Seneviratne S, Poon YF, Wong CSC, Ma VWS (1994). Lack of evidence of pathogenetic role of epstein-barr virus in thymic lymphoid hyperplasia and thymomas in the chinese population of Hong Kong. Int J Surg Pathol 2: 17-22.
329. Chan KL, Veinot J, Leach A, Bedard P, Smith S, Marquis JF (2001). Diagnosis of left atrial sarcoma by transvenous endocardial biopsy. Can J Cardiol 17: 206-208.
330. Chang YL, Lee YC, Shih JY, Wu CT (2001). Pulmonary pleomorphic (spindle) cell carcinoma: peculiar clinicopathologic manifestations different from ordinary non-small cell carcinoma. Lung Cancer 34: 91-97.
331. Chang YL, Wu CT, Shih JY, Lee YC (2002). New aspects in clinicopathologic and oncogene studies of 23 pulmonary lymphoepithelioma-like carcinomas. Am J Surg Pathol 26: 715-723.
332. Chang YS, Kong G, Sun S, Liu D, el Naggar AK, Khuri FR, Hong WK, Lee HY, Gong K (2002). Clinical significance of insulin-like growth factor-binding protein-3 expression in stage I non-small cell lung cancer. Clin Cancer Res 8: 3796-3802.
333. Chapman AD, Kerr KM (2000). The association between atypical adenomatous hyperplasia and primary lung cancer. Br J Cancer 83: 632-636.
334. Chapman AD, Thetford D, Kerr KM (2000). Pathological and clinical investigation of pulmonary atypical adenomatous hyperplasia and its association with primary lung adenocarcinoma. Lung Cancer 29(S1): 215-216.
335. Chariot P, Monnet I, Gaulard P, Abd-Alsamad I, Ruffie P, De Cremoux H (1993). Systemic mastocytosis following mediastinal germ cell tumor: an association confirmed. Hum Pathol 24: 111-112.
336. Charloux A, Quoix E, Wolkove N, Small D, Pauli G, Kreisman H (1997). The increasing incidence of lung adenocarcinoma: reality or artefact? A review of the epidemiology of lung adenocarcinoma. Int J Epidemiol 26: 14-23.
337. Chejfec G, Candel A, Jansson DS, Warren WH, Koukoulis GK, Gould JE, Manderino GL, Gooch GT, Gould VE (1991). Immunohistochemical features of giant cell carcinoma of the lung: patterns of expression of cytokeratins, vimentin, and the mucinous glycoprotein recognized by monoclonal antibody A-80. Ultrastruct Pathol 15: 131-138.
338. Chen FF, Yan JJ, Chang KC, Lai WW, Chen RM, Jin YT (1996). Immunohistochemical localization of Mcl-1 and bcl-2 proteins in thymic epithelial tumours. Histopathology 29: 541-547.
339. Chen FF, Yan JJ, Jin YT, Su IJ (1996). Detection of bcl-2 and p53 in thymoma: expression of bcl-2 as a reliable marker of tumor aggressiveness. Hum Pathol 27: 1089-1092.
340. Chen FF, Yan JJ, Lai WW, Jin YT, Su IJ (1998). Epstein-Barr virus-associated nonsmall cell lung carcinoma: undifferentiated "lymphoepithelioma-like" carcinoma as a distinct entity with better prognosis. Cancer 82: 2334-2342.
341. Chen G, Marx A, Wen-Hu C, Yong J, Puppe B, Stroebel P, Mueller-Hermelink HK (2002). New WHO histologic classification predicts prognosis of thymic epithelial tumors: a clinicopathologic study of 200 thymoma cases from China. Cancer 95: 420-429.
342. Chen HM, Chiu CC, Lee CS, Lai WD, Lin YT (2001). Intractable ventricular tachycardia in a patient with left ventricular epicardial lipoma. J Formos Med Assoc 100: 339-342.
343. Chen PC, Pan CC, Yang AH, Wang LS, Chiang H (2002). Detection of Epstein-Barr virus genome within thymic epithelial tumours in Taiwanese patients by nested PCR, PCR in situ hybridization, and RNA in situ hybridization. J Pathol 197: 684-688.
344. Chen W, Chan CW, Mok C (1982). Malignant fibrous histiocytoma of the mediastinum. Cancer 50: 797-800.
345. Cheng JQ, Jhanwar SC, Klein WM, Bell DW, Lee WC, Altomare DA, Nobori T, Olopade OI, Buckler AJ, Testa JR (1994). p16 alterations and deletion mapping of 9p21-p22 in malignant mesothelioma. Cancer Res 54: 5547-5551.
346. Cheng JQ, Lee WC, Klein MA, Cheng GZ, Jhanwar SC, Testa JR (1999). Frequent mutations of NF2 and allelic loss from chromosome band 22q12 in malignant mesothelioma: evidence for a two-hit mechanism of NF2 inactivation. Genes Chromosomes Cancer 24: 238-242.
347. Cheng TO (2000). Role of selective coronary arteriography in patients with cardiac myxoma. Cardiology 94: 263.
348. Cheng YL, Lee SC, Harn HJ, Chen CJ, Chang YC, Chen JC, Yu CP (2003). Prognostic prediction of the immunohistochemical expression of p53 and p16 in resected non-small cell lung cancer. Eur J Cardiothorac Surg 23: 221-228.
349. Chetty R, Batitang S, Govender D (1997). Large cell neuroendocrine carcinoma of the thymus. Histopathology 31: 274-276.
350. Chetty R, Bhana B, Batitang S, Govender D (1997). Lung carcinomas composed of rhabdoid cells. Eur J Surg Oncol 23: 432-434.
351. Cheuk W, Kwan MY, Suster S, Chan JK (2001). Immunostaining for thyroid transcription factor 1 and cytokeratin 20 aids the distinction of small cell carcinoma from Merkel cell carcinoma, but not pulmonary from extrapulmonary small cell carcinomas. Arch Pathol Lab Med 125: 228-231.
352. Chhieng DC, Cangiarella JF, Zakowski MF, Goswami S, Cohen JM, Yee HT (2001). Use of thyroid transcription factor 1, PE-10, and cytokeratins 7 and 20 in discriminating between primary lung carcinomas and metastatic lesions in fine-needle aspiration biopsy specimens. Cancer 93: 330-336.
353. Chibon F, Mairal A, Freneaux P, Terrier P, Coindre JM, Sastre X, Aurias A (2000). The RB1 gene is the target of chromosome 13 deletions in malignant fibrous histiocytoma. Cancer Res 60: 6339-6345.
354. Chilosi M, Castelli P, Martignoni G, Pizzolo G, Montresor E, Facchetti F, Truini M, Mombello A, Lestani M, Scarpa A (1992). Neoplastic epithelial cells in a subset of human thymomas express the B cell-associated CD20 antigen. Am J Surg Pathol 16: 988-997.
355. Chilosi M, Doglioni C, Yan Z, Lestani M, Menestrina F, Sorio C, Benedetti A, Vinante F, Pizzolo G, Inghirami G (1998). Differential expression of cyclin-dependent kinase 6 in cortical thymocytes and T-cell lymphoblastic lymphoma/leukemia. Am J Pathol 152: 209-217.
356. Chitwood WRJr (1988). Cardiac neoplasms: current diagnosis, pathology, and therapy. J Card Surg 3: 119-154.
357. Chiyo M, Fujisawa T, Yasukawa T, Shiba M, Shibuya K, Sekine Y, Hiroshima K, Ohwada H (2001). Successful resection of a primary liposarcoma in the anterior mediastinum in a child: report of a case. Surg Today 31: 230-232.
358. Cho KJ, Ha CW, Koh JS, Zo JI, Jang JJ (1993). Thymic carcinoid tumor combined with thymoma—neuroendocrine differentiation in thymoma? J Korean Med Sci 8: 458-463.
359. Choi PC, To KF, Lai FM, Lee TW, Yim AP, Chan JK (2000). Follicular dendritic cell sarcoma of the neck: report of two cases complicated by pulmonary metastases. Cancer 89: 664-672.
360. Choi WW, Lui YH, Lau WH, Crowley P, Khan A, Chan JK (2003). Adenocarcinoma of the thymus: report of two cases, including a previously undescribed mucinous subtype. Am J Surg Pathol 27: 124-130.
361. Chopra P, Ray R, Airan B, Talwar KK, Venugopal P (1999). Appraisal of histogenesis of cardiac myxoma: our experience of 78 cases and review of literature. Indian Heart J 51: 69-74.
362. Chopra P, Ray R, Singh MK, Venugopal P (2003). Cardiac myxoma with glandular elements: a histologic, histochemical and immunohistochemical evaluation. Indian Heart J 55: 182-184.
363. Chou ST, Arkles LB, Gill GD, Pinkus N, Parkin A, Hicks JD (1983). Primary lymphoma of the heart. A case report. Cancer 52: 744-747.

364. Chow LT, Chow WH, Tsui WM, Chan SK, Lee JC (1995). Fine-needle aspiration cytologic diagnosis of lymphoepithelioma-like carcinoma of the lung. Report of two cases with immunohistochemical study. Am J Clin Pathol 103: 35-40.
365. Christiansen S, Stypmann J, Baba HA, Hammel D, Scheld HH (2000). Surgical management of extensive lipomatous hypertrophy of the right atrium. Cardiovasc Surg 8: 88-90.
366. Chu P, Wu E, Weiss LM (2000). Cytokeratin 7 and cytokeratin 20 expression in epithelial neoplasms: a survey of 435 cases. Mod Pathol 13: 962-972.
367. Chu PG, Weiss LM (2002). Expression of cytokeratin 5/6 in epithelial neoplasms: an immunohistochemical study of 509 cases. Mod Pathol 15: 6-10.
368. Chu PG, Weiss LM (2002). Keratin expression in human tissues and neoplasms. Histopathology 40: 403-439.
369. Chubachi A, Miura I, Takahashi N, Nimura T, Imai H, Miura AB (1993). Acute myelogenous leukemia associated with a mediastinal tumor. Leuk Lymphoma 12: 143-146.
370. Chujo M, Noguchi T, Miura T, Arinaga M, Uchida Y, Tagawa Y (2002). Comparative genomic hybridization analysis detected frequent overrepresentation of chromosome 3q in squamous cell carcinoma of the lung. Lung Cancer 38: 23-29.
371. Chung CK, Zaino R, Stryker JA, O'Neill MJr, DeMuth WEJr (1982). Carcinoma of the lung: evaluation of histological grade and factors influencing prognosis. Ann Thorac Surg 33: 599-604.
372. Churg A, Johnston WH, Stulbarg M (1980). Small cell squamous and mixed small cell squamous—small cell anaplastic carcinomas of the lung. Am J Surg Pathol 4: 255-263.
373. Churg A, Warnock ML (1976). Pulmonary tumorlet. A form of peripheral carcinoid. Cancer 37: 1469-1477.
374. Cicala C, Pompetti F, Carbone M (1993). SV40 induces mesotheliomas in hamsters. Am J Pathol 142: 1524-1533.
375. Clark J, Rocques PJ, Crew AJ, Gill S, Shipley J, Chan AM, Gusterson BA, Cooper CS (1994). Identification of novel genes, SYT and SSX, involved in the t(X;18)(p11.2;q11.2) translocation found in human synovial sarcoma. Nat Genet 7: 502-508.
376. Clark OH (1988). Mediastinal parathyroid tumors. Arch Surg 123: 1096-1100.
377. Clement PB, Young RH, Scully RE (1987). Endometrioid-like variant of ovarian yolk sac tumor. A clinicopathological analysis of eight cases. Am J Surg Pathol 11: 767-778.
378. Close PM, Kirchner T, Uys CJ, Muller-Hermelink HK (1995). Reproducibility of a histogenetic classification of thymic epithelial tumours. Histopathology 26: 339-343.
379. Cobo F, Hernandez S, Hernandez L, Pinyol M, Bosch F, Esteve J, Lopez-Guillermo A, Palacin A, Raffeld M, Montserrat E, Jaffe ES, Campo E (1999). Expression of potentially oncogenic HHV-8 genes in an EBV-negative primary effusion lymphoma occurring in an HIV-seronegative patient. J Pathol 189: 288-293.
380. Codish S, Abu-Shakra M, Ariad S, Zirkin HJ, Yermiyahu T, Dupin N, Boshoff C, Sukenik S (2000). Manifestations of three HHV-8-related diseases in an HIV-negative patient: immunoblastic variant multicentric Castleman's disease, primary effusion lymphoma, and Kaposi's sarcoma. Am J Hematol 65: 310-314.
381. Coffin CM, Humphrey PA, Dehner LP (1998). Extrapulmonary inflammatory myofibroblastic tumor: a clinical and pathological survey. Semin Diagn Pathol 15: 85-101.
382. Coffin CM, Jaszcz W, O'Shea PA, Dehner LP (1994). So-called congenital-infantile fibrosarcoma: does it exist and what is it? Pediatr Pathol 14: 133-150.
383. Coffin CM, Patel A, Perkins S, Elenitoba-Johnson KS, Perlman E, Griffin CA (2001). ALK1 and p80 expression and chromosomal rearrangements involving 2p23 in inflammatory myofibroblastic tumor. Mod Pathol 14: 569-576.
384. Coffin CM, Watterson J, Priest JR, Dehner LP (1995). Extrapulmonary inflammatory myofibroblastic tumor (inflammatory pseudotumor). A clinicopathologic and immunohistochemical study of 84 cases. Am J Surg Pathol 19: 859-872.
385. Cohen-Barak O, Hagiwara N, Arlt MF, Horton JP, Brilliant MH (2001). Cloning, characterization and chromosome mapping of the human SOX6 gene. Gene 265: 157-164.
386. Cohen MB, Friend DS, Molnar JJ, Talerman A (1987). Gonadal endodermal sinus (yolk sac) tumor with pure intestinal differentiation: a new histologic type. Pathol Res Pract 182: 609-616.
387. Coindre JM, Terrier P, Bui NB, Bonichon F, Collin F, Le Doussal V, Mandard AM, Vilain MO, Jacquemier J, Duplay H, Sastre X, Barlier C, Henry-Amar M, Mace-Lesech J, Contesso G (1996). Prognostic factors in adult patients with locally controlled soft tissue sarcoma. A study of 546 patients from the French Federation of Cancer Centers Sarcoma Group. J Clin Oncol 14: 869-877.
388. Coindre JM, Terrier P, Guillou L, Le Doussal V, Collin F, Ranchere D, Sastre X, Vilain MO, Bonichon F, N'Guyen Bui B (2001). Predictive value of grade for metastasis development in the main histologic types of adult soft tissue sarcomas: a study of 1240 patients from the French Federation of Cancer Centers Sarcoma Group. Cancer 91: 1914-1926.
389. Coindre JM, Trojani M, Contesso G, David M, Rouesse J, Bui NB, Bodaert A, de Mascarel I, de Mascarel A, Goussot JF (1986). Reproducibility of a histopathologic grading system for adult soft tissue sarcoma. Cancer 58: 306-309.
390. Colby TV (1995). Malignancies in the lung and pleura mimicking benign processes. Semin Diagn Pathol 12: 30-44.
391. Colby TV, Koss M, Travis WD (1995). Tumors of the Lower Respiratory Tract. 3rd ed. Armed Forces Institute of Pathology: Washington, DC.
392. Colby TV, Wistuba II, Gazdar A (1998). Precursors to pulmonary neoplasia. Adv Anat Pathol 5: 205-215.
393. Colley MH, Geppert E, Franklin WA (1989). Immunohistochemical detection of steroid receptors in a case of pulmonary lymphangioleiomyomatosis. Am J Surg Pathol 13: 803-807.
394. Colwell AS, D'Cunha J, Vargas SO, Parker B, Cin PD, Maddaus MA (2002). Synovial sarcoma of the pleura: a clinical and pathologic study of three cases. J Thorac Cardiovasc Surg 124: 828-832.
395. Comin CE, Novelli L, Boddi V, Paglierani M, Dini S (2001). Calretinin, thrombomodulin, CEA, and CD15: a useful combination of immunohistochemical markers for differentiating pleural epithelial mesothelioma from peripheral pulmonary adenocarcinoma. Hum Pathol 32: 529-536.
396. Comings DE, Ferry L, Bradshaw-Robinson S, Burchette R, Chiu C, Muhleman D (1996). The dopamine D2 receptor (DRD2) gene: a genetic risk factor in smoking. Pharmacogenetics 6: 73-79.
397. Comiter CV, Kibel AS, Richie JP, Nucci MR, Renshaw AA (1998). Prognostic features of teratomas with malignant transformation: a clinicopathological study of 21 cases. J Urol 159: 859-863.
398. Conlan AA, Payne WS, Woolner LB, Sanderson DR (1978). Adenoid cystic carcinoma (cylindroma) and mucoepidermoid carcinoma of the bronchus. Factors affecting survival. J Thorac Cardiovasc Surg 76: 369-377.
399. Conn JM, Goncalves MA, Mansour KA, McGarity WC (1991). The mediastinal parathyroid. Am Surg 57: 62-66.
400. Constantinou LL, Charitos CE, Lariou CM, Garyphalos DJ, Douras AL, Vichas GJ, Livathinos AJ, Moraitis SD, Antonatos PG (1996). Primary synovial cardiac sarcoma: a rare cause of tamponade. Eur Heart J 17: 1766-1768.
401. Cook JR, Dehner LP, Collins MH, Ma Z, Morris SW, Coffin CM, Hill DA (2001). Anaplastic lymphoma kinase (ALK) expression in the inflammatory myofibroblastic tumor: a comparative immunohistochemical study. Am J Surg Pathol 25: 1364-1371.
402. Cooper CA, Carby FA, Bubb VJ, Lamb D, Kerr KM, Wyllie AH (1997). The pattern of K-ras mutation in pulmonary adenocarcinoma defines a new pathway of tumour development in the human lung. J Pathol 181: 401-404.
403. Copeland JN, Amin MB, Humphrey PA, Tamboli P, Ro JY, Gal AA (2002). The morphologic spectrum of metastatic prostatic adenocarcinoma to the lung: special emphasis on histologic features overlapping with other pulmonary neoplasms. Am J Clin Pathol 117: 552-557.
404. Copie-Bergman C, Gaulard P, Maouche-Chretien L, Briere J, Haioun C, Alonso MA, Romeo PH, Leroy K (1999). The MAL gene is expressed in primary mediastinal large B-cell lymphoma. Blood 94: 3567-3575.
405. Copie-Bergman C, Wotherspoon AC, Norton AJ, Diss TC, Isaacson PG (1998). True histiocytic lymphoma: a morphologic, immunohistochemical, and molecular genetic study of 13 cases. Am J Surg Pathol 22: 1386-1392.
406. Corbett R, Carter R, MacVicar D, Horwich A, Pinkerton R (1994). Embryonal rhabdomyosarcoma arising in a germ cell tumour. Med Pediatr Oncol 23: 497-502.
407. Cordier JF, Chailleux E, Lauque D, Reynaud-Gaubert M, Dietemann-Molard A, Dalphin JC, Blanc-Jouvan F, Loire R (1993). Primary pulmonary lymphomas. A clinical study of 70 cases in nonimmunocompromised patients. Chest 103: 201-208.
408. Corrin B (2000). Pathology of Lung Tumours. Churchill Livingstone: New York.
409. Corrin B, Harrison WJ, Wright DH (1983). The so-called intravascular bronchioloalveolar tumour of lung (low grade sclerosing angiosarcoma): presentation with extrapulmonary deposits. Diagn Histopathol 6: 229-237.
410. Corson JM, Weiss LM, Banks-Schlegel SP, Pinkus GS (1984). Keratin proteins and carcinoembryonic antigen in synovial sarcomas: an immunohistochemical study of 24 cases. Hum Pathol 15: 615-621.
411. Coskun U, Gunel N, Yildirim Y, Memis L, Boyacioglu ZM (2002). Primary mediastinal yolk sac tumor in a 66-year-old woman. Med Princ Pract 11: 218-220.
412. Costa J (1990). The grading and staging of soft tissue sarcomas. In: Pathobiology of Soft Tissue Tumors, Fletcher CD, McKee PH, eds., Churchill Livingstone: Edinburg , pp. 221-238.
413. Costa J, Wesley RA, Glatstein E, Rosenberg SA (1984). The grading of soft tissue sarcomas. Results of a clinicohistopathologic correlation in a series of 163 cases. Cancer 53: 530-541.
414. Costello LC, Hartman TE, Ryu JH (2000). High frequency of pulmonary lymphangioleiomyomatosis in women with tuberous sclerosis complex. Mayo Clin Proc 75: 591-594.
415. Costes V, Faumont N, Cesarman E, Rousset T, Meggetto F, Delsol G, Brousset P (2002). Human herpesvirus-8-associated lymphoma of the bowel in human immunodeficiency virus-positive patients without history of primary effusion lymphoma. Hum Pathol 33: 846-849.
416. Costes V, Marty-Ane C, Picot MC, Serre I, Pujol JL, Mary H, Baldet P (1995). Typical and atypical bronchopulmonary carcinoid tumors: a clinicopathologic and KI-67-labeling study. Hum Pathol 26: 740-745.
417. Cote RJ, Jhanwar SC, Novick S, Pellicer A (1991). Genetic alterations of the p53 gene are a feature of malignant mesotheliomas. Cancer Res 51: 5410-5416.
418. Cotton JL, Kavey RE, Palmier CE, Tunnessen WWJr (1991). Cardiac tumors and the nevoid basal cell carcinoma syndrome. Pediatrics 87: 725-728.
419. Cox JE, Chiles C, Aquino SL, Savage P, Oaks T (1997). Pulmonary artery sarcomas: a review of clinical and radiologic features. J Comput Assist Tomogr 21: 750-755.
420. Craig ID, Desrosiers P, Lefcoe MS (1983). Giant-cell carcinoma of the lung. A cytologic study. Acta Cytol 27: 293-298.
421. Craig ID, Finley RJ (1982). Spindle-cell carcinoid tumor of lung. Cytologic, histopathologic and ultrastructural features. Acta Cytol 26: 495-498.
422. Crespo C, Navarro M, Gonzalez I, Lorente MF, Gonzalez R, Mayol MJ (2001). Intracranial and mediastinal inflammatory myofibroblastic tumour. Pediatr Radiol 31: 600-602.
423. Crist W, Gehan EA, Ragab AH, Dickman PS, Donaldson SS, Fryer C, Hammond D, Hays DM, Herrmann J, Heyn R (1995). The Third Intergroup Rhabdomyosarcoma Study. J Clin Oncol 13: 610-630.
424. Crotty EJ, McAdams HP, Erasmus JJ, Sporn TA, Roggli VL (2000). Epithelioid hemangioendothelioma of the pleura: clinical and radiologic features. AJR Am J Roentgenol 175: 1545-1549.
425. Crotty TB, Myers JL, Katzenstein AL, Tazelaar HD, Swensen SJ, Churg A (1994). Localized malignant mesothelioma. A clinicopathologic and flow cytometric study. Am J Surg Pathol 18: 357-363.
426. Crow J, Slavin G, Kreel L (1981). Pulmonary metastasis: a pathologic and radiologic study. Cancer 47: 2595-2602.
427. Curran WJJr (2001). Therapy of limited stage small cell lung cancer. Cancer Treat Res 105: 229-252.
428. Cushing B, Bhanot PK, Watts FBJr, Hertzler JH, Brough AJ (1983). Rhabdomyosarcoma and benign teratoma. Pediatr Pathol 1: 345-348.

429. Cwierzyk TA, Glasberg SS, Virshup MA, Cranmer JC (1985). Pulmonary oncocytoma. Report of a case with cytologic, histologic and electron microscopic study. Acta Cytol 29: 620-623.

430. Dacic S, Colby TV, Yousem SA (2000). Nodular amyloidoma and primary pulmonary lymphoma with amyloid production: a differential diagnostic problem. Mod Pathol 13: 934-940.

431. Dacic S, Finkelstein SD, Sasatomi E, Swalsky PA, Yousem SA (2002). Molecular pathogenesis of pulmonary carcinosarcoma as determined by microdissection-based allelotyping. Am J Surg Pathol 26: 510-516.

432. Dai Y, Morishita Y, Mase K, Sato N, Akaogi E, Mitsui T, Noguchi M (2000). Application of the p53 and K-ras gene mutation patterns for cytologic diagnosis of recurrent lung carcinomas. Cancer 90: 258-263.

433. Daibata M, Taguchi T, Nemoto Y, Saito T, Machida H, Imai S, Miyoshi I, Taguchi H (2002). Epstein-Barr virus (EBV)-positive pyothorax-associated lymphoma (PAL): chromosomal integration of EBV in a novel CD2-positive PAL B-cell line. Br J Haematol 117: 546-557.

434. Dail DH, Hammar SP (1994). Pulmonary Pathology. 2nd Edition ed. Springler Verlag: New York.

435. Dail DH, Liebow AA, Gmelich JT, Friedman PJ, Miyai K, Myer W, Patterson SD, Hammar SP (1983). Intravascular, bronchiolar, and alveolar tumor of the lung (IVBAT). An analysis of twenty cases of a peculiar sclerosing endothelial tumor. Cancer 51: 452-464.

436. Dal Cin P, Sciot R, Fletcher CD, Hilliker C, de Wever I, Van Damme B, van den Berghe H (1996). Trisomy 21 in solitary fibrous tumor. Cancer Genet Cytogenet 86: 58-60.

437. Dal Cin P, Wolf-Peeters C, Aly MS, Deneffe G, Van Mieghem W, van den Berghe H (1993). Ring chromosome 6 as the only change in a thymoma. Genes Chromosomes Cancer 6: 243-244.

438. Dal Cin P, Wolf-Peeters C, Deneffe G, Fryns JP, van den Berghe H (1996). Thymoma with a t(15;22)(p11;q11). Cancer Genet Cytogenet 89: 181-183.

439. Dang TP, Gazdar AF, Virmani AK, Sepetavec T, Hande KR, Minna JD, Roberts JR, Carbone DP (2000). Chromosome 19 translocation, overexpression of Notch3, and human lung cancer. J Natl Cancer Inst 92: 1355-1357.

440. Daugaard G, Rorth M, von der Maase H, Skakkebaek NE (1992). Management of extragonadal germ-cell tumors and the significance of bilateral testicular biopsies. Ann Oncol 3: 283-289.

441. Daugaard G, von der Maase H, Olsen J, Rorth M, Skakkebaek NE (1987). Carcinoma-in-situ testis in patients with assumed extragonadal germ-cell tumours. Lancet 2: 528-530.

442. Davidson RS, Nwogu CE, Brentjens MJ, Anderson TM (2001). The surgical management of pulmonary metastasis: current concepts. Surg Oncol 10: 35-42.

443. Davis MP, Eagan RT, Weiland LH, Pairolero PC (1984). Carcinosarcoma of the lung: Mayo Clinic experience and response to chemotherapy. Mayo Clin Proc 59: 598-603.

444. Daya D, McCaughey WT (1990). Well-differentiated papillary mesothelioma of the peritoneum. A clinicopathologic study of 22 cases. Cancer 65: 292-296.

445. de Jong D, Richel DJ, Schenkeveld C, Boerrigter L, van't Veer LJ (1997). Oligoclonal peripheral T-cell lymphocytosis as a result of aberrant T-cell development in a cortical thymoma. Diagn Mol Pathol 6: 244-248.

446. de Leon GA, Zaeri N, Donner RM, Karmazin N (1990). Cerebral rhinocele, hydrocephalus, and cleft lip and palate in infants with cardiac fibroma. J Neurol Sci 99: 27-36.

447. de Leval L, Defraigne JO, Hermans G, Dome F, Boniver J, Herens C (2003). Malignant solitary fibrous tumor of the pleura: report of a case with cytogenetic analysis. Virchows Arch 442: 388-392.

448. de Leval L, Ferry JA, Falini B, Shipp M, Harris NL (2001). Expression of bcl-6 and CD10 in primary mediastinal large B-cell lymphoma: evidence for derivation from germinal center B cells? Am J Surg Pathol 25: 1277-1282.

449. de Montpreville VT, Dulmet EM, Chapelier AR, Dartevelle PG, Verley JM (1993). Extramedullary hematopoietic tumors of the posterior mediastinum related to asymptomatic refractory anemia. Chest 104: 1623-1624.

450. de Montpreville VT, Macchiarini P, Dulmet E (1996). Thymic neuroendocrine carcinoma (carcinoid): a clinicopathologic study of fourteen cases. J Thorac Cardiovasc Surg 111: 134-141.

451. de Montpreville VT, Serraf A, Aznag H, Nashashibi N, Planche C, Dulmet E (2001). Fibroma and inflammatory myofibroblastic tumor of the heart. Ann Diagn Pathol 5: 335-342.

452. de Montpreville VT, Zemoura L, Dulmet E (2002). [Thymoma with epithelial micronodules and lymphoid hyperplasia: six cases of a rare and equivocal subtype]. Ann Pathol 22: 177-182.

453. de Nictolis M, Brancorsini D, Goteri G, Prat J (1996). Epithelioid haemangioma of the heart. Virchows Arch 428: 119-123.

454. de Nictolis M, Goteri G, Brancorsini D, Giannulis I, Prete E, Fabris G (1995). Extraskeletal osteosarcoma of the mediastinum associated with long-term patient survival. A case report. Anticancer Res 15: 2785-2789.

455. de Nictolis M, Goteri G, Campanati G, Prat J (1995). Elastofibrolipoma of the mediastinum. A previously undescribed benign tumor containing abnormal elastic fibers. Am J Surg Pathol 19: 364-367.

456. de Perrot M, Spiliopoulos A, Fischer S, Totsch M, Keshavjee S (2002). Neuroendocrine carcinoma (carcinoid) of the thymus associated with Cushing's syndrome. Ann Thorac Surg 73: 675-681.

457. De Rienzo A, Balsara BR, Apostolou S, Jhanwar SC, Testa JR (2001). Loss of heterozygosity analysis defines a 3-cM region of 15q commonly deleted in human malignant mesothelioma. Oncogene 20: 6245-6249.

458. De Rienzo A, Jhanwar SC, Testa JR (2000). Loss of heterozygosity analysis of 13q and 14q in human malignant mesothelioma. Genes Chromosomes Cancer 28: 337-341.

459. de Saint Aubain Somerhausen N, Rubin BP, Fletcher CD (1999). Myxoid solitary fibrous tumor: a study of seven cases with emphasis on differential diagnosis. Mod Pathol 12: 463-471.

460. De Santis M, Bokemeyer C, Becherer A, Stoiber F, Oechsle K, Kletter K, Dohmen BM, Dittrich C, Pont J (2001). Predictive impact of 2-18fluoro-2-deoxy-D-glucose positron emission tomography for residual postchemotherapy masses in patients with bulky seminoma. J Clin Oncol 19: 3740-3744.

461. De Toma G, Plocco M, Nicolanti V, Brozzetti S, Letizia C, Cavallaro A (2001). Type B1 thymoma in multiple endocrine neoplasia type 1 (MEN-1) syndrome. Tumori 87: 266-268.

462. De Young BR, Frierson HFJr, Ly MN, Smith D, Swanson PE (1998). CD31 immunoreactivity in carcinomas and mesotheliomas. Am J Clin Pathol 110: 374-377.

463. Debelenko LV, Brambilla E, Agarwal SK, Swalwell JI, Kester MB, Lubensky IA, Zhuang Z, Guru SC, Manickam P, Olufemi SE, Chandrasekharappa SC, Crabtree JS, Kim YS, Heppner C, Burns AL, Spiegel AM, Marx SJ, Liotta LA, Collins FS, Travis WD, Emmert-Buck MR (1997). Identification of MEN1 gene mutations in sporadic carcinoid tumors of the lung. Hum Mol Genet 6: 2285-2290.

464. Debelenko LV, Swalwell JI, Kelley MJ, Brambilla E, Manickam P, Baibakov G, Agarwal SK, Spiegel AM, Marx SJ, Chandrasekharappa SC, Collins FS, Travis WD, Emmert-Buck MR (2000). MEN1 gene mutation analysis of high-grade neuroendocrine lung carcinoma. Genes Chromosomes Cancer 28: 58-65.

465. Deenadayalu RP, Tuuri D, Dewall RA, Johnson GF (1974). Intrapericardial teratoma and bronchogenic cyst. Review of literature and report of successful surgery in infant with intrapericardial teratoma. J Thorac Cardiovasc Surg 67: 945-952.

466. Dehner LP (1990). Germ cell tumors of the mediastinum. Semin Diagn Pathol 7: 266-284.

467. Dehner LP, Coffin CM (1998). Idiopathic fibrosclerotic disorders and other inflammatory pseudotumors. Semin Diagn Pathol 15: 161-173.

468. Dehner LP, Watterson J, Priest J (1995). Pleuropulmonary blastoma: a unique intratoracic-pulmonary neoplasm of childhood. Perspect Pediatr Pathol 18: 214-226.

469. Dei Tos AP, Wadden C, Calonje E, Sciot R, Pauwels P, Knight JC, Dal Cin P, Fletcher CD (1995). Immunohistochemical demonstratioin of glycoprotein p30/32 mic2 (CD99) in synovial sarcoma: a potential cause of diagnostic confusion. Appl Immunohistochem 3: 168-173.

470. Dein JR, Frist WH, Stinson EB, Miller DC, Baldwin JC, Oyer PE, Jamieson S, Mitchell RS, Shumway NE (1987). Primary cardiac neoplasms. Early and late results of surgical treatment in 42 patients. J Thorac Cardiovasc Surg 93: 502-511.

471. DeLellis RA (2001). The neuroendocrine system and its tumors: an overview. Am J Clin Pathol 115 Suppl: S5-16.

472. Delpiano C, Claren R, Sironi M, Cenacchi G, Spinelli M (2000). Cytological appearance of papillary mucous gland adenoma of the left lobar bronchus with histological confirmation. Cytopathology 11: 193-196.

473. deMent SH (1990). Association between mediastinal germ cell tumors and hematologic malignancies: an update. Hum Pathol 21: 699-703.

474. deMent SH, Eggleston JC, Spivak JL (1985). Association between mediastinal germ cell tumors and hematologic malignancies. Report of two cases and review of the literature. Am J Surg Pathol 9: 23-30.

475. Demirer T, Ravits J, Aboulafia D (1994). Myasthenic (Eaton-Lambert) syndrome associated with pulmonary large-cell neuroendocrine carcinoma. South Med J 87: 1186-1189.

476. Denayer MA, Rao KR, Wirz D, McNally D (1986). Hepatic metastatic thymoma and myasthenia gravis twenty-two years after the apparent cure of an invasive thymoma. A case report and review of the literature. J Neurol Sci 76: 23-30.

477. Denissenko MF, Pao A, Tang M, Pfeifer GP (1996). Preferential formation of benzo[a]pyrene adducts at lung cancer mutational hotspots in P53. Science 274: 430-432.

478. Denning K, Sehmann G, Richter T (2000). The angiosarcoma in the left atrium. N Engl J Med 443-444.

479. DePond W, Said JW, Tasaka T, de Vos S, Kahn D, Cesarman E, Knowles DM, Koeffler HP (1997). Kaposi's sarcoma-associated herpesvirus and human herpesvirus 8 (KSHV/HHV8)-associated lymphoma of the bowel. Report of two cases in HIV-positive men with secondary effusion lymphomas. Am J Surg Pathol 21: 719-724.

480. Derenoncourt AN, Castro-Magana M, Jones KL (1995). Mediastinal teratoma and precocious puberty in a boy with mosaic Klinefelter syndrome. Am J Med Genet 55: 38-42.

481. Dermer GB (1982). Origin of bronchioloalveolar carcinoma and peripheral bronchial adenocarcinoma. Cancer 49: 881-887.

482. Desai SB, Pradhan SA, Chinoy RF (2000). Mediastinal Castleman's disease complicated by follicular dendritic cell tumour. Indian J Cancer 37: 129-132.

483. Deshpande A, Kumar S, Chopra P (1994). Recurrent, biatrial, familial cardiac myxomas. Int J Cardiol 47: 71-73.

484. Dessy E, Braidotti P, Del Curto B, Falleni M, Coggi G, Santa Cruz G, Carai A, Versace R, Pietra GG (2000). Peripheral papillary tumor of type-II pneumocytes: a rare neoplasm of undetermined malignant potential. Virchows Arch 436: 289-295.

485. Devendra G, Mo M, Kerr KM, Fedullo PF, Yi J, Kapelanski D, Jamieson S, Auger WR (2002). Pulmonary artery sarcomas: the UCSD experience. Am J Respir Crit Care Med 165: A24.

486. Devesa SS, Grauman DJ, Blot WJ, Fraumeni JFJr (1999). Cancer surveillance series: changing geographic patterns of lung cancer mortality in the United States, 1950 through 1994. J Natl Cancer Inst 91: 1040-1050.

487. Devesa SS, Shaw GL, Blot WJ (1991). Changing patterns of lung cancer incidence by histological type. Cancer Epidemiol Biomarkers Prev 1: 29-34.

488. Devouassoux-Shisheboran M, Hayashi T, Linnoila RI, Koss MN, Travis WD (2000). A clinicopathologic study of 100 cases of pulmonary sclerosing hemangioma with immunohistochemical studies: TTF-1 is expressed in both round and surface cells, suggesting an origin from primitive respiratory epithelium. Am J Surg Pathol 24: 906-916.

489. Dewald GW, Dahl RJ, Spurbeck JL, Carney JA, Gordon H (1987). Chromosomally abnormal clones and nonrandom telomeric translocations in cardiac myxomas. Mayo Clin Proc 62: 558-567.

490. Dexeus FH, Logothetis CJ, Chong C, Sella A, Ogden S (1988). Genetic abnormalities in men with germ cell tumors. J Urol 140: 80-84.

491. Di Cataldo A, Villari L, Milone P, Miano

AE, Sambataro MP, Florio G, Petrillo G (2000). Thymic carcinoma, systemic lupus erythematosus, and hypertrophic pulmonary osteoarthropathy in an 11-year-old boy: a novel association. Pediatr Hematol Oncol 17: 701-706.
492. Di Liang C, Ko SF, Huang SC (2000). Echocardiographic evaluation of cardiac rhabdomyoma in infants and children. J Clin Ultrasound 28: 381-386.
493. Di Loreto C, Mariuzzi L, De Grassi A, Beltrami CA (1996). B cell lymphoma of the thymus and salivary gland. J Clin Pathol 49: 595-597.
494. Di Tullio MT, Indolfi P, Casale F, Pettinato G, Martone A, Morgera C (1999). Pleuropulmonary blastoma: survival after intraocular recurrence. Med Pediatr Oncol 33: 588-590.
495. Diehl V, Franklin J, Hasenclever D, Tesch H, Pfreundschuh M, Lathan B, Paulus U, Sieber M, Rueffer JU, Sextro M, Engert A, Wolf J, Hermann R, Holmer L, Stappert-Jahn U, Winnerlein-Trump E, Wulf G, Krause S, Glunz A, von Kalle K, Bischoff H, Haedicke C, Duehmke E, Georgii A, Loeffler M (1998). BEACOPP, a new dose-escalated and accelerated regimen, is at least as effective as COPP/ABVD in patients with advanced-stage Hodgkin's lymphoma: interim report from a trial of the German Hodgkin's Lymphoma Study Group. J Clin Oncol 16: 3810-3821.
496. Diehl V, Sextro M, Franklin J, Hansmann ML, Harris N, Jaffe E, Poppema S, Harris M, Franssila K, van Krieken J, Marafioti T, Anagnostopoulos I, Stein H (1999). Clinical presentation, course, and prognostic factors in lymphocyte-predominant Hodgkin's disease and lymphocyte-rich classical Hodgkin's disease: report from the European Task Force on Lymphoma Project on Lymphocyte-Predominant Hodgkin's Disease. J Clin Oncol 17: 776-783.
497. Dijkhuizen T, de Jong B, Meuzelaar JJ, Molenaar WM, van den Berg E (2001). No cytogenetic evidence for involvement of gene(s) at 2p16 in sporadic cardiac myxomas: cytogenetic changes in ten sporadic cardiac myxomas. Cancer Genet Cytogenet 126: 162-165.
498. Dijkhuizen T, van den Berg E, Molenaar WM, Meuzelaar JJ, de Jong B (1995). Rearrangements involving 12p12 in two cases of cardiac myxoma. Cancer Genet Cytogenet 82: 161-162.
499. Dillon KM, Hill CM, Cameron CH, Attanoos RL, McCluggage WG (2002). Mediastinal mixed dendritic cell sarcoma with hybrid features. J Clin Pathol 55: 791-794.
500. Dishop MK, O'Connor WN, Abraham S, Cottrill CM (2001). Primary cardiac lipoblastoma. Pediatr Dev Pathol 4: 276-280.
500A. Divine KK, Gilliland FD, Crowell RE, Stidley CA, Bocklage TJ, Cook DL, Belinski SA (2001). The XRCC1 399 glutamine allele is a risk factor for adenocarcinoma of the lung. Mutat Res 461: 273-278
501. Do YS, Im JG, Lee BH, Kim KH, Oh YW, Chin SY, Zo JI, Jang JJ (1995). CT findings in malignant tumors of thymic epithelium. J Comput Assist Tomogr 19: 192-197.
502. Dobin S, Speights VOJr, Donner LR (1997). Addition (1)(q32) as the sole clonal chromosomal abnormality in a case of cardiac myxoma. Cancer Genet Cytogenet 96: 181-182.
503. Doglioni C, Bontempini L, Iuzzolino P, Furlan G, Rosai J (1988). Ependymoma of the mediastinum. Arch Pathol Lab Med 112: 194-196.
504. Doll R, Hill AB (1950). Smoking and cancer of the lung; preliminary report. Br Med J 4682: 739-748.
505. Doll R, Peto R (1981). The causes of cancer: quantitative estimates of avoidable risks of cancer in the United States today. J Natl Cancer Inst 66: 1191-1308.
506. Domingo A, Romagosa V, Callis M, Vivancos P, Guionnet N, Soler J (1989). Mediastinal germ cell tumor and acute megakaryoblastic leukemia. Ann Intern Med 111: 539.
507. Dominguez-Malagon H, Guerrero-Medrano J, Suster S (1995). Ectopic poorly differentiated (insular) carcinoma of the thyroid. Report of a case presenting as an anterior mediastinal mass. Am J Clin Pathol 104: 408-412.
508. Donner LR, Silva MT, Dobin SM (1999). Solitary fibrous tumor of the pleura: a cytogenetic study. Cancer Genet Cytogenet 111: 169-171.
509. Donsbeck AV, Ranchere D, Coindre JM, Le Gall F, Cordier JF, Loire R (1999). Primary cardiac sarcomas: an immunohistochemical and grading study with long-term follow-up of 24 cases. Histopathology 34: 295-304.
510. Dorfler H, Permanetter W, Kuffer G, Haussinger K, Zollner N (1990). Sclerosing epitheloid angiosarcoma of bone and lung—intravascular sclerosing bronchioloalveolar tumor. Klin Wochenschr 68: 388-392.
511. Dorfman DM, Shahsafaei A, Chan JK (1997). Thymic carcinomas, but not thymomas and carcinomas of other sites, show CD5 immunoreactivity. Am J Surg Pathol 21: 936-940.
512. Dotti G, Fiocchi R, Motta T, Facchinetti B, Chiodini B, Borleri GM, Gavazzeni G, Barbui T, Rambaldi A (1999). Primary effusion lymphoma after heart transplantation: a new entity associated with human herpesvirus-8. Leukemia 13: 664-670.
513. Downes KA, Goldblum JR, Montgomery EA, Fisher C (2001). Pleomorphic liposarcoma: a clinicopathologic analysis of 19 cases. Mod Pathol 14: 179-184.
514. Drexler HG, Meyer C, Gaidano G, Carbone A (1999). Constitutive cytokine production by primary effusion (body cavity-based) lymphoma-derived cell lines. Leukemia 13: 634-640.
515. Duarte IG, Gal AA, Mansour KA (1998). Primary malignant melanoma of the trachea. Ann Thorac Surg 65: 559-560.
516. Dubost C, Guilmet D, de Parades B, Pedeferri G (1966). [New technic of opening of the left auricle in open-heart surgery: the transseptal bi-auricular approach]. Presse Med 74: 1607-1608.
517. Dudgeon DL, Haller JAJr (1984). Pediatric lipoblastomatosis: two unusual cases. Surgery 95: 371-373.
518. Dueland S, Stenwig AE, Heilo A, Hoie J, Ous S, Fossa SD (1998). Treatment and outcome of patients with extragonadal germ cell tumours—the Norwegian Radium Hospital's experience 1979-94. Br J Cancer 77: 329-335.
519. Dulmet-Brender E, Jaubert F, Huchon G (1986). Exophytic endobronchial epidermoid carcinoma. Cancer 57: 1358-1364.
520. Dulmet EM, Macchiarini P, Suc B, Verley JM (1993). Germ cell tumors of the mediastinum. A 30-year experience. Cancer 72: 1894-1901.
521. Dunn PJ (1984). Pancreatic endocrine tissue in benign mediastinal teratoma. J Clin Pathol 37: 1105-1109.
522. Dupin N, Fisher C, Kellam P, Ariad S, Tulliez M, Franck N, van Marck E, Salmon D, Gorin I, Escande JP, Weiss RA, Alitalo K, Boshoff C (1999). Distribution of human herpesvirus-8 latently infected cells in Kaposi's sarcoma, multicentric Castleman's disease, and primary effusion lymphoma. Proc Natl Acad Sci U S A 96: 4546-4551.
523. Duray PH, Mark EJ, Barwick KW, Madri JA, Strom RL (1985). Congenital polycystic tumor of the atrioventricular node. Autopsy study with immunohistochemical findings suggesting endodermal derivation. Arch Pathol Lab Med 109: 30-34.
524. Durgut K, Gormus N, Ozulku M, Ozergin U, Ozpinar C (2002). Clinical features and surgical treatment of cardiac myxoma: report of 18 cases. Asian Cardiovasc Thorac Ann 10: 111-114.
525. Dyamenahalli U, Black MD, Boutin C, Gow RM, Freedom RM (1998). Obstructive rhabdomyoma and univentricular physiology: a rare combination. Ann Thorac Surg 65: 835-837.
526. Eble JN, Sauter G, Epstein J, Sesterhenn IA (2003). Wolrd Health Organization Classification of Tumours. Pathology and Genetics of Tumours of the Urinary System and Male Genital Organs. IARC Press: Lyon.
527. Economides EG, Singh A (1998). Case of tumor neovascularization demonstrated by cardiac catheterization. Cathet Cardiovasc Diagn 43: 451-453.
528. Economopoulos GC, Lewis JWJr, Lee MW, Silverman NA (1990). Carcinoid tumors of the thymus. Ann Thorac Surg 50: 58-61.
529. Edmonson JH, Ryan LM, Blum RH, Brooks JS, Shiraki M, Frytak S, Parkinson DR (1993). Randomized comparison of doxorubicin alone versus ifosfamide plus doxorubicin or mitomycin, doxorubicin, and cisplatin against advanced soft tissue sarcomas. J Clin Oncol 11: 1269-1275.
530. Edwards A, Bermudez C, Piwonka G, Berr ML, Zamorano J, Larrain E, Franck R, Gonzalez M, Alvarez E, Maiers E (2002). Carney's syndrome: complex myxomas. Report of four cases and review of the literature. Cardiovasc Surg 10: 264-275.
531. Edwards FH, Hale D, Cohen A, Thompson L, Pezzella AT, Virmani R (1991). Primary cardiac valve tumors. Ann Thorac Surg 52: 1127-1131.
532. Edwards SL, Roberts C, McKean ME, Cockburn JS, Jeffrey RR, Kerr KM (2000). Preoperative histological classification of primary lung cancer: accuracy of diagnosis and use of the non-small cell category. J Clin Pathol 53: 537-540.
533. Eggleston JC (1985). The intravascular bronchioloalveolar tumor and the sclerosing hemangioma of the lung: misnomers of pulmonary neoplasia. Semin Diagn Pathol 2: 270-280.
534. Eimoto T, Kitaoka M, Ogawa H, Niwa H, Murase T, Tateyama H, Inagaki H, Soji T, Wang HJ (2002). Thymic sarcomatoid carcinoma with skeletal muscle differentiation: report of two cases, one with cytogenetic analysis. Histopathology 40: 46-57.
535. Eisen MB, Spellman PT, Brown PO, Botstein D (1998). Cluster analysis and display of genome-wide expression patterns. Proc Natl Acad Sci U S A 95: 14863-14868.
536. Ekfors TO, Joensuu K, Toivio I, Laurinen P, Pelttari L (1986). Fatal epithelioid haemangioendothelioma presenting in the lung and liver. Virchows Arch A Pathol Anat Histopathol 410: 9-16.
537. el Gatit A, al Kaisi N, Moftah S, Olling S, al Khaja N, Belboul A, Roberts D (1994). Atypical bronchial carcinoid tumour with amyloid deposition. Eur J Surg Oncol 20: 586-587.
538. Elderkin RA, Radford DJ (2002). Primary cardiac tumours in a paediatric population. J Paediatr Child Health 38: 173-177.
539. Emanuel RL, Torday JS, Mu Q, Asokananthan N, Sikorski KA, Sunday ME (1999). Bombesin-like peptides and receptors in normal fetal baboon lung: roles in lung growth and maturation. Am J Physiol 277: L1003-L1017.
540. Eng J, Ruiz K, Kay PH (1992). Giant epicardial lipoma. Int J Cardiol 37: 115-117.
541. Engel P, Marx A, Muller-Hermelink HK (1999). Thymic tumours in Denmark. A retrospective study of 213 cases from 1970-1993. Pathol Res Pract 195: 565-570.
542. Engels EA, Katki HA, Nielsen NM, Winther JF, Hjalgrim H, Gjerris F, Rosenberg PS, Frisch M (2003). Cancer incidence in Denmark following exposure to poliovirus vaccine contaminated with simian virus 40. J Natl Cancer Inst 95: 532-539.
543. England DM, Hochholzer L (1995). Truly benign "bronchial adenoma". Report of 10 cases of mucous gland adenoma with immunohistochemical and ultrastructural findings. Am J Surg Pathol 19: 887-899.
544. England DM, Hochholzer L, McCarthy MJ (1989). Localized benign and malignant fibrous tumors of the pleura. A clinicopathologic review of 223 cases. Am J Surg Pathol 13: 640-658.
545. Enzinger FM, Weiss SW (1988). Malignant vascular tumors. In: Soft Tissue Tumors, Enzinger FM, Weiss SW, eds., 2nd ed. Mosby: St Louis , pp. 545-554.
546. Essary LR, Vargas SO, Fletcher CD (2002). Primary pleuropulmonary synovial sarcoma: reappraisal of a recently described anatomic subset. Cancer 94: 459-469.
547. Evans DG, Ladusans EJ, Rimmer S, Burnell LD, Thakker N, Farndon PA (1993). Complications of the naevoid basal cell carcinoma syndrome: results of a population based study. J Med Genet 30: 460-464.
548. Ewing J (1928). A Treatise on Tumors. WB Saunders: Philadelphia.
549. Eymin B, Gazzeri S, Brambilla C, Brambilla E (2001). Distinct pattern of E2F1 expression in human lung tumours: E2F1 is upregulated in small cell lung carcinoma. Oncogene 20: 1678-1687.
550. Eymin B, Karayan L, Seite P, Brambilla C, Brambilla E, Larsen CJ, Gazzeri S (2001). Human ARF binds E2F1 and inhibits its transcriptional activity. Oncogene 20: 1033-1041.
551. Eymin B, Leduc C, Coll JL, Brambilla E, Gazzeri S (2003). p14ARF induces G2 arrest and apoptosis independently of p53 leading to regression of tumours established in nude mice. Oncogene 22: 1822-1835.
552. Falini B, Mason DY (2002). Proteins encoded by genes involved in chromosomal alterations in lymphoma and leukemia: clinical value of their detection by immunocytochemistry. Blood 99: 409-426.
553. Falleni M, Roz E, Dessy E, Del Curto B, Braidotti P, Gianelli U, Pietra GG (2001). Primary intrathoracic meningioma: histopathological, immunohistochemical and ultrastructural study of two cases. Virchows Arch 439: 196-200.
554. Fan R, Wu MT, Miller D, Wain JC,

Kelsey KT, Wiencke JK, Christiani DC (2000). The p53 codon 72 polymorphism and lung cancer risk. Cancer Epidemiol Biomarkers Prev 9: 1037-1042.
555. Fantone JC, Geisinger KR, Appelman HD (1982). Papillary adenoma of the lung with lamellar and electron dense granules. An ultrastructural study. Cancer 50: 2839-2844.
556. Farooki ZQ, Ross RD, Paridon SM, Humes RA, Karpawich PP, Pinsky WW (1991). Spontaneous regression of cardiac rhabdomyoma. Am J Cardiol 67: 897-899.
557. Farrell DJ, Cooper PN, Malcolm AJ (1995). Carcinosarcoma of lung associated with asbestosis. Histopathology 27: 484-486.
558. Farrell JFJ (1935). Pulmonary metastasis: a pathologic, clinical roentgenologic study based on 78 cases seen at necroscopy. Radiology 24: 444-451.
559. Fasching K, Panzer S, Haas OA, Marschalek R, Gadner H, Panzer-Grumayer ER (2000). Presence of clone-specific antigen receptor gene rearrangements at birth indicates an in utero origin of diverse types of early childhood acute lymphoblastic leukemia. Blood 95: 2722-2724.
560. Fassina A, Marino F, Poletti A, Rea F, Pennelli N, Ninfo V (2001). Follicular dendritic cell tumor of the mediastinum. Ann Diagn Pathol 5: 361-367.
561. Fassone L, Bhatia K, Gutierrez M, Capello D, Gloghini A, Dolcetti R, Vivenza D, Ascoli V, Lo Coco F, Pagani L, Dotti G, Rambaldi A, Raphael M, Tirelli U, Saglio G, Magrath IT, Carbone A, Gaidano G (2000). Molecular profile of Epstein-Barr virus infection in HHV-8-positive primary effusion lymphoma. Leukemia 14: 271-277.
562. Fauci AS, Haynes BF, Costa J, Katz P, Wolff SM (1982). Lymphomatoid Granulomatosis. Prospective clinical and therapeutic experience over 10 years. N Engl J Med 306: 68-74.
563. Faul JL, Berry GJ, Colby TV, Ruoss SJ, Walter MB, Rosen GD, Raffin TA (2000). Thoracic lymphangiomas, lymphangiectasis, lymphangiomatosis, and lymphatic dysplasia syndrome. Am J Respir Crit Care Med 161: 1037-1046.
564. Feder M, Siegfried JM, Balshem A, Litwin S, Keller SM, Liu Z, Testa JR (1998). Clinical relevance of chromosome abnormalities in non-small cell lung cancer. Cancer Genet Cytogenet 102: 25-31.
565. Federici S, Domenichelli V, Tani G, Sciutti R, Burnelli R, Zanetti G, Domini R (2001). Pleuropulmonary blastoma in congenital cystic adenomatoid malformation: report of a case. Eur J Pediatr Surg 11: 196-199.
566. Fekete PS, Cohen C, DeRose PB (1990). Pulmonary spindle cell carcinoid. Needle aspiration biopsy, histologic and immunohistochemical findings. Acta Cytol 34: 50-56.
567. Fekete PS, Nassar VH, Talley JD, Boedecker EA (1983). Cardiac papilloma. A case report with evidence of thrombotic origin. Arch Pathol Lab Med 107: 246-248.
568. Feld R, Sagman U, Leblanc M (2000). Staging and prognosic factors for small cell carcinoma. In: Lung Cancer, Principles and Practice, Pass HI, Mitchell JB, Johnson DH, Turrisi AT, Minna JD, eds., Lippincott Williams and Wilkins: Philadelphia , pp. 967-980.
569. Feltkamp CA, van Heerde P, Feltkamp-Vroom TM, Koudstaal J (1981). A malignant tumor arising from interdigitating cells; light microscopical, ultrastructural, immuno-and enzyme-histochemical characteristics. Virchows Arch A Pathol Anat Histol 393: 183-192.
570. Felton WL, Liebow AA, Lindskog GE (1953). Peripheral and multiple bronchial adenomas. Cancer 6: 555-567.
571. Fenoglio JJJr, McAllister HAJr, Ferrans VJ (1976). Cardiac rhabdomyoma: a clinicopathologic and electron microscopic study. Am J Cardiol 38: 241-251.
Ferguson HL, Hawkins EP, Cooley LD (1996). Infant cardiac fibroma with clonal t(1;9)(q32;q22) and review of benign fibrous tissue cytogenetics. Cancer Genet Cytogenet 87: 34-37.
572. A. Ferlay J, Bray F, Pisani P, Parkin DM (2001). Globocan 2000: Cancer incidence, mortality and prevalence worldwide. IARC Press: Lyon.
573. Fernandes F, Soufen HN, Ianni BM, Arteaga E, Ramires FJ, Mady C (2001). Primary neoplasms of the heart. Clinical and histological presentation of 50 cases. Arq Bras Cardiol 76: 231-237.
574. Ferry JA, Linggood RM, Convery KM, Efird JT, Eliseo R, Harris NL (1993). Hodgkin disease, nodular sclerosis type. Implications of histologic subclassification. Cancer 71: 457-463.
575. Fetsch JF, Montgomery EA, Meis JM (1993). Calcifying fibrous pseudotumor. Am J Surg Pathol 17: 502-508.
576. Feyler A, Voho A, Bouchardy C, Kuokkanen K, Dayer P, Hirvonen A, Benhamou S (2002). Point: myeloperoxidase -463G —> a polymorphism and lung cancer risk. Cancer Epidemiol Biomarkers Prev 11: 1550-1554.
577. Fiche M, Caprons F, Berger F, Galateau F, Cordier JF, Loire R, Diebold J (1995). Primary pulmonary non-Hodgkin's lymphomas. Histopathology 26: 529-537.
578. Filderman AE, Coppage L, Shaw C, Matthay RA (1989). Pulmonary and pleural manifestations of extrathoracic malignancies. Clin Chest Med 10: 747-807.
579. Fine G, Chang CH (1991). Adenoma of type 2 pneumocytes with oncocytic features. Arch Pathol Lab Med 115: 797-801.
580. Fink G, Krelbaum T, Yellin A, Bendayan D, Saute M, Glazer M, Kramer MR (2001). Pulmonary carcinoid: presentation, diagnosis, and outcome in 142 cases in Israel and review of 640 cases from the literature. Chest 119: 1647-1651.
581. Finkelstein SD, Hasegawa T, Colby T, Yousem SA (1999). 11q13 allelic imbalance discriminates pulmonary carcinoids from tumorlets. A microdissection-based genotyping approach useful in clinical practice. Am J Pathol 155: 633-640.
582. Finley JL, Silverman JF, Dabbs DJ (1988). Fine-needle aspiration cytology of pulmonary carcinosarcoma with immunocytochemical and ultrastructural observations. Diagn Cytopathol 4: 239-243.
583. Fischer DR, Beerman LB, Park SC, Bahnson HT, Fricker FJ, Mathews RA (1984). Diagnosis of intracardiac rhabdomyoma by two-dimensional echocardiography. Am J Cardiol 53: 978-979.
584. Fishback NF, Travis WD, Moran CA, Guinee DGJr, McCarthy WF, Koss MN (1994). Pleomorphic (spindle/giant cell) carcinoma of the lung. A clinicopathologic correlation of 78 cases. Cancer 73: 2936-2945.
585. Fisher C, Schofield JB (1991). S-100 protein positive synovial sarcoma. Histopathology 19: 375-377.
586. Fitzgibbons PL, Kern WH (1985). Adenosquamous carcinoma of the lung: a clinical and pathologic study of seven cases. Hum Pathol 16: 463-466.
587. Fizazi K, Culine S, Droz JP, Kramar A, Theodore C, Ruffie P, Le Chevalier T (1998). Primary mediastinal nonseminomatous germ cell tumors: results of modern therapy including cisplatin-based chemotherapy. J Clin Oncol 16: 725-732.
588. Fizazi K, Tjulandin S, Salvioni R, Germa-Lluch JR, Bouzy J, Ragan D, Bokemeyer C, Gerl A, Flechon A, de Bono JS, Stenning S, Horwich A, Pont J, Albers P, De Giorgi U, Bower M, Bulanov A, Pizzocaro G, Aparicio J, Nichols CR, Theodore C, Hartmann JT, Schmoll HJ, Kaye SB, Culine S, Droz JP, Mahe C (2001). Viable malignant cells after primary chemotherapy for disseminated nonseminomatous germ cell tumors: prognostic factors and role of postsurgery chemotherapy—results from an international study group. J Clin Oncol 19: 2647-2657.
589. Fleming MV, Guinee DGJr, Chu WS, Freedman AN, Caporaso NE, Bennett WP, Colby TV, Tazelaar H, Abbondanzo SL, Jett J, Pairolero P, Trastek V, Liotta LA, Harris CC, Travis WD (1998). Bcl-2 immunohistochemistry in a surgical series of non-small cell lung cancer patients. Hum Pathol 29: 60-64.
590. Fletcher CDM, Unni KK, Mertens F (2002). World Health Organization Classification of Tumours. Pathology and Genetics of Tumours of Soft Tissue and Bone. IARC Press: Lyon.
591. Fletcher JA, Longtine J, Wallace K, Mentzer SJ, Sugarbaker DJ (1995). Cytogenetic and histologic findings in 17 pulmonary chondroid hamartomas: evidence for a pathogenetic relationship with lipomas and leiomyomas. Genes Chromosomes Cancer 12: 220-223.
592. Flieder DB, Koss MN, Nicholson A, Sesterhenn IA, Petras RE, Travis WD (1998). Solitary pulmonary papillomas in adults: a clinicopathologic and in situ hybridization study of 14 cases combined with 27 cases in the literature. Am J Surg Pathol 22: 1328-1342.
593. Flieder DB, Moran CA, Suster S (1997). Primary alveolar soft-part sarcoma of the mediastinum: a clinicopathological and immunohistochemical study of two cases. Histopathology 31: 469-473.
594. Flieder DB, Travis WD (1997). Clear cell "sugar" tumor of the lung: association with lymphangioleiomyomatosis and multifocal micronodular pneumocyte hyperplasia in a patient with tuberous sclerosis. Am J Surg Pathol 21: 1242-1247.
595. Flint A, Lloyd RV (1992). Pulmonary metastases of colonic carcinoma. Distinction from pulmonary adenocarcinoma. Arch Pathol Lab Med 116: 39-42.
596. Flint A, Weiss SW (1995). CD-34 and keratin expression distinguishes solitary fibrous tumor (fibrous mesothelioma) of pleura from desmoplastic mesothelioma. Hum Pathol 26: 428-431.
597. Flotte T, Pinar H, Feiner H (1980). Papillary elastofibroma of the left ventricular septum. Am J Surg Pathol 4: 585-588.
598. Fogt F, Zimmerman RL, Hartmann CJ, Brown CA, Narula N (2002). Genetic alterations of Carney complex are not present in sporadic cardiac myxomas. Int J Mol Med 9: 59-60.
599. Folpe AL, Chand EM, Goldblum JR, Weiss SW (2001). Expression of Fli-1, a nuclear transcription factor, distinguishes vascular neoplasms from potential mimics. Am J Surg Pathol 25: 1061-1066.
600. Folpe AL, Gown AM, Lamps LW, Garcia R, Dail DH, Zarbo RJ, Schmidt RA (1999). Thyroid transcription factor-1: immunohistochemical evaluation in pulmonary neuroendocrine tumors. Mod Pathol 12: 5-8.
601. Folpe AL, Weiss SW (2002). Lipoleiomyosarcoma (well-differentiated liposarcoma with leiomyosarcomatous differentiation): a clinicopathologic study of nine cases including one with dedifferentiation. Am J Surg Pathol 26: 742-749.
602. Fontanini G, Calcinai A, Boldrini L, Lucchi M, Mussi A, Angeletti CA, Cagno C, Tognetti MA, Basolo F (1999). Modulation of neoangiogenesis in bronchial preneoplastic lesions. Oncol Rep 6: 813-817.
603. Fontham ET, Correa P, Reynolds P, Wu-Williams A, Buffler PA, Greenberg RS, Chen VW, Alterman T, Boyd P, Austin DF, Liff J (1994). Environmental tobacco smoke and lung cancer in nonsmoking women. A multicenter study. JAMA 271: 1752-1759.
604. Foroulis CN, Iliadis KH, Mauroudis PM, Kosmidis PA (2002). Basaloid carcinoma, a rare primary lung neoplasm: report of a case and review of the literature. Lung Cancer 35: 335-338.
605. Francis D, Jacobsen M (1983). Pulmonary blastoma. Curr Top Pathol 73: 265-294.
606. Franke A, Strobel P, Fackeldey V, Schafer R, Goller T, Becker HP, Schoneich R, Muller-Hermelink HK, Marx A (2004). Hepatoid thymic carcinoma: report of a case. Am J Surg Pathol 28: 250-256.
607. Franklin WA (1994). Immunophenotypic changes associated with neoplastic transformation of human respiratory tract epithelium. Lung Cancer 5: 15-36.
608. Franklin WA, Veve R, Hirsch FR, Helfrich BA, Bunn PAJr (2002). Epidermal growth factor receptor family in lung cancer and premalignancy. Semin Oncol 29: 3-14.
609. Franklin WA, Waintrub M, Edwards D, Christensen K, Prendegrast P, Woods J, Bunn PA, Kolhouse JF (1994). New anti-lung-cancer antibody cluster 12 reacts with human folate receptors present on adenocarcinoma. Int J Cancer Suppl 8: 89-95.
610. Franz DN, Brody A, Meyer C, Leonard J, Chuck G, Dabora S, Sethuraman G, Colby TV, Kwiatkowski DJ, McCormack FX (2001). Mutational and radiographic analysis of pulmonary disease consistent with lymphangioleiomyomatosis and micronodular pneumocyte hyperplasia in women with tuberous sclerosis. Am J Respir Crit Care Med 164: 661-668.
611. Fraser RS, Muller NL, Colman N, Pare PD (1999). Lymphoproliferative disorders and leukemia. In: Fraser and Paré's Diagnosis of Diseases of the Chest, Fraser RS, Muller NL, Colman N, Pare PD, eds., 4th ed. WB Saunders: Philadelphia .
612. Fraser RS, Müller NL, Colman N, Pare PD (1999). Neoplasms of the tracheobronchial glands. In: Fraser and Pare's Diagnosis of the Chest, Fraser RS, Müller NL, Colman N, Pare PD, eds., WB Saunders: Philadelphia , pp. 1251-1261.
613. Fraser RS, Müller NL, Colman N, Pare PD (1999). Neuroendocrine neoplasms. In: Fraser and Pare's Diagnosis of Diseases of the Chest, Fraser RS, Müller NL, Colman N, Pare PD, eds., WB Saunders: Philadelphia pp. 1229-1251.
614. Fraser RS, Müller NL, Colman N, Pare PD (1999). Pulmonary carcinoma. In: Fraser's and Pare's Diagnosis of Diseases

of the Chest, Fraser RS, Müller NL, Colman N, Pare PD, eds., WB Saunders: Philadelphia , pp. 1069-1228.
615. Freedom RM, Lee KJ, MacDonald C, Taylor G (2000). Selected aspects of cardiac tumors in infancy and childhood. Pediatr Cardiol 21: 299-316.
616. French CA, Miyoshi I, Aster JC, Kubonishi I, Kroll TG, Dal Cin P, Vargas SO, Perez-Atayde AR, Fletcher JA (2001). BRD4 bromodomain gene rearrangement in aggressive carcinoma with translocation t(15;19). Am J Pathol 159: 1987-1992.
617. French CA, Miyoshi I, Kubonishi I, Grier HE, Perez-Atayde AR, Fletcher JA (2003). BRD4-NUT Fusion Oncogene: A Novel Mechanism in Aggressive Carcinoma. Cancer Res 63: 304-307.
618. Friedman M, Forgione H, Shanbhag V (1980). Needle aspiration of metastatic melanoma. Acta Cytol 24: 7-15.
619. Frierson HFJr, Covell JL, Mills SE (1987). Fine needle aspiration cytology of atypical carcinoid of the lung. Acta Cytol 31: 471-475.
620. Frost JK, Ball WCJr, Levin ML, Tockman MS, Erozan YS, Gupta PK, Eggleston JC, Pressman NJ, Donithan MP, Kimball AWJr (1986). Sputum cytopathology: use and potential in monitoring the workplace environment by screening for biological effects of exposure. J Occup Med 28: 692-703.
621. Frost JK, Erozan YS, Gupta PK, Carter D (1983). Cytopathology. In: National Cancer Institute. Atlas of Early Lung Cancer, National Cancer Institute. Atlas of Early Lung Cancer, Igaku-Shoin: Tokyo .
622. Fu K, Moran CA, Suster S (2002). Primary mediastinal giant cell tumors: a clinicopathologic and immunohistochemical study of two cases. Ann Diagn Pathol 6: 100-105.
623. Fujii T, Dracheva T, Player A, Chacko S, Clifford R, Strausberg RL, Buetow K, Azumi N, Travis WD, Jen J (2002). A preliminary transcriptome map of non-small cell lung cancer. Cancer Res 62: 3340-3346.
624. Fujimoto K, Muller NL, Sadohara J, Harada H, Hayashi A, Hayabuchi N (2002). Alveolar adenoma of the lung: computed tomography and magnetic resonance imaging findings. J Thorac Imaging 17: 163-166.
625. Fujino S, Nojima T, Asakura S, Onoe M, Watarida S, Mori A (1991). [Complete resection of thymic carcinoma supported by cardiopulmonary bypass]. Nippon Kyobu Geka Gakkai Zasshi 39: 1188-1193.
626. Fujita Y, Shimizu T, Yamazaki K, Hirose T, Murayama M, Yamazaki Y, Matsumoto H, Tobise K (2000). Bronchial brushing cytology features of primary malignant fibrous histiocytoma of the lung. A case report. Acta Cytol 44: 227-231.
627. Fujiyoshi F, Ichinari N, Fukukura Y, Sasaki M, Hiraki Y, Nakajo M (1998). Sclerosing hemangioma of the lung: MR findings and correlation with pathological features. J Comput Assist Tomogr 22: 1006-1008.
628. Fukai I, Masaoka A, Fujii Y, Yamakawa Y, Yokoyama T, Murase T, Eimoto T (1999). Thymic neuroendocrine tumor (thymic carcinoid): a clinicopathologic study in 15 patients. Ann Thorac Surg 67: 208-211.
629. Fukasawa Y, Takada A, Tateno M, Sato H, Koizumi M, Tanaka A, Sato T (1998). Solitary fibrous tumor of the pleura causing recurrent hypoglycemia by secretion of insulin-like growth factor II. Pathol Int 48: 47-52.
630. Fukayama M, Hayashi Y, Shiozawa Y, Maeda Y, Koike M (1990). Human chorionic gonadotropin in the thymus. An immunocytochemical study on discordant expression of subunits. Am J Pathol 136: 123-129.
631. Fukayama M, Ibuka T, Hayashi Y, Ooba T, Koike M, Mizutani S (1993). Epstein-Barr virus in pyothorax-associated pleural lymphoma. Am J Pathol 143: 1044-1049.
632. Fukayama M, Maeda Y, Funata N, Koike M, Saito K, Sakai T, Ikeda T (1988). Pulmonary and pleural thymoma. Diagnostic application of lymphocyte markers to the thymoma of unusual site. Am J Clin Pathol 89: 617-621.
633. Fukayama M, Nihei Z, Takizawa T, Koike M, Ikeda T (1984). A case of squamous cell carcinoma of the thymus, probably originating from thymic cyst. Lung Cancer 24: 415-420.
634. Fukino S, Hayashi E, Fukata T, Okada M, Okada K, Makihara K, Morio S (1998). Primary clear cell carcinoma of the lung: report of an operative case. Kyobu Geka 51: 513-516.
635. Fukuda T, Ohnishi Y, Kanai I, Emura I, Watanabe T, Kitazawa M, Okamura A (1992). Papillary adenoma of the lung. Histological and ultrastructural findings in two cases. Acta Pathol Jpn 42: 56-61.
636. Fukunaga M, Ushigome S (1998). Giant cell angiofibroma of the mediastinum. Histopathology 32: 187-189.
637. Fukushima K, Yamaguchi T, Take A, Ohara T, Hasegawa T, Mochizuki M (1992). [A case report of so-called solitary fibrous tumor of the mediastinum]. Nippon Kyobu Geka Gakkai Zasshi 40: 978-982.
638. Fukushima KK, Mitani T, Hashimoto K, Hosogi S, Emori T, Morita H, Fujimoto Y, Nakamura K, Yamanari H, Ohe T (1999). Ventricular tachycardia in a patient with cardiac lipoma. J Cardiovasc Electrophysiol 10: 1161.
639. Fulford LG, Kamata Y, Okudera K, Dawson A, Corrin B, Sheppard MN, Ibrahim NB, Nicholson AG (2001). Epithelial-myoepithelial carcinomas of the bronchus. Am J Surg Pathol 25: 1508-1514.
640. Funai K, Yokose T, Ishii G, Araki K, Yoshida J, Nishimura M, Nagai K, Nishiwaki Y, Ochiai A (2003). Clinicopathologic characteristics of peripheral squamous cell carcinoma of the lung. Am J Surg Pathol 27: 978-984.
641. Funai K, Yokose T, Ishii G, Araki K, Yoshida J, Nishimura M, Nagai K, Nishiwaki Y, Ochiai A (2003). Clinicopathologic characteristics of peripheral squamous cell carcinoma of the lung. Am J Surg Pathol 27: 978-984.
642. Fushimi H, Kotoh K, Watanabe D, Tanio Y, Ogawa T, Miyoshi S (2000). Malignant melanoma in the thymus. Am J Surg Pathol 24: 1305-1308.
643. Gabe ED, Rodriguez Correa C, Vigliano C, San Martino J, Wisner JN, Gonzalez P, Boughen RP, Torino A, Suarez LD (2002). [Cardiac myxoma. Clinical-pathological correlation]. Rev Esp Cardiol 55: 505-513.
644. Gaertner E, Zeren EH, Fleming MV, Colby TV, Travis WD (1996). Biphasic synovial sarcomas arising in the pleural cavity. A clinicopathologic study of five cases. Am J Surg Pathol 20: 36-45.
645. Gaertner EM, Steinberg DM, Huber M, Hayashi T, Tsuda N, Askin FB, Bell SW, Nguyen B, Colby TV, Nishimura SL, Miettinen M, Travis WD (2000). Pulmonary and mediastinal glomus tumors—report of five cases including a pulmonary glomangiosarcoma: a clinicopathologic study with literature review. Am J Surg Pathol 24: 1105-1114.
646. Gaffey MJ, Mills SE, Askin FB, Ross GW, Sale GE, Kulander BG, Visscher DW, Yousem SA, Colby TV (1990). Clear cell tumor of the lung. A clinicopathologic, immunohistochemical, and ultrastructural study of eight cases. Am J Surg Pathol 14: 248-259.
647. Gaffey MJ, Mills SE, Frierson HFJr, Askin FB, Maygarden SJ (1998). Pulmonary clear cell carcinoid tumor: another entity in the differential diagnosis of pulmonary clear cell neoplasia. Am J Surg Pathol 22: 1020-1025.
648. Gaffey MJ, Mills SE, Zarbo RJ, Weiss LM, Gown AM (1991). Clear cell tumor of the lung. Immunohistochemical and ultrastructural evidence of melanogenesis. Am J Surg Pathol 15: 644-653.
649. Gaidano G, Capello D, Cilia AM, Gloghini A, Perin T, Quattrone S, Migliazza A, Lo Coco F, Saglio G, Ascoli V, Carbone A (1999). Genetic characterization of HHV-8/KSHV-positive primary effusion lymphoma reveals frequent mutations of BCL6: implications for disease pathogenesis and histogenesis. Genes Chromosomes Cancer 24: 16-23.
650. Gaidano G, Gloghini A, Gattei V, Rossi MF, Cilia AM, Godeas C, Degan M, Perin T, Canzonieri V, Aldinucci D, Saglio G, Carbone A, Pinto A (1997). Association of Kaposi's sarcoma-associated herpesvirus-positive primary effusion lymphoma with expression of the CD138/syndecan-1 antigen. Blood 90: 4894-4900.
651. Gajra A, Tatum AH, Newman N, Gamble GP, Lichtenstein S, Rooney MT, Graziano SL (2002). The predictive value of neuroendocrine markers and p53 for response to chemotherapy and survival in patients with advanced non-small cell lung cancer. Lung Cancer 36: 159-165.
652. Gal AA, Koss MN, Hochholzer L, Chejfec G (1991). An immunohistochemical study of benign clear cell ('sugar') tumor of the lung. Arch Pathol Lab Med 115: 1034-1038.
653. Gal AA, Koss MN, Hochholzer L, DeRose PB, Cohen C (1993). Pigmented pulmonary carcinoid tumor. An immunohistochemical and ultrastructural study. Arch Pathol Lab Med 117: 832-836.
654. Gal AA, Koss MN, McCarthy WF, Hochholzer L (1994). Prognostic factors in pulmonary fibrohistiocytic lesions. Cancer 73: 1817-1824.
655. Gal AA, Nassar VH, Miller JI (2002). Cytopathologic diagnosis of pulmonary sclerosing hemangioma. Diagn Cytopathol 26: 163-166.
656. Galateau-Salle F (2002). Well differentiated papillary mesothelioma. Histopathology 41 Supplement 2: 154-156.
657. Galateau-Salle FB, Luna RE, Horiba K, Sheppard MN, Hayashi T, Fleming MV, Colby TV, Bennett W, Harris CC, Stetler-Stevenson WG, Liotta L, Ferrans VJ, Travis WD (2000). Matrix metalloproteinases and tissue inhibitors of metalloproteinases in bronchial squamous preinvasive lesions. Hum Pathol 31: 296-305.
658. Galili N, Davis RJ, Fredericks WJ, Mukhopadhyay S, Rauscher FJ, III, Emanuel BS, Rovera G, Barr FG (1993). Fusion of a fork head domain gene to PAX3 in the solid tumour alveolar rhabdomyosarcoma. Nat Genet 5: 230-235.
659. Gallo R, Kumar N, Prabhakar G, Awada A, Maalouf Y, Duran CM (1993). Papillary fibroelastoma of mitral valve chorda. Ann Thorac Surg 55: 1576-1577.
660. Ganjoo KN, Rieger KM, Kesler KA, Sharma M, Heilman DK, Einhorn LH (2000). Results of modern therapy for patients with mediastinal nonseminomatous germ cell tumors. Cancer 88: 1051-1056.
661. Garber ME, Troyanskaya OG, Schluens K, Petersen S, Thaesler Z, Pacyna-Gengelbach M, van de Rijn M, Rosen GD, Perou CM, Whyte RI, Altman RB, Brown PO, Botstein D, Petersen I (2001). Diversity of gene expression in adenocarcinoma of the lung. Proc Natl Acad Sci U S A 98: 13784-13789.
662. Garcia JM, Gonzalez R, Silva JM, Dominguez G, Vegazo IS, Gamallo C, Provencio M, Espana P, Bonilla F (2000). Mutational status of K-ras and TP53 genes in primary sarcomas of the heart. Br J Cancer 82: 1183-1185.
663. Garnick MB, Griffin JD (1983). Idiopathic thrombocytopenia in association with extragonadal germ cell cancer. Ann Intern Med 98: 926-927.
664. Garson AJr, Gillette PC, Titus JL, Hawkins E, Kearney D, Ott D, Cooley DA, McNamara DG (1984). Surgical treatment of ventricular tachycardia in infants. N Engl J Med 310: 1443-1445.
665. Garson AJr, Smith RTJr, Moak JP, Kearney DL, Hawkins EP, Titus JL, Cooley DA, Ott DA (1987). Incessant ventricular tachycardia in infants: myocardial hamartomas and surgical cure. J Am Coll Cardiol 10: 619-626.
666. Gartner LA, Voorhess ML (1993). Adrenocorticotropic hormone—producing thymic carcinoid in a teenager. Cancer 71: 106-111.
667. Gaumann A, Petrow P, Mentzel T, Mayer E, Dahm M, Otto M, Kirkpatrick CJ, Kriegsmann J (2001). Osteopontin expression in primary sarcomas of the pulmonary artery. Virchows Arch 439: 668-674.
668. Gazdar AF, Carbone M (2003). Molecular pathogenesis of malignant mesothelioma and its relationship to simian virus 40. Clin Lung Cancer 5: 177-181.
669. Gazzeri S, Della Valle V, Chaussade L, Brambilla C, Larsen CJ, Brambilla E (1998). The human p19ARF protein encoded by the beta transcript of the p16INK4a gene is frequently lost in small cell lung cancer. Cancer Res 58: 3926-3931.
670. Gazzeri S, Gouyer V, Vour'ch C, Brambilla C, Brambilla E (1998). Mechanisms of p16INK4A inactivation in non small-cell lung cancers. Oncogene 16: 497-504.
671. Gebauer C (1982). The postoperative prognosis of primary pulmonary sarcomas. A review with a comparison between the histological forms and the other primary endothoracal sarcomas based on 474 cases. Scand J Thorac Cardiovasc Surg 16: 91-97.
672. Geisinger K, Silverman J, Wakely PJr (1994). Pediatric Cytopathology. American Society for Clinical Pathology Press (ASCP Press): Chicago.
673. Geisinger KR, Stanley MW, Raab SS, Silverman JF, Abati A (2003). Modern Cytopathology. Churchill Livingstone: New York.
674. Gels ME (1997). Testicular Germ Cell Tumors. Development in Surgery and Follow-up. University of Groningen, The Netherlands: Groningen.
675. Gengenbach S, Ridker PM (1991). Left ventricular hemangioma in Kasabach-Merritt syndrome. Am Heart J 121: 202-203.
676. Geradts J, Fong KM, Zimmerman PV,

Minna JD (2000). Loss of Fhit expression in non-small-cell lung cancer: correlation with molecular genetic abnormalities and clinicopathological features. Br J Cancer 82: 1191-1197.

677. Gerald WL, Ladanyi M, de Alava E, Cuatrecasas M, Kushner BH, LaQuaglia MP, Rosai J (1998). Clinical, pathologic, and molecular spectrum of tumors associated with t(11;22)(p13;q12): desmoplastic small round-cell tumor and its variants. J Clin Oncol 16: 3028-3036.

678. Gharagozloo F, Porter CJ, Tazelaar HD, Danielson GK (1994). Multiple myocardial hamartomas causing ventricular tachycardia in young children: combined surgical modification and medical treatment. Mayo Clin Proc 69: 262-267.

679. Giatromanolaki A, Gorgoulis V, Chetty R, Koukourakis MI, Whitehouse R, Kittas C, Veslemes M, Gatter KC, Iordanoglou I (1996). C-erbB-2 oncoprotein expression in operable non-small cell lung cancer. Anticancer Res 16: 987-993.

680. Gibas Z, Miettinen M (1992). Recurrent parapharyngeal rhabdomyoma. Evidence of neoplastic nature of the tumor from cytogenetic study. Am J Surg Pathol 16: 721-728.

681. Gibril F, Chen YJ, Schrump DS, Vortmeyer A, Zhuang Z, Lubensky IA, Reynolds JC, Louie A, Entsuah LK, Huang K, Asgharian B, Jensen RT (2003). Prospective study of thymic carcinoids in patients with multiple endocrine neoplasia type 1. J Clin Endocrinol Metab 88: 1066-1081.

682. Gilbert-Barness E, Barness LA (1999). Nonmalformative cardiovascular pathology in infants and children. Pediatr Dev Pathol 2: 499-530.

683. Gilcrease MZ, Rajan B, Ostrowski ML, Ramzy I, Schwartz MR (1997). Localized thymic Langerhans' cell histiocytosis and its relationship with myasthenia gravis. Immunohistochemical, ultrastructural, and cytometric studies. Arch Pathol Lab Med 121: 134-138.

684. Gill J, Malin M, Hollander GA, Boyd R (2002). Generation of a complete thymic microenvironment by MTS24(+) thymic epithelial cells. Nat Immunol 3: 635-642.

685. Gilliland FD, Samet JM (1994). Lung cancer. Cancer Surv 19-20: 175-195.

686. Ginsberg SS, Buzaid AC, Stern H, Carter D (1992). Giant cell carcinoma of the lung. Cancer 70: 606-610.

687. Girard L, Zochbauer-Muller S, Virmani AK, Gazdar AF, Minna JD (2000). Genome-wide allelotyping of lung cancer identifies new regions of allelic loss, differences between small cell lung cancer and non-small cell lung cancer, and loci clustering. Cancer Res 60: 4894-4906.

688. Gisselsson D, Pettersson L, Hoglund M, Heidenblad M, Gorunova L, Wiegant J, Mertens F, Dal Cin P, Mitelman F, Mandahl N (2000). Chromosomal breakage-fusion-bridge events cause genetic intratumor heterogeneity. Proc Natl Acad Sci U S A 97: 5357-5362.

689. Gjevre JA, Myers JL, Prakash UB (1996). Pulmonary hamartomas. Mayo Clin Proc 71: 14-20.

690. Gladish GW, Sabloff BM, Munden RF, Truong MT, Erasmus JJ, Chasen MH (2002). Primary thoracic sarcomas. Radiographics 22: 621-637.

691. Glancy DL, Morales JBJr, Roberts WC (1968). Angiosarcoma of the heart. Am J Cardiol 21: 413-419.

692. Glaser SL, Lin RJ, Stewart SL,

Ambinder RF, Jarrett RF, Brousset P, Pallesen G, Gulley ML, Khan G, O'Grady J, Hummel M, Preciado MV, Knecht H, Chan JK, Claviez A (1997). Epstein-Barr virus-associated Hodgkin's disease: epidemiologic characteristics in international data. Int J Cancer 70: 375-382.

693. Glatstein E, Levinson BS (1995). Malignancies of the Thymus. Thoracic Oncology. 2nd ed. WB Saunders: Philadelphia.

694. Glehen A, Allias F, Patricot LM, Thivolet-Bejui F (2000). [Primary pulmonary synovial sarcoma. Apropos of 1 case with cytogenetic study]. Ann Pathol 20: 620-622.

695. Gobel U, Calaminus G, Engert J, Kaatsch P, Gadner H, Bokkerink JP, Hass RJ, Waag K, Blohm ME, Dippert S, Teske C, Harms D (1998). Teratomas in infancy and childhood. Med Pediatr Oncol 31: 8-15.

696. Gobel U, Schneider DT, Calaminus G, Haas RJ, Schmidt P, Harms D (2000). Germ-cell tumors in childhood and adolescence. GPOH MAKEI and the MAHO study groups. Ann Oncol 11: 263-271.

697. Godschalk RW, Schooten FJ, Bartsch H (2003). A critical evaluation of DNA adducts as biological markers for human exposure to polycyclic aromatic compounds. J Biochem Mol Biol 36: 1-11.

698. Goeze A, Schluns K, Wolf G, Thasler Z, Petersen S, Petersen I (2002). Chromosomal imbalances of primary and metastatic lung adenocarcinomas. J Pathol 196: 8-16.

699. Goh SGN, Lau LC, Sivaswaren C, Chuah KL, Tan PH, Lai D (2001). Pseudodicentric (16;12)(q11;p11.2) in a type AB (mixed) thymoma. Cancer Genet Cytogenet 131: 42-47.

700. Goldsmith JD, Pawel B, Goldblum JR, Pasha TL, Roberts S, Nelson P, Khurana JS, Barr FG, Zhang PJ (2002). Detection and diagnostic utilization of placental alkaline phosphatase in muscular tissue and tumors with myogenic differentiation. Am J Surg Pathol 26: 1627-1633.

701. Goldstein DJ, Oz MC, Rose EA, Fisher P, Michler RE (1995). Experience with heart transplantation for cardiac tumors. J Heart Lung Transplant 14: 382-386.

702. Goldstein LS, Kavuru MS, Meli Y, Tuthill RJ, Mehta AC (1999). Uterine rhabdomyosarcoma metastatic to mediastinal lymph nodes: diagnosis by transbronchial needle aspiration. South Med J 92: 84-87.

703. Goldstein NS, Mani A, Chmielewski G, Welsh R, Pursel S (2000). Immunohistochemically detected micrometastases in peribronchial and mediastinal lymph nodes from patients with T1, N0, M0 pulmonary adenocarcinomas. Am J Surg Pathol 24: 274-279.

704. Goldstein NS, Thomas M (2001). Mucinous and nonmucinous bronchioloalveolar adenocarcinomas have distinct staining patterns with thyroid transcription factor and cytokeratin 20 antibodies. Am J Clin Pathol 116: 319-325.

705. Gologorsky E, Gologorsky A (2002). Aortic valve fibroelastomas as an incidental intraoperative transesophageal echocardiographic finding. Anesth Analg 95: 1198-9, table.

706. Golub TR, Slonim DK, Tamayo P, Huard C, Gaasenbeek M, Mesirov JP, Coller H, Loh ML, Downing JR, Caligiuri MA, Bloomfield CD, Lander ES (1999). Molecular classification of cancer: class discovery and class prediction by gene expression monitoring. Science 286: 531-537.

707. Gomez-Roman JJ, Sanchez-Velasco P,

Ocejo-Vinyals G, Hernandez-Nieto E, Leyva-Cobian F, Val-Bernal JF (2001). Human herpesvirus-8 genes are expressed in pulmonary inflammatory myofibroblastic tumor (inflammatory pseudotumor). Am J Surg Pathol 25: 624-629.

708. Gonzalez-Crussi F (1982). Teratomas of the mediastinum. In: Extragonadal Teratomas, Hartmann WA, Cowan WR, eds., Armed Forces Institute of Pathology: Washington, DC .

709. Gonzalez-Vela JL, Savage PD, Manivel JC, Torkelson JL, Kennedy BJ (1990). Poor prognosis of mediastinal germ cell cancers containing sarcomatous components. Cancer 66: 1114-1116.

710. Gonzalez CL, Medeiros LJ, Jaffe ES (1991). Composite lymphoma. A clinicopathologic analysis of nine patients with Hodgkin's disease and B-cell non-Hodgkin's lymphoma. Am J Clin Pathol 96: 81-89.

711. Gonzalez S, von Bassewitz DB, Grundmann E, Nakhosteen JA, Muller KM (1985). Atypical cilia in hyperplastic, metaplastic, and dysplastic human bronchial mucosa. Ultrastruct Pathol 8: 345-356.

712. Gonzalez S, von Bassewitz DB, Grundmann E, Nakhosteen JA, Muller KM (1986). The ultrastructural heterogeneity of potentially preneoplastic lesions in the human bronchial mucosa. Pathol Res Pract 181: 408-417.

713. Gopal A, Li Mandri G, King DL, Marboe C, Homma S (1994). Aortic valve papillary fibroelastoma. A diagnosis by transthoracic echocardiography. Chest 105: 1885-1887.

714. Gordon GJ, Jensen RV, Hsiao LL, Gullans SR, Blumenstock JE, Richards WG, Jaklitsch MT, Sugarbaker DJ, Bueno R (2003). Using gene expression ratios to predict outcome among patients with mesothelioma. J Natl Cancer Inst 95: 598-605.

715. Gordon GJ, Richards WG, Sugarbaker DJ, Jaklitsch MT, Bueno R (2003). A prognostic test for adenocarcinoma of the lung from gene expression profiling data. Cancer Epidemiol Biomarkers Prev 12: 905-910.

716. Gorlin RJ, Goltz RW (1960). Multiple nevoid basal-cell epithelioma, jaw cysts and bifid rib - a syndrome. N Engl J Med 262: 908-912.

717. Gosney JR (1997). Pulmonary neuroendocrine cell system in pediatric and adult lung disease. Microsc Res Tech 37: 107-113.

718. Gosney JR, Denley H, Resl M (1999). Sustentacular cells in pulmonary neuroendocrine tumours. Histopathology 34: 211-215.

719. Gosney JR, Sissons MC, Allibone RO (1988). Neuroendocrine cell populations in normal human lungs: a quantitative study. Thorax 43: 878-882.

720. Gosney JR, Sissons MC, Allibone RO, Blakey AF (1989). Pulmonary endocrine cells in chronic bronchitis and emphysema. J Pathol 157: 127-133.

721. Goss PE, Schwertfeger L, Blackstein ME, Iscoe NA, Ginsberg RJ, Simpson WJ, Jones DP, Shepherd FA (1994). Extragonadal germ cell tumors. A 14-year Toronto experience. Cancer 73: 1971-1979.

722. Goswami KC, Shrivastava S, Bahl VK, Saxena A, Manchanda SC, Wasir HS (1998). Cardiac myxomas: clinical and echocardiographic profile. Int J Cardiol 63: 251-259.

723. Goto K, Kodama T, Matsuno Y, Yokose

T, Asamura H, Kamiya N, Shimosato Y (2001). Clinicopathologic and DNA cytometric analysis of carcinoid tumors of the thymus. Mod Pathol 14: 985-994.

724. Gotz M, Brunner P (1985). Micropapillomatosis of the bronchial basement membrane: pathogenesis and types. Zentralbl Allg Pathol 130: 375-381.

725. Gouttefangeas C, Bensussan A, Boumsell L (1990). Study of the CD3-associated T-cell receptors reveals further differences between T-cell acute lymphoblastic lymphoma and leukemia. Blood 75: 931-934.

726. Gouyer V, Gazzeri S, Bolon I, Drevet C, Brambilla C, Brambilla E (1998). Mechanism of retinoblastoma gene inactivation in the spectrum of neuroendocrine lung tumors. Am J Respir Cell Mol Biol 18: 188-196.

727. Gouyer V, Gazzeri S, Brambilla E, Bolon I, Moro D, Perron P, Benabid AL, Brambilla C (1994). Loss of heterozygosity at the RB locus correlates with loss of RB protein in primary malignant neuro-endocrine lung carcinomas. Int J Cancer 58: 818-824.

728. Govender D, Pillay SV (2001). Right pulmonary artery sarcoma. Pathology 33: 243-245.

729. Govender D, Pillay SV (2002). Mediastinal immature teratoma with yolk sac tumor and myelomonocytic leukemia associated with Klinefelter's syndrome. Int J Surg Pathol 10: 157-162.

730. Gowarf FJS (1978). Unusual mucous cyst of the lung. Thorax 33: 796-799.

731. Gowdamarajan A, Michler RE (2000). Therapy for primary cardiac tumors: is there a role for heart transplantation? Curr Opin Cardiol 15: 121-125.

732. Granata C, Battistini E, Toma P, Balducci T, Mattioli G, Fregonese B, Gambini C, Rossi GA (1997). Mucoepidermoid carcinoma of the bronchus: a case report and review of the literature. Pediatr Pulmonol 23: 226-232.

733. Grandmougin D, Fayad G, Decoene C, Pol A, Warembourg H (2001). Total orthotopic heart transplantation for primary cardiac rhabdomyosarcoma: factors influencing long-term survival. Ann Thorac Surg 71: 1438-1441.

734. Grandmougin D, Fayad G, Moukassa D, Decoene C, Abolmaali K, Bodart JC, Limousin M, Warembourg H (2000). Cardiac valve papillary fibroelastomas: clinical, histological and immunohistochemical studies and a physiopathogenic hypothesis. J Heart Valve Dis 9: 832-841.

735. Graziano SL, Mazid R, Newman N, Tatum A, Oler A, Mortimer JA, Gullo JJ, DiFino SM, Scalzo AJ (1989). The use of neuroendocrine immunoperoxidase markers to predict chemotherapy response in patients with non-small-cell lung cancer. J Clin Oncol 7: 1398-1406.

736. Grebenc ML, Rosado-de-Christenson ML, Green CE, Burke AP, Galvin JR (2002). Cardiac myxoma: imaging features in 83 patients. Radiographics 22: 673-689.

737. Grebenc ML, Rosado de Christenson ML, Burke AP, Green CE, Galvin JR (2000). Primary cardiac and pericardial neoplasms: radiologic-pathologic correlation. Radiographics 20: 1073-1103.

738. Greene FL, Page DL, Fleming ID, Fritz AG, Balch CM, Haller DG, Morrow M (2002). AJCC Cancer Staging Manual. Sixth ed. Springer: New York.

739. Greenwood SM, Meschter SC (1989). Extraskeletal osteogenic sarcoma of the mediastinum. Arch Pathol Lab Med 113: 430-433.

740. Grewal RG, Prager K, Austin JH, Rotterdam H (1993). Long term survival in non-encapsulated primary liposarcoma of the mediastinum. Thorax 48: 1276-1277.

741. Griffin CA, Hawkins AL, Dvorak C, Henkle C, Ellingham T, Perlman EJ (1999). Recurrent involvement of 2p23 in inflammatory myofibroblastic tumors. Cancer Res 59: 2776-2780.

742. Grinda JM, Couetil JP, Chauvaud S, D'Attellis N, Berrebi A, Fabiani JN, Deloche A, Carpentier A (1999). Cardiac valve papillary fibroelastoma: surgical excision for revealed or potential embolization. J Thorac Cardiovasc Surg 117: 106-110.

743. Gschwendtner A, Fend F, Hoffmann Y, Krugmann J, Klingler PJ, Mairinger T (1999). DNA-ploidy analysis correlates with the histogenetic classification of thymic epithelial tumours. J Pathol 189: 576-580.

744. Gu J, Spitz MR, Yang F, Wu X (1999). Ethnic differences in poly(ADP-ribose) polymerase pseudogene genotype distribution and association with lung cancer risk. Carcinogenesis 20: 1465-1469.

745. Guarino M, Micheli P, Pallotti F, Giordano F (1999). Pathological relevance of epithelial and mesenchymal phenotype plasticity. Pathol Res Pract 195: 379-389.

746. Gugger M, Burckhardt E, Kappeler A, Hirsiger H, Laissue JA, Mazzucchelli L (2002). Quantitative expansion of structural genomic alterations in the spectrum of neuroendocrine lung carcinomas. J Pathol 196: 408-415.

747. Guillou L, Coindre J, Gallagher G, Terrier P, Gebhard S, de Saint Aubain Somerhausen N, Michels J, Jundt G, Vince DR, Collin F, Trassard M, Le Doussal V, Benhattar J (2001). Detection of the synovial sarcoma translocation t(X;18) (SYT;SSX) in paraffin-embedded tissues using reverse transcriptase-polymerase chain reaction: a reliable and powerful diagnostic tool for pathologists. A molecular analysis of 221 mesenchymal tumors fixed in different fixatives. Hum Pathol 32: 105-112.

748. Guillou L, Coindre JM, Bonichon F, Nguyen BB, Terrier P, Collin F, Vilain MO, Mandard AM, Le Doussal V, Leroux A, Jacquemier J, Duplay H, Sastre-Garau X, Costa J (1997). Comparative study of the National Cancer Institute and French Federation of Cancer Centers Sarcoma Group grading systems in a population of 410 adult patients with soft tissue sarcoma. J Clin Oncol 15: 350-362.

749. Guillou L, Wadden C, Kraus MD, Dei Tos AP, Fletcher CDM (1996). S-100 protein reactivity in synovial sarcomas - A potentially frequent diagnostic pitfall - Immunohistochemical analysis of 100 cases. Appl Immunohistochem 4: 167-175.

750. Guinee DGJr, Fishback NF, Koss MN, Abbondanzo SL, Travis WD (1994). The spectrum of immunohistochemical staining of small-cell lung carcinoma in specimens from transbronchial and open-lung biopsies. Am J Clin Pathol 102: 406-414.

751. Guinee DGJr, Perkins SL, Travis WD, Holden JA, Tripp SR, Koss MN (1998). Proliferation and cellular phenotype in lymphomatoid granulomatosis: implications of a higher proliferation index in B cells. Am J Surg Pathol 22: 1093-1100.

752. Guinee DJr, Jaffe E, Kingma D, Fishback N, Wallberg K, Krishnan J, Frizzera G, Travis W, Koss M (1994). Pulmonary lymphomatoid granulomatosis. Evidence for a proliferation of Epstein-Barr virus infected B-lymphocytes with a promi-

nent T-cell component and vasculitis. Am J Surg Pathol 18: 753-764.

753. Gupta D, Holden J, Layfield L (2001). Topoisomerase alpha II, retinoblastoma gene product, and p53: potential relationships with aggressive behavior and malignant transformation in recurrent respiratory papillomatosis. Appl Immunohistochem Mol Morphol 9: 86-91.

754. Hackshaw AK, Law MR, Wald NJ (1997). The accumulated evidence on lung cancer and environmental tobacco smoke. BMJ 315: 980-988.

755. Hagberg H, Gustavson KH, Sundstrom C, Gerdes U (1983). Blastic phase of myeloproliferative syndrome coexisting with a malignant teratoma. Scand J Haematol 30: 36-42.

756. Hahn H, Wicking C, Zaphiropoulous PG, Gailani MR, Shanley S, Chidambaram A, Vorechovsky I, Holmberg E, Unden AB, Gillies S, Negus K, Smyth I, Pressman C, Leffell DJ, Gerrard B, Goldstein AM, Dean M, Toftgard R, Chenevix-Trench G, Wainwright B, Bale AE (1996). Mutations of the human homolog of Drosophila patched in the nevoid basal cell carcinoma syndrome. Cell 85: 841-851.

757. Hailemariam S, Engeler DS, Bannwart F, Amin MB (1997). Primary mediastinal germ cell tumor with intratubular germ cell neoplasia of the testis—further support for germ cell origin of these tumors: a case report. Cancer 79: 1031-1036.

758. Hainaut P, Lesage V, Weynand B, Coche E, Noirhomme P (1999). Calcifying fibrous pseudotumor (CFPT): a patient presenting with multiple pleural lesions. Acta Clin Belg 54: 162-164.

759. Hainsworth JD, Greco FA (2001). Germ cell neoplasms and other malignancies of the mediastinum. Cancer Treat Res 105: 303-325.

760. Hajar R, Roberts WC, Folger GMJr (1986). Embryonal botryoid rhabdomyosarcoma of the mitral valve. Am J Cardiol 57: 376.

761. Haley KJ, Drazen JM, Osathanondh R, Sunday ME (1997). Comparison of the ontogeny of protein gene product 9.5, chromogranin A and proliferating cell nuclear antigen in developing human lung. Microsc Res Tech 37: 62-68.

762. Halicek F, Rosai J (1984). Histioeosinophilic granulomas in the thymuses of 29 myasthenic patients: a complication of pneumomediastinum. Hum Pathol 15: 1137-1144.

763. Hall GFM (1949). A case of thymolipoma with observations on a possible relationship to intrathoracic lipomata. Br J Surg 36: 321-324.

764. Hallahan DE, Vogelzang NJ, Borow KM, Bostwick DG, Simon MA (1986). Cardiac metastases from soft-tissue sarcomas. J Clin Oncol 4: 1662-1669.

765. Halliday BE, Slagel DD, Elsheikh TE, Silverman JF (1998). Diagnostic utility of MIC-2 immunocytochemical staining in the differential diagnosis of small blue cell tumors. Diagn Cytopathol 19: 410-416.

766. Hamakawa H, Bao Y, Takarada M, Fukuzumi M, Tanioka H (1998). Cytokeratin expression in squamous cell carcinoma of the lung and oral cavity: an immunohistochemical study with possible clinical relevance. Oral Surg Oral Med Oral Pathol Oral Radiol Endod 85: 438-443.

767. Hammar S (1987). The use of electron microscopy and immunohistochemistry in the diagnosis and understanding of lung neoplasms. Clin Lab Med 7: 1-30.

768. Hammar SP (1994). Common neoplasms. In: Pulmonary Pathology, Dail DH, Hammar SP, eds., 2nd ed. Springer-Verlag: New York , pp. 1123-1278.

769. Hammond ME, Sause WT (1985). Large cell neuroendocrine tumors of the lung. Clinical significance and histopathologic definition. Cancer 56: 1624-1629.

770. Han AJ, Xiong M, Gu YY, Lin SX, Xiong M (2001). Lymphoepithelioma-like carcinoma of the lung with a better prognosis. A clinicopathologic study of 32 cases. Am J Clin Pathol 115: 841-850.

771. Han AJ, Xiong M, Zong YS (2000). Association of Epstein-Barr virus with lymphoepithelioma-like carcinoma of the lung in southern China. Am J Clin Pathol 114: 220-226.

772. Hanau CA, Miettinen M (1995). Solitary fibrous tumor: histological and immunohistochemical spectrum of benign and malignant variants presenting at different sites. Hum Pathol 26: 440-449.

773. Hanly AJ, Elgart GW, Jorda M, Smith J, Nadji M (2000). Analysis of thyroid transcription factor-1 and cytokeratin 20 separates merkel cell carcinoma from small cell carcinoma of lung. J Cutan Pathol 27: 118-120.

774. Hanson CA, Jaszcz W, Kersey JH, Astorga MG, Peterson BA, Gajl-Peczalska KJ, Frizzera G (1989). True histiocytic lymphoma: histopathologic, immunophenotypic and genotypic analysis. Br J Haematol 73: 187-198.

775. Happle R (1993). Klippel-Trenaunay syndrome: is it a paradominant trait? Br J Dermatol 128: 465-466.

776. Haque AK, Myers JL, Hudnall SD, Gelman BB, Lloyd RV, Payne D, Borucki M (1998). Pulmonary lymphomatoid granulomatosis in acquired immunodeficiency syndrome: lesions with Epstein-Barr virus infection. Mod Pathol 11: 347-356.

777. Harding CO, Pagon RA (1990). Incidence of tuberous sclerosis in patients with cardiac rhabdomyoma. Am J Med Genet 37: 443-446.

778. Harigae H, Ichinohasama R, Miura I, Kameoka J, Meguro K, Miyamura K, Sasaki O, Ishikawa I, Takahashi S, Kaku M, Sasaki T (2002). Primary marginal zone lymphoma of the thymus accompanied by chromosomal anomaly 46,X,dup(X)(p11p22). Cancer Genet Cytogenet 133: 142-147.

779. Harkness EF, Brewster DH, Kerr KM, Fergusson RJ, MacFarlane GJ (2002). Changing trends in incidence of lung cancer by histologic type in Scotland. Int J Cancer 102: 179-183.

780. Harper PG, Houang M, Spiro SG, Geddes D, Hodson M, Souhami RL (1981). Computerized axial tomography in the pretreatment assessment of small-cell carcinoma of the bronchus. Cancer 47: 1775-1780.

781. Harpole DHJr, Johnson CM, Wolfe WG, George SL, Seigler HF (1992). Analysis of 945 cases of pulmonary metastatic melanoma. J Thorac Cardiovasc Surg 103: 743-748.

782. Harris NL (1998). The many faces of Hodgkin's disease around the world: what have we learned from its pathology? Ann Oncol 9 Suppl 5: S45-S56.

783. Harris NL, Jaffe ES, Stein H, Banks PM, Chan JK, Cleary ML, Delsol G, Wolf-Peeters C, Falini B, Gatter KC (1994). A revised European-American classification of lymphoid neoplasms: a proposal from the International Lymphoma Study Group. Blood 84: 1361-1392.

784. Harris NL, Muller-Hermelink HK (1999). Thymoma classification. A siren's song of simplicity. Am J Clin Pathol 112: 299-303.

785. Hartmann CA, Roth C, Minck C, Niedobitek G (1990). Thymic carcinoma. Report of five cases and review of the literature. J Cancer Res Clin Oncol 116: 69-82.

786. Hartmann JT, Einhorn L, Nichols CR, Droz JP, Horwich A, Gerl A, Fossa SD, Beyer J, Pont J, Schmoll HJ, Kanz L, Bokemeyer C (2001). Second-line chemotherapy in patients with relapsed extragonadal nonseminomatous germ cell tumors: results of an international multicenter analysis. J Clin Oncol 19: 1641-1648.

787. Hartmann JT, Fossa SD, Nichols CR, Droz JP, Horwich A, Gerl A, Beyer J, Pont J, Fizazi K, Hecker H, Kanz L, Einhorn L, Bokemeyer C (2001). Incidence of metachronous testicular cancer in patients with extragonadal germ cell tumors. J Natl Cancer Inst 93: 1733-1738.

788. Hartmann JT, Nichols CR, Droz JP, Horwich A, Gerl A, Fossa SD, Beyer J, Pont J, Einhorn L, Kanz L, Bokemeyer C (2000). The relative risk of second nongerminal malignancies in patients with extragonadal germ cell tumors. Cancer 88: 2629-2635.

789. Hartmann JT, Nichols CR, Droz JP, Horwich A, Gerl A, Fossa SD, Beyer J, Pont J, Fizazi K, Einhorn L, Kanz L, Bokemeyer C (2000). Hematologic disorders associated with primary mediastinal nonseminomatous germ cell tumors. J Natl Cancer Inst 92: 54-61.

790. Hartmann JT, Nichols CR, Droz JP, Horwich A, Gerl A, Fossa SD, Beyer J, Pont J, Kanz L, Einhorn L, Bokemeyer C (2002). Prognostic variables for response and outcome in patients with extragonadal germ-cell tumors. Ann Oncol 13: 1017-1028.

791. Hasegawa T, Matsuno Y, Shimoda T, Hirohashi S, Hirose T, Sano T (1998). Frequent expression of bcl-2 protein in solitary fibrous tumors. Jpn J Clin Oncol 28: 86-91.

792. Haskovcova I, Povysil C, Pafko P (1997). [Alveolar adenoma of the lung (case report)]. Cesk Patol 33: 49-52.

793. Hasle H, Jacobsen BB (1995). Origin of male mediastinal germ-cell tumours. Lancet 345: 1046.

794. Hasle H, Jacobsen BB, Asschenfeldt P, Andersen K (1992). Mediastinal germ cell tumour associated with Klinefelter syndrome. A report of case and review of the literature. Eur J Pediatr 151: 735-739.

795. Hasle H, Mellemgaard A, Nielsen J, Hansen J (1995). Cancer incidence in men with Klinefelter syndrome. Br J Cancer 71: 416-420.

796. Hasleton PS (1996). Pleural disease. In: Spencer's pathology of the lung, Hasleton PS, ed., 5th ed. McGraw Hill: New York .

797. Hasserjian RP, Klimstra DS, Rosai J (1995). Carcinoma of the thymus with clear-cell features. Report of eight cases and review of the literature. Am J Surg Pathol 19: 835-841.

798. Hattori H, Tateyama H, Tada T, Saito Y, Yamakawa Y, Eimoto T (2000). PE-35-related antigen expression and CD1a-positive lymphocytes in thymoma subtypes based on Muller-Hermelink classification.An immunohistochemical study using catalyzed signal amplification. Virchows Arch 436: 20-27.

799. Hattori Y, Iriyama T, Watanabe K, Negi K, Takeda I, Sugimura S (2000). Primary cardiac sarcoma: two case reports. Jpn Circ J 64: 222-224.

800. Have-Opbroek AA, Benfield JR, van

Krieken JH, Dijkman JH (1997). The alveolar type II cell is a pluripotential stem cell in the genesis of human adenocarcinomas and squamous cell carcinomas. Histol Histopathol 12: 319-336.
801. Havlicek F, Rosai J (1984). A sarcoma of thymic stroma with features of liposarcoma. Am J Clin Pathol 82: 217-224.
802. Hayashi H, Miyamoto H, Ito T, Kameda Y, Nakamura N, Kubota Y, Kitamura H (1997). Analysis of p21Waf1/Cip1 expression in normal, premalignant, and malignant cells during the development of human lung adenocarcinoma. Am J Pathol 151: 461-470.
803. Hayes MMM, Vanderwesthuizen NG, Forgie R (1993). Malignant mixed tumor of bronchus - a biphasic neoplasm of epithelial and myoepethelial cells. Mod Pathol 6: 85-88.
804. Heard BE, Corrin B, Dewar A (1985). Pathology of seven mucous cell adenomas of the bronchial glands with particular reference to ultrastructure. Histopathology 9: 687-701.
805. Heath AC, Cates R, Martin NG, Meyer J, Hewitt JK, Neale MC, Eaves LJ (1993). Genetic contribution to risk of smoking initiation: comparisons across birth cohorts and across cultures. J Subst Abuse 5: 221-246.
806. Heath AC, Martin NG (1993). Genetic models for the natural history of smoking: evidence for a genetic influence on smoking persistence. Addict Behav 18: 19-34.
807. Hecht SS (2002). Cigarette smoking and lung cancer: chemical mechanisms and approaches to prevention. Lancet Oncol 3: 461-469.
808. Hegg CA, Flint A, Singh G (1992). Papillary adenoma of the lung. Am J Clin Pathol 97: 393-397.
809. Heilbrun A, Crosby IK (1972). Adenocystic carcinoma and mucoepidermoid carcinoma of tracheobronchial tree. Chest 61: 145-&.
810. Heintz NH, Janssen YM, Mossman BT (1993). Persistent induction of c-fos and c-jun expression by asbestos. Proc Natl Acad Sci U S A 90: 3299-3303.
811. Heitmiller RF, Mathisen DJ, Ferry JA, Mark EJ, Grillo HC (1989). Mucoepidermoid lung tumors. Ann Thorac Surg 47: 394-399.
812. Hekimgil M, Hamulu F, Cagirici U, Karabulut B, Ozgen AG, Soydan S, Yilmaz C (2001). Small cell neuroendocrine carcinoma of the thymus complicated by Cushing's syndrome. Report of a 58-year-old woman with a 3-year history of hypertension. Pathol Res Pract 197: 129-133.
813. Helfritzsch H, Junker K, Bartel M, Scheele J (2002). Differentiation of positive autofluorescence bronchoscopy findings by comparative genomic hybridization. Oncol Rep 9: 697-701.
814. Helman LJ, Ozols RF, Longo DL (1984). Thrombocytopenia and extragonadal germ-cell neoplasm. Ann Intern Med 101: 280.
815. Henderson DW, Shilkin KB, Whitaker D, Atwood HD, Constance TJ, Steele RH, Leppard PJ (1992). The pathology of malignant mesothelioma, including immunohistology and ultrastructure. In: Malignant Mesothelioma, Henderson DW, Shilkin KB, Langlois SL, Whitaker D, eds., Hemisphere Publishing Corporation: New York , pp. 69-139.
816. Henley JD, Cummings OW, Loehrer PJ, Sr. (2004). Tyrosine kinase receptor expression in thymomas. J Cancer Res Clin Oncol 130: 222-224.
817. Henschke CI (2003). I-ELCAP protocol. International Collaboration to Screen for Lung Cancer http://ICScreen.med.cornell.edu/.
818. Henschke CI, McCauley DI, Yankelevitz DF, Naidich DP, McGuinness G, Miettinen OS, Libby DM, Pasmantier MW, Koizumi J, Altorki NK, Smith JP (1999). Early Lung Cancer Action Project: overall design and findings from baseline screening. Lancet 354: 99-105.
819. Henschke CI, Yankelevitz DF, Mirtcheva R, McGuinness G, McCauley D, Miettinen OS (2002). CT screening for lung cancer: frequency and significance of part-solid and nonsolid nodules. AJR Am J Roentgenol 178: 1053-1057.
820. Herbst WM, Kummer W, Hofmann W, Otto H, Heym C (1987). Carcinoid tumors of the thymus. An immunohistochemical study. Cancer 60: 2465-2470.
821. Hermine O, Michel M, Buzyn-Veil A, Gessain A (1996). Body-cavity-based lymphoma in an HIV-seronegative patient without Kaposi's sarcoma-associated herpesvirus-like DNA sequences. N Engl J Med 334: 272-273.
822. Herndon JE, Green MR, Chahinian AP, Corson JM, Suzuki Y, Vogelzang NJ (1998). Factors predictive of survival among 337 patients with mesothelioma treated between 1984 and 1994 by the Cancer and Leukemia Group B. Chest 113: 723-731.
823. Herrmann MA, Shankerman RA, Edwards WD, Shub C, Schaff HV (1992). Primary cardiac angiosarcoma: a clinicopathologic study of six cases. J Thorac Cardiovasc Surg 103: 655-664.
824. Hess JL (1998). Chromosomal translocations in benign tumors: the HMGI proteins. Am J Clin Pathol 109: 251-261.
825. Hess JL, Bodis S, Pinkus G, Silver B, Mauch P (1994). Histopathologic grading of nodular sclerosis Hodgkin's disease. Lack of prognostic significance in 254 surgically staged patients. Cancer 74: 708-714.
826. Hibi K, Trink B, Patturajan M, Westra WH, Caballero OL, Hill DE, Ratovitski EA, Jen J, Sidransky D (2000). AIS is an oncogene amplified in squamous cell carcinoma. Proc Natl Acad Sci U S A 97: 5462-5467.
827. Hida T, Yatabe Y, Achiwa H, Muramatsu H, Kozaki K, Nakamura S, Ogawa M, Mitsudomi T, Sugiura T, Takahashi T (1998). Increased expression of cyclooxygenase 2 occurs frequently in human lung cancers, specifically in adenocarcinomas. Cancer Res 58: 3761-3764.
828. Higgins JP, Montgomery K, Wang L, Domanay E, Warnke RA, Brooks JD, van de Rijn M (2003). Expression of FKBP12 in benign and malignant vascular endothelium: an immunohistochemical study on conventional sections and tissue microarrays. Am J Surg Pathol 27: 58-64.
829. Higgins JP, Warnke RA (1999). CD30 expression is common in mediastinal large B-cell lymphoma. Am J Clin Pathol 112: 241-247.
830. Hill KA, Gonzalez-Crussi F, Chou PM (2001). Calcifying fibrous pseudotumor versus inflammatory myofibroblastic tumor: a histological and immunohistochemical comparison. Mod Pathol 14: 784-790.
831. Hillerdal G (1983). Malignant mesothelioma 1982: review of 4710 published cases. Br J Dis Chest 77: 321-343.
832. Hilliard RI, McKendry JB, Phillips MJ (1990). Congenital abnormalities of the lymphatic system: a new clinical classification. Pediatrics 86: 988-994.
833. Hills EA (1971). Cylindroma of the trachea and left main bronchus. Proc R Soc Med 64: 221-222.
834. Hines GL (1993). Paravertebral extramedullary hematopoiesis (as a posterior mediastinal tumor) associated with congenital dyserythropoietic anemia. J Thorac Cardiovasc Surg 106: 760-761.
835. Hirabayashi H, Fujii Y, Sakaguchi M, Tanaka H, Yoon HE, Komoto Y, Inoue M, Miyoshi S, Matsuda H (1997). p16INK4, pRB, p53 and cyclin D1 expression and hypermethylation of CDKN2 gene in thymoma and thymic carcinoma. Int J Cancer 73: 639-644.
836. Hirabayashi H, Ohta M, Tanaka H, Sakaguchi M, Fujii Y, Miyoshi S, Matsuda H (2002). Prognostic significance of p27KIP1 expression in resected non-small cell lung cancers: analysis in combination with expressions of p16INK4A, pRB, and p53. J Surg Oncol 81: 177-184.
837. Hiraga H, Nojima T, Abe S, Sawa H, Yamashiro K, Yamawaki S, Kaneda K, Nagashima K (1998). Diagnosis of synovial sarcoma with the reverse transcriptase-polymerase chain reaction: analyses of 84 soft tissue and bone tumors. Diagn Mol Pathol 7: 102-110.
838. Hiraiwa H, Hamazaki M, Tsuruta S, Hattori H, Mimaya J, Hasegawa S, Kohno S, Aoki K (1998). Infantile hemangioendothelioma of the thymus with massive pleural effusion and Kasabach—Merritt syndrome: histopathological, flow cytometrical analysis of the tumor. Acta Paediatr Jpn 40: 604-607.
839. Hirao T, Bueno R, Chen CJ, Gordon GJ, Heilig E, Kelsey KT (2002). Alterations of the p16(INK4) locus in human malignant mesothelial tumors. Carcinogenesis 23: 1127-1130.
840. Hiroshima K, Ishibashi M, Ohwada H, Kawano Y, Mizutani F, Hayashi Y (1992). A case of adenocarcinoma of the lung with a spindle cell component. Acta Pathol Jpn 42: 841-846.
841. Hiroshima K, Iyoda A, Shibuya K, Toyozaki T, Haga Y, Fujisawa T, Ohwada H (2002). Prognostic significance of neuroendocrine differentiation in adenocarcinoma of the lung. Ann Thorac Surg 73: 1732-1735.
842. Hirota J, Akiyama K, Ookado A, Takiguchi M, Oosawa S, Hashimoto A (1996). [A case report of papillary fibroelastoma of the aortic valve]. Nippon Kyobu Geka Gakkai Zasshi 44: 705-708.
843. Hirota T, Konno K, Fujimoto T, Ohta H, Kato S, Hara K (1999). Unusual late extrapulmonary metastasis in osteosarcoma. Pediatr Hematol Oncol 16: 545-549.
844. Hirsch FR, Franklin WA, Gazdar AF, Bunn PAJr (2001). Early detection of lung cancer: clinical perspectives of recent advances in biology and radiology. Clin Cancer Res 7: 5-22.
845. Hirsch FR, Franklin WA, Veve R, Varella-Garcia M, Bunn PAJr (2002). HER2/neu expression in malignant lung tumors. Semin Oncol 29: 51-58.
846. Hirsch FR, Matthews MJ, Yesner R (1982). Histopathologic classification of small cell carcinoma of the lung: comments based on an interobserver examination. Cancer 50: 1360-1366.
847. Hirsch FR, Osterlind K, Jensen LI, Thomsen C, Peters K, Jensen F, Hansen HH (1992). The impact of abdominal computerized tomography on the pretreatment staging and prognosis of small cell lung cancer. Ann Oncol 3: 469-474.
848. Hirsch FR, Paulson OB, Hansen HH, Vraa-Jensen J (1982). Intracranial metastases in small cell carcinoma of the lung: correlation of clinical and autopsy findings. Cancer 50: 2433-2437.
849. Hirsch FR, Prindiville SA, Miller YE, Franklin WA, Dempsey EC, Murphy JR, Bunn PAJr, Kennedy TC (2001). Fluorescence versus white-light bronchoscopy for detection of preneoplastic lesions: a randomized study. J Natl Cancer Inst 93: 1385-1391.
850. Hisaoka M, Hashimoto H, Iwamasa T, Ishikawa K, Aoki T (1999). Primary synovial sarcoma of the lung: report of two cases confirmed by molecular detection of SYT-SSX fusion gene transcripts. Histopathology 34: 205-210.
851. Hishima T, Fukayama M, Fujisawa M, Hayashi Y, Arai K, Funata N, Koike M (1994). CD5 expression in thymic carcinoma. Am J Pathol 145: 268-275.
852. Hishima T, Fukayama M, Hayashi Y, Fujii T, Arai K, Shiozawa Y, Funata N, Koike M (1997). Neuroendocrine differentiation in thymic epithelial tumors. Immunohistochemical studies. In: Epithelial Tumors of the Thymus. Pathology, Biology, Treatment, Marx A, Muller-Hermelink HK, eds., Plenum Press: New York , pp. 67-73.
853. Hishima T, Fukayama M, Hayashi Y, Fujii T, Arai K, Shiozawa Y, Funata N, Koike M (1998). Neuroendocrine differentiation in thymic epithelial tumors with special reference to thymic carcinoma and atypical thymoma. Hum Pathol 29: 330-338.
854. Hishima T, Fukayama M, Hayashi Y, Fujii T, Ooba T, Funata N, Koike M (2000). CD70 expression in thymic carcinoma. Am J Surg Pathol 24: 742-746.
855. Hittmair A, Rogatsch H, Hobisch A, Mikuz G, Feichtinger H (1996). CD30 expression in seminoma. Hum Pathol 27: 1166-1171.
856. Ho FC, Fu KH, Lam SY, Chiu SW, Chan AC, Muller-Hermelink HK (1994). Evaluation of a histogenetic classification for thymic epithelial tumours. Histopathology 25: 21-29.
857. Ho FC, Ho JC (1977). Pigmented carcinoid tumour of the thymus. Histopathology 1: 363-369.
858. Hodgson JT, Darnton A (2000). The quantitative risks of mesothelioma and lung cancer in relation to asbestos exposure. Ann Occup Hyg 44: 565-601.
859. Hoffacker V, Schultz A, Tiesinga JJ, Gold R, Schalke B, Nix W, Kiefer R, Muller-Hermelink HK, Marx A (2000). Thymomas alter the T-cell subset composition in the blood: a potential mechanism for thymoma-associated autoimmune disease. Blood 96: 3872-3879.
860. Hoffner L, Deka R, Chakravarti A, Surti U (1994). Cytogenetics and origins of pediatric germ cell tumors. Cancer Genet Cytogenet 74: 54-58.
861. Hofmann W, Moller P, Manke HG, Otto HF (1985). Thymoma. A clinicopathologic study of 98 cases with special reference to three unusual cases. Pathol Res Pract 179: 337-353.
862. Hofmann WJ, Momburg F, Moller P (1988). Thymic medullary cells expressing B lymphocyte antigens. Hum Pathol 19: 1280-1287.
863. Holley DG, Martin GR, Brenner JI, Fyfe DA, Huhta JC, Kleinman CS, Ritter SB, Silverman NH (1995). Diagnosis and management of fetal cardiac tumors: a multicenter experience and review of published reports. J Am Coll Cardiol 26: 516-520.
864. Hollinger P, Gaeng D (1997).

Simultaneous bilateral spontaneous pneumothorax in a patient with peritoneal and pleural papillary mesothelioma. Respiration 64: 233-235.
865. Hollingsworth HC, Stetler-Stevenson M, Gagneten D, Kingma DW, Raffeld M, Jaffe ES (1994). Immunodeficiency-associated malignant lymphoma. Three cases showing genotypic evidence of both T- and B-cell lineages. Am J Surg Pathol 18: 1092-1101.
866. Holst VA, Finkelstein S, Colby TV, Myers JL, Yousem SA (1997). p53 and K-ras mutational genotyping in pulmonary carcinosarcoma, spindle cell carcinoma, and pulmonary blastoma: implications for histogenesis. Am J Surg Pathol 21: 801-811.
867. Hongyo T, Kurooka M, Taniguchi E, Iuchi K, Nakajima Y, Aozasa K, Nomura T (1998). Frequent p53 mutations at dipyrimidine sites in patients with pyothorax-associated lymphoma. Cancer Res 58: 1105-1107.
868. Horenstein MG, Nador RG, Chadburn A, Hyjek EM, Inghirami G, Knowles DM, Cesarman E (1997). Epstein-Barr virus latent gene expression in primary effusion lymphomas containing Kaposi's sarcoma-associated herpesvirus/human herpesvirus-8. Blood 90: 1186-1191.
869. Hou SM, Falt S, Nyberg F (2001). Glutathione S-transferase T1-null genotype interacts synergistically with heavy smoking on lung cancer risk. Environ Mol Mutagen 38: 83-86.
870. Houlston RS (2000). CYP1A1 polymorphisms and lung cancer risk: a meta-analysis. Pharmacogenetics 10: 105-114.
871. Hsieh PP, Ho WL, Peng HC, Lee T (2002). Synovial sarcoma of the mediastinum. Zhonghua Yi Xue Za Zhi (Taipei) 65: 83-85.
872. Hsu FJ, Levy R (1995). Preferential use of the VH4 Ig gene family by diffuse large-cell lymphoma. Blood 86: 3072-3082.
873. Hsueh C, Kuo TT, Tsang NM, Lin JN, Yang CP (2002). Thymic lymphoepithelioma-like carcinoma in children: detection of EBV encoded latent membrane protein-1 gene without 30-bp deletion. Mod Pathol 15.
874. Hu J, Schuster AE, Fritsch MK, Schneider DT, Lauer S, Perlman EJ (2001). Deletion mapping of 6q21-26 and frequency of 1p36 deletion in childhood endodermal sinus tumors by microsatellite analysis. Oncogene 20: 8042-8044.
875. Huang CI, Taki T, Higashiyama M, Kohno N, Miyake M (2000). p16 protein expression is associated with a poor prognosis in squamous cell carcinoma of the lung. Br J Cancer 82: 374-380.
876. Huang MN, Edgerton F, Takita H, Douglas HOJr, Karakousis C (1978). Lung resection for metastatic sarcoma. Am J Surg 135: 804-806.
877. Huang Q, Chang KL, Gaal K, Arber DA (2002). Primary effusion lymphoma with subsequent development of a small bowel mass in an HIV-seropositive patient: a case report and literature review. Am J Surg Pathol 26: 1363-1367.
878. Hummel P, Cangiarella JF, Cohen JM, Yang G, Waisman J, Chhieng DC (2001). Transthoracic fine-needle aspiration biopsy of pulmonary spindle cell and mesenchymal lesions: a study of 61 cases. Cancer 93: 187-198.
879. Hurt RD, Bruckman JE, Farrow GM, Bernatz PE, Hahn RG, Earle JD (1982). Primary anterior mediastinal seminoma. Cancer 49: 1658-1663.
880. Hussain SP, Amstad P, Raja K, Sawyer M, Hofseth L, Shields PG, Hewer A, Phillips DH, Ryberg D, Haugen A, Harris CC (2001). Mutability of p53 hotspot codons to benzo(a)pyrene diol epoxide (BPDE) and the frequency of p53 mutations in nontumorous human lung. Cancer Res 61: 6350-6355.
881. Hussain SP, Hofseth LJ, Harris CC (2001). Tumor suppressor genes: at the crossroads of molecular carcinogenesis, molecular epidemiology and human risk assessment. Lung Cancer 34 Suppl 2: S7-15.
882. Hussong JW, Brown M, Perkins SL, Dehner LP, Coffin CM (1999). Comparison of DNA ploidy, histologic, and immunohistochemical findings with clinical outcome in inflammatory myofibroblastic tumors. Mod Pathol 12: 279-286.
883. Huszar M, Suster S, Herczeg E, Geiger B (1986). Sclerosing hemangioma of the lung. Immunohistochemical demonstration of mesenchymal origin using antibodies to tissue-specific intermediate filaments. Cancer 58: 2422-2427.
884. IARC (2003). IARC Monographs on the Evaluation of Carcinogenic Risks to Humans. Volume 83. Tobacco smoke and involuntary smoking. IARC Monographs .
885. Iezzoni JC, Gaffey MJ, Weiss LM (1995). The role of Epstein-Barr virus in lymphoepithelioma-like carcinomas. Am J Clin Pathol 103: 308-315.
886. Iezzoni JC, Nass LB (1996). Thymic basaloid carcinoma: a case report and review of the literature. Mod Pathol 9: 21-25.
887. Ihde DC, Dunnick NR, Johnston-Early A, Bunn PA, Cohen MH, Minna JD (1982). Abdominal computed tomography in small cell lung cancer: assessment of extent of disease and response to therapy. Cancer 49: 1485-1490.
888. Ikeda T, Ishihara T, Yoshimatsu H, Kikuchi K, Murakami M (1974). Primary osteogenic sarcoma of the mediastinum. Thorax 29: 582-588.
889. Ilhan I, Kutluk T, Gogus S, Besim A, Buyukpamukcu M (1994). Hypertrophic pulmonary osteoarthropathy in a child with thymic carcinoma: an unusual presentation in childhood. Med Pediatr Oncol 23: 140-143.
890. Im JG, Kim WH, Han MC, Han YM, Chung JW, Ahn JM, Do YS (1994). Sclerosing hemangiomas of the lung and interlobar fissures: CT findings. J Comput Assist Tomogr 18: 34-38.
891. Inagaki H, Chan JK, Ng JW, Okabe M, Yoshino T, Okamoto M, Ogawa H, Matsushita H, Yokose T, Matsuno Y, Nakamura N, Nagasaka T, Ueda R, Eimoto T, Nakamura S (2002). Primary thymic extranodal marginal-zone B-cell lymphoma of mucosa-associated lymphoid tissue type exhibits distinctive clinicopathological and molecular features. Am J Pathol 160: 1435-1443.
892. Indolfi P, Casale F, Carli M, Bisogno G, Ninfo V, Cecchetto G, Bagnulo S, Santoro N, Giuliano M, Di Tullio MT (2000). Pleuropulmonary blastoma: management and prognosis of 11 cases. Cancer 89: 1396-1401.
893. Ingham PW, Nystedt S, Nakano Y, Brown W, Stark D, van den Heuvel M, Taylor AM (2000). Patched represses the Hedgehog signalling pathway by promoting modification of the Smoothened protein. Curr Biol 10: 1315-1318.
894. Inghirami G, Chilosi M, Knowles DM (1990). Western thymomas lack Epstein-Barr virus by Southern blotting analysis and by polymerase chain reaction. Am J Pathol 136: 1429-1436.
895. Inoue H, Ishii H, Alder H, Snyder E, Druck T, Huebner K, Croce CM (1997). Sequence of the FRA3B common fragile region: implications for the mechanism of FHIT deletion. Proc Natl Acad Sci U S A 94: 14584-14589.
896. Inoue M, Marx A, Zettl A, Strobel P, Muller-Hermelink HK, Starostik P (2002). Chromosome 6 suffers frequent and multiple aberrations in thymoma. Am J Pathol 161: 1507-1513.
897. Inoue M, Starostik P, Zettl A, Strobel P, Schwarz S, Scaravilli F, Henry K, Willcox N, Muller-Hermelink HK, Marx A (2003). Correlating genetic aberrations with WHO-defined histology and stage across the spectrum of thymomas. Cancer Res 63: 3708-3715.
898. Institute of Pathology "Rudolf-Virchow-Haus" (2003). Comparative Genomic Hybridization (CGH). University Hospital Charité Humboldt-University of Berlin. http://amba charite de/cgh/
899. International Union Against Cancer (UICC) (2003). TNM Supplement. A Commentary on Uniform Use. 3rd ed. Wiley-Liss: New York.
900. Inzucchi SE, Pfaff-Amesse T (1998). Ectopic thymic carcinoid masquerading as a thyroid nodule. Thyroid 8: 589-595.
901. Iolascon A, Faienza MF, Coppola B, della Ragione F, Schettini F, Biondi A (1996). Homozygous deletions of cyclin-dependent kinase inhibitor genes, p16(INK4A) and p18, in childhood T cell lineage acute lymphoblastic leukemias. Leukemia 10: 255-260.
902. Iribarren C, Tekawa IS, Sidney S, Friedman GD (1999). Effect of cigar smoking on the risk of cardiovascular disease, chronic obstructive pulmonary disease, and cancer in men. N Engl J Med 340: 1773-1780.
903. Isaacs H (2002). Tumors of the Fetus and Infant. Springer Verlag: New York.
904. Isaacson PG (1990). Lymphomas of mucosa-associated lymphoid tissue (MALT). Histopathology 16: 617-619.
905. Isaacson PG, Chan JK, Tang C, Addis BJ (1990). Low-grade B-cell lymphoma of mucosa-associated lymphoid tissue arising in the thymus. A thymic lymphoma mimicking myoepithelial sialadenitis. Am J Surg Pathol 14: 342-351.
906. Isaacson PG, Norton AJ, Addis BJ (1987). The human thymus contains a novel population of B lymphocytes. Lancet 2: 1488-1491.
907. Iseki M, Tsuda N, Kishikawa M, Shimada O, Hayashi T, Kawahara K, Tomita M (1990). Thymolipoma with striated myoid cells. Histological, immunohistochemical, and ultrastructural study. Am J Surg Pathol 14: 395-398.
908. Ishibashi H, Shimoyama T, Akamatsu H, Sunamori M, Ohtani T, Imai K (2002). [A successfully resected case of giant malignant mediastinal germ cell tumor]. Kyobu Geka 55: 815-818.
909. Ishida T, Kaneko S, Yokoyama H, Inoue T, Sugio K, Sugimachi K (1992). Adenosquamous carcinoma of the lung. Clinicopathologic and immunohistochemical features. Am J Clin Pathol 97: 678-685.
910. Ishida Y, Kato K, Kigasawa H, Ohama Y, Ijiri R, Tanaka Y (2000). Synchronous occurrence of pleuropulmonary blastoma and cystic nephroma: possible genetic link in cystic lesions of the lung and the kidney. Med Pediatr Oncol 35: 85-87.
911. Ishihara T, Kikuchi K, Ikeda T, Yamazaki S (1973). Metastatic pulmonary diseases: biologic factors and modes of treatment. Chest 63: 227-232.
912. Ishiwa N, Ogawa N, Shoji A, Maehara T, Hayashi Y, Takanashi Y, Yazawa T, Ito T (2003). Correlation between lymph node micrometastasis and histologic classification of small lung adenocarcinomas, in considering the indication of limited surgery. Lung Cancer 39: 159-164.
913. Israel DH, Sherman W, Ambrose JA, Sharma S, Harpaz N, Robbins M (1991). Dynamic coronary ostial obstruction due to papillary fibroelastoma leading to myocardial ischemia and infarction. Am J Cardiol 67: 104-105.
914. Ito H, Hamajima N, Takezaki T, Matsuo K, Tajima K, Hatooka S, Mitsudomi T, Suyama M, Sato S, Ueda R (2002). A limited association of OGG1 Ser326Cys polymorphism for adenocarcinoma of the lung. J Epidemiol 12: 258-265.
915. Iuchi K, Ichimiya A, Akashi A, Mizuta T, Lee YE, Tada H, Mori T, Sawamura K, Lee YS, Furuse K, Yamamoto S, Aozasa K (1987). Non-Hodgkin's lymphoma of the pleural cavity developing from long-standing pyothorax. Cancer 60: 1771-1775.
916. Iyoda A, Hiroshima K, Toyozaki T, Haga Y, Fujisawa T, Ohwada H (2001). Clinical characterization of pulmonary large cell neuroendocrine carcinoma and large cell carcinoma with neuroendocrine morphology. Cancer 91: 1992-2000.
917. Jacobsen M, Francis D (1980). Pulmonary blastoma. A clinico-pathological study of eleven cases. Acta Pathol Microbiol Scand [A] 88: 151-160.
918. Jacobson JO, Aisenberg AC, Lamarre L, Willett CG, Linggood RM, Miketic LM, Harris NL (1988). Mediastinal large cell lymphoma. An uncommon subset of adult lymphoma curable with combined modality therapy. Cancer 62: 1893-1898.
919. Jaffe ES, Harris NL, Stein H, Vardiman JW (2001). World Health Organization Classification of Tumours. Pathology and Genetics of Tumours of Haematopoietic and Lymphoid Tissues. 1st ed. IARC Press: Lyon.
920. Jaffe ES, Wilson WH (1997). Lymphomatoid granulomatosis: pathogenesis, pathology and clinical implications. Cancer Surv 30: 233-248.
921. Janigan DT, Husain A, Robinson NA (1986). Cardiac angiosarcomas. A review and a case report. Cancer 57: 852-859.
922. Janower ML, Blennerhassett JB (1971). Lymphangitic spread of metastatic cancer to the lung. A radiologic-pathologic classification. Radiology 101: 267-273.
923. Janssen-Heijnen ML, Nab HW, van Reek J, van der Heijden LH, Schipper R, Coebergh JW (1995). Striking changes in smoking behaviour and lung cancer incidence by histological type in south-east Netherlands, 1960-1991. Eur J Cancer 31A: 949-952.
924. Jansson JO, Svensson J, Bengtsson BA, Frohman LA, Ahlman H, Wangberg B, Nilsson O, Nilsson M (1998). Acromegaly and Cushing's syndrome due to ectopic production of GHRH and ACTH by a thymic carcinoid tumour: in vitro responses to GHRH and GHRP-6. Clin Endocrinol (Oxf) 48: 243-250.
925. Javett SN, Braudo JL, Webster I (1963). Congenital Dilation of Pulmonary Lymphatics. Pediatrics 31: 416-&.

926. Jeanmart M, Lantuejoul S, Fievet F, Moro D, Sturm N, Brambilla C, Brambilla E (2003). Value of immunohistochemical markers in preinvasive bronchial lesions in risk assessment of lung cancer. Clin Cancer Res 9: 2195-2203.

927. Jedrychowski W, Becher H, Wahrendorf J, Basa-Cierpialek Z, Gomola K (1992). Effect of tobacco smoking on various histological types of lung cancer. J Cancer Res Clin Oncol 118: 276-282.

928. Jennings TA, Axiotis CA, Kress Y, Carter D (1990). Primary malignant melanoma of the lower respiratory tract. Report of a case and literature review. Am J Clin Pathol 94: 649-655.

929. Jeong HS, Lee GK, Sung R, Ahn JH, Song HG (1997). Calcifying fibrous pseudo-tumor of mediastinum—a case report. J Korean Med Sci 12: 58-62.

930. Jimenez JF, Uthman EO, Townsend JW, Gloster ES, Seibert JJ (1986). Primary bronchopulmonary leiomyosarcoma in childhood. Arch Pathol Lab Med 110: 348-351.

931. Johnson BE, Russell E, Simmons AM, Phelps R, Steinberg SM, Ihde DC, Gazdar AF (1996). MYC family DNA amplification in 126 tumor cell lines from patients with small cell lung cancer. J Cell Biochem Suppl 24: 210-217.

932. Johnson DE, Appelt G, Samuels ML, Luna M (1976). Metastases from testicular carcinoma. Study of 78 autopsied cases. Urology 8: 234-239.

933. Johnson DH (1999). Management of small cell lung cancer: current state of the art. Chest 116: 525S-530S.

934. Johnson RL, Donnell RM (1979). Diffuse granulocytic infiltration of giant cell carcinoma of the lung: a distinctive histologic finding with clinical significance. Lab Invest 40: 262.

935. Johnson RM, Lindskog GE (1967). 100 cases of tumor metastatic to lung and mediastinum. Treatment and results. JAMA 202: 94-98.

936. Johnston WW, Elson CE (1997). Respiratory tract. In: Comprehensive Cytopathology, Bibbo M, Day L, eds., 2nd ed. WB Saunders: Philadelphia , pp. 325-402.

937. Jones D, Ballestas ME, Kaye KM, Gulizia JM, Winters GL, Fletcher J, Scadden DT, Aster JC (1998). Primary-effusion lymphoma and Kaposi's sarcoma in a cardiac-transplant recipient. N Engl J Med 339: 444-449.

938. Jones H, Yaman M, Penn CR, Clarke T (1993). Primary stromal sarcoma of the thymus with areas of liposarcoma. Histopathology 23: 81-82.

939. Joos S, Granzow M, Holtgreve-Grez H, Siebert R, Harder L, Martin-Subero JI, Wolf J, Adamowicz M, Barth TF, Lichter P, Jauch A (2003). Hodgkin's lymphoma cell lines are characterized by frequent aberrations on chromosomes 2p and 9p including REL and JAK2. Int J Cancer 103: 489-495.

940. Joos S, Menz CK, Wrobel G, Siebert R, Gesk S, Ohl S, Mechtersheimer G, Trumper L, Moller P, Lichter P, Barth TF (2002). Classical Hodgkin lymphoma is characterized by recurrent copy number gains of the short arm of chromosome 2. Blood 99: 1381-1387.

941. Joos S, Otano-Joos MI, Ziegler S, Bruderlein S, du Manoir S, Bentz M, Moller P, Lichter P (1996). Primary mediastinal (thymic) B-cell lymphoma is characterized by gains of chromosomal material including 9p and amplification of the REL gene.

Blood 87: 1571-1578.

942. Jordan AG, Predmore L, Sullivan MM, Memoli VA (1987). The cytodiagnosis of well-differentiated neuroendocrine carcinoma. A distinct clinicopathologic entity. Acta Cytol 31: 464-470.

943. Jordan KG, Kwong JS, Flint J, Muller NL (1997). Surgically treated pneumothorax. Radiologic and pathologic findings. Chest 111: 280-285.

944. Jourenkova-Mironova N, Wikman H, Bouchardy C, Voho A, Dayer P, Benhamou S, Hirvonen A (1998). Role of glutathione S-transferase GSTM1, GSTM3, GSTP1 and GSTT1 genotypes in modulating susceptibility to smoking-related lung cancer. Pharmacogenetics 8: 495-502.

945. Junewick JJ, Fitzgerald NE (1999). The thymus in Langerhans' cell histiocytosis. Pediatr Radiol 29: 904-907.

946. Jung KJ, Lee KS, Han J, Kim J, Kim TS, Kim EA (2001). Malignant thymic epithelial tumors: CT-pathologic correlation. AJR Am J Roentgenol 176: 433-439.

947. Jurkovich D, de Marchena E, Bilsker M, Fierro-Renoy C, Temple D, Garcia H (2000). Primary cardiac lymphoma diagnosed by percutaneous intracardiac biopsy with combined fluoroscopic and transesophageal echocardiographic imaging. Catheter Cardiovasc Interv 50: 226-233.

948. Kamby C, Vejborg I, Kristensen B, Olsen LO, Mouridsen HT (1988). Metastatic pattern in recurrent breast cancer. Special reference to intrathoracic recurrences. Cancer 62: 2226-2233.

949. Kamel OW, Gocke CD, Kell DL, Cleary ML, Warnke RA (1995). True histiocytic lymphoma: a study of 12 cases based on current definition. Leuk Lymphoma 18: 81-86.

950. Kamimura K, Nakamura N, Ishibashi T, Maruyama Y, Abe M (2002). Somatic hypermutation of immunoglobulin heavy chain variable region genes in thymic marginal zone B-cell lymphoma of MALT type of a patient with Sjogren's syndrome. Histopathology 40: 294-296.

951. Kaminishi Y, Watanabe Y, Nakata H, Shimokama T, Jikuya T (2002). Cystic tumor of the atrioventricular nodal region. Jpn J Thorac Cardiovasc Surg 50: 37-39.

952. Kamiya H, Yasuda T, Nagamine H, Sakakibara N, Nishida S, Kawasuji M, Watanabe G (2001). Surgical treatment of primary cardiac tumors: 28 years' experience in Kanazawa University Hospital. Jpn Circ J 65: 315-319.

953. Kanavaros P, Gaulard P, Charlotte F, Martin N, Ducos C, Lebezu M, Mason DY (1995). Discordant expression of immunoglobulin and its associated molecule mb-1/CD79a is frequently found in mediastinal large B cell lymphomas. Am J Pathol 146: 735-741.

954. Kanno H, Aozasa K (1998). Mechanism for the development of pyothorax-associated lymphoma. Pathol Int 48: 653-664.

955. Kanno H, Naka N, Yasunaga Y, Iuchi K, Yamauchi S, Hashimoto M, Aozasa K (1997). Production of the immunosuppressive cytokine interleukin-10 by Epstein-Barr-virus-expressing pyothorax-associated lymphoma: possible role in the development of overt lymphoma in immunocompetent hosts. Am J Pathol 150: 349-357.

956. Kanno H, Yasunaga Y, Iuchi K, Yamauchi S, Tatekawa T, Sugiyama H, Aozasa K (1996). Interleukin-6-mediated growth enhancement of cell lines derived from pyothorax-associated lymphoma. Lab Invest 75: 167-173.

957. Kaplan MA, Goodman MD, Satish J, Bhagavan BS, Travis WD (1996). Primary pulmonary sarcoma with morphologic features of monophasic synovial sarcoma and chromosome translocation t(X; 18). Am J Clin Pathol 105: 195-199.

958. Kaplan MA, Tazelaar HD, Hayashi T, Schroer KR, Travis WD (1996). Adenomatoid tumors of the pleura. Am J Surg Pathol 20: 1219-1223.

959. Kaplinsky EJ, Favaloro RR, Pombo G, Perrone SV, Vigliano CA, Schnidt JL, Boughen RP (2000). Primary pulmonary artery sarcoma resembling chronic thromboembolic pulmonary disease. Eur Respir J 16: 1202-1204.

960. Karakoca Y, Emri S, Bagci T, Demir A, Erdem Y, Baris E, Sahin AA (1998). Environmentally-induced malignant pleural mesothelioma and HLA distribution in Turkey. Int J Tuberc Lung Dis 2: 1017-1022.

961. Karbowniczek M, Astrindis A, Balsara BR, Testa JR, Lium JH, Colby TV, McCormack FX, Henske EP (2003). Recurrent lymphangiomyomatosis after transplantation: genetic analyses reveal a metastatic mechanism. Am J Respir Crit Care Med 167: 976-982.

962. Kardamakis D, Bouboulis N, Ravazoula P, Dimopoulos P, Dougenis D (1996). Primary hemangiosarcoma of the mediastinum. Lung Cancer 16: 81-86.

963. Karl SR, Dunn J (1985). Posterior mediastinal teratomas. J Pediatr Surg 20: 508-510.

964. Kasai K, Kuwao S, Sato Y, Murayama M, Harano Y, Kameya T (1992). Case report of primary cardiac lymphoma. The applications of PCR to the diagnosis of primary cardiac lymphoma. Acta Pathol Jpn 42: 667-671.

965. Katial RK, Ranlett R, Whitlock WL (1994). Human papilloma virus associated with solitary squamous papilloma complicated by bronchiectasis and bronchial stenosis. Chest 106: 1887-1889.

966. Katlic MR, Grillo HC, Wang CA (1985). Substernal goiter. Analysis of 80 patients from Massachusetts General Hospital. Am J Surg 149: 283-287.

967. Kato H, Okunaka T, Shimatani H (1996). Photodynamic therapy for early stage bronchogenic carcinoma. J Clin Laser Med Surg 14: 235-238.

968. Katz A, Lattes R (1969). Granulomatous thymoma or Hodgkin's disease of thymus? A clinical and histologic study and a re-evaluation. Cancer 23: 1-15.

969. Katzenstein AL, Carrington CB, Liebow AA (1979). Lymphomatoid granulomatosis: a clinicopathologic study of 152 cases. Cancer 43: 360-373.

970. Katzenstein AL, Gmelich JT, Carrington CB (1980). Sclerosing hemangioma of the lung: a clinicopathologic study of 51 cases. Am J Surg Pathol 4: 343-356.

971. Katzenstein AL, Prioleau PG, Askin FB (1980). The histologic spectrum and significance of clear-cell change in lung carcinoma. Cancer 45: 943-947.

972. Katzenstein AL, Weise DL, Fulling K, Battifora H (1983). So-called sclerosing hemangioma of the lung. Evidence for mesothelial origin. Am J Surg Pathol 7: 3-14.

973. Kauczor HU, Schwickert HC, Mayer E, Kersjes W, Moll R, Schweden F (1994). Pulmonary artery sarcoma mimicking chronic thromboembolic disease: computed tomography and magnetic resonance imaging findings. Cardiovasc Intervent Radiol 17: 185-189.

974. Kauffman SL (1981). Histogenesis of the papillary Clara cell adenoma. Am J Pathol 103: 174-180.

975. Kaufmann O, Dietel M (2000). Expression of thyroid transcription factor-1 in pulmonary and extrapulmonary small cell carcinomas and other neuroendocrine carcinomas of various primary sites. Histopathology 36: 415-420.

976. Kaufmann O, Kother S, Dietel M (1998). Use of antibodies against estrogen and progesterone receptors to identify metastatic breast and ovarian carcinomas by conventional immunohistochemical and tyramide signal amplification methods. Mod Pathol 11: 357-363.

977. Kawada M, Oda K, Hirose K, Fukutomi T, Yamashiro T, Ogoshi S (1996). [A case report of surgical treatment for left ventricular papillary fibroelastoma]. Nippon Kyobu Geka Gakkai Zasshi 44: 1159-1162.

978. Kawajiri K, Nakachi K, Imai K, Watanabe J, Hayashi S (1993). Germ line polymorphisms of p53 and CYP1A1 genes involved in human lung cancer. Carcinogenesis 14: 1085-1089.

979. Kawakami S, Sone S, Takashima S, Li F, Yang ZG, Maruyama Y, Honda T, Hasegawa M, Wang JC (2001). Atypical adenomatous hyperplasia of the lung: correlation between high-resolution CT findings and histopathologic features. Eur Radiol 11: 811-814.

980. Kawashima O, Kamiyoshihara M, Sakata S, Kurihara T, Ishikawa S, Morishita Y (1999). Basaloid carcinoma of the thymus. Ann Thorac Surg 68: 1863-1865.

981. Kaye FJ (2002). RB and cyclin dependent kinase pathways: defining a distinction between RB and p16 loss in lung cancer. Oncogene 21: 6908-6914.

982. Kazmierczak B, Meyer-Bolte K, Tran KH, Wockel W, Breightman I, Rosigkeit J, Bartnitzke S, Bullerdiek J (1999). A high frequency of tumors with rearrangements of genes of the HMGI(Y) family in a series of 191 pulmonary chondroid hamartomas. Genes Chromosomes Cancer 26: 125-133.

983. Kazmierczak B, Wanschura S, Rommel B, Bartnitzke S, Bullerdiek J (1996). Ten pulmonary chondroid hamartomas with chromosome 6p21 breakpoints within the HMG-I(Y) gene or its immediate surroundings. J Natl Cancer Inst 88: 1234-1236.

984. Kearney DL, Titus JL, Hawkins EP, Ott DA, Garson AJr (1987). Pathologic features of myocardial hamartomas causing childhood tachyarrhythmias. Circulation 75: 705-710.

985. Kees UR, Mulcahy MT, Willoughby ML (1991). Intrathoracic carcinoma in an 11-year-old girl showing a translocation t(15;19). Am J Pediatr Hematol Oncol 13: 459-464.

986. Keith RL, Miller YE, Gemmill RM, Drabkin HA, Dempsey EC, Kennedy TC, Prindiville S, Franklin WA (2000). Angiogenic squamous dysplasia in bronchi of individuals at high risk for lung cancer. Clin Cancer Res 6: 1616-1625.

987. Kelleher P, Misbah SA (2003). What is Good's syndrome? Immunological abnormalities in patients with thymoma. J Clin Pathol 56: 12-16.

988. Keller AR, Castleman B (1974). Hodgkin's disease of the thymus gland. Cancer 33: 1615-1623.

989. Keller SA, Schattner EJ, Cesarman E (2000). Inhibition of NF-kappaB induces apoptosis of KSHV-infected primary effusion lymphoma cells. Blood 96: 2537-2542.

990. Kelly MD, Sheridan BF, Farnsworth AE,

Palfreeman S (1994). Parathyroid carcinoma in a mediastinal sixth parathyroid gland. Aust N Z J Surg 64: 446-449.
991. Kelsey AM, McNally K, Birch J, Mitchell EL (1997). Case of extra pulmonary, pleuro-pulmonary blastoma in a child: pathological and cytogenetic findings. Med Pediatr Oncol 29: 61-64.
992. Kennedy A (1973). "Sclerosing haemangioma" of the lung: an alternative view of its development. J Clin Pathol 26: 792-799.
993. Kennedy TC, Proudfoot SP, Franklin WA, Merrick TA, Saccomanno G, Corkill ME, Mumma DL, Sirgi KE, Miller YE, Archer PG, Prochazka A (1996). Cytopathological analysis of sputum in patients with airflow obstruction and significant smoking histories. Cancer Res 56: 4673-4678.
994. Kerr KM (2001). Pulmonary preinvasive neoplasia. J Clin Pathol 54: 257-271.
995. Kerr KM, Carey FA, King G, Lamb D (1994). Atypical alveolar hyperplasia: relationship with pulmonary adenocarcinoma, p53, and c-erbB-2 expression. J Pathol 174: 249-256.
996. Kesler KA, Brooks JA, Rieger KM, Fineberg NS, Einhorn LH, Brown JW (2003). Mediastinal metastases from testicular nonseminomatous germ cell tumors: patterns of dissemination and predictors of long-term survival with surgery. J Thorac Cardiovasc Surg 125: 913-923.
997. Kesler KA, Rieger KM, Ganjoo KN, Sharma M, Fineberg NS, Einhorn LH, Brown JW (1999). Primary mediastinal nonseminomatous germ cell tumors: the influence of postchemotherapy pathology on long-term survival after surgery. J Thorac Cardiovasc Surg 118: 692-700.
998. Khalidi HS, Chang KL, Medeiros LJ, Brynes RK, Slovak ML, Murata-Collins JL, Arber DA (1999). Acute lymphoblastic leukemia. Survey of immunophenotype, French-American-British classification, frequency of myeloid antigen expression, and karyotypic abnormalities in 210 pediatric and adult cases. Am J Clin Pathol 111: 467-476.
999. Khalifa MA, Montgomery EA, Azumi N, Gomes MN, Zeman RK, Min KW, Lack EE (1997). Solitary fibrous tumors: a series of lesions, some in unusual sites. South Med J 90: 793-799.
1000. Khalifa MA, Montgomery EA, Ismiil N, Azumi N (2000). What are the CD34+ cells in benign peripheral nerve sheath tumors? Double immunostaining study of CD34 and S-100 protein. Am J Clin Pathol 114: 123-126.
1001. Khong TY, Keeling JW (1990). Massive congenital mesenchymal malformation of the lung: another cause of non-immune hydrops. Histopathology 16: 609-611.
1002. Khuder SA (2001). Effect of cigarette smoking on major histological types of lung cancer: a meta-analysis. Lung Cancer 31: 139-148.
1003. Kiaffas MG, Powell AJ, Geva T (2002). Magnetic resonance imaging evaluation of cardiac tumor characteristics in infants and children. Am J Cardiol 89: 1229-1233.
1004. Kierszenbaum AL, Tres LL (2001). Primordial germ cell-somatic cell partnership: a balancing cell signaling act. Mol Reprod Dev 60: 277-280.
1005. Kiffer JD, Sandeman TF (1999). Primary malignant mediastinal germ cell tumours: a literature review and a study of 18 cases. Australas Radiol 43: 58-68.
1006. Kihara M, Kihara M, Noda K (1999). Lung cancer risk of the GSTM1 null genotype is enhanced in the presence of the GSTP1 mutated genotype in male Japanese smokers. Cancer Lett 137: 53-60.
1007. Kim DH, Nelson HH, Wiencke JK, Zheng S, Christiani DC, Wain JC, Mark EJ, Kelsey KT (2001). p16(INK4a) and histology-specific methylation of CpG islands by exposure to tobacco smoke in non-small cell lung cancer. Cancer Res 61: 3419-3424.
1008. Kim K, Koo BC, Davis JT, Franco-Saenz R (1984). Primary myelolipoma of mediastinum. J Comput Tomogr 8: 119-123.
1009. Kim KH, Sul HJ, Kang DY (2003). Sclerosing hemangioma with lymph node metastasis. Yonsei Med J 44: 150-154.
1010. Kim TH, Kim YM, Han MY, Kim WH, Oh MH, Han KS (2002). Perinatal sonographic diagnosis of cardiac fibroma with MR imaging correlation. AJR Am J Roentgenol 178: 727-729.
1011. Kim TS, Lee KS, Han J, Im JG, Seo JB, Kim JS, Kim HY, Han SW (1999). Mucoepidermoid carcinoma of the tracheobronchial tree: radiographic and CT findings in 12 patients. Radiology 212: 643-648.
1012. Kim YC, Park KO, Kern JA, Park CS, Lim SC, Jang AS, Yang JB (1998). The interactive effect of Ras, HER2, P53 and Bcl-2 expression in predicting the survival of non-small cell lung cancer patients. Lung Cancer 22: 181-190.
1013. Kimura N, Ishikawa T, Sasaki Y, Sasano N, Onodera K, Shimizu Y, Kimura I, Steiner DF, Nagura H (1996). Expression of prohormone convertase, PC2, in adrenocorticotropin-producing thymic carcinoid with elevated plasma corticotropin-releasing hormone. J Clin Endocrinol Metab 81: 390-395.
1014. King LJ, Padley SP, Wotherspoon AC, Nicholson AG (2000). Pulmonary MALT lymphoma: imaging findings in 24 cases. Eur Radiol 10: 1932-1938.
1015. Kirchner T, Hoppe F, Marx A, Papadopoulos T, Muller-Hermelink HK (1988). [Histogenic and functional markers of epithelial differentiation in thymomas and thymus carcinomas]. Verh Dtsch Ges Pathol 72: 349-353.
1016. Kirchner T, Schalke B, Buchwald J, Ritter M, Marx A, Muller-Hermelink HK (1992). Well-differentiated thymic carcinoma. An organotypical low-grade carcinoma with relationship to cortical thymoma. Am J Surg Pathol 16: 1153-1169.
1017. Kirchner T, Schalke B, Marx A, Muller-Hermelink HK (1989). Evaluation of prognostic features in thymic epithelial tumors. Thymus 14: 195-203.
1018. Kirschner LS, Carney JA, Pack SD, Taymans SE, Giatzakis C, Cho YS, Cho-Chung YS, Stratakis CA (2000). Mutations of the gene encoding the protein kinase A type I-alpha regulatory subunit in patients with the Carney complex. Nat Genet 26: 89-92.
1019. Kitaichi M, Nishimura K, Itoh H, Izumi T (1995). Pulmonary lymphangioleiomyomatosis: a report of 46 patients including a clinicopathologic study of prognostic factors. Am J Respir Crit Care Med 151: 527-533.
1020. Kitamura F, Araki S, Suzuki Y, Yokoyama K, Tanigawa T, Iwasaki R (2002). Assessment of the mutations of p53 suppressor gene and Ha- and Ki-ras oncogenes in malignant mesothelioma in relation to asbestos exposure: a study of 12 American patients. Ind Health 40: 175-181.
1021. Kitamura H, Kameda Y, Ito T, Hayashi H (1999). Atypical adenomatous hyperplasia of the lung. Implications for the pathogenesis of peripheral lung adenocarcinoma. Am J Clin Pathol 111: 610-622.
1022. Kitamura H, Kameda Y, Ito T, Hayashi H, Nakamura N, Nakatani Y, Inayama Y, Kanisawa M (1997). Cytodifferentiation of atypical adenomatous hyperplasia and bronchioloalveolar lung carcinoma: immunohistochemical and ultrastructural studies. Virchows Arch 431: 415-424.
1023. Kitamura H, Kameda Y, Nakamura N, Inayama Y, Nakatani Y, Shibagaki T, Ito T, Hayashi H, Kimura H, Kanisawa M (1996). Atypical adenomatous hyperplasia and bronchoalveolar lung carcinoma. Analysis by morphometry and the expressions of p53 and carcinoembryonic antigen. Am J Surg Pathol 20: 553-562.
1024. Kiyohara C, Yamamura KI, Nakanishi Y, Takayama K, Hara N (2000). Polymorphism in GSTM1, GSTT1, and GSTP1 and Susceptibility to Lung Cancer in a Japanese Population. Asian Pac J Cancer Prev 1: 293-298.
1025. Kiziltepe TT, Patrick E, Alvarado C, Parker P, Winn K (1999). Pleuropulmonary blastoma and ovarian teratoma. Pediatr Radiol 29: 901-903.
1026. Kleihues P, Sobin LH (2000). World Health Organization Classification of Tumours. Pathology and Genetics of Tumours of the Nervous System. IARC Press: Lyon.
1027. Klein U, Gloghini A, Gaidano G, Chadburn A, Cesarman E, Dalla-Favera R, Carbone A (2003). Gene expression profile analysis of AIDS-related primary effusion lymphoma (PEL) suggests a plasmablastic derivation and identifies PEL-specific transcripts. Blood 101: 4115-4121.
1028. Klemm KM, Moran CA, Suster S (1999). Pigmented thymic carcinoids: a clinicopathological and immunohistochemical study of two cases. Mod Pathol 12: 946-948.
1029. Klepfish A, Sarid R, Shtalrid M, Shvidel L, Berrebi A, Schattner A (2001). Primary effusion lymphoma (PEL) in HIV-negative patients—a distinct clinical entity. Leuk Lymphoma 41: 439-443.
1030. Klimstra DS, Moran CA, Perino G, Koss MN, Rosai J (1995). Liposarcoma of the anterior mediastinum and thymus. A clinicopathologic study of 28 cases. Am J Surg Pathol 19: 782-791.
1031. Kline ME, Patel BU, Agosti SJ (1990). Noninfiltrating angiolipoma of the mediastinum. Radiology 175: 737-738.
1032. Knapp RH, Fritz SR, Reiman HM (1982). Primary embryonal carcinoma and choriocarcinoma of the mediastinum. A case report. Arch Pathol Lab Med 106: 507-509.
1033. Knapp RH, Hurt RD, Payne WS, Farrow GM, Lewis BD, Hahn RG, Muhm JR, Earle JD (1985). Malignant germ cell tumors of the mediastinum. J Thorac Cardiovasc Surg 89: 82-89.
1034. Knobel B, Rosman P, Kishon Y, Husar M (1992). Intracardiac primary fibrosarcoma. Case report and literature review. Thorac Cardiovasc Surg 40: 227-230.
1035. Knudson AG (2000). On a new genetic syndrome. Med Pediatr Oncol 35: 428.
1036. Kocak Z, Adli M, Erdir O, Erekul S, Cakmak A (2000). Intrathoracic desmoid tumor of the posterior mediastinum with transdiaphragmatic extension. Report of a case. Tumori 86: 489-491.
1037. Kodama H, Hirotani T, Suzuki Y, Ogawa S, Yamazaki K (2002). Cardiomyogenic differentiation in cardiac myxoma expressing lineage-specific transcription factors. Am J Pathol 161: 381-389.
1038. Kodama K, Higashiyama M, Yokouchi H, Takami K, Kuriyama K, Kusunoki Y, Nakayama T, Imamura F (2002). Natural history of pure ground-glass opacity after long-term follow-up of more than 2 years. Ann Thorac Surg 73: 386-392.
1039. Kodama K, Higashiyama M, Yokouchi H, Takami K, Kuriyama K, Mano M, Nakayama T (2001). Prognostic value of ground-glass opacity found in small lung adenocarcinoma on high-resolution CT scanning. Lung Cancer 33: 17-25.
1040. Kodama T, Biyajima S, Watanabe S, Shimosato Y (1986). Morphometric study of adenocarcinomas and hyperplastic epithelial lesions in the peripheral lung. Am J Clin Pathol 85: 146-151.
1041. Kodama T, Nishiyama H, Nishiwaki Y, Takanashi K, Kuroki M, Hayashibe A, Nukariya N, Kitaya T, Matussuyama T (1988). Histopathological study of adenocarcinoma and hyperplastic epithelial lesions of the lung. Lung Cancer (Haigan) 8: 325-333.
1042. Kodama T, Shimosato Y, Koide T, Watanabe S, Yoneyama T (1984). Endobronchial polypoid adenocarcinoma of the lung. Histological and ultrastructural studies of five cases. Am J Surg Pathol 8: 845-854.
1043. Koga K, Matsuno Y, Noguchi M, Mukai K, Asamura H, Goya T, Shimosato Y (1994). A review of 79 thymomas: modification of staging system and reappraisal of conventional division into invasive and non-invasive thymoma. Pathol Int 44: 359-367.
1044. Kohno H, Hiroshima K, Toyozaki T, Fujisawa T, Ohwada H (1999). p53 mutation and allelic loss of chromosome 3p, 9p of preneoplastic lesions in patients with non-small cell lung carcinoma. Cancer 85: 341-347.
1045. Kohno T, Shinmura K, Tosaka M, Tani M, Kim SR, Sugimura H, Nohmi T, Kasai H, Yokota J (1998). Genetic polymorphisms and alternative splicing of the hOGG1 gene, that is involved in the repair of 8-hydroxyguanine in damaged DNA. Oncogene 16: 3219-3225.
1046. Koita H, Suzumiya J, Ohshima K, Takeshita M, Kimura N, Kikuchi M, Koono M (1997). Lymphoblastic lymphoma expressing natural killer cell phenotype with involvement of the mediastinum and nasal cavity. Am J Surg Pathol 21: 242-248.
1047. Kollmannsberger C, Beyer J, Droz JP, Harstrick A, Hartmann JT, Biron P, Flechon A, Schoffski P, Kuczyk M, Schmoll HJ, Kanz L, Bokemeyer C (1998). Secondary leukemia following high cumulative doses of etoposide in patients treated for advanced germ cell tumors. J Clin Oncol 16: 3386-3391.
1048. Komaki R, Cox JD, Whitson W (1981). Risk of brain metastasis from small cell carcinoma of the lung related to length of survival and prophylactic irradiation. Cancer Treat Rep 65: 811-814.
1049. Kondo K, Monden Y (2001). A questionaire about thymic epithelial tumors as compared to pulmonary atypical carcinoids. Nihon Kokyuki Geka Gakkai Zasshi 15: 633-642.
1050. Kondo T, Yamada K, Noda K, Nakayama H, Kameda Y (2002). Radiologic-prognostic correlation in patients with small pulmonary adenocarcinomas. Lung Cancer 36: 49-57.

1051. Kontny HU, Sleasman JW, Kingma DW, Jaffe ES, Avila NA, Pizzo PA, Mueller BU (1997). Multilocular thymic cysts in children with human immunodeficiency virus infection: clinical and pathologic aspects. J Pediatr 131: 264-270.

1052. Koo CH, Reifel J, Kogut N, Cove JK, Rappaport H (1992). True histiocytic malignancy associated with a malignant teratoma in a patient with 46XY gonadal dysgenesis. Am J Surg Pathol 16: 175-183.

1053. Kooijman CD (1988). Immature teratomas in children. Histopathology 12: 491-502.

1054. Koppl H, Freudenberg N, Berwanger I, Frenzer K, Bohm N (1996). Type II pneumocytic differentiation in an alveolar adenoma of the lung. An immunohistochemical study. Pathologe 17: 150-153.

1055. Koprowska I, An SH, Corsey D, Dracopoulos I, Vaskelis PS (1965). Cytologic patterns of developing bronchogenic carcinoma. Acta Cytol 9: 424-430.

1056. Korbmacher B, Doering C, Schulte HD, Hort W (1992). Malignant fibrous histiocytoma of the heart—case report of a rare left-atrial tumor. Thorac Cardiovasc Surg 40: 303-307.

1057. Korn WM, Oide Weghuis DE, Suijkerbuijk RF, Schmidt U, Otto T, du Manoir S, Geurts van Kessel A, Harstrick A, Seeber S, Becher R (1996). Detection of chromosomal DNA gains and losses in testicular germ cell tumors by comparative genomic hybridization. Genes Chromosomes Cancer 17: 78-87.

1058. Kornstein MJ (1999). Thymoma classification: my opinion. Am J Clin Pathol 112: 304-307.

1059. Kornstein MJ, Rosai J (1998). CD5 labeling of thymic carcinomas and other nonlymphoid neoplasms. Am J Clin Pathol 109: 722-726.

1060. Koss M, Travis W, Moran C, Hochholzer L (1992). Pseudomesotheliomatous adenocarcinoma: a reappraisal. Semin Diagn Pathol 9: 117-123.

1061. Koss MN, Hochholzer L, Frommelt RA (1999). Carcinosarcomas of the lung: a clinicopathologic study of 66 patients. Am J Surg Pathol 23: 1514-1526.

1062. Koss MN, Hochholzer L, Langloss JM, Wehunt WD, Lazarus AA, Nichols PW (1986). Lymphomatoid granulomatosis: a clinicopathologic study of 42 patients. Pathology 18: 283-288.

1063. Koss MN, Hochholzer L, Nichols PW, Wehunt WD, Lazarus AA (1983). Primary non-Hodgkin's lymphoma and pseudolymphoma of lung: a study of 161 patients. Hum Pathol 14: 1024-1038.

1064. Koss MN, Hochholzer L, O'Leary T (1991). Pulmonary blastomas. Cancer 67: 2368-2381.

1065. Koutras P, Urschel HCJr, Paulson DL (1971). Hamartoma of the lung. J Thorac Cardiovasc Surg 61: 768-776.

1066. Kradin RL, Mark EJ (1983). Benign lymphoid disorders of the lung, with a theory regarding their development. Hum Pathol 14: 857-867.

1067. Kragel PJ, Devaney KO, Meth BM, Linnoila RI, Frierson HF, Travis WD (1990). Mucinous cystadenoma of the lung - a report of 2 cases with immunohistochemical and ultrastructural analysis . Arch Pathol Lab Med 114: 1053-1056.

1068. Kragel PJ, Devaney KO, Travis WD (1991). Mucinous Cystadenoma of the Lung - Reply. Arch Pathol Lab Med 115: 740-741.

1069. Kralstein J, Frishman W (1987). Malignant pericardial diseases: diagnosis and treatment. Am Heart J 113: 785-790.

1070. Krapp M, Baschat AA, Gembruch U, Gloeckner K, Schwinger E, Reusche E (1999). Tuberous sclerosis with intracardiac rhabdomyoma in a fetus with trisomy 21: case report and review of literature. Prenat Diagn 19: 610-613.

1071. Kratzke RA, Otterson GA, Lincoln CE, Ewing S, Oie H, Geradts J, Kaye FJ (1995). Immunohistochemical analysis of the p16INK4 cyclin-dependent kinase inhibitor in malignant mesothelioma. J Natl Cancer Inst 87: 1870-1875.

1072. Kreyberg L (1981). World Health Organization Classification of Tumours. Histological Typing of Lung Tumours. 2nd ed. World Health Organization: Geneva.

1073. Krismann M, Adams H, Jaworska M, Muller KM, Johnen G (2000). Patterns of chromosomal imbalances in benign solitary fibrous tumours of the pleura. Virchows Arch 437: 248-255.

1074. Krismann M, Muller KM (2000). [Malignant mesothelioma of the pleura, pericardium and peritoneum. 1: Etiology, pathogenesis, pathology]. Chirurg 71: 877-886.

1075. Krismann M, Muller KM, Jaworska M, Johnen G (2002). Molecular cytogenetic differences between histological subtypes of malignant mesotheliomas: DNA cytometry and comparative genomic hybridization of 90 cases. J Pathol 197: 363-371.

1076. Kristoffersson U, Heim S, Mandahl N, Akerman M, Mitelman F (1989). Multiple clonal chromosome-aberrations in 2 thymomas. Cancer Genet Cytogenet 41: 93-98.

1077. Kroe DJ, Pitcock JA (1967). Benign mucous gland adenoma of the bronchus. Arch Pathol 84: 539-542.

1078. Krompecher E (1900). Der drusernartige oberflachen-epitheliakrebscarcinom epitheliale adenoides. Beitr Pathol 28: 1-41.

1079. Kruger I, Borowski A, Horst M, de Vivie ER, Theissen P, Gross-Fengels W (1990). Symptoms, diagnosis, and therapy of primary sarcomas of the pulmonary artery. Thorac Cardiovasc Surg 38: 91-95.

1080. Krugmann J, Feichtinger H, Greil R, Fend F (1999). Thymic Hodgkin's disease— a histological and immunohistochemical study of three cases. Pathol Res Pract 195: 681-687.

1081. Kubonishi I, Takehara N, Iwata J, Sonobe H, Ohtsuki Y, Abe T, Miyoshi I (1991). Novel t(15;19)(q15;p13) chromosome abnormality in a thymic carcinoma. Cancer Res 51: 3327-3328.

1082. Kuhnen C, Harms D, Niessen KH, Diehm T, Muller KM (2001). [Congenital pulmonary fibrosarcoma. Differential diagnosis of infantile pulmonary spindle cell tumors]. Pathologe 22: 151-156.

1083. Kuhnen C, Preisler K, Muller KM (2001). Pulmonary lymphangioleiomyomatosis. Morphologic and immunohistochemical findings. Pathologe 22: 197-204.

1084. Kumaki F, Matsui K, Kawai T, Ozeki Y, Yu ZX, Ferrans VJ, Travis WD (2001). Expression of matrix metalloproteinases in invasive pulmonary adenocarcinoma with bronchioloalveolar component and atypical adenomatous hyperplasia. Am J Pathol 159: 2125-2135.

1085. Kuo T (1994). Sclerosing thymoma—a possible phenomenon of regression. Histopathology 25: 289-291.

1086. Kuo T (2000). Cytokeratin profiles of the thymus and thymomas: histogenetic correlations and proposal for a histological classification of thymomas. Histopathology 36: 403-414.

1087. Kuo T, Lo SK (1997). Immunohistochemical metallothionein expression in thymoma: correlation with histological types and cellular origin. Histopathology 30: 243-248.

1088. Kuo T, Shih LY (2001). Histologic types of thymoma associated with pure red cell aplasia: a study of five cases including a composite tumor of organoid thymoma associated with an unusual lipofibroadenoma. Int J Surg Pathol 9: 29-35.

1089. Kuo T, Tsang NM (2001). Salivary gland type nasopharyngeal carcinoma: a histologic, immunohistochemical, and Epstein-Barr virus study of 15 cases including a psammomatous mucoepidermoid carcinoma. Am J Surg Pathol 25: 80-86.

1090. Kuo TT (1994). Carcinoid tumor of the thymus with divergent sarcomatoid differentiation: report of a case with histogenetic consideration. Hum Pathol 25: 319-323.

1091. Kuo TT (2000). Frequent presence of neuroendocrine small cells in thymic carcinoma: a light microscopic and immunohistochemical study. Histopathology 37: 19-26.

1092. Kuo TT (2002). Pigmented spindle cell carcinoid tumour of the thymus with ectopic adrenocorticotropic hormone secretion: report of a rare variant and differential diagnosis of mediastinal spindle cell neoplasms. Histopathology 40: 159-165.

1093. Kuo TT, Chan JK (1998). Thymic carcinoma arising in thymoma is associated with alterations in immunohistochemical profile. Am J Surg Pathol 22: 1474-1481.

1094. Kuo TT, Chang JP, Lin FJ, Wu WC, Chang CH (1990). Thymic carcinomas: histopathological varieties and immunohistochemical study. Am J Surg Pathol 14: 24-34.

1095. Kuo TT, Lo SK (1993). Thymoma: a study of the pathologic classification of 71 cases with evaluation of the Muller-Hermelink system. Hum Pathol 24: 766-771. Kuo TT, Shih LY (2001). Histologic types of thymoma associated with pure red cell aplasia: a study of five cases including a composite tumor of organoid thymoma associated with an unusual lipofibroadenoma. Int J Surg Pathol 9: 29-35.

1096. A. Kuppers R, Hansmann ML, Rajewsky K (1998). Clonality and germinal centre B-cell derivation of Hodgkin/Reed-Sternberg cells in Hodgkin's disease. Ann Oncol 9 Suppl 5: S17-S20.

1097. Kuppers R, Kanzler H, Hansmann ML, Rajewsky K (1996). Single cell analysis of Hodgkin/Reed-Sternberg cells. Ann Oncol 7 Suppl 4: 27-30.

1098. Kuppers R, Rajewsky K, Hansmann ML (1997). Diffuse large cell lymphomas are derived from mature B cells carrying V region genes with a high load of somatic mutation and evidence of selection for antibody expression. Eur J Immunol 27: 1398-1405.

1099. Kuppers R, Rajewsky K, Zhao M, Simons G, Laumann R, Fischer R, Hansmann ML (1994). Hodgkin disease: Hodgkin and Reed-Sternberg cells picked from histological sections show clonal immunoglobulin gene rearrangements and appear to be derived from B cells at various stages of development. Proc Natl Acad Sci U S A 91: 10962-10966.

1100. Kurasono Y, Ito T, Kameda Y, Nakamura N, Kitamura H (1998). Expression of cyclin D1, retinoblastoma gene protein, and p16 MTS1 protein in atypical adenomatous hyperplasia and adenocarcinoma of the lung. An immuno-histochemical analysis. Virchows Arch 432: 207-215.

1101. Kurie JM, Shin HJ, Lee JS, Morice RC, Ro JY, Lippman SM, Hittelman WN, Yu R, Lee JJ, Hong WK (1996). Increased epidermal growth factor receptor expression in metaplastic bronchial epithelium. Clin Cancer Res 2: 1787-1793.

1102. Kurman RJ, Norris HJ (1976). Endodermal sinus tumor of the ovary: a clinical and pathologic analysis of 71 cases. Cancer 38: 2404-2419.

1103. Kurotaki H, Kamata Y, Kimura M, Nagai K (1993). Multiple papillary adenomas of type II pneumocytes found in a 13-year-old boy with von Recklinghausen's disease. Virchows Arch A Pathol Anat Histol 423: 319-322.

1104. Kurtin PJ, Myers JL, Adlakha H, Strickler JG, Lohse C, Pankratz VS, Inwards DJ (2001). Pathologic and clinical features of primary pulmonary extranodal marginal zone B-cell lymphoma of MALT type. Am J Surg Pathol 25: 997-1008.

1105. Kurup AN, Tazelaar HD, Edwards WD, Burke AP, Virmani R, Klarich KW, Orszulak TA (2002). Iatrogenic cardiac papillary fibroelastoma: a study of 12 cases (1990 to 2000). Hum Pathol 33: 1165-1169.

1106. Kurzrock EA, Tunuguntla HS, Busby JE, Gandour-Edwards R, Goldman LA (2002). Klinefelter's syndrome and precocious puberty: a harbinger for tumor. Urology 60: 514.

1107. Kusafuka T, Kuroda S, Inoue M, Ara T, Yoneda A, Oue T, Udatsu Y, Osugi Y, Okada A (2002). P53 gene mutations in pleuropulmonary blastomas. Pediatr Hematol Oncol 19: 117-128.

1108. Kushihashi T, Munechika H, Ri K, Kubota H, Ukisu R, Satoh S, Motoya H, Kurashita Y, Soejima K, Kadokura M (1994). Bronchioloalveolar adenoma of the lung: CT-pathologic correlation. Radiology 193: 789-793.

1109. Kwon JW, Goo JM, Seo JB, Seo JW, Im JG (1999). Mucous gland adenoma of the bronchus: CT findings in two patients. J Comput Assist Tomogr 23: 758-760.

1110. Laberge-le Couteulx S, Jung HH, Labauge P, Houtteville JP, Lescoat C, Cecillon M, Marechal E, Joutel A, Bach JF, Tournier-Lasserve E (1999). Truncating mutations in CCM1, encoding KRIT1, cause hereditary cavernous angiomas. Nat Genet 23: 189-193.

1111. Lack EE, Weinstein HJ, Welch KJ (1985). Mediastinal germ cell tumors in childhood. A clinical and pathological study of 21 cases. J Thorac Cardiovasc Surg 89: 826-835.

1112. Ladanyi M, Roy I, Landanyi M (1988). Mediastinal germ cell tumors and histiocytosis. Hum Pathol 19: 586-590.

1113. Ladanyi M, Samaniego F, Reuter VE, Motzer RJ, Jhanwar SC, Bosl GJ, Chaganti RS (1990). Cytogenetic and immunohistochemical evidence for the germ cell origin of a subset of acute leukemias associated with mediastinal germ cell tumors. J Natl Cancer Inst 82: 221-227.

1114. Lagrange W, Dahm HH, Karstens J, Feichtinger J, Mittermayer C (1987). Melanocytic neuroendocrine carcinoma of the thymus. Cancer 59: 484-488.

1115. Lallier M, Bouchard S, Di Lorenzo M, Youssef S, Blanchard H, Lapierre JG, Vischoff D, Tucci M, Brochu P (1999). Pleuropulmonary blastoma: a rare pathology with an even rarer presentation. J Pediatr Surg 34: 1057-1059.

1116. Lam KY, Dickens P, Chan AC (1993).

Tumors of the heart. A 20-year experience with a review of 12,485 consecutive autopsies. Arch Pathol Lab Med 117: 1027-1031.
1117. Lam S, Kennedy T, Unger M, Miller YE, Gelmont D, Rusch V, Gipe B, Howard D, LeRiche JC, Coldman A, Gazdar AF (1998). Localization of bronchial intraepithelial neoplastic lesions by fluorescence bronchoscopy. Chest 113: 696-702.
1118. Lam S, LeRiche JC, Zheng Y, Coldman A, MacAulay C, Hawk E, Kelloff G, Gazdar AF (1999). Sex-related differences in bronchial epithelial changes associated with tobacco smoking. J Natl Cancer Inst 91: 691-696.
1119. Lam S, MacAulay C, Hung J, LeRiche J, Profio AE, Palcic B (1993). Detection of dysplasia and carcinoma in situ with a lung imaging fluorescence endoscope device. J Thorac Cardiovasc Surg 105: 1035-1040.
1120. Lam S, MacAulay C, LeRiche JC, Palcic B (2000). Detection and localization of early lung cancer by fluorescence bronchoscopy. Cancer 89: 2468-2473.
1121. Lamarre L, Jacobson JO, Aisenberg AC, Harris NL (1989). Primary large cell lymphoma of the mediastinum. A histologic and immunophenotypic study of 29 cases. Am J Surg Pathol 13: 730-739.
1122. Lamy A, Sesboue R, Bourguignon J, Dautreaux B, Metayer J, Frebourg T, Thiberville L (2002). Aberrant methylation of the CDKN2a/p16INK4a gene promoter region in preinvasive bronchial lesions: a prospective study in high-risk patients without invasive cancer. Int J Cancer 100: 189-193.
1123. Lamy AL, Fradet GJ, Luoma A, Nelems B (1994). Anterior and middle mediastinum paraganglioma: complete resection is the treatment of choice. Ann Thorac Surg 57: 249-252.
1124. Lancaster KJ, Liang CY, Myers JC, McCabe KM (1997). Goblet cell carcinoid arising in a mature teratoma of the mediastinum. Am J Surg Pathol 21: 109-113.
1125. Lang-Lazdunski L, Oroudji M, Pansard Y, Vissuzaine C, Hvass U (1994). Successful resection of giant intrapericardial lipoma. Ann Thorac Surg 58: 238-240.
1126. Lantuejoul S, Constantin B, Drabkin H, Brambilla C, Roche J, Brambilla E (2003). Expression of VEGF, semaphorin SEMA3F, and their common receptors neuropilins NP1 and NP2 in preinvasive bronchial lesions, lung tumours, and cell lines. J Pathol 200: 336-347.
1127. Lantuejoul S, Isaac S, Pinel N, Negoescu A, Guibert B, Brambilla E (1997). Clear cell tumor of the lung: an immunohistochemical and ultrastructural study supporting a pericytic differentiation. Mod Pathol 10: 1001-1008.
Lantuejoul S, Moro D, Michalides RJ, Brambilla C, Brambilla E (1998). Neural cell adhesion molecules (NCAM) and NCAM-PSA expression in neuroendocrine lung tumors. Am J Surg Pathol 22: 1267-1276.
1128. A. Lantz DA, Dougherty TH, Lucca MJ (1989). Primary angiosarcoma of the heart causing cardiac rupture. Am Heart J 118: 186-188.
1129. Laquay N, Ghazouani S, Vaccaroni L, Vouhe P (2003). Intrapericardial teratoma in newborn babies. Eur J Cardiothorac Surg 23: 642-644.
1130. Lardinois D, Rechsteiner R, Lang RH, Gugger M, Betticher D, von Briel C, Krueger T, Ris HB (2000). Prognostic relevance of Masaoka and Muller-Hermelink classification in patients with thymic tumors. Ann Thorac Surg 69: 1550-1555.
1131. Larramendy ML, Tarkkanen M, Blomqvist C, Virolainen M, Wiklund T, Asko-Seljavaara S, Elomaa I, Knuutila S (1997). Comparative genomic hybridization of malignant fibrous histiocytoma reveals a novel prognostic marker. Am J Pathol 151: 1153-1161.
1132. Larsen M, Evans WK, Shepherd FA, Phillips MJ, Bailey D, Messner H (1984). Acute lymphoblastic leukemia. Possible origin from a mediastinal germ cell tumor. Cancer 53: 441-444.
1133. Larsson S, Lepore V, Kennergren C (1989). Atrial myxomas: results of 25 years' experience and review of the literature. Surgery 105: 695-698.
1134. Lattes R (1962). Thymoma and other tumors of the thymus - an analysis of 107 cases. Cancer 15: 1224-1260.
1135. Latza U, Foss HD, Durkop H, Eitelbach F, Dieckmann KP, Loy V, Unger M, Pizzolo G, Stein H (1995). CD30 antigen in embryonal carcinoma and embryogenesis and release of the soluble molecule. Am J Pathol 146: 463-471.
1136. Lau SK, Desrochers MJ, Luthringer DJ (2002). Expression of thyroid transcription factor-1, cytokeratin 7, and cytokeratin 20 in bronchioloalveolar carcinomas: an immunohistochemical evaluation of 67 cases. Mod Pathol 15: 538-542.
1137. Lau SK, Luthringer DJ, Eisen RN (2002). Thyroid transcription factor-1: a review. Appl Immunohistochem Mol Morphol 10: 97-102.
1138. Laurino L, Furlanetto A, Orvieto E, Del Tos AP (2001). Well-differentiated liposarcoma (atypical lipomatous tumors). Semin Diagn Pathol 18: 258-262.
1139. Lauriola L, Erlandson RA, Rosai J (1998). Neuroendocrine differentiation is a common feature of thymic carcinoma. Am J Surg Pathol 22: 1059-1066.
1140. Lauritzen AF, Delsol G, Hansen NE, Horn T, Ersboll J, Hou-Jensen K, Ralfkiaer E (1994). Histiocytic sarcomas and monoblastic leukemias. A clinical, histologic, and immunophenotypical study. Am J Clin Pathol 102: 45-54.
1141. Lauweryns JM, Goddeeris P (1975). Neuroepithelial bodies in the human child and adult lung. Am Rev Respir Dis 111: 469-476.
1142. Laya MB, Mailliard JA, Bewtra C, Levin HS (1987). Malignant fibrous histiocytoma of the heart. A case report and review of the literature. Cancer 59: 1026-1031.
1143. Lazzarino M, Orlandi E, Paulli M, Strater J, Klersy C, Gianelli U, Gargantini L, Rousset MT, Gambacorta M, Marra E, Lavabre-Bertrand T, Magrini U, Manegold C, Bernasconi C, Moller P (1997). Treatment outcome and prognostic factors for primary mediastinal (thymic) B-cell lymphoma: a multicenter study of 106 patients. J Clin Oncol 15: 1646-1653.
1144. Le Marc'hadour F, Peoc'h M, Pasquier B, Leroux D (1994). Cardiac synovial sarcoma with translocation (X;18) associated with asbestos exposure. Cancer 74: 986.
1145. Le Marchand L, Donlon T, Lum-Jones A, Seifried A, Wilkens LR (2002). Association of the hOGG1 Ser326Cys polymorphism with lung cancer risk. Cancer Epidemiol Biomarkers Prev 11: 409-412.
1146. Lechapt-Zalcman E, Challine D, Delfau-Larue MH, Haioun C, Desvaux D, Gaulard P (2001). Association of primary pleural effusion lymphoma of T-cell origin and human herpesvirus 8 in a human immunodeficiency virus-seronegative man. Arch Pathol Lab Med 125: 1246-1248.
1147. Lechner JF, Neft RE, Gilliland FD, Crowell RE, Auckley DH, Temes RT, Belinsky SA (1998). Individuals at high risk for lung cancer have airway epithelial cells with chromosome aberrations frequently found in lung tumor cells. In Vivo 12: 23-26.
1148. Lee AC, Kwong YI, Fu KH, Chan GC, Ma L, Lau YL (1993). Disseminated mediastinal carcinoma with chromosomal translocation (15;19). A distinctive clinicopathologic syndrome. Cancer 72: 2273-2276.
1149. Lee JJ, Liu D, Lee JS, Kurie JM, Khuri FR, Ibarguen H, Morice RC, Walsh G, Ro JY, Broxson A, Hong WK, Hittelman WN (2001). Long-term impact of smoking on lung epithelial proliferation in current and former smokers. J Natl Cancer Inst 93: 1081-1088.
1150. Lee JS, Brown KK, Cool C, Lynch DA (2002). Diffuse pulmonary neuroendocrine cell hyperplasia: radiologic and clinical features. J Comput Assist Tomogr 26: 180-184.
1151. Lee KS, Topol EJ, Stewart WJ (1993). Atypical presentation of papillary fibroelastoma mimicking multiple vegetations in suspected subacute bacterial endocarditis. Am Heart J 125: 1443-1445.
1152. Lee PN, Fry JS, Forey BA (1990). Trends in lung cancer, chronic obstructive lung disease, and emphysema death rates for England and Wales 1941-85 and their relation to trends in cigarette smoking. Thorax 45: 657-665.
1153. Lee ST, Lee YC, Hsu CY, Lin CC (1992). Bilateral multiple sclerosing hemangiomas of the lung. Chest 101: 572-573.
1154. Lee WJ, Brennan P, Boffetta P, London SJ, Benhamou S, Rannug A, To-Figueras J, Ingelman-Sundberg M, Shields P, Gaspari L, Taioli E (2002). Microsomal epoxide hydrolase polymorphisms and lung cancer risk: a quantitative review. Biomarkers 7: 230-241.
1155. Lee YC, Chang YL, Luh SP, Lee JM, Chen JS (1999). Significance of P53 and Rb protein expression in surgically treated non-small cell lung cancers. Ann Thorac Surg 68: 343-347.
1156. Leigh J, Davidson P, Hendrie L, Berry D (2002). Malignant mesothelioma in Australia, 1945-2000. Am J Ind Med 41: 188-201.
1157. Leighton J, Hurst JW, Crawford JD (1950). Squamous epithelial cysts in the heart of an infant, with coincident cystic changes in the ovaries and breasts. Arch Pathol 632-643.
1158. Leithauser F, Bauerle M, Huynh MQ, Moller P (2001). Isotype-switched immunoglobulin genes with a high load of somatic hypermutation and lack of ongoing mutational activity are prevalent in mediastinal B-cell lymphoma. Blood 98: 2762-2770.
1159. Lemarie E, Assouline PS, Diot P, Regnard JF, Levasseur P, Droz JP, Ruffie P (1992). Primary mediastinal germ cell tumors. Results of a French retrospective study. Chest 102: 1477-1483.
1160. Lemos LB, Hamoudi AB (1978). Malignant thymic tumor in an infant (malignant histiocytoma). Arch Pathol Lab Med 102: 84-89.
1161. Leong AS, Brown JH (1984). Malignant transformation in a thymic cyst. Am J Surg Pathol 8: 471-475.
1162. Lepper W, Shivalkar B, Rinkevich D, Belcik T, Wei K (2002). Assessment of the vascularity of a left ventricular mass using myocardial contrast echocardiography. J Am Soc Echocardiogr 15: 1419-1422.
1163. Lerman C, Caporaso N, Main D, Audrain J, Boyd NR, Bowman ED, Shields PG (1998). Depression and self-medication with nicotine: the modifying influence of the dopamine D4 receptor gene. Health Psychol 17: 56-62.
1164. Lerman C, Caporaso NE, Audrain J, Main D, Bowman ED, Lockshin B, Boyd NR, Shields PG (1999). Evidence suggesting the role of specific genetic factors in cigarette smoking. Health Psychol 18: 14-20.
1165. Lerman C, Shields PG, Audrain J, Main D, Cobb B, Boyd NR, Caporaso N (1998). The role of the serotonin transporter gene in cigarette smoking. Cancer Epidemiol Biomarkers Prev 7: 253-255.
1166. Lerman C, Shields PG, Main D, Audrain J, Roth J, Boyd NR, Caporaso NE (1997). Lack of association of tyrosine hydroxylase genetic polymorphism with cigarette smoking. Pharmacogenetics 7: 521-524.
1167. Lerman MI, Minna JD (2000). The 630-kb lung cancer homozygous deletion region on human chromosome 3p21.3: identification and evaluation of the resident candidate tumor suppressor genes. The International Lung Cancer Chromosome 3p21.3 Tumor Suppressor Gene Consortium. Cancer Res 60: 6116-6133.
1168. Letendre L (1989). Treatment of lymphomatoid granulomatosis-old and new perspectives. Semin Respir Med 10: 178-181.
1169. Levine GD, Rosai J (1976). A spindle cell varient of thymic carcinoid tumor. A clinical, histologic, and fine structural study with emphasis on its distinction from spindle cell thymoma. Arch Pathol Lab Med 100: 293-300.
1170. Levine GD, Rosai J (1978). Thymic hyperplasia and neoplasia: a review of current concepts. Hum Pathol 9: 495-515.
1171. Lewis BD, Hurt RD, Payne WS, Farrow GM, Knapp RH, Muhm JR (1983). Benign teratomas of the mediastinum. J Thorac Cardiovasc Surg 86: 727-731.
1172. Lewis JE, Wick MR, Scheithauer BW, Bernatz PE, Taylor WF (1987). Thymoma. A clinicopathologic review. Cancer 60: 2727-2743.
1173. Lewman LV, Demany MA, Zimmerman HA (1972). Congenital tumor of atrioventricular node with complete heart block and sudden death. Mesothelioma or lymphangio-endothelioma of atrioventricular node. Am J Cardiol 29: 554-557.
1174. Leyvraz S, Henle W, Chahinian AP, Perlmann C, Klein G, Gordon RE, Rosenblum M, Holland JF (1985). Association of Epstein-Barr virus with thymic carcinoma. N Engl J Med 312: 1296-1299.
1175. Li FP, Lokich J, Lapey J, Neptune WB, Wilkins EWJr (1978). Familial mesothelioma after intense asbestos exposure at home. JAMA 240: 467.
1176. Li G, Hansmann ML, Zwingers T, Lennert K (1990). Primary lymphomas of the lung: morphological, immunohistochemical and clinical features. Histopathology 16: 519-531.
1177. Li L, Cerilli LA, Wick MR (2002). Inflammatory pseudotumor (myofibroblastic tumor) of the heart. Ann Diagn Pathol 6: 116-121.
1178. Liang TC, Lu MY, Chen SJ, Lu FL, Lin KH (2002). Cardiac tamponade caused by intrapericardial yolk sac tumor in a boy. J

Formos Med Assoc 101: 355-358.

1179. Lichtenstein HL, Lee JC, Stewart S (1979). Papillary tumor of the heart: incidental finding at surgery. Hum Pathol 10: 473-475.

1180. Lie JT (1993). Gamma-Gandy body of the heart - petrified cardiac myxoma mimicking atrial thrombus. Cardiovasc Pathol 2: 97-98.

1181. Lieberman PH, Jones CR, Steinman RM, Erlandson RA, Smith J, Gee T, Huvos A, Garin-Chesa P, Filippa DA, Urmacher C, Gangi MD, Sperber M (1996). Langerhans cell (eosinophilic) granulomatosis. A clinicopathologic study encompassing 50 years. Am J Surg Pathol 20: 519-552.

1182. Liebow AA, Carrington CR, Friedman PJ (1972). Lymphomatoid granulomatosis. Hum Pathol 3: 457-558.

1183. Liebow AA, Hubbell DS (1956). Sclerosing Hemangioma (Histiocytoma,Xanthoma) of the Lung. Cancer 9: 53-75.

1184. Lin BT, Colby T, Gown AM, Hammar SP, Mertens RB, Churg A, Battifora H (1996). Malignant vascular tumors of the serous membranes mimicking mesothelioma. A report of 14 cases. Am J Surg Pathol 20: 1431-1439.

1185. Lin KL, Chen CY, Hsu HH, Kao PF, Huang MJ, Wang HS (1999). Ectopic ACTH syndrome due to thymic carcinoid tumor in a girl. J Pediatr Endocrinol Metab 12: 573-578.

1186. Lin O, Frizzera G (1997). Angiomyoid and follicular dendritic cell proliferative lesions in Castleman's disease of hyaline-vascular type: a study of 10 cases. Am J Surg Pathol 21: 1295-1306.

1187. Lin O, Harkin TJ, Jagirdar J (1995). Basaloid-squamous cell carcinoma of the bronchus. Report of a case with review of the literature. Arch Pathol Lab Med 119: 1167-1170.

1188. Lindell MM, Doubleday LC, von Eschenbach AC, Libshitz HI (1982). Mediastinal metastases from prostatic carcinoma. J Urol 128: 331-334.

1189. Linder J, Shelburne JD, Sorge JP, Whalen RE, Hackel DB (1984). Congenital endodermal heterotopia of the atrioventricular node: evidence for the endodermal origin of so-called mesotheliomas of the atrioventricular node. Hum Pathol 15: 1093-1098.

1190. Lindner V, Edah-Tally S, Chakfe N, Onody T, Eisenmann B, Walter P (1999). Cardiac myxoma with glandular component: case report and review of the literature. Pathol Res Pract 195: 267-272.

1191. Lindskog BI, Malm A (1965). Diagnostic and surgical considerations on mediastinal (intrathoracic) goiter. Dis Chest 47: 201-207.

1192. Lipford EHJr, Margolick JB, Longo DL, Fauci AS, Jaffe ES (1988). Angiocentric immunoproliferative lesions: a clinicopathologic spectrum of post-thymic T-cell proliferations. Blood 72: 1674-1681.

1193. Liu G, Miller DP, Zhou W, Thurston SW, Fan R, Xu LL, Lynch TJ, Wain JC, Su L, Christiani DC (2001). Differential association of the codon 72 p53 and GSTM1 polymorphisms on histological subtype of non-small cell lung carcinoma. Cancer Res 61: 8718-8722.

1194. Llombart-Cussac A, Pivot X, Contesso G, Rhor-Alvarado A, Delord JP, Spielmann M, Tursz T, Le Cesne A (1998). Adjuvant chemotherapy for primary cardiac sarcomas: the IGR experience. Br J Cancer 78: 1624-1628.

1195. Loehrer PJSr, Hui S, Clark S, Seal M, Einhorn LH, Williams SD, Ulbright T, Mandelbaum I, Rowland R, Donohue JP (1986). Teratoma following cisplatin-based combination chemotherapy for nonseminomatous germ cell tumors: a clinicopathological correlation. J Urol 135: 1183-1189.

1196. Loehrer PJSr, Wick MR (2001). Thymic malignancies. Cancer Treat Res 105: 277-302.

1197. Loffler H, Grille W (2003). Classification of malignant cardiac tumors with respect to oncological treatment. Thorac Cardiovasc Surg 38: 196-199.

1198. Logan PM, Miller RR, Evans K, Muller NL (1996). Bronchogenic carcinoma and coexistent bronchioloalveolar cell adenomas. Assessment of radiologic detection and follow-up in 28 patients. Chest 109: 713-717.

1199. Logothetis CJ, Samuels ML, Trindade A, Johnson DE (1982). The growing teratoma syndrome. Cancer 50: 1629-1635.

1200. Loire R, Donsbeck AV, Nighoghossian N, Perinetti M, Le Gall F (1999). [Papillary fibroelastoma of the heart. A review of 20 cases]. Arch Anat Cytol Pathol 47: 19-25.

1201. Loire R, Hellal H (1993). [Neoplastic pericarditis. Study by thoracotomy and biopsy in 80 cases]. Presse Med 22: 244-248.

1202. Loire R, Tabib A (1994). [Malignant mesothelioma of the pericardium. An anatomo-clinical study of 10 cases]. Arch Mal Coeur Vaiss 87: 255-262.

1203. Longo DL, Glatstein E, Duffey PL, Ihde DC, Hubbard SM, Fisher RI, Jaffe ES, Gilliom M, Young RC, DeVita VTJr (1989). Treatment of localized aggressive lymphomas with combination chemotherapy followed by involved-field radiation therapy. J Clin Oncol 7: 1295-1302.

1204. Looijenga LH, Oosterhuis JW (2002). Pathobiology of testicular germ cell tumors: views and news. Anal Quant Cytol Histol 24: 263-279.

1205. Looijenga LH, Rosenberg C, van Gurp RJ, Geelen E, Echten-Arends J, de Jong B, Mostert M, Wolter Oosterhuis J (2000). Comparative genomic hybridization of microdissected samples from different stages in the development of a seminoma and a non-seminoma. J Pathol 191: 187-192.

1206. Lopez-Abente G, Pollan M, de la Iglesia P, Ruiz M (1995). Characterization of the lung cancer epidemic in the European Union (1970-1990). Cancer Epidemiol Biomarkers Prev 4: 813-820.

1207. Lopez-Andreu JA, Ferris-Tortajada J, Gomez J (1996). Pleuropulmonary blastoma and congenital cystic malformations. J Pediatr 129: 773-775.

1208. Loriot MA, Rebuissou S, Oscarson M, Cenee S, Miyamoto M, Ariyoshi N, Kamataki T, Hemon D, Beaune P, Stucker I (2001). Genetic polymorphisms of cytochrome P450 2A6 in a case-control study on lung cancer in a French population. Pharmacogenetics 11: 39-44.

1209. Lorsbach RB, Pinkus GS, Shahsafaei A, Dorfman DM (2000). Primary marginal zone lymphoma of the thymus. Am J Clin Pathol 113: 784-791.

1210. Lu YJ, Dong XY, Shipley J, Zhang RG, Cheng SJ (1999). Chromosome 3 imbalances are the most frequent aberration found in non-small cell lung carcinoma. Lung Cancer 23: 61-66.

1211. Lubin JH, Blot WJ (1984). Assessment of lung cancer risk factors by histologic category. J Natl Cancer Inst 73: 383-389.

1212. Luburich P, Ayuso MC, Picado C, Serra-Batlles J, Ramirez JF, Sole M (1994). CT of pulmonary epithelioid hemangioendothelioma. J Comput Assist Tomogr 18: 562-565.

1213. Ludwigsen E (1977). Endobronchial carcinosarcoma. A case with osteosarcoma of pulmonary invasive part, and a review with respect to prognosis. Virchows Arch A Pathol Anat Histol 373: 293-302.

1214. Lumadue JA, Askin FB, Perlman EJ (1994). MIC2 analysis of small cell carcinoma. Am J Clin Pathol 102: 692-694.

1215. Lund JT, Ehman RL, Julsrud PR, Sinak LJ, Tajik AJ (1989). Cardiac masses: assessment by MR imaging. AJR Am J Roentgenol 152: 469-473.

1216. Lyda MH, Weiss LM (2000). Immunoreactivity for epithelial and neuroendocrine antibodies are useful in the differential diagnosis of lung carcinomas. Hum Pathol 31: 980-987.

1217. Lynch TJ, Bell DW, Sordella R, Gurubhagavatula S, Okimoto RA, Brannigan BW, Harris PL, Haserlat SM, Supko JG, Haluska FG, Louis DN, Christiani DC, Settleman J, Haber DA (2004). Activating Mutations in the Epidermal Growth Factor Receptor Underlying Responsiveness of Non-Small-Cell Lung Cancer to Gefitinib. N Engl J Med .

1218. MacDonald LL, Yazdi HM (2001). Fine-needle aspiration biopsy of bronchioloalveolar carcinoma. Cancer 93: 29-34.

1219. Machin T, Mashiyama ET, Henderson JA, McCaughey WT (1988). Bony metastases in desmoplastic pleural mesothelioma. Thorax 43: 155-156.

1220. Mackay B, Lukeman JM, Ordonez NG (1991). Tumors of the Lung. WB Saunders: Philadelphia.

1221. MacLennan KA, Bennett MH, Tu A, Hudson BV, Easterling MJ, Hudson GV, Jelliffe AM (1989). Relationship of histopathologic features to survival and relapse in nodular sclerosing Hodgkin's disease. A study of 1659 patients. Cancer 64: 1686-1693.

1222. Maeshima AM, Niki T, Maeshima A, Yamada T, Kondo H, Matsuno Y (2002). Modified scar grade: a prognostic indicator in small peripheral lung adenocarcinoma. Cancer 95: 2546-2554.

1223. Magid MS, Chen YT, Soslow RA, Boulad F, Kernan NA, Szabolcs P (1998). Juvenile-onset recurrent respiratory papillomatosis involving the lung: A case report and review of the literature. Pediatr Dev Pathol 1: 157-163.

1224. Mairal A, Terrier P, Chibon F, Sastre X, Lecesne A, Aurias A (1999). Loss of chromosome 13 is the most frequent genomic imbalance in malignant fibrous histiocytomas. A comparative genomic hybridization analysis of a series of 30 cases. Cancer Genet Cytogenet 111: 134-138.

1225. Majano-Lainez RA (1997). Cardiac tumors: a current clinical and pathological perspective. Crit Rev Oncog 8: 293-303.

1226. Majumdar N, Ray R, Venugopal P, Chopra P (1998). DNA ploidy and proliferative index of cardiac myxoma. Indian Heart J 50: 535-538.

1227. Makhlouf HR, Ishak KG, Goodman ZD (1999). Epithelioid hemangioendothelioma of the liver: a clinicopathologic study of 137 cases. Cancer 85: 562-582.

1228. Malats N, Camus-Radon AM, Nyberg F, Ahrens W, Constantinescu V, Mukeria A, Benhamou S, Batura-Gabryel H, Bruske-Hohlfeld I, Simonato L, Menezes A, Lea S, Lang M, Boffetta P (2000). Lung cancer risk in nonsmokers and GSTM1 and GSTT1 genetic polymorphism. Cancer Epidemiol Biomarkers Prev 9: 827-833.

1229. Mangano WE, Cagle PT, Churg A, Vollmer RT, Roggli VL (1998). The diagnosis of desmoplastic malignant mesothelioma and its distinction from fibrous pleurisy: a histologic and immunohistochemical analysis of 31 cases including p53 immunostaining. Am J Clin Pathol 110: 191-199.

1230. Manivel C, Wick MR, Abenoza P, Rosai J (1986). The occurrence of sarcomatous components in primary mediastinal germ cell tumors. Am J Surg Pathol 10: 711-717.

1231. Manivel JC, Priest JR, Watterson J, Steiner M, Woods WG, Wick MR, Dehner LP (1988). Pleuropulmonary blastoma. The so-called pulmonary blastoma of childhood. Cancer 62: 1516-1526.

1232. Mann JR, Pearson D, Barrett A, Raafat F, Barnes JM, Wallendszus KR (1989). Results of the United Kingdom Children's Cancer Study Group's malignant germ cell tumor studies. Cancer 63: 1657-1667.

1233. Mann JR, Raafat F, Robinson K, Imeson J, Gornall P, Phillips M, Sokal M, Gray E, McKeever P, Oakhill A (1998). UKCCSG's germ cell tumour (GCT) studies: improving outcome for children with malignant extracranial non-gonadal tumours—carboplatin, etoposide, and bleomycin are effective and less toxic than previous regimens. United Kingdom Children's Cancer Study Group. Med Pediatr Oncol 30: 217-227.

1234. Mann RB, Wu TC, MacMahon EM, Ling Y, Charache P, Ambinder RF (1992). In situ localization of Epstein-Barr virus in thymic carcinoma. Mod Pathol 5: 363-366.

1235. Mao L (2001). Molecular abnormalities in lung carcinogenesis and their potential clinical implications. Lung Cancer 34 Suppl 2: S27-S34.

1236. Mao L, Lee JS, Kurie JM, Fan YH, Lippman SM, Lee JJ, Ro JY, Broxson A, Yu R, Morice RC, Kemp BL, Khuri FR, Walsh GL, Hittelman WN, Hong WK (1997). Clonal genetic alterations in the lungs of current and former smokers. J Natl Cancer Inst 89: 857-862.

1237. Marafioti T, Hummel M, Anagnostopoulos I, Foss HD, Falini B, Delsol G, Isaacson PG, Pileri S, Stein H (1997). Origin of nodular lymphocyte-predominant Hodgkin's disease from a clonal expansion of highly mutated germinal-center B cells. N Engl J Med 337: 453-458.

1238. Marchevsky AM (1995). Lung tumors derived from ectopic tissues. Semin Diagn Pathol 12: 172-184.

1239. Marchevsky AM, Dikman SH (1979). Mediastinal carcinoid with an incomplete Sipple's syndrome. Cancer 43: 2497-2501.

1240. Marchevsky AM, Gal AA, Shah S, Koss MN (2001). Morphometry confirms the presence of considerable nuclear size overlap between "small cells" and "large cells" in high-grade pulmonary neuroendocrine neoplasms. Am J Clin Pathol 116: 466-472.

1241. Marchiano D, Fisher F, Hofstetter S (1993). Epithelioid hemangioendothelioma of the heart with distant metastases. A case report and literature review. J Cardiovasc Surg (Torino) 34: 529-533.

1242. Marci M, Ziino O, D'Angelo P, Miranda G, Pappone C, Battaglia A (2001). Fibroma of the left ventricle in a patient with Sotos syndrome. Echocardiography

18: 171-173.
1243. Margolin K, Traweek T (1992). The unique association of malignant histiocytosis and a primary gonadal germ cell tumor. Med Pediatr Oncol 20: 162-164.
1244. Marina NM, Cushing B, Giller R, Cohen L, Lauer SJ, Ablin A, Weetman R, Cullen J, Rogers P, Vinocur C, Stolar C, Rescorla F, Hawkins E, Heifetz S, Rao PV, Krailo M, Castleberry RP (1999). Complete surgical excision is effective treatment for children with immature teratomas with or without malignant elements: A Pediatric Oncology Group/Children's Cancer Group Intergroup Study. J Clin Oncol 17: 2137-2143.
1245. Marino M, Muller-Hermelink HK (1985). Thymoma and thymic carcinoma. Relation of thymoma epithelial cells to the cortical and medullary differentiation of thymus. Virchows Arch A Pathol Anat Histol 407: 119-149.
1246. Mark EJ, Quay SC, Dickersin GR (1981). Papillary carcinoid tumor of the lung. Cancer 48: 316-324.
1247. Markhede G, Angervall L, Stener B (1982). A multivariate analysis of the prognosis after surgical treatment of malignant soft-tissue tumors. Cancer 49: 1721-1733.
1248. Marrogi AJ, Travis WD, Welsh JA, Khan MA, Rahim H, Tazelaar H, Pairolero P, Trastek V, Jett J, Caporaso NE, Liotta LA, Harris CC (2000). Nitric oxide synthase, cyclooxygenase 2, and vascular endothelial growth factor in the angiogenesis of non-small cell lung carcinoma. Clin Cancer Res 6: 4739-4744.
1249. Martin-Subero JI, Gesk S, Harder L, Sonoki T, Tucker PW, Schlegelberger B, Grote W, Novo FJ, Calasanz MJ, Hansmann ML, Dyer MJ, Siebert R (2002). Recurrent involvement of the REL and BCL11A loci in classical Hodgkin lymphoma. Blood 99: 1474-1477.
1250. Martin A, Capron F, Liguory-Brunaud MD, De Frejacques C, Pluot M, Diebold J (1994). Epstein-Barr virus-associated primary malignant lymphomas of the pleural cavity occurring in longstanding pleural chronic inflammation. Hum Pathol 25: 1314-1318.
1251. Martin B, Verdebout JM, Mascaux C, Paesmans M, Rouas G, Verhest A, Ninane V, Sculier JP (2002). Expression of p53 in preneoplastic and early neoplastic bronchial lesions. Oncol Rep 9: 223-229.
1252. Martinet N, Alla F, Farre G, Labib T, Drouot H, Vidili R, Picard E, Gaube MP, Le Faou D, Siat J, Borelly J, Vermylen P, Bazarbachi T, Vignaud JM, Martinet Y (2000). Retinoic acid receptor and retinoid X receptor alterations in lung cancer precursor lesions. Cancer Res 60: 2869-2875.
1253. Marx A, Muller-Hermelink HK (1999). Thymoma and thymic carcinoma. Am J Surg Pathol 23: 739-742.
1254. Marx GR, Bierman FZ, Matthews E, Williams R (1984). Two-dimensional echocardiographic diagnosis of intracardiac masses in infancy. J Am Coll Cardiol 3: 827-832.
1255. Masaoka A, Monden Y, Nakahara K, Tanioka T (1981). Follow-up study of thymomas with special reference to their clinical stages. Cancer 48: 2485-2492.
1256. Massard G, Eichler F, Gasser B, Bergerat JP, Wihlm JM (1998). Recurrence of the mediastinal growing teratoma syndrome. Ann Thorac Surg 66: 605-606.
1257. Mathur A, Airan B, Bhan A, Sharma R, Sampath Kumar A, Talwar KK, Chopra P, Venugopal P (2000). Non-myxomatous cardiac tumours: twenty-year experience. Indian Heart J 52: 319-323.
1258. Matolcsy A, Nador RG, Cesarman E, Knowles DM (1998). Immunoglobulin VH gene mutational analysis suggests that primary effusion lymphomas derive from different stages of B cell maturation. Am J Pathol 153: 1609-1614.
1259. Matsubara O, Tan-Liu NS, Kenney RM, Mark EJ (1988). Inflammatory pseudotumors of the lung: progression from organizing pneumonia to fibrous histiocytoma or to plasma cell granuloma in 32 cases. Hum Pathol 19: 807-814.
1260. Matsui K, Beasley MB, Nelson WK, Barnes PM, Bechtle J, Falk R, Ferrans VJ, Moss J, Travis WD (2001). Prognostic significance of pulmonary lymphangioleiomyomatosis histologic score. Am J Surg Pathol 25: 479-484.
1261. Matsui K, Kitagawa M (1991). Spindle cell carcinoma of the lung. A clinicopathologic study of three cases. Cancer 67: 2361-2367.
1262. Matsui K, Kitagawa M, Wakaki K, Masuda S (1993). Lung carcinoma mimicking malignant lymphoma: report of three cases. Acta Pathol Jpn 43: 608-614.
1263. Matsuno Y, Morozumi N, Hirohashi S, Shimosato Y, Rosai J (1998). Papillary carcinoma of the thymus: report of four cases of a new microscopic type of thymic carcinoma. Am J Surg Pathol 22: 873-880.
1264. Matsuno Y, Mukai K, Noguchi M, Sato Y, Shimosato Y (1989). Histochemical and immunohistochemical evidence of glandular differentiation in thymic carcinoma. Acta Pathol Jpn 39: 433-438.
1265. Matsuno Y, Mukai K, Uhara H, Akao I, Furuya S, Sato Y, Hirohashi S, Shimosato Y (1992). Detection of Epstein-Barr virus DNA in a Japanese case of lymphoepithelioma-like thymic carcinoma. Jpn J Cancer Res 83: 127-130.
1266. Matsuo T, Hayashida R, Kobayashi K, Tanaka Y, Ohtsuka S (2002). Thymic basaloid carcinoma with hepatic metastasis. Ann Thorac Surg 74: 579-582.
1267. Mattoo A, Fedullo PF, Kapelanski D, Ilowite JS (2002). Pulmonary artery sarcoma: a case report of surgical cure and 5-year follow-up. Chest 122: 745-747.
1268. Matturri L, Lavezzi AM (1994). Recurrent chromosome alterations in non-small cell lung cancer. Eur J Histochem 38: 53-58.
1269. Matturri L, Varesi C, Cuttin MS, Nappo A (1998). [Anatomopathological and immunohistochemical findings in 6 cardiac myxomas]. Minerva Med 89: 335-339.
1270. Mauch P, Armitage J, Diehl V, Hoppe RT, Weiss LM (1999). The Epidemiology of Hodgkin's Disease. Lippencott Williams & Wilkins: Philadelphia.
1271. Maziak DE, Todd TR, Keshavjee SH, Winton TL, Van Nostrand P, Pearson FG (1996). Adenoid cystic carcinoma of the airway: thirty-two-year experience. J Thorac Cardiovasc Surg 112: 1522-1531.
1272. Mazieres J, Daste G, Molinier L, Berjaud J, Dahan M, Delsol M, Carles P, Didier A, Bachaud JM (2002). Large cell neuroendocrine carcinoma of the lung: pathological study and clinical outcome of 18 resected cases. Lung Cancer 37: 287-292.
1273. Mazumdar M, Bajorin DF, Bacik J, Higgins G, Motzer RJ, Bosl GJ (2001). Predicting outcome to chemotherapy in patients with germ cell tumors: the value of the rate of decline of human chorionic gonadotrophin and alpha-fetoprotein during therapy. J Clin Oncol 19: 2534-2541.
1274. McAllister HA, Fenoglio JJ (1978). Atlas of Tumor Pathology. 2nd ed. Armed Forces Institute of Pathology: Washington, DC.
1275. McCarthy PM, Piehler JM, Schaff HV, Pluth JR, Orszulak TA, Vidaillet HJJr, Carney JA (1986). The significance of multiple, recurrent, and "complex" cardiac myxomas. J Thorac Cardiovasc Surg 91: 389-396.
1276. McCarthy PM, Schaff HV, Winkler HZ, Lieber MM, Carney JA (1989). Deoxyribonucleic acid ploidy pattern of cardiac myxomas. Another predictor of biologically unusual myxomas. J Thorac Cardiovasc Surg 98: 1083-1086.
1277. McCaughey WT, Dardick I, Barr JR (1983). Angiosarcoma of serous membranes. Arch Pathol Lab Med 107: 304-307.
1278. McCluggage WG, Boyd HK, Jones FG, Mayne EE, Bharucha H (1998). Mediastinal granulocytic sarcoma: a report of two cases. Arch Pathol Lab Med 122: 545-547.
1279. McCluggage WG, McManus K, Qureshi R, McAleer S, Wotherspoon AC (2000). Low-grade B-cell lymphoma of mucosa-associated lymphoid tissue (MALT) of thymus. Hum Pathol 31: 255-259.
1280. McDonnell PJ, Mann RB, Bulkley BH (1982). Involvement of the heart by malignant lymphoma: a clinicopathologic study. Cancer 49: 944-951.
1281. McDowell EM, Barrett LA, Glavin F, Harris CC, Trump BF (1978). The respiratory epithelium. I. Human bronchus. J Natl Cancer Inst 61: 539-549.
1282. McDowell EM, Trump BF (1981). Pulmonary smell cell carcinoma showing tripartite differentiation in individual cells. Hum Pathol 12: 286-294.
1283. McDowell EM, Wilson TS, Trump BF (1981). Atypical endocrine tumors of the lung. Arch Pathol Lab Med 105: 20-28.
1284. McGinnis M, Jacobs G, el Naggar A, Redline RW (1993). Congenital peribronchial myofibroblastic tumor (so-called "congenital leiomyosarcoma"). A distinct neonatal lung lesion associated with nonimmune hydrops fetalis. Mod Pathol 6: 487-492.
1285. McGlennen RC, Manivel JC, Stanley SJ, Slater DL, Wick MR, Dehner LP (1989). Pulmonary artery trunk sarcoma: a clinicopathologic, ultrastructural, and immunohistochemical study of four cases. Mod Pathol 2: 486-494.
1286. McGregor CG, Gibson A, Caves P (1984). Infantile cardiomyopathy with histiocytoid change in cardiac muscle cells: successful surgical intervention and prolonged survival. Am J Cardiol 53: 982-983.
1287. McLoud TC, Kalisher L, Stark P, Greene R (1978). Intrathoracic lymph node metastases from extrathoracic neoplasms. AJR Am J Roentgenol 131: 403-407.
1288. McLoud TC, Meyer JE (1982). Mediastinal metastases. Radiol Clin North Am 20: 453-468.
1289. McMahon CJ, Ayres NA, Lewin MB (2001). Cardiac rhabdomyoma: a report of alternative strategies to surgical resection. Cardiol Young 11: 670-672.
1290. McNeil MM, Leong AS, Sage RE (1981). Primary mediastinal embryonal carcinoma in association with Klinefelter's syndrome. Cancer 47: 343-345.
1291. Meis-Kindblom JM, Kindblom LG (1998). Angiosarcoma of soft tissue: a study of 80 cases. Am J Surg Pathol 22: 683-697.
1292. Meis-Kindblom JM, Kjellstrom C, Kindblom LG (1998). Inflammatory fibrosarcoma: update, reappraisal, and perspective on its place in the spectrum of inflammatory myofibroblastic tumors. Semin Diagn Pathol 15: 133-143.
1293. Meissner A, Kirsch W, Regensburger D, Mayer-Eichberger S, Ohnhaus EE (1988). Intrapericardial teratoma in an adult. Am J Med 84: 1089-1090.
1294. Mende S, Moschopulos M, Marx A, Laeng RH (2004). Ectopic micronodular thymoma with lymphoid stroma. Virchows Arch .
1295. Mendlick MR, Nelson M, Pickering D, Johansson SL, Seemayer TA, Neff JR, Vergara G, Rosenthal H, Bridge JA (2001). Translocation t(1;3)(p36.3;q25) is a nonrandom aberration in epithelioid hemangioendothelioma. Am J Surg Pathol 25: 684-687.
1296. Menestrina F, Chilosi M, Bonetti F, Lestani M, Scarpa A, Novelli P, Doglioni C, Todeschini G, Ambrosetti A, Fiore-Donati L (1986). Mediastinal large-cell lymphoma of B-type, with sclerosis: histopathological and immunohistochemical study of eight cases. Histopathology 10: 589-600.
1297. Menet E, Etchandy-Laclau K, Corbi P, Levillain P, Babin P (1999). [Alveolar adenoma: a rare peripheral pulmonary tumor]. Ann Pathol 19: 325-328.
1298. Meng Q, Lai H, Lima J, Tong W, Qian Y, Lai S (2002). Echocardiographic and pathologic characteristics of primary cardiac tumors: a study of 149 cases. Int J Cardiol 84: 69-75.
1299. Merlo A, Gabrielson E, Askin F, Sidransky D (1994). Frequent loss of chromosome 9 in human primary non-small cell lung cancer. Cancer Res 54: 640-642.
1300. Merlo A, Herman JG, Mao L, Lee DJ, Gabrielson E, Burger PC, Baylin SB, Sidransky D (1995). 5' CpG island methylation is associated with transcriptional silencing of the tumour suppressor p16/CDKN2/MTS1 in human cancers. Nat Med 1: 686-692.
1301. Mertens F, Johansson B, Hoglund M, Mitelman F (1997). Chromosomal imbalance maps of malignant solid tumors: a cytogenetic survey of 3185 neoplasms. Cancer Res 57: 2765-2780.
1302. Metcalf RA, Welsh JA, Bennett WP, Seddon MB, Lehman TA, Pelin K, Linnainmaa K, Tammilehto L, Mattson K, Gerwin BI, Harris CC (1992). p53 and Kirsten-ras mutations in human mesothelioma cell lines. Cancer Res 52: 2610-2615.
1303. Meurman LO, Kiviluoto R, Hakama M (1979). Combined effect of asbestos exposure and tobacco smoking on Finnish anthophyllite miners and millers. Ann N Y Acad Sci 330: 491-495.
1304. Michal M, Havlicek F (1993). Immunohistochemical phenotypes of histioeosinophilic granulomas of thymus and reactive eosinophilic pleuritis. Acta Histochem 94: 97-101.
1305. Middleton G (1966). Involvement of the thymus by metastic neoplasms. Br J Cancer 20: 41-46.
1306. Miettinen M (1991). Keratin subsets in spindle cell sarcomas. Keratins are widespread but synovial sarcoma contains a distinctive keratin polypeptide pattern and desmoplakins. Am J Pathol 138: 505-513.
1307. Miettinen M (1993). Keratin immunohistochemistry: update of applications and pitfalls. Pathol Annu 28 Pt 2: 113-143.
1308. Miettinen M, Fetsch JF (2000). Distribution of keratins in normal endothelial cells and a spectrum of vascular tumors: implications in tumor diagnosis. Hum Pathol 31: 1062-1067.

1309. Miettinen M, Fletcher CD, Lasota J (1993). True histiocytic lymphoma of small intestine. Analysis of two S-100 protein-positive cases with features of interdigitating reticulum cell sarcoma. Am J Clin Pathol 100: 285-292.

1310. Miettinen M, Limon J, Niezabitowski A, Lasota J (2001). Calretinin and other mesothelioma markers in synovial sarcoma: analysis of antigenic similarities and differences with malignant mesothelioma. Am J Surg Pathol 25: 610-617.

1311. Miettinen MM, el Rifai W, Sarlomo-Rikala M, Andersson LC, Knuutila S (1997). Tumor size-related DNA copy number changes occur in solitary fibrous tumors but not in hemangiopericytomas. Mod Pathol 10: 1194-1200.

1312. Miller DP, De Vivo I, Neuberg D, Wain JC, Lynch TJ, Su L, Christiani DC (2003). Association between self-reported environmental tobacco smoke exposure and lung cancer: modification by GSTP1 polymorphism. Int J Cancer 104: 758-763.

1313. Miller DP, Liu G, De Vivo I, Lynch TJ, Wain JC, Su L, Christiani DC (2002). Combinations of the variant genotypes of GSTP1, GSTM1, and p53 are associated with an increased lung cancer risk. Cancer Res 62: 2819-2823.

1314. Miller MA, Mark GJ, Kanarek D (1978). Multiple peripheral pulmonary carcinoids and tumorlets of carcinoid type, with restrictive and obstructive lung disease. Am J Med 65: 373-378.

1315. Miller R, Kurtz SM, Powers JM (1978). Mediastinal rhabdomyoma. Cancer 42: 1983-1988.

1316. Miller RR (1990). Bronchioloalveolar cell adenomas. Am J Surg Pathol 14: 904-912.

1317. Miller RR, Muller NL (1995). Neuroendocrine cell hyperplasia and obliterative bronchiolitis in patients with peripheral carcinoid tumors. Am J Surg Pathol 19: 653-658.

1318. Miller RR, Nelems B, Evans KG, Muller NL, Ostrow DN (1988). Glandular neoplasia of the lung. A proposed analogy to colonic tumors. Cancer 61: 1009-1014.

1319. Miller SU, Pruett HJ, Long A (1959). Fatal Chylopericardium caused by hamartomatous lymphangiomatosis - case report and review of the literature. Am J Med 26: 951-956.

1320. Miller TP, Jones SE (1983). Initial chemotherapy for clinically localized lymphomas of unfavorable histology. Blood 62: 413-418.

1321. Miller VA, Kris MG, Shah N, Patel J, Azzoli C, Gomez J, Krug LM, Pao W, Rizvi N, Pizzo B, Tyson L, Venkatraman E, Ben Porat L, Memoli N, Zakowski M, Rusch V, Heelan RT (2004). Bronchioloalveolar pathologic subtype and smoking history predict sensitivity to gefitinib in advanced non-small-cell lung cancer. J Clin Oncol 22: 1103-1109.

1322. Mills NE, Fishman CL, Scholes J, Anderson SE, Rom WN, Jacobson DR (1995). Detection of K-ras oncogene mutations in bronchoalveolar lavage fluid for lung cancer diagnosis. J Natl Cancer Inst 87: 1056-1060.

1323. Minna JD, Roth JA, Gazdar AF (2002). Focus on lung cancer. Cancer Cell 1: 49-52.

1324. Mirtcheva RM, Vazquez M, Yankelevitz DF, Henschke CI (2002). Bronchioloalveolar carcinoma and adenocarcinoma with bronchioloalveolar features presenting as ground-glass opacities on CT. Clin Imaging 26: 95-100.

1325. Mirza I, Kazimi SN, Ligi R, Burns J, Braza F (2000). Cytogenetic profile of a thymoma. A case report and review of the literature. Arch Pathol Lab Med 124: 1714-1716.

1326. Mishalani SH, Lones MA, Said JW (1995). Multilocular thymic cyst. A novel thymic lesion associated with human immunodeficiency virus infection. Arch Pathol Lab Med 119: 467-470.

1327. Mishina T, Dosaka-Akita H, Hommura F, Nishi M, Kojima T, Ogura S, Shimizu M, Katoh H, Kawakami Y (2000). Cyclin E expression, a potential prognostic marker for non-small cell lung cancers. Clin Cancer Res 6: 11-16.

1328. Mishriki YY, Lane BP, Lozowski MS, Epstein H (1983). Hurthle-cell tumor arising in the mediastinal ectopic thyroid and diagnosed by fine needle aspiration. Light microscopic and ultrastructural features. Acta Cytol 27: 188-192.

1329. Mitchell ML, Parker FP (1991). Capillaries. A cytologic feature of pulmonary carcinoid tumors. Acta Cytol 35: 183-185.

1330. Mitelman F, Johansson B, Mertens F (2003). Mitelman Database of Chromosome Aberrations in Cancer. http://cgap nci nih gov/Chromosomes/Mitelman http://cgap.nci.nih.gov/Chromosomes/Mitelman.

1331. Mitsudomi T, Hamajima N, Ogawa M, Takahashi T (2000). Prognostic significance of p53 alterations in patients with non-small cell lung cancer: a meta-analysis. Clin Cancer Res 6: 4055-4063.

1332. Miura K, Bowman ED, Simon R, Peng AC, Robles AI, Jones RT, Katagiri T, He P, Mizukami H, Charboneau L, Kikuchi T, Liotta LA, Nakamura Y, Harris CC (2002). Laser capture microdissection and microarray expression analysis of lung adenocarcinoma reveals tobacco smoking- and prognosis-related molecular profiles. Cancer Res 62: 3244-3250.

1333. Miwa H, Takakuwa T, Nakatsuka S, Tomita Y, Iuchi K, Aozasa K (2002). DNA sequences of the immunoglobulin heavy chain variable region gene in pyothorax-associated lymphoma. Oncology 62: 241-250.

1334. Miyagawa-Hayashino A, Tazelaar HD, Langel DJ, Colby TV (2003). Pulmonary sclerosing hemangioma with lymph node metastases: report of 4 cases. Arch Pathol Lab Med 127: 321-325.

1335. Miyoshi T, Satoh Y, Okumura S, Nakagawa K, Shirakusa T, Tsuchiya E, Ishikawa Y (2003). Early-stage lung adenocarcinomas with a micropapillary pattern, a distinct pathologic marker for a significantly poor prognosis. Am J Surg Pathol 27: 101-109.

1336. Mizuno T, Masaoka A, Hashimoto T, Shibata K, Yamakawa Y, Torii K, Fukai I, Ito K (1990). Coexisting thymic carcinoid tumor and thymoma. Ann Thorac Surg 50: 650-652.

1337. Moeller KH, Rosado-de-Christenson ML, Templeton PA (1997). Mediastinal mature teratoma: imaging features. AJR Am J Roentgenol 169: 985-990.

1338. Molina JE, Edwards JE, Ward HB (1990). Primary cardiac tumors: experience at the University of Minnesota. Thorac Cardiovasc Surg 38 Suppl 2: 183-191.

1339. Molinie V, Pouchot J, Navratil E, Aubert F, Vinceneux P, Barge J (1996). Primary Epstein-Barr virus-related non-Hodgkin's lymphoma of the pleural cavity following long-standing tuberculous empyema. Arch Pathol Lab Med 120: 288-291.

1340. Moller P, Bruderlein S, Strater J, Leithauser F, Hasel C, Bataille F, Moldenhauer G, Pawlita M, Barth TF (2001). MedB-1, a human tumor cell line derived from a primary mediastinal large B-cell lymphoma. Int J Cancer 92: 348-353.

1341. Moller P, Lammler B, Eberlein-Gonska M, Feichter GE, Hofmann WJ, Schmitteckert H, Otto HF (1986). Primary mediastinal clear cell lymphoma of B-cell type. Virchows Arch A Pathol Anat Histol 409: 79-92.

1342. Moller P, Lammler B, Herrmann B, Otto HF, Moldenhauer G, Momburg F (1986). The primary mediastinal clear cell lymphoma of B-cell type has variable defects in MHC antigen expression. Immunology 59: 411-417.

1343. Moller P, Matthaei-Maurer DU, Hofmann WJ, Dorken B, Moldenhauer G (1989). Immunophenotypic similarities of mediastinal clear-cell lymphoma and sinusoidal (monocytoid) B cells. Int J Cancer 43: 10-16.

1344. Moller P, Moldenhauer G, Momburg F, Lammler B, Eberlein-Gonska M, Kiesel S, Dorken B (1987). Mediastinal lymphoma of clear cell type is a tumor corresponding to terminal steps of B cell differentiation. Blood 69: 1087-1095.

1345. Monma N, Satodate R, Tashiro A, Segawa I (1991). Origin of so-called mesothelioma of the atrioventricular node. An immunohistochemical study. Arch Pathol Lab Med 115: 1026-1029.

1346. Montanaro F, Bray F, Gennaro V, Merler E, Tyczynski JE, Parkin DM, Strnad M, Jechov'a M, Storm HH, Aareleid T, Hakulinen T, Velten M, Lef'evre H, Danzon A, Buemi A, Daur'es JP, Menegoz F, Raverdy N, Sauvage M, Ziegler H, Comber H, Paci E, Vercelli M, De Lisi V, Tumino R, Zanetti R, Berrino F, Stanta G, Langmark F, Rachtan J, Mezyk R, Blaszczyk J, Ivan P, Primic-Zakelj M, Martinez AC, Izarzugaza I, Borras J, Garcia CM, Garau I, Sanchez NC, Aicua A, Barlow L, Torhorst J, Bouchardy C, Levi F, Fisch T, Probst N, Visser O, Quinn M, Gavin A, Brewster D, Mikov M (2003). Pleural mesothelioma incidence in Europe: evidence of some deceleration in the increasing trends. Cancer Causes Control 14: 791-803.

1347. Montanaro F, Bray F, Gennaro V, Merler E, Tyczynski JE, Parkin DM, Strnad M, Jechov'a M, Storm HH, Aareleid T, Hakulinen T, Velten M, Lef'evre H, Danzon A, Buemi A, Daur'es JP, Menegoz F, Raverdy N, Sauvage M, Ziegler H, Comber H, Paci E, Vercelli M, De Lisi V, Tumino R, Zanetti R, Berrino F, Stanta G, Langmark F, Rachtan J, Mezyk R, Blaszczyk J, Ivan P, Primic-Zakelj M, Martinez AC, Izarzugaza I, Borras J, Garcia CM, Garau I, Sanchez NC, Aicua A, Barlow L, Torhorst J, Bouchardy C, Levi F, Fisch T, Probst N, Visser O, Quinn M, Gavin A, Brewster D, Mikov M (2003). Pleural mesothelioma incidence in Europe: evidence of some deceleration in the increasing trends. Cancer Causes Control 14: 791-803.

1348. Mooi WJ (1996). Common lung cancers. In: Spencer's Pathology of the Lung, Hasleton PS, ed., 5th ed. McGraw-Hill: New York, pp. 1009-1064.

1349. Moran CA (1999). Germ cell tumors of the mediastinum. Pathol Res Pract 195: 583-587.

1350. Moran CA, Albores-Saavedra J, Wenig BM, Mena H (1997). Pigmented extraadrenal paragangliomas. A clinico-pathologic and immunohistochemical study of five cases. Cancer 79: 398-402.

1351. Moran CA, Koss MN (1993). Rhabdomyomatous thymoma. Am J Surg Pathol 17: 633-636.

1352. Moran CA, Rosado-de-Christenson M, Suster S (1995). Thymolipoma: clinicopathologic review of 33 cases. Mod Pathol 8: 741-744.

1353. Moran CA, Suster S (1995). Mediastinal hemangiomas: a study of 18 cases with emphasis on the spectrum of morphological features. Hum Pathol 26: 416-421.

1354. Moran CA, Suster S (1995). Mediastinal seminomas with prominent cystic changes. A clinicopathologic study of 10 cases. Am J Surg Pathol 19: 1047-1053.

1355. Moran CA, Suster S (1997). Hepatoid yolk sac tumors of the mediastinum: a clinicopathologic and immunohistochemical study of four cases. Am J Surg Pathol 21: 1210-1214.

1356. Moran CA, Suster S (1997). Primary germ cell tumors of the mediastinum: I. Analysis of 322 cases with special emphasis on teratomatous lesions and a proposal for histopathologic classification and clinical staging. Cancer 80: 681-690.

1357. Moran CA, Suster S (1997). Primary mediastinal choriocarcinomas: a clinicopathologic and immunohistochemical study of eight cases. Am J Surg Pathol 21: 1007-1012.

1358. Moran CA, Suster S (1997). Yolk sac tumors of the mediastinum with prominent spindle cell features: a clinicopathologic study of three cases. Am J Surg Pathol 21: 1173-1177.

1359. Moran CA, Suster S (1998). Germ-cell tumors of the mediastinum. Adv Anat Pathol 5: 1-15.

1360. Moran CA, Suster S (1999). Angiomatoid neuroendocrine carcinoma of the thymus: report of a distinctive morphological variant of neuroendocrine tumor of the thymus resembling a vascular neoplasm. Hum Pathol 30: 635-639.

1361. Moran CA, Suster S (2000). Neuroendocrine carcinomas (carcinoid tumor) of the thymus. A clinicopathologic analysis of 80 cases. Am J Clin Pathol 114: 100-110.

1362. Moran CA, Suster S (2000). Primary neuroendocrine carcinoma (thymic carcinoid) of the thymus with prominent oncocytic features: a clinicopathologic study of 22 cases. Mod Pathol 13: 489-494.

1363. Moran CA, Suster S (2000). Thymic neuroendocrine carcinomas with combined features ranging from well-differentiated (carcinoid) to small cell carcinoma. A clinicopathologic and immunohistochemical study of 11 cases. Am J Clin Pathol 113: 345-350.

1364. Moran CA, Suster S, Askin FB, Koss MN (1994). Benign and malignant salivary gland-type mixed tumors of the lung. Clinicopathologic and immunohistochemical study of eight cases. Cancer 73: 2481-2490.

1365. Moran CA, Suster S, Fishback N, Koss MN (1993). Mediastinal paragangliomas. A clinicopathologic and immunohistochemical study of 16 cases. Cancer 72: 2358-2364.

1366. Moran CA, Suster S, Fishback N, Koss MN (1995). Extramedullary hematopoiesis presenting as posterior mediastinal mass: a study of four cases. Mod Pathol 8: 249-251.

1367. Moran CA, Suster S, Fishback NF,

Koss MN (1995). Primary intrapulmonary thymoma. A clinicopathologic and immunohistochemical study of eight cases. Am J Surg Pathol 19: 304-312.
1368. Moran CA, Suster S, Koss MN (1994). Primary adenoid cystic carcinoma of the lung. A clinicopathologic and immunohistochemical study of 16 cases. Cancer 73: 1390-1397.
1369. Moran CA, Suster S, Koss MN (1997). Primary germ cell tumors of the mediastinum: III. Yolk sac tumor, embryonal carcinoma, choriocarcinoma, and combined nonteratomatous germ cell tumors of the mediastinum—a clinicopathologic and immunohistochemical study of 64 cases. Cancer 80: 699-707.
1370. Moran CA, Suster S, Perino G, Kaneko M, Koss MN (1994). Malignant smooth muscle tumors presenting as mediastinal soft tissue masses. A clinicopathologic study of 10 cases. Cancer 74: 2251-2260.
1371. Moran CA, Suster S, Przygodzki RM, Koss MN (1997). Primary germ cell tumors of the mediastinum: II. Mediastinal seminomas—a clinicopathologic and immunohistochemical study of 120 cases. Cancer 80: 691-698.
1372. Moran CA, Zeren H, Koss MN (1994). Thymofibrolipoma. A histologic variant of thymolipoma. Arch Pathol Lab Med 118: 281-282.
1373. Morgan DE, Sanders C, McElvein RB, Nath H, Alexander CB (1992). Intrapulmonary teratoma: a case report and review of the literature. J Thorac Imaging 7: 70-77.
1374. Mori K, Cho H, Som M (1977). Primary "flat" melanoma of the trachea. J Pathol 121: 101-105.
1375. Mori M, Chiba R, Takahashi T (1993). Atypical adenomatous hyperplasia of the lung and its differentiation from adenocarcinoma. Characterization of atypical cells by morphometry and multivariate cluster analysis. Cancer 72: 2331-2340.
1376. Mori M, Chiba R, Tezuka F, Kaji M, Kobubo T, Nukiwa T, Takahashi T (1996). Papillary adenoma of type II pneumocytes might have malignant potential. Virchows Arch 428: 195-200.
1377. Mori M, Kaji M, Tezuka F, Takahashi T (1998). Comparative ultrastructural study of atypical adenomatous hyperplasia and adenocarcinoma of the human lung. Ultrastruct Pathol 22: 459-466.
1378. Mori M, Rao SK, Popper HH, Cagle PT, Fraire AE (2001). Atypical adenomatous hyperplasia of the lung: a probable forerunner in the development of adenocarcinoma of the lung. Mod Pathol 14: 72-84.
1379. Mori M, Tezuka F, Chiba R, Funae Y, Watanabe M, Nukiwa T, Takahashi T (1996). Atypical adenomatous hyperplasia and adenocarcinoma of the human lung: their heterology in form and analogy in immunohistochemical characteristics. Cancer 77: 665-674.
1380. Mori N, Yatabe Y, Narita M, Kobayashi T, Asai J (1996). Pyothorax-associated lymphoma. An unusual case with biphenotypic character of T and B cells. Am J Surg Pathol 20: 760-766.
1381. Mori T, Hongo H, Kondo K, Akamine T, Hanada N, Toyota N, Yoshioka M, Tabira Y, Hiraoka T, Kitamura N (1998). [Successful chemotherapy based on in vitro chemosensitivity testing in a case of recurrent thymic carcinoma]. Kyobu Geka 51: 235-238.
1382. Morice WG, Kurtin PJ, Myers JL (2002). Expression of cytolytic lymphocyte-associated antigens in pulmonary lymphomatoid granulomatosis. Am J Clin Pathol 118: 391-398.
1383. Morikami Y, Higashi T, Isomura T, Hirano A, Tanaka K, Hisatomi K, Ohishi K (1994). Cardiac lipoma with changes of ST segment and T wave on electrocardiogram. Jpn Circ J 58: 733-736.
1384. Morimitsu Y, Nakajima M, Hisaoka M, Hashimoto H (2000). Extrapleural solitary fibrous tumor: clinicopathologic study of 17 cases and molecular analysis of the p53 pathway. APMIS 108: 617-625.
1385. Morinaga S, Nomori H, Kobayashi R, Atsumi Y (1994). Well-differentiated adenocarcinoma arising from mature cystic teratoma of the mediastinum (teratoma with malignant transformation). Report of a surgical case. Am J Clin Pathol 101: 531-534.
1386. Morinaga S, Sato Y, Shimosato Y, Sinkai T, Tsuchiya R (1987). Multiple thymic squamous cell carcinomas associated with mixed type thymoma. Am J Surg Pathol 11: 982-988.
1387. Morinaga S, Shimosato Y (1987). Pathology of the microadenocarcinoma in the periphery of the lung. Pathol Clin Med Jpn 5: 74-80.
1388. Morishita Y, Fukasawa M, Takeuchi M, Inadome Y, Matsuno Y, Noguchi M (2001). Small-sized adenocarcinoma of the lung. Cytologic characteristics and clinical behavior. Cancer 93: 124-131.
1389. Moro-Sibilot D, Jeanmart M, Lantuejoul S, Arbib F, Laverriere MH, Brambilla E, Brambilla C (2002). Cigarette smoking, preinvasive bronchial lesions, and autofluorescence bronchoscopy. Chest 122: 1902-1908.
1390. Moro D, Brichon PY, Brambilla E, Veale D, Labat F, Brambilla C (1994). Basaloid bronchial carcinoma. A histologic group with a poor prognosis. Cancer 73: 2734-2739.
1391. Moss J, Avila NA, Barnes PM, Litzenberger RA, Bechtle J, Brooks PG, Hedin CJ, Hunsberger S, Kristof AS (2001). Prevalence and clinical characteristics of lymphangioleiomyomatosis (LAM) in patients with tuberous sclerosis complex. Am J Respir Crit Care Med 164: 669-671.
1392. Mostert M, Rosenberg C, Stoop H, Schuyer M, Timmer A, Oosterhuis W, Looijenga L (2000). Comparative genomic and in situ hybridization of germ cell tumors of the infantile testis. Lab Invest 80: 1055-1064.
1393. Mott BD, Canver CC, Nazeer T, Buchan A, Ilves R (2001). Staged resection of bilateral pleuropulmonary blastoma in a two-month old girl. J Cardiovasc Surg (Torino) 42: 135-137.
1394. Motzer RJ, Amsterdam A, Prieto V, Sheinfeld J, Murty VV, Mazumdar M, Bosl GJ, Chaganti RS, Reuter VE (1998). Teratoma with malignant transformation: diverse malignant histologies arising in men with germ cell tumors. J Urol 159: 133-138.
1395. Moysset I, Lloreta J, Miguel A, Vadell C, Ribalta T, Estrach T, Serrano S (1997). Thymoma associated with CD4+ lymphopenia, cytomegalovirus infection, and Kaposi's sarcoma. Hum Pathol 28: 1211-1213.
1396. Muir CS, Fraumeni JFJr, Doll R (1994). The interpretation of time trends. Cancer Surv 19-20: 5-21.
1397. Muir KW, McNeish I, Grosset DG, Metcalfe M (1996). Visualization of cardiac emboli from mitral valve papillary fibroelastoma. Stroke 27: 1133-1134.
Mukai K, Shinkai T, Tominaga K, Shimosato Y (1988). The incidence of secondary tumors of the heart and pericardium: a 10-year study. Jpn J Clin Oncol 18: 195-201.
1398. A. Mukohara N, Tobe S, Azami T (2001). Angiosarcoma causing cardiac rupture. Jpn J Thorac Carciovasc Surg 49: 516-518.
1399. Mukundan G, Urban BA, Askin FB, Fishman EK (2000). Pulmonary epithelioid hemangioendothelioma: atypical radiologic findings of a rare tumor with pathologic correlation. J Comput Assist Tomogr 24: 719-720.
1400. Mulder H, Schlangen JT, van Voorthuisen AE (1975). Extramedullary hematopoiesis in the posterior mediastinum. Radiol Clin (Basel) 44: 550-556.
1401. Mullaney BP, Ng VL, Herndier BG, McGrath MS, Pallavicini MG (2000). Comparative genomic analyses of primary effusion lymphoma. Arch Pathol Lab Med 124: 824-826.
1402. Muller-Hermelink HK (2002). Case no 2 Slide workshop. V Annual Meeting of the Japanese German pathologists .
1403. Muller-Hermelink HK, Marx A (1999). Pathological aspects of malignant and benign thymic disorders. Ann Med 31 Suppl 2: 5-14.
1404. Muller-Hermelink HK, Marx A (2000). Thymoma. Curr Opin Oncol 12: 426-433.
1405. Muller-Hermelink HK, Marx A (2000). Towards a histogenetic classification of thymic epithelial tumours? Histopathology 36: 466-469.
1406. Muller-Tidow C, Metzger R, Kugler K, Diederichs S, Idos G, Thomas M, Dockhorn-Dworniczak B, Schneider PM, Koeffler HP, Berdel WE, Serve H (2001). Cyclin E is the only cyclin-dependent kinase 2-associated cyclin that predicts metastasis and survival in early stage non-small cell lung cancer. Cancer Res 61: 647-653.
1407. Muller KM, Muller G (1983). The ultrastructure of preneoplastic changes in the bronchial mucosa. In: Current Topics of Pathology, Current Topics of Pathology, Springer Verlag: Berlin Heidelberg , pp. 233-263.
1408. Muller KM, Nakhosteen JA, Khanavkar B, Fisseler-Eckhoff A (1998). [Bronchopulmonary preneoplasia. Diagnosis using LIFE system and pathology panel of the European Early Lung Cancer Study Group (EELCSG)]. Pathologe 19: 388-394.
1409. Mulliken JB, Young AE (1988). Vascular Birthmarks: Hemangiomas and Malformations. WB Saunders: Philadelphia.
1410. Mullins RK, Thompson SK, Coogan PS, Shurbaji MS (1994). Paranuclear blue inclusions: an aid in the cytopathologic diagnosis of primary and metastatic pulmonary small-cell carcinoma. Diagn Cytopathol 10: 332-335.
1411. Murphy MC, Sweeney MS, Putnam JBJr, Walker WE, Frazier OH, Ott DA, Cooley DA (1990). Surgical treatment of cardiac tumors: a 25-year experience. Ann Thorac Surg 49: 612-617.
1412. Murphy MN, Glennon PG, Diocee MS, Wick MR, Cavers DJ (1986). Nonsecretory parathyroid carcinoma of the mediastinum. Light microscopic, immunocytochemical, and ultrastructural features of a case, and review of the literature. Cancer 58: 2468-2476.
1413. Murthy SS, Shen T, De Rienzo A, Lee WC, Ferriola PC, Jhanwar SC, Mossman BT, Filmus J, Testa JR (2000). Expression of GPC3, an X-linked recessive overgrowth gene, is silenced in malignant mesothelioma. Oncogene 19: 410-416.
1414. Muschen M, Rajewsky K, Brauninger A, Baur AS, Oudejans JJ, Roers A, Hansmann ML, Kuppers R (2000). Rare occurrence of classical Hodgkin's disease as a T cell lymphoma. J Exp Med 191: 387-394.
1415. Musk AW, Dewar J, Shilkin KB, Whitaker D (1991). Miliary spread of malignant pleural mesothelioma without a clinically identifiable pleural tumour. Aust N Z J Med 21: 460-462.
1416. Musso P, Ronzani G, Ravera A, Comoglio C, Motta M, Dalmasso M (2002). [Primary cardiac lymphoma presenting with complete atrioventricular block. Case report and review of the literature]. Ital Heart J 3: 1047-1050.
1417. Myers JL, Kurtin PJ, Katzenstein AL, Tazelaar HD, Colby TV, Strickler JG, Lloyd RV, Isaacson PG (1995). Lymphomatoid granulomatosis. Evidence of immunophenotypic diversity and relationship to Epstein-Barr virus infection. Am J Surg Pathol 19: 1300-1312.
1418. Myhre-Jensen O, Kaae S, Madsen EH, Sneppen O (1983). Histopathological grading in soft-tissue tumours. Relation to survival in 261 surgically treated patients. Acta Pathol Microbiol Immunol Scand [A] 91: 145-150.
1419. Myojin M, Choi NC, Wright CD, Wain JC, Harris N, Hug EB, Mathisen DJ, Lynch T, Carey RW, Grossbard M, Finkelstein DM, Grillo HC (2000). Stage III thymoma: pattern of failure after surgery and postoperative radiotherapy and its implication for future study. Int J Radiat Oncol Biol Phys 46: 927-933.
1420. Nacht M, Dracheva T, Gao Y, Fujii T, Chen Y, Player A, Akmaev V, Cook B, Dufault M, Zhang M, Zhang W, Guo M, Curran J, Han S, Sidransky D, Buetow K, Madden SL, Jen J (2001). Molecular characteristics of non-small cell lung cancer. Proc Natl Acad Sci U S A 98: 15203-15208.
1421. Nador RG, Cesarman E, Chadburn A, Dawson DB, Ansari MQ, Sald J, Knowles DM (1996). Primary effusion lymphoma: a distinct clinicopathologic entity associated with the Kaposi's sarcoma-associated herpes virus. Blood 88: 645-656.
1422. Nador RG, Cesarman E, Knowles DM, Said JW (1995). Herpes-like DNA sequences in a body-cavity-based lymphoma in an HIV-negative patient. N Engl J Med 333: 943.
1423. Nagamoto N, Saito Y, Imai T, Suda H, Hashimoto K, Nakada T, Sato H (1986). Roentgenographically occult bronchogenic squamous cell carcinoma: location in the bronchi, depth of invasion and length of axial involvement of the bronchus. Tohoku J Exp Med 148: 241-256.
1424. Nagamoto N, Saito Y, Suda H, Imai T, Sato M, Ohta S, Kanma K, Sagawa M, Takahashi S, Usuda K (1989). Relationship between length of longitudinal extension and maximal depth of transmural invasion in roentgenographically occult squamous cell carcinoma of the bronchus (nonpolypoid type). Am J Surg Pathol 13: 11-20.
1425. Nagao M, Murase K, Yasuhara Y, Ikezoe J, Eguchi K, Mogami H, Mandai K, Nakata M, Ooshiro Y (2002). Measurement of localized ground-glass attenuation on thin-section computed tomography images: correlation with the progression of

bronchioloalveolar carcinoma of the lung. Invest Radiol 37: 692-697.

1426. Nagasaka T, Lai R, Harada T, Chen YY, Chen WG, Arber DA, Weiss LM (2000). Coexisting thymic and gastric lymphomas of mucosa-associated lymphoid tissues in a patient with Sjogren syndrome. Arch Pathol Lab Med 124: 770-773.

1427. Nagel H, Schulten HJ, Gunawan B, Brinck U, Fuzesi L (2002). The potential value of comparative genomic hybridization analysis in effusion-and fine needle aspiration cytology. Mod Pathol 15: 818-825.

1428. Naka N, Tomita Y, Nakanishi H, Araki N, Hongyo T, Ochi T, Aozasa K (1997). Mutations of p53 tumor-suppressor gene in angiosarcoma. Int J Cancer 71: 952-955.

1429. Nakahara R, Yokose T, Nagai K, Nishiwaki Y, Ochiai A (2001). Atypical adenomatous hyperplasia of the lung: a clinicopathological study of 118 cases including cases with multiple atypical adenomatous hyperplasia. Thorax 56: 302-305.

1430. Nakajima M, Kasai T, Hashimoto H, Iwata Y, Manabe H (1999). Sarcomatoid carcinoma of the lung: a clinicopathologic study of 37 cases. Cancer 86: 608-616.

1431. Nakajima R, Yokose T, Kakinuma R, Nagai K, Nishiwaki Y, Ochiai A (2002). Localized pure ground-glass opacity on high-resolution CT: histologic characteristics. J Comput Assist Tomogr 26: 323-329.

1432. Nakamura H, Saji H, Ogata A, Hosaka M, Hagiwara M, Kawasaki N, Kato H (2003). Correlation between encoded protein over-expression and copy number of the HER2 gene with survival in non-small cell lung cancer. Int J Cancer 103: 61-66.

1433. Nakamura S, Sasajima Y, Koshikawa T, Kitoh K, Kato M, Ueda R, Mori S, Suchi T (1995). Ki-1 (CD30) positive anaplastic large cell lymphoma of T-cell phenotype developing in association with long-standing tuberculous pyothorax: report of a case with detection of Epstein-Barr virus genome in the tumor cells. Hum Pathol 26: 1382-1385.

1434. Nakanishi K (1990). Alveolar epithelial hyperplasia and adenocarcinoma of the lung. Arch Pathol Lab Med 114: 363-368.

1435. Nakatani Y, Dickersin GR, Mark EJ (1990). Pulmonary endodermal tumor resembling fetal lung: a clinicopathologic study of five cases with immunohistochemical and ultrastructural characterization. Hum Pathol 21: 1097-1107.

1436. Nakatani Y, Kitamura H, Inayama Y, Kamijo S, Nagashima Y, Shimoyama K, Nakamura N, Sano J, Ogawa N, Shibagaki T, Resl M, Mark EJ (1998). Pulmonary adenocarcinomas of the fetal lung type: a clinicopathologic study indicating differences in histology, epidemiology, and natural history of low-grade and high-grade forms. Am J Surg Pathol 22: 399-411.

1437. Nakatsuka S, Yao M, Hoshida Y, Yamamoto S, Iuchi K, Aozasa K (2002). Pyothorax-associated lymphoma: a review of 106 cases. J Clin Oncol 20: 4255-4260.

1438. Nakayama H, Noguchi M, Tsuchiya R, Kodama T, Shimosato Y (1990). Clonal growth of atypical adenomatous hyperplasia of the lung: cytofluorometric analysis of nuclear DNA content. Mod Pathol 3: 314-320.

1439. Nakhoul F, Kerner H, Levin M, Best LA, Better OS (1994). Carcinoid tumor of the lung and type-1 multiple endocrine neoplasia associated with persistent hypercalcemia: a case report. Miner Electrolyte Metab 20: 107-111.

1440. Nappi O, Glasner SD, Swanson PE, Wick MR (1994). Biphasic and monophasic sarcomatoid carcinomas of the lung. A reappraisal of 'carcinosarcomas' and 'spindle-cell carcinomas'. Am J Clin Pathol 102: 331-340.

1441. Nappi O, Swanson PE, Wick MR (1994). Pseudovascular adenoid squamous cell carcinoma of the lung: clinicopathologic study of three cases and comparison with true pleuropulmonary angiosarcoma. Hum Pathol 25: 373-378.

1442. Nappi O, Wick MR (1993). Sarcomatoid neoplasms of the respiratory tract. Semin Diagn Pathol 10: 137-147.

1443. Nascimento AF, Ruiz R, Hornick JL, Fletcher CD (2002). Calcifying fibrous 'pseudotumor': clinicopathologic study of 15 cases and analysis of its relationship to inflammatory myofibroblastic tumor. Int J Surg Pathol 10: 189-196.

1444. Nathaniels EK, Nathaniels AM, Wang CA (1970). Mediastinal parathyroid tumors: a clinical and pathological study of 84 cases. Ann Surg 171: 165-170.

1445. Naunheim KS, Taylor JR, Skosey C, Hoffman PC, Ferguson MK, Golomb HM, Little AG (1987). Adenosquamous lung carcinoma: clinical characteristics, treatment, and prognosis. Ann Thorac Surg 44: 462-466.

1446. Naylor SL, Johnson BE, Minna JD, Sakaguchi AY (1987). Loss of heterozygosity of chromosome 3p markers in small-cell lung cancer. Nature 329: 451-454.

1447. Nazar-Stewart V, Vaughan TL, Stapleton P, Van Loo J, Nicol-Blades B, Eaton DL (2003). A population-based study of glutathione S-transferase M1, T1 and P1 genotypes and risk for lung cancer. Lung Cancer 40: 247-258.

1448. Neal MH, Kosinski R, Cohen P, Orenstein JM (1986). Atypical endocrine tumors of the lung: a histologic, ultrastructural, and clinical study of 19 cases. Hum Pathol 17: 1264-1277.

1449. Neft RE, Crowell RE, Gilliland FD, Murphy MM, Lane JL, Harms H, Coons T, Heaphy E, Belinsky SA, Lechner JF (1998). Frequency of trisomy 20 in nonmalignant bronchial epithelium from lung cancer patients and cancer-free former uranium miners and smokers. Cancer Epidemiol Biomarkers Prev 7: 1051-1054.

1450. Neiman RS, Orazi A (1999). Mediastinal non-seminomatous germ cell tumours: their association with non-germ cell malignancies. Pathol Res Pract 195: 589-594.

1451. Nemunaitis J, Klemow S, Tong A, Courtney A, Johnston W, Mack M, Taylor W, Solano M, Stone M, Mallams J, Mues G (1998). Prognostic value of K-ras mutations, ras oncoprotein, and c-erb B-2 oncoprotein expression in adenocarcinoma of the lung. Am J Clin Oncol 21: 155-160.

1452. Nenninger R, Schultz A, Vandekerckhove B, Hunig T, Muller-Hermelink HK, Marx A (1997). Abnormal T lymphocyte development in myasthenia gravis-associated thymomas. In: Epithelial Tumors of the Thymus: Pathology, Biology, Treatment, Epithelial Tumors of the Thymus, Pathology, Biology, Treatment, Plenum Pub Corp: New York, London .

1453. Nerlich A, Berndt R, Schleicher E (1991). Differential basement membrane composition in multiple epithelioid haemangioendotheliomas of liver and lung. Histopathology 18: 303-307.

1454. Newman HA, Cordell AR, Prichard RW (1966). Intracardiac myxomas. Literature review and report of six cases, one successfully treated. Am Surg 32: 219-230.

1455. Ng AK, Bernardo MV, Weller E, Backstrand K, Silver B, Marcus KC, Tarbell NJ, Stevenson MA, Friedberg JW, Mauch PM (2002). Second malignancy after Hodgkin disease treated with radiation therapy with or without chemotherapy: long-term risks and risk factors. Blood 100: 1989-1996.

1456. Ng WL, Ma L (1983). Is sclerosing hemangioma of lung an alveolar mixed tumour? Pathology 15: 205-211.

1457. Nguyen GK (1995). Cytopathology of pulmonary carcinoid tumors in sputum and bronchial brushings. Acta Cytol 39: 1152-1160.

1458. Nichols CR (1991). Mediastinal germ cell tumors. Clinical features and biologic correlates. Chest 99: 472-479.

1459. Nichols CR, Heerema NA, Palmer C, Loehrer PJSr, Williams SD, Einhorn LH (1987). Klinefelter's syndrome associated with mediastinal germ cell neoplasms. J Clin Oncol 5: 1290-1294.

1460. Nichols CR, Hoffman R, Einhorn LH, Williams SD, Wheeler LA, Garnick MB (1985). Hematologic malignancies associated with primary mediastinal germ-cell tumors. Ann Intern Med 102: 603-609.

1461. Nichols CR, Roth BJ, Heerema N, Griep J, Tricot G (1990). Hematologic neoplasia associated with primary mediastinal germ-cell tumors. N Engl J Med 322: 1425-1429.

1462. Nichols CR, Saxman S, Williams SD, Loehrer PJ, Miller ME, Wright C, Einhorn LH (1990). Primary mediastinal nonseminomatous germ cell tumors. A modern single institution experience. Cancer 65: 1641-1646.

1463. Nicholson AG, Goldstraw P, Fisher C (1998). Synovial sarcoma of the pleura and its differentiation from other primary pleural tumours: a clinicopathological and immunohistochemical review of three cases. Histopathology 33: 508-513.

1464. Nicholson AG, Magkou C, Snead D, Vohra HA, Sheppard MN, Goldstraw P, Beddow E, Hansell DM, Travis WD, Corrin B (2002). Unusual sclerosing haemangiomas and sclerosing haemangioma-like lesions, and the value of TTF-1 in making the diagnosis. Histopathology 41: 404-413.

1465. Nicholson AG, Perry LJ, Cury PM, Jackson P, McCormick CM, Corrin B, Wells AU (2001). Reproducibility of the WHO/IASLC grading system for pre-invasive squamous lesions of the bronchus: a study of inter-observer and intra-observer variation. Histopathology 38: 202-208.

1466. Nicholson AG, Rigby M, Lincoln C, Meller S, Fisher C (1997). Synovial sarcoma of the heart. Histopathology 30: 349-352.

1467. Nicholson AG, Wotherspoon AC, Diss TC, Butcher DN, Sheppard MN, Isaacson PG, Corrin B (1995). Pulmonary B-cell non-Hodgkin's lymphomas. The value of immunohistochemistry and gene analysis in diagnosis. Histopathology 26: 395-403.

1468. Nicholson AG, Wotherspoon AC, Diss TC, Singh N, Butcher DN, Pan LX, Isaacson PG, Corrin B (1996). Lymphomatoid granulomatosis: evidence that some cases represent Epstein-Barr virus-associated B-cell lymphoma. Histopathology 29: 317-324.

1469. Nicholson AG, Wotherspoon AC, Jones AL, Sheppard MN, Isaacson PG, Corrin B (1996). Pulmonary B-cell non-Hodgkin's lymphoma associated with autoimmune disorders: a clinicopathologi-cal review of six cases. Eur Respir J 9: 2022-2025.

1470. Nicholson SA, Beasley MB, Brambilla E, Hasleton PS, Colby TV, Sheppard MN, Falk R, Travis WD (2002). Small cell lung carcinoma (SCLC): a clinicopathologic study of 100 cases with surgical specimens. Am J Surg Pathol 26: 1184-1197.

1471. Nicholson SA, Okby NT, Khan MA, Welsh JA, McMenamin MG, Travis WD, Jett JR, Tazelaar HD, Trastek V, Pairolero PC, Corn PG, Herman JG, Liotta LA, Caporaso NE, Harris CC (2001). Alterations of p14ARF, p53, and p73 genes involved in the E2F-1-mediated apoptotic pathways in non-small cell lung carcinoma. Cancer Res 61: 5636-5643.

1472. Niehues T, Harms D, Jurgens H, Gobel U (1996). Treatment of pediatric malignant thymoma: long-term remission in a 14-year-old boy with EBV-associated thymic carcinoma by aggressive, combined modality treatment. Med Pediatr Oncol 26: 419-424.

1473. Nielsen GP, O'Connell JX, Dickersin GR, Rosenberg AE (1997). Solitary fibrous tumor of soft tissue: a report of 15 cases, including 5 malignant examples with light microscopic, immunohistochemical, and ultrastructural data. Mod Pathol 10: 1028-1037.

1474. Niho S, Suzuki K, Yokose T, Kodama T, Nishiwaki Y, Esumi H (1998). Monoclonality of both pale cells and cuboidal cells of sclerosing hemangioma of the lung. Am J Pathol 152: 1065-1069.

1475. Niho S, Yokose T, Suzuki K, Kodama T, Nishiwaki Y, Mukai K (1999). Monoclonality of atypical adenomatous hyperplasia of the lung. Am J Pathol 154: 249-254.

1476. Nind NR, Attanoos RL, Gibbs AR (2003). Unusual intraparenchymal growth patterns of malignant pleural mesothelioma. Histopathology 42: 150-155.

1477. Nine JS, Yousem SA, Paradis IL, Keenan R, Griffith BP (1994). Lymphangioleiomyomatosis: recurrence after lung transplantation. J Heart Lung Transplant 13: 714-719.

1478. Nishimura M, Kodama T, Nishiyama H, Nishiwaki Y, Yokose T, Shimosato Y (1997). A case of sarcomatoid carcinoma of the thymus. Pathol Int 47: 260-263.

1479. Nishio M, Koshikawa T, Yatabe Y, Kuroishi T, Suyama M, Nagatake M, Sugiura T, Ariyoshi Y, Mitsudomi T, Takahashi T (1997). Prognostic significance of cyclin D1 and retinoblastoma expression in combination with p53 abnormalities in primary, resected non-small cell lung cancers. Clin Cancer Res 3: 1051-1058.

1480. Nistal M, Garcia-Viera M, Martinez-Garcia C, Paniagua R (1994). Epithelial-myoepithelial tumor of the bronchus. Am J Surg Pathol 18: 421-425.

1481. Niwa K, Tanaka T, Mori H, Takahashi M (1987). Extramedullary plasmacytoma of the mediastinum. Jpn J Clin Oncol 17: 95-100.

1482. Noble EP, St Jeor ST, Ritchie T, Syndulko K, St Jeor SC, Fitch RJ, Brunner RL, Sparkes RS (1994). D2 dopamine receptor gene and cigarette smoking: a reward gene? Med Hypotheses 42: 257-260.

1483. Noguchi M, Kodama T, Shimosato Y, Koide T, Naruke T, Singh G, Katyal SL (1986). Papillary adenoma of type 2 pneumocytes. Am J Surg Pathol 10: 134-139.

1484. Noguchi M, Morikawa A, Kawasaki M, Matsuno Y, Yamada T, Hirohashi S, Kondo H, Shimosato Y (1995). Small adeno-

carcinoma of the lung. Histologic characteristics and prognosis. Cancer 75: 2844-2852.
1485. Noh TW, Kim SH, Lim BJ, Yang WI, Chung KY (2001). Thymoma with pseudosarcomatous stroma. Yonsei Med J 42: 571-575.
1486. Nolan LP, Heatley MK (2001). The value of immunocytochemistry in distinguishing between clear cell carcinoma of the kidney and ovary. Int J Gynecol Pathol 20: 155-159.
1487. Nomori H, Kaseda S, Kobayashi K, Ishihara T, Yanai N, Torikata C (1988). Adenoid cystic carcinoma of the trachea and main-stem bronchus. A clinical, histopathologic, and immunohistochemical study. J Thorac Cardiovasc Surg 96: 271-277.
1488. Nonomura A, Kurumaya H, Kono N, Nakanuma Y, Ohta G, Terahata S, Matsubara F, Matsuda T, Asaka T, Nishino T (1988). Primary pulmonary artery sarcoma. Report of two autopsy cases studied by immunohistochemistry and electron microscopy, and review of 110 cases reported in the literature. Acta Pathol Jpn 38: 883-896.
1489. Nonomura A, Mizukami Y, Shimizu J, Watanabe Y, Kobayashi T, Kamimura R, Takashima T, Nakamura S, Tanimoto K (1995). Small giant cell carcinoma of the lung diagnosed preoperatively by transthoracic aspiration cytology. A case report. Acta Cytol 39: 129-133.
1490. Notohara K, Hsueh CL, Awai M (1990). Glial fibrillary acidic protein immunoreactivity of chondrocytes in immature and mature teratomas. Acta Pathol Jpn 40: 335-342.
1491. Novak L, Castro CY, Listinsky CM (2003). Multiple Langerhans cell nodules in an incidental thymectomy. Arch Pathol Lab Med 127: 218-220.
1492. Novak R, Dasu S, Agamanolis D, Herold W, Malone J, Waterson J (1997). Trisomy 8 is a characteristic finding in pleuropulmonary blastoma. Pediatr Pathol Lab Med 17: 99-103.
1493. Nugent JL, Bunn PAJr, Matthews MJ, Ihde DC, Cohen MH, Gazdar A, Minna JD (1979). CNS metastases in small cell bronchogenic carcinoma: increasing frequency and changing pattern with lengthening survival. Cancer 44: 1885-1893.
1494. Null JA, Livolsi VA, Glenn WW (1977). Hodgkin's disease of the thymus (granulomatous thymoma) and myasthenia gravis: a unique association. Am J Clin Pathol 67: 521-525.
1495. O'Brien JD, Lium JH, Parosa JF, Deyoung BR, Wick MR, Trulock EP (1995). Lymphangiomyomatosis recurrence in the allograft after single-lung transplantation. Am J Respir Crit Care Med 151: 2033-2036.
1496. O'Donovan M, Silva I, Uhlmann V, Bermingham N, Luttich K, Martin C, Sheils O, Killalea A, Kenny C, Pileri S, O'Leary JJ (2001). Expression profile of human herpesvirus 8 (HHV-8) in pyothorax associated lymphoma and in effusion lymphoma. Mol Pathol 54: 80-85.
1497. O'Neill JH, Murray NM, Newsom-Davis J (1988). The Lambert-Eaton myasthenic syndrome. A review of 50 cases. Brain 111 (Pt 3): 577-596.
1498. Obedian E, Fischer DB, Haffty BG (2000). Second malignancies after treatment of early-stage breast cancer: lumpectomy and radiation therapy versus mastectomy. J Clin Oncol 18: 2406-2412.
1499. Oh KY, Shimizu M, Edwards WD, Tazelaar HD, Danielson GK (2001). Surgical pathology of the parietal pericardium: a study of 344 cases (1993-1999). Cardiovasc Pathol 10: 157-168.
1500. Oh YL, Ko YH, Ree HJ (1998). Aspiration cytology of ectopic cervical thymoma mimicking a thyroid mass. A case report. Acta Cytol 42: 1167-1171.
1501. Ohchi T, Tanaka H, Shibuya Y, Shibusa T, Inuzuka M, Satoh M, Abe S (1998). Thymic carcinoid with mucinous stroma: a case report. Respir Med 92: 880-882.
1502. Ohgaki H, Kros JM, Okamoto Y, Gaspert A, Huang H, Kurrer MO (2004). APC mutations are infrequent but present in human lung cancer. Cancer Lett 207: 197-203.
1503. Ohsawa M, Tomita Y, Kanno H, Iuchi K, Kawabata Y, Nakajima Y, Komatsu H, Mukai K, Shimoyama M, Aozasa K (1995). Role of Epstein-Barr virus in pleural lymphomagenesis. Mod Pathol 8: 848-853.
1504. Ohshima K, Muta H, Kawasaki C, Muta K, Deyev V, Kanda M, Kumano Y, Podack ER, Kikuchi M (2001). Bcl10 expression, rearrangement and mutation in MALT lymphoma: correlation with expression of nuclear factor-kappaB. Int J Oncol 19: 283-289.
1505. Ohtsuka M, Satoh H, Inoue M, Yazawa T, Yamashita YT, Sekizawa K, Hasegawa S (2000). Disseminated metastasis of neuroblastomatous component in immature mediastinal teratoma: a case report. Anticancer Res 20: 527-530.
1506. Oizumi S, Igarashi K, Takenaka T, Yamashiro K, Hiraga H, Fujino T, Horimoto M (1999). Primary pericardial synovial sarcoma with detection of the chimeric transcript SYT-SSX. Jpn Circ J 63: 330-332.
1507. Okada S, Ohshima K, Mori M (1994). The Cushing syndrome induced by atrial natriuretic peptide-producing thymic carcinoid. Ann Intern Med 121: 75-76.
1508. Okamoto K, Kato S, Katsuki S, Wada Y, Toyozumi Y, Morimatsu M, Aoyagi S, Imaizumi T (2001). Malignant fibrous histiocytoma of the heart: case report and review of 46 cases in the literature. Intern Med 40: 1222-1226.
1509. Okudela K, Nakamura N, Sano J, Ito T, Kitamura H (2001). Thymic carcinosarcoma consisting of squamous cell carcinomatous and embryonal rhabdomyosarcomatous components. Report of a case and review of the literature. Pathol Res Pract 197: 205-210.
1510. Okumura M, Miyoshi S, Fujii Y, Takeuchi Y, Shiono H, Inoue M, Fukuhara K, Kadota Y, Tateyama H, Eimoto T, Matsuda H (2001). Clinical and functional significance of WHO classification on human thymic epithelial neoplasms: a study of 146 consecutive tumors. Am J Surg Pathol 25: 103-110.
1511. Okumura M, Ohta M, Tateyama H, Nakagawa K, Matsumura A, Maeda H, Tada H, Eimoto T, Matsuda H, Masaoka A (2002). The World Health Organization histologic classification system reflects the oncologic behavior of thymoma: a clinical study of 273 patients. Cancer 94: 624-632.
1512. Oliai BR, Tazelaar HD, Lloyd RV, Doria MI, Trastek VF (1999). Leiomyosarcoma of the pulmonary veins. Am J Surg Pathol 23: 1082-1088.
1513. Oliveira AM, Tazelaar HD, Myers JL, Erickson LA, Lloyd RV (2001). Thyroid transcription factor-1 distinguishes metastatic pulmonary from well-differentiated neuroendocrine tumors of other sites. Am J Surg Pathol 25: 815-819.
1514. Oliveira P, Moura Nunes JF, Clode AL, da Costa JD, Almeida MO (1996). Alveolar adenoma of the lung: further characterization of this uncommon tumour. Virchows Arch 429: 101-108.
1515. Omezzine N, Khouatra C, Larive S, Freyer G, Isaac-Pinet S, Geriniere L, Droz JP, Souquet PJ (2002). Rhabdomyosarcoma arising in mediastinal teratoma in an adult man: a case report. Ann Oncol 13: 323-326.
1516. Onuki N, Wistuba II, Travis WD, Virmani AK, Yashima K, Brambilla E, Hasleton P, Gazdar AF (1999). Genetic changes in the spectrum of neuroendocrine lung tumors. Cancer 85: 600-607.
1517. Oosterhuis JW, Rammeloo RH, Cornelisse CJ, de Jong B, Dam A, Sleijfer DT (1990). Ploidy of malignant mediastinal germ-cell tumors. Hum Pathol 21: 729-732.
1518. Orazi A, Neiman RS, Ulbright TM, Heerema NA, John K, Nichols CR (1993). Hematopoietic precursor cells within the yolk sac tumor component are the source of secondary hematopoietic malignancies in patients with mediastinal germ cell tumors. Cancer 71: 3873-3881.
1519. Ordonez NG (2000). Localized (solitary) fibrous tumor of the pleura. Adv Anat Pathol 7: 327-340.
1520. Osada H, Tatematsu Y, Yatabe Y, Nakagawa T, Konishi H, Harano T, Tezel E, Takada M, Takahashi T (2002). Frequent and histological type-specific inactivation of 14-3-3sigma in human lung cancers. Oncogene 21: 2418-2424.
1521. Osanai M, Igarashi T, Yoshida Y (2001). Unique cellular features in atypical adenomatous hyperplasia of the lung: ultrastructural evidence of its cytodifferentiation. Ultrastruct Pathol 25: 367-373.
1522. Ost D, Joseph C, Sogoloff H, Menezes G (1999). Primary pulmonary melanoma: case report and literature review. Mayo Clin Proc 74: 62-66.
1523. Osterlind K, Andersen PK (1986). Prognostic factors in small cell lung cancer: multivariate model based on 778 patients treated with chemotherapy with or without irradiation. Cancer Res 46: 4189-4194.
1524. Ostoros G, Orosz Z, Kovacs G, Soltesz I (2002). Desmoplastic small round cell tumour of the pleura: a case report with unusual follow-up. Lung Cancer 36: 333-336.
1525. Otani Y, Morishita Y, Yoshida I, Ishikawa S, Otaki A, Aihara T, Nakajima T (1996). A malignant Triton tumor in the anterior mediastinum requiring emergency surgery: report of a case. Surg Today 26: 834-836.
1526. Ovcak Z, Masera A, Lamovec J (1992). Malignant fibrous histiocytoma of the heart. Arch Pathol Lab Med 116: 872-874.
1527. Ovrum E, Birkeland S (1979). Mediastinal tumours and cysts. A review of 91 cases. Scand J Thorac Cardiovasc Surg 13: 161-168.
1528. Oyaizu T, Arita S, Hatano T, Tsubura A (1996). Immunohistochemical detection of estrogen and progesterone receptors performed with an antigen-retrieval technique on methacarn-fixed paraffin-embedded breast cancer tissues. J Surg Res 60: 69-73.
1529. Pachter MR, Lattes R (1963). Mesenchymal tumors of mediastinum. 1. Tumors of fibrous tissue, adipose tissue, smooth muscle, and striated muscle. Cancer 16: 74-&.
1530. Paez JG, Janne PA, Lee JC, Tracy S, Greulich H, Gabriel S, Herman P, Kaye FJ, Lindeman N, Boggon TJ, Naoki K, Sasaki H, Fujii Y, Eck MJ, Sellers WR, Johnson BE, Meyerson M (2004). EGFR Mutations in Lung Cancer: Correlation with Clinical Response to Gefitinib Therapy. Science .
1531. Paget S (1989). The distribution of secondary growths in cancer of the breast. 1889. Cancer Metastasis Rev 8: 98-101.
1532. Palanisamy N, Abou-Elella AA, Chaganti SR, Houldsworth J, Offit K, Louie DC, Terayu-Feldstein J, Cigudosa JC, Rao PH, Sanger WG, Weisenburger DD, Chaganti RS (2002). Similar patterns of genomic alterations characterize primary mediastinal large-B-cell lymphoma and diffuse large-B-cell lymphoma. Genes Chromosomes Cancer 33: 114-122.
1533. Palcic B, Garner DM, Beveridge J, Sun XR, Doudkine A, MacAulay C, Lam S, Payne PW (2002). Increase of sensitivity of sputum cytology using high-resolution image cytometry: field study results. Cytometry 50: 168-176.
1534. Pallesen G, Hamilton-Dutoit SJ (1988). Ki-1 (CD30) antigen is regularly expressed by tumor cells of embryonal carcinoma. Am J Pathol 133: 446-450.
1535. Palmer FJ, Sawyers TM (1978). Hyperparathyroidism, chemodectoma, thymoma, and myasthenia gravis. Arch Intern Med 138: 1402-1403.
1536. Palmer PE, Safaii H, Wolfe HJ (1976). Alpha1-antitrypsin and alpha-fetoprotein. Protein markers in endodermal sinus (yolk sac) tumors. Am J Clin Pathol 65: 575-582.
1537. Pan CC, Chen PC, Wang LS, Chi KH, Chiang H (2001). Thymoma is associated with an increased risk of second malignancy. Cancer 92: 2406-2411.
1538. Pan CC, Chen WY, Chiang H (2001). Spindle cell and mixed spindle/lymphocytic thymomas: an integrated clinicopathologic and immunohistochemical study of 81 cases. Am J Surg Pathol 25: 111-120.
1539. Pan CC, Ho DM, Chen WY, Huang CW, Chiang H (1998). Ki67 labelling index correlates with stage and histology but not significantly with prognosis in thymoma. Histopathology 33: 453-458.
1540. Pan CC, Wu HP, Yang CF, Chen WY, Chiang H (1994). The clinicopathological correlation of epithelial subtyping in thymoma: a study of 112 consecutive cases. Hum Pathol 25: 893-899.
1541. Paniagua JR, Sadaba JR, Davidson LA, Munsch CM (2000). Cystic tumour of the atrioventricular nodal region: report of a case successfully treated with surgery. Heart 83: E6.
1542. Panos A, Kalangos A, Sztajzel J (1997). Left atrial myxoma presenting with myocardial infarction. Case report and review of the literature. Int J Cardiol 62: 73-75.
1543. Papadimitriou A, Neustein HB, Dimauro S, Stanton R, Bresolin N (1984). Histiocytoid cardiomyopathy of infancy: deficiency of reducible cytochrome b in heart mitochondria. Pediatr Res 18: 1023-1028.
1544. Papagiannopoulos K, Hughes S, Nicholson AG, Goldstraw P (2002). Cystic lung lesions in the pediatric and adult population: surgical experience at the Brompton Hospital. Ann Thorac Surg 73: 1594-1598.
1545. Papagiannopoulos KA, Sheppard M, Bush AP, Goldstraw P (2001). Pleuropulmonary blastoma: is prophylactic resection of congenital lung cysts effective? Ann Thorac Surg 72: 604-605.

1546. Parente F, Grosgeorge J, Coindre JM, Terrier P, Vilain O, Turc-Carel C (1999). Comparative genomic hybridization reveals novel chromosome deletions in 90 primary soft tissue tumors. Cancer Genet Cytogenet 115: 89-95.
1547. Parish JM, Rosenow ECI, Swensen SJ, Crotty TB (1996). Pulmonary artery sarcoma. Clinical features. Chest 110: 1480-1488.
1548. Park HK, Park CM, Ko KH, Rim MS, Kim YI, Hwang JH, Im SC, Kim YC, Park KO (2000). A case of Cushing's syndrome in ACTH-secreting mediastinal paraganglioma. Korean J Intern Med 15: 142-146.
1549. Park IW, Wistuba II, Maitra A, Milchgrub S, Virmani AK, Minna JD, Gazdar AF (1999). Multiple clonal abnormalities in the bronchial epithelium of patients with lung cancer. J Natl Cancer Inst 91: 1863-1868.
1550. Park MJ, Shimizu K, Nakano T, Park YB, Kohno T, Tani M, Yokota J (2003). Pathogenetic and biologic significance of TP14ARF alterations in nonsmall cell lung carcinoma. Cancer Genet Cytogenet 141: 5-13.
1551. Parkash V, Gerald WL, Parma A, Miettinen M, Rosai J (1995). Desmoplastic small round cell tumor of the pleura. Am J Surg Pathol 19: 659-665.
1552. Parker JR, Ro JY, Ordonez NG (1999). Benign nevus cell aggregates in the thymus: a case report. Mod Pathol 12: 329-332.
1553. Parkin DM, Pisani P, Lopez AD, Masuyer E (1994). At least one in seven cases of cancer is caused by smoking. Global estimates for 1985. Int J Cancer 59: 494-504.
1554. Parkin DM, Whelan SL, Ferlay J, Teppo L, Thomas DB (2002). Cancer Incidence in Five Continents, Vol. VIII. IARC Scientific Publications No. 155. IARCPress: Lyon.
1555. Parravicini C, Chandran B, Corbellino M, Berti E, Paulli M, Moore PS, Chang Y (2000). Differential viral protein expression in Kaposi's sarcoma-associated herpesvirus-infected diseases: Kaposi's sarcoma, primary effusion lymphoma, and multicentric Castleman's disease. Am J Pathol 156: 743-749.
1556. Parrens M, Dubus P, Danjoux M, Jougon J, Brousset P, Velly JF, de Mascarel A, Merlio JP (2002). Mucosa-associated lymphoid tissue of the thymus hyperplasia vs lymphoma. Am J Clin Pathol 117: 51-56.
1557. Paties C, Zangrandi A, Vassallo G, Rindi G, Solcia E (1991). Multidirectional carcinoma of the thymus with neuroendocrine and sarcomatoid components and carcinoid syndrome. Pathol Res Pract 187: 170-177.
1558. Paulli M, Strater J, Gianelli U, Rousset MT, Gambacorta M, Orlandi E, Klersy C, Lavabre-Bertrand T, Morra E, Manegold C, Lazzarino M, Magrini U, Moller P (1999). Mediastinal B-cell lymphoma: a study of its histomorphologic spectrum based on 109 cases. Hum Pathol 30: 178-187.
1559. Paulsen SM, Egeblad K (1983). Sarcoma of the pulmonary artery. A light and electron microscopic study. J Submicrosc Cytol 15: 811-821.
1560. Payne WS, Ellis FH, Woolner LB, Moersch HJ (1959). The surgical treatment of cylindroma (adenoid cystic carcinoma) and muco-epidermoid tumors of the bronchus. J Thorac Cardiovasc Surg 38: 709-726.
1561. Payne WS, Woolner LB, Fontana RS (1964). Bronchial tumors originating from mucous glands - current classification and unusual manifestations. Med Clin North Am 48: 945-960.
1562. Pederzolli C, Terrini A, Ricci A, Motta A, Martinelli L, Graffigna A (2002). Pulmonary valve lipoma presenting as syncope. Ann Thorac Surg 73: 1305-1306.
1563. Pelosi G, Fraggetta F, Maffini F, Solli P, Cavallon A, Viale G (2001). Pulmonary epithelial-myoepithelial tumor of unproven malignant potential: report of a case and review of the literature. Mod Pathol 14: 521-526.
1564. Pelosi G, Fraggetta F, Pasini F, Maisonneuve P, Sonzogni A, Iannucci A, Terzi A, Bresaola E, Valduga F, Lupo C, Viale G (2001). Immunoreactivity for thyroid transcription factor-1 in stage I non-small cell carcinomas of the lung. Am J Surg Pathol 25: 363-372.
1565. Pelosi G, Fraggetta F, Sonzogni A, Fazio N, Cavallon A, Viale G (2000). CD99 immunoreactivity in gastrointestinal and pulmonary neuroendocrine tumours. Virchows Arch 437: 270-274.
1566. Pelosi G, Pasini F, Sonzogni A, Maffini F, Maisonneuve P, Iannucci A, Terzi A, De Manzoni G, Bresaola E, Viale G (2003). Prognostic implications of neuroendocrine differentiation and hormone production in patients with Stage I nonsmall cell lung carcinoma. Cancer 97: 2487-2497.
1567. Penzel R, Hoegel J, Schmitz W, Blaeker H, Morresi-Hauf A, Aulmann S, Hecker E, Mechtersheimer G, Otto HF, Rieker RJ (2003). Clusters of chromosomal imbalances in thymic epithelial tumours are associated with the WHO classification and the staging system according to Masaoka. Int J Cancer 105: 494-498.
1568. Perchinsky MJ, Lichtenstein SV, Tyers GF (1997). Primary cardiac tumors: forty years' experience with 71 patients. Cancer 79: 1809-1815.
1569. Perdikogianni C, Stiakaki E, Danilatou V, Delides G, Kalmanti M (2001). Pleuropulmonary blastoma: an aggressive intrathoracic neoplasm of childhood. Pediatr Hematol Oncol 18: 259-266.
1570. Perera FP, Mooney LA, Stampfer M, Phillips DH, Bell DA, Rundle A, Cho S, Tsai WY, Ma J, Blackwood A, Tang D (2002). Associations between carcinogen-DNA damage, glutathione S-transferase genotypes, and risk of lung cancer in the prospective Physicians' Health Cohort Study. Carcinogenesis 23: 1641-1646.
1571. Perez-Ordonez B, Erlandson RA, Rosai J (1996). Follicular dendritic cell tumor: report of 13 additional cases of a distinctive entity. Am J Surg Pathol 20: 944-955.
1572. Perlman EJ, Cushing B, Hawkins E, Griffin CA (1994). Cytogenetic analysis of childhood endodermal sinus tumors: a Pediatric Oncology Group study. Pediatr Pathol 14: 695-708.
1573. Perlman EJ, Hu J, Ho D, Cushing B, Lauer S, Castleberry RP (2000). Genetic analysis of childhood endodermal sinus tumors by comparative genomic hybridization. J Pediatr Hematol Oncol 22: 100-105.
1574. Perlman EJ, Valentine MB, Griffin CA, Look AT (1996). Deletion of 1p36 in childhood endodermal sinus tumors by two-color fluorescence in situ hybridization: a pediatric oncology group study. Genes Chromosomes Cancer 16: 15-20.
1575. Perrone T, Frizzera G, Rosai J (1986). Mediastinal diffuse large-cell lymphoma with sclerosis. A clinicopathologic study of 60 cases. Am J Surg Pathol 10: 176-191.
1576. Perry L, Florio R, Dewar A, Nicholson A (2000). Giant lamellar bodies as a feature of pulmonary low-grade MALT lymphomas. Histopathology 36: 240-244.
1577. Pescarmona E, Giardini R, Brisigotti M, Callea F, Pisacane A, Baroni CD (1992). Thymoma in childhood: a clinicopathological study of five cases. Histopathology 21: 65-68.
1578. Pescarmona E, Rendina EA, Ricci C, Baroni CD (1989). Histiocytosis X and lymphoid follicular hyperplasia of the thymus in myasthenia gravis. Histopathology 14: 465-470.
1579. Pescarmona E, Rendina EA, Venuta F, D'Arcangelo E, Pagani M, Ricci C, Ruco LP, Baroni CD (1990). Analysis of prognostic factors and clinicopathological staging of thymoma. Ann Thorac Surg 50: 534-538.
1580. Pescarmona E, Rosati S, Pisacane A, Rendina EA, Venuta F, Baroni CD (1992). Microscopic thymoma: histological evidence of multifocal cortical and medullary origin. Histopathology 20: 263-266.
1581. Petersen I (2003). Chromosome numbers, ploidy and DNA imbalances of human lung cancer. //SUBMITTED// submitted.
1582. Petersen I, Bujard M, Petersen S, Wolf G, Goeze A, Schwendel A, Langreck H, Gellert K, Reichel M, Just K, du Manoir S, Cremer T, Dietel M, Ried T (1997). Patterns of chromosomal imbalances in adenocarcinoma and squamous cell carcinoma of the lung. Cancer Res 57: 2331-2335.
1583. Petersen I, Hidalgo A, Petersen S, Schluns K, Schewe C, Pacyna-Gengelbach M, Goeze A, Krebber B, Knosel T, Kaufmann O, Szymas J, von Deimling A (2000). Chromosomal imbalances in brain metastases of solid tumors. Brain Pathol 10: 395-401.
1584. Petersen S, Aninat-Meyer M, Schluns K, Gellert K, Dietel M, Petersen I (2000). Chromosomal alterations in the clonal evolution to the metastatic stage of squamous cell carcinomas of the lung. Br J Cancer 82: 65-73.
1585. Petersen S, Wolf G, Bockmuhl U, Gellert K, Dietel M, Petersen I (1998). Allelic loss on chromosome 10q in human lung cancer: association with tumour progression and metastatic phenotype. Br J Cancer 77: 270-276.
1586. Petitjean B, Jardin F, Joly B, Martin-Garcia N, Tilly H, Picquenot JM, Briere J, Danel C, Mehaut S, Abd-Al-Samad I, Copie-Bergman C, Delfau-Larue MH, Gaulard P (2002). Pyothorax-associated lymphoma: a peculiar clinicopathologic entity derived from B cells at late stage of differentiation and with occasional aberrant dual B- and T-cell phenotype. Am J Surg Pathol 26: 724-732.
1587. Peto J, Decarli A, La Vecchia C, Levi F, Negri E (1999). The European mesothelioma epidemic. Br J Cancer 79: 666-672.
Peto J, Hodgson JT, Matthews FE, Jones JR (1995). Continuing increase in mesothelioma mortality in Britain. Lancet 345: 535-539.
1588. A. Peto R, Darby S, Deo H, Silcocks P, Whitley E, Doll R (2000). Smoking, smoking cessation, and lung cancer in the UK since 1950: combination of national statistics with two case-control studies. BMJ 321: 323-329.
Peto R, Lopez AD, Boreham J, Thun M, Heath CJr, Doll R (1994). Mortality from Smoking in Developed Countries 1950-2000: Iindirect estimates from national vital statistics. Oxford University Press: Oxford.
1589. A. Peto R (2004). WHO Mortality statistics with UN population estimates, 1950-2000. www.ctsu.ox.ac.uk.
1590. Petruzzelli GJ (2001). The biology of distant metastases in head and neck cancer. ORL J Otorhinolaryngol Relat Spec 63: 192-201.
1591. Pfeifer GP, Denissenko MF, Olivier M, Tretyakova N, Hecht SS, Hainaut P (2002). Tobacco smoke carcinogens, DNA damage and p53 mutations in smoking-associated cancers. Oncogene 21: 7435-7451.
1592. Phillips GW, Choong M (1991). Chondrosarcoma presenting as an anterior mediastinal mass. Clin Radiol 43: 63-64.
1593. Picaud JC, Levrey H, Bouvier R, Chappuis JP, Louis D, Frappaz D, Claris O, Bellon G (2000). Bilateral cystic pleuropulmonary blastoma in early infancy. J Pediatr 136: 834-836.
1594. Pich A, Chiarle R, Chiusa L, Ponti R, Geuna M, Casadio C, Maggi G, Palestro G (1995). Long-term survival of thymoma patients by histologic pattern and proliferative activity. Am J Surg Pathol 19: 918-926.
1595. Pileri SA, Gaidano G, Zinzani PL, Falini B, Gaulard P, Zucca E, Pieri F, Berra E, Sabattini E, Ascani S, Piccioli M, Johnson PW, Giardini R, Pescarmona E, Novero D, Piccaluga PP, Marafioti T, Alonso MA, Cavalli F (2003). Primary mediastinal B-cell lymphoma: high frequency of BCL-6 mutations and consistent expression of the transcription factors OCT-2, BOB.1, and PU.1 in the absence of immunoglobulins. Am J Pathol 162: 243-253.
1596. Pileri SA, Grogan TM, Harris NL, Banks P, Campo E, Chan JK, Favera RD, Delsol G, Wolf-Peeters C, Falini B, Gascoyne RD, Gaulard P, Gatter KC, Isaacson PG, Jaffe ES, Kluin P, Knowles DM, Mason DY, Mori S, Muller-Hermelink HK, Piris MA, Ralfkiaer E, Stein H, Su IJ, Warnke RA, Weiss LM (2002). Tumours of histiocytes and accessory dendritic cells: an immunohistochemical approach to classification from the International Lymphoma Study Group based on 61 cases. Histopathology 41: 1-29.
1597. Pimpec-Barthes F, Martinod E, Riquet M, Saint-Blancard P, Jancovici R (1998). [Tumors of the phrenic nerve]. Rev Mal Respir 15: 93-95.
1598. Pinede L, Duhaut P, Loire R (2001). Clinical presentation of left atrial cardiac myxoma. A series of 112 consecutive cases. Medicine (Baltimore) 80: 159-172.
1599. Pinkard NB, Wilson RW, Lawless N, Dodd LG, McAdams HP, Koss MN, Travis WD (1996). Calcifying fibrous pseudotumor of pleura. A report of three cases of a newly described entity involving the pleura. Am J Clin Pathol 105: 189-194.
1600. Pinkus GS, Pinkus JL, Langhoff E, Matsumura F, Yamashiro S, Mosialos G, Said JW (1997). Fascin, a sensitive new marker for Reed-Sternberg cells of hodgkin's disease. Evidence for a dendritic or B cell derivation? Am J Pathol 150: 543-562.
1601. Pinyol M, Cobo F, Bea S, Jares P, Nayach I, Fernandez PL, Montserrat E, Cardesa A, Campo E (1998). p16(INK4a) gene inactivation by deletions, mutations, and hypermethylation is associated with transformed and aggressive variants of non-Hodgkin's lymphomas. Blood 91: 2977-2984.
1602. Pipitone S, Mongiovi M, Grillo R, Gagliano S, Sperandeo V (2002). Cardiac rhabdomyoma in intrauterine life: clinical features and natural history. A case series

and review of published reports. Ital Heart J 3: 48-52.
1603. Pisani RJ, DeRemee RA (1990). Clinical implications of the histopathologic diagnosis of pulmonary lymphomatoid granulomatosis. Mayo Clin Proc 65: 151-163.
1604. Pittaluga S, Uppenkamp M, Cossman J (1987). Development of T3/T cell receptor gene expression in human pre-T neoplasms. Blood 69: 1062-1067.
1605. Pogrebniak HW, Haas G, Linehan WM, Rosenberg SA, Pass HI (1992). Renal cell carcinoma: resection of solitary and multiple metastases. Ann Thorac Surg 54: 33-38.
1606. Poletti V, Casadei G, Boaron M, Bertanti T, Venturi P, Colinelli C, Baruzzi G (1997). Epithelioid haemangioendothelioma of the lung imitating clinical features of pulmonary histiocytosis X. Monaldi Arch Chest Dis 52: 346-348.
1607. Poletti V, Romagna M, Allen KA, Gasponi A, Spiga L (1995). Bronchoalveolar lavage in the diagnosis of disseminated lung tumors. Acta Cytol 39: 472-477.
1608. Polskj JM, Evans HL, Grosso LE, Popovic WJ, Taylor L, Dunphy CH (2000). CD7 and CD56-positive primary effusion lymphoma in a human immunodeficiency virus-negative host. Leuk Lymphoma 39: 633-639.
1609. Pomplun S, Wotherspoon AC, Shah G, Goldstraw P, Ladas G, Nicholson AG (2002). Immunohistochemical markers in the differentiation of thymic and pulmonary neoplasms. Histopathology 40: 152-158.
1610. Poppema S (1994). Case no D2 Slide workshop T-cell lymphomas: Compariosn of Eastern and Western Experience. Pre-Congress Meeting of XX International Congress of The International Academy of Pathology
1611. Popper HH, el Shabrawi Y, Wockel W, Hofler G, Kenner L, Juttner-Smolle FM, Pongratz MG (1994). Prognostic importance of human papilloma virus typing in squamous cell papilloma of the bronchus: comparison of in situ hybridization and the polymerase chain reaction. Hum Pathol 25: 1191-1197.
1612. Popper HH, Wirnsberger G, Juttner-Smolle FM, Pongratz MG, Sommersgutter M (1992). The predictive value of human papilloma virus (HPV) typing in the prognosis of bronchial squamous cell papillomas. Histopathology 21: 323-330.
1613. Povey S, Burley MW, Attwood J, Benham F, Hunt D, Jeremiah SJ, Franklin D, Gillett G, Malas S, Robson EB (1994). Two loci for tuberous sclerosis: one on 9q34 and one on 16p13. Ann Hum Genet 58 (Pt 2): 107-127.
1614. Prat J, Bhan AK, Dickersin GR, Robboy SJ, Scully RE (1982). Hepatoid yolk sac tumor of the ovary (endodermal sinus tumor with hepatoid differentiation): a light microscopic, ultrastructural and immunohistochemical study of seven cases. Cancer 50: 2355-2368.
1615. Pratt JW, Cohen DM, Mutabagani KH, Davis JT, Wheller JJ (2000). Neonatal intrapericardial teratomas: clinical and surgical considerations. Cardiol Young 10: 27-31.
1616. Premaratne S, Hasaniya NW, Arakaki HY, Mugiishi MM, Mamiya RT, McNamara JJ (1995). Atrial myxomas: experiences with 35 patients in Hawaii. Am J Surg 169: 600-603.
1617. Prichard RW (1951). Tumors of the Heart. Arch Pathol 98-128.
1618. Prichard RW (1951). Tumors of the heart - review of the subject and report of 150 cases. AMA Arch Pathol 51: 98-128.
1619. Priest JR, McDermott MB, Bhatia S, Watterson J, Manivel JC, Dehner LP (1997). Pleuropulmonary blastoma: a clinicopathologic study of 50 cases. Cancer 80: 147-161.
1620. Priest JR, Watterson J, Strong L, Huff V, Woods WG, Byrd RL, Friend SH, Newsham I, Amylon MD, Pappo A, Mahoney DH, Langston C, Heyn R, Kohut G, Freyer DR, Bostrom B, Richardson MS, Barredo J, Dehner LP (1996). Pleuropulmonary blastoma: a marker for familial disease. J Pediatr 128: 220-224.
1621. Prommegger R, Salzer GM (1998). Long-term results of surgery for adenoid cystic carcinoma of the trachea and bronchi. Eur J Surg Oncol 24: 440-444.
1622. Przygodzki RM, Finkelstein SD, Langer JC, Swalsky PA, Fishback N, Bakker A, Guinee DG, Koss M, Travis WD (1996). Analysis of p53, K-ras-2, and C-raf-1 in pulmonary neuroendocrine tumors. Correlation with histological subtype and clinical outcome. Am J Pathol 148: 1531-1541.
1623. Przygodzki RM, Hubbs AE, Zhao FQ, O'Leary TJ (2002). Primary mediastinal seminomas: evidence of single and multiple KIT mutations. Lab Invest 82: 1369-1375.
1624. Przygodzki RM, Koss MN, O'Leary TJ (2001). Pleomorphic (giant and/or spindle cell) carcinoma of lung shows a high percentage of variant CYP1A12. Mol Diagn 6: 109-115.
1625. Pucci A, Gagliardotto P, Zanini C, Pansini S, di Summa M, Mollo F (2000). Histopathologic and clinical characterization of cardiac myxoma: review of 53 cases from a single institution. Am Heart J 140: 134-138.
1626. Puglisi F, Finato N, Mariuzzi L, Marchini C, Floretti G, Beltrami CA (1995). Microscopic thymoma and myasthenia gravis. J Clin Pathol 48: 682-683.
1627. Putnam JBJr, Schantz SP, Pugh WC, Hickey RC, Samaan NA, Garza R, Suda RW (1990). Extended en bloc resection of a primary mediastinal parathyroid carcinoma. Ann Thorac Surg 50: 138-140.
1628. Puvaneswary M, Edwards JR, Bastian BC, Khatri SK (2000). Pericardial lipoma: ultrasound, computed tomography and magnetic resonance imaging findings. Australas Radiol 44: 321-324.
1629. Quint LE, Tummala S, Brisson LJ, Francis IR, Krupnick AS, Kazerooni EA, Iannettoni MD, Whyte RI, Orringer MB (1996). Distribution of distant metastases from newly diagnosed non-small cell lung cancer. Ann Thorac Surg 62: 246-250.
1630. Quintanilla-Martinez L, Wilkins EWJr, Choi N, Efird J, Hug E, Harris NL (1994). Thymoma. Histologic subclassification is an independent prognostic factor. Cancer 74: 606-617.
1631. Quintanilla-Martinez L, Wilkins EWJr, Ferry JA, Harris NL (1993). Thymoma—morphologic subclassification correlates with invasiveness and immunohistologic features: a study of 122 cases. Hum Pathol 24: 958-969.
1632. Quintanilla-Martinez L, Zukerberg LR, Harris NL (1992). Prethymic adult lymphoblastic lymphoma. A clinicopathologic and immunohistochemical analysis. Am J Surg Pathol 16: 1075-1084.
1633. Raab SS, Berg LC, Swanson PE, Wick MR (1993). Adenocarcinoma in the lung in patients with breast cancer. A prospective analysis of the discriminatory value of immunohistology. Am J Clin Pathol 100: 27-35.
1634. Raaf HN, Raaf JH (1994). Sarcomas related to the heart and vasculature. Semin Surg Oncol 10: 374-382.
1635. Rabkin MS, Kjeldsberg CR, Hammond ME, Wittwer CT, Nathwani B (1988). Clinical, ultrastructural immunohistochemical and DNA content analysis of lymphomas having features of interdigitating reticulum cells. Cancer 61: 1594-1601.
1636. Ramachandra S, Hollowood K, Bisceglia M, Fletcher CD (1995). Inflammatory pseudotumour of soft tissues: a clinicopathological and immunohistochemical analysis of 18 cases. Histopathology 27: 313-323.
1637. Ramani P, Shah A (1993). Lymphangiomatosis. Histologic and immunohistochemical analysis of four cases. Am J Surg Pathol 17: 329-335.
1638. Ramaswamy S, Ross KN, Lander ES, Golub TR (2003). A molecular signature of metastasis in primary solid tumors. Nat Genet 33: 49-54.
1639. Ramos-Nino ME, Timblin CR, Mossman BT (2002). Mesothelial cell transformation requires increased AP-1 binding activity and ERK-dependent Fra-1 expression. Cancer Res 62: 6065-6069.
1640. Rao SK, Fraire AE (1995). Alveolar Cell Hyperplasia in Association with Adenocarcinoma of Lung. Mod Pathol 8: 165-169.
1641. Ratnasinghe D, Yao SX, Tangrea JA, Qiao YL, Andersen MR, Barrett MJ, Giffen CA, Erozan Y, Tockman MS, Taylor PR (2001). Polymorphisms of the DNA repair gene XRCC1 and lung cancer risk. Cancer Epidemiol Biomarkers Prev 10: 119-123.
1642. Raunio H, Rautio A, Gullsten H, Pelkonen O (2001). Polymorphisms of CYP2A6 and its practical consequences. Br J Clin Pharmacol 52: 357-363.
1643. Ravandi-Kashani F, Cortes J, Giles FJ (2000). Myelodysplasia presenting as granulocytic sarcoma of mediastinum causing superior vena cava syndrome. Leuk Lymphoma 36: 631-637.
1644. Refior M, Mees K (2000). [Coexistence of bilateral paraganglioma of the A. carotis, thymoma and thyroid adenoma: a chance finding?]. Laryngorhinootologie 79: 337-340.
1645. Regnard JF, Magdeleinat P, Dromer C, Dulmet E, de Montpreville V, Levi JF, Levasseur P (1996). Prognostic factors and long-term results after thymoma resection: a series of 307 patients. J Thorac Cardiovasc Surg 112: 376-384.
1646. Reichle FA, Rosemond GP (1966). Mucoepidermoid tumors of the bronchus. J Thorac Cardiovasc Surg 51: 443-448.
1647. Reid AH, Tsai MM, Venzon DJ, Wright CF, Lack EE, O'Leary TJ (1996). MDM2 amplification, P53 mutation, and accumulation of the P53 gene product in malignant fibrous histiocytoma. Diagn Mol Pathol 5: 65-73.
1648. Reimer D, Singh SM (1981). A kindred with 5 cases of multiple endocrine adenomatosis type I. Hum Hered 31: 84-88.
1649. Reis-Filho JS, Pope LZ, Milanezi F, Balderrama CM, Serapiao MJ, Schmitt FC (2002). Primary epithelial malignant mesothelioma of the pericardium with deciduoid features: cytohistologic and immunohistochemical study. Diagn Cytopathol 26: 117-122.
1650. Reix P, Levrey H, Parret M, Louis D, Bellon G (2000). [Pulmonary cystic images as a presentation of a pleuropulmonary blastoma]. Arch Pediatr 7: 287-289.
1651. Rendina EA, Pescarmona EO, Venuta F, Nardi S, De Rosa G, Martelli M, Ricci C (1988). Thymoma: a clinico-pathologic study based on newly developed morphologic criteria. Tumori 74: 79-84.
1652. Renshaw AA (1995). O-13 (CD99) in spindle-cell tumors - reactivity with hemangiopericytoma, solitary fibrous tumor, synovial sarcoma, and meningioma but rarely with sarcomatoid mesothelioma. Appl Immunohistochem 3: 250-256.
1653. Rettmar K, Stierle U, Sheikhzadeh A, Diederich KW (1993). Primary angiosarcoma of the heart. Report of a case and review of the literature. Jpn Heart J 34: 667-683.
1654. Rettmar K, Stierle U, Sheikhzadeh A, Diederich KW (1993). Primary angiosarcoma of the heart. Report of a case and review of the literature. Jpn Heart J 34: 667-683.
1655. Reuter VE (2002). The pre and post chemotherapy pathologic spectrum of germ cell tumors. Chest Surg Clin N Am 12: 673-694.
1656. Reynen K (1996). Frequency of primary tumors of the heart. Am J Cardiol 77: 107.
1657. Rhodes A, Jasani B, Balaton AJ, Miller KD (2000). Immunohistochemical demonstration of oestrogen and progesterone receptors: correlation of standards achieved on in house tumours with that achieved on external quality assessment material in over 150 laboratories from 26 countries. J Clin Pathol 53: 292-301.
1658. Richkind KE, Wason D, Vidaillet HJ (1994). Cardiac myxoma characterized by clonal telomeric association. Genes Chromosomes Cancer 9: 68-71.
1659. Richmond I, Pritchard GE, Ashcroft T, Avery A, Corris PA, Walters EH (1993). Bronchus associated lymphoid tissue (BALT) in human lung: its distribution in smokers and non-smokers. Thorax 48: 1130-1134.
1660. Rienmuller R, Lloret JL, Tiling R, Groh J, Manert W, Muller KD, Seifert K (1989). MR imaging of pediatric cardiac tumors previously diagnosed by echocardiography. J Comput Assist Tomogr 13: 621-626.
1661. Rigaud G, Moore PS, Taruscio D, Scardoni M, Montresor M, Menestrina F, Scarpa A (2001). Alteration of chromosome arm 6p is characteristic of primary mediastinal B-cell lymphoma, as identified by genome-wide allelotyping. Genes Chromosomes Cancer 31: 191-195.
1662. Ritter JH, Mills SE, Nappi O, Wick MR (1995). Angiosarcoma-like neoplasms of epithelial organs: true endothelial tumors or variants of carcinoma? Semin Diagn Pathol 12: 270-282.
1663. Ritter JH, Wick MR (1999). Primary carcinomas of the thymus gland. Semin Diagn Pathol 16: 18-31.
1664. Ro JY, Chen JL, Lee JS, Sahin AA, Ordonez NG, Ayala AG (1992). Sarcomatoid carcinoma of the lung. Immunohistochemical and ultrastructural studies of 14 cases. Cancer 69: 376-386.
1665. Robert J, Pache JC, Seium Y, de Perrot M, Spiliopoulos A (2002). Pulmonary blastoma: report of five cases and identification of clinical features suggestive of the disease. Eur J Cardiothorac Surg 22: 708-711.
1666. Robles AI, Linke SP, Harris CC (2002). The p53 network in lung carcinogenesis. Oncogene 21: 6898-6907.
1667. Rodenburg CJ, Kluin P, Maes A, Paul

LC (1985). Malignant lymphoma confined to the heart, 13 years after a cadaver kidney transplant. N Engl J Med 313: 122.
1668. Rodenhuis S, Slebos RJ (1990). The ras oncogenes in human lung cancer. Am Rev Respir Dis 142: S27-S30.
1669. Rodenhuis S, Slebos RJ (1992). Clinical significance of ras oncogene activation in human lung cancer. Cancer Res 52: 2665s-2669s.
1670. Rodenhuis S, Slebos RJ, Boot AJ, Evers SG, Mooi WJ, Wagenaar SS, van Bodegom PC, Bos JL (1988). Incidence and possible clinical significance of K-ras oncogene activation in adenocarcinoma of the human lung. Cancer Res 48: 5738-5741.
1671. Rodewald HR, Paul S, Haller C, Bluethmann H, Blum C (2001). Thymus medulla consisting of epithelial islets each derived from a single progenitor. Nature 414: 763-768.
1672. Rodriguez Blanco V, Barriales Alvarez V, Puebla Rojo V, Moller Bustinza I, Castellanos Martinez E, Cortina Llosa A (1997). [Primary cardiac tumors: a review of 29 cases]. Rev Port Cardiol 16: 985-9, 956.
1673. Rodriguez E, Mathew S, Reuter V, Ilson DH, Bosl GJ, Chaganti RS (1992). Cytogenetic analysis of 124 prospectively ascertained male germ cell tumors. Cancer Res 52: 2285-2291.
1674. Rodriguez I, Ayala E, Caballero C, De Miguel C, Matias-Guiu X, Cubilla AL, Rosai J (2001). Solitary fibrous tumor of the thyroid gland: report of seven cases. Am J Surg Pathol 25: 1424-1428.
1675. Roeyen G, Van Schil P, Somville J, Colpaert C, Van Oosterom A (1999). Chordoma of the mediastinum. Eur J Surg Oncol 25: 224-225.
1676. Roggli VL, Vollmer RT, Greenberg SD, McGavran MH, Spjut HJ, Yesner R (1985). Lung cancer heterogeneity: a blinded and randomized study of 100 consecutive cases. Hum Pathol 16: 569-579.
1677. Roglic M, Jukic S, Damjanov I (1975). Cytology of the solitary papilloma of the bronchus. Acta Cytol 19: 11-13.
1678. Rojas M, Godschalk R, Alexandrov K, Cascorbi I, Kriek E, Ostertag J, Van Schooten FJ, Bartsch H (2001). Myeloperoxidase—463A variant reduces benzo[a]pyrene diol epoxide DNA adducts in skin of coal tar treated patients. Carcinogenesis 22: 1015-1018.
1679. Rolla G, Bertero MT, Pastena G, Tartaglia N, Corradi F, Casabona R, Motta M, Caligaris-Cappio F (2002). Primary lymphoma of the heart. A case report and review of the literature. Leuk Res 26: 117-120.
1680. Roller MB, Manoharan A, Lvoff R (1991). Primary cardiac lymphoma. Acta Haematol 85: 47-48.
1681. Rolston R, Sasatomi E, Hunt J, Swalsky PA, Finkelstein SD (2001). Distinguishing de novo second cancer formation from tumor recurrence: mutational fingerprinting by microdissection genotyping. J Mol Diagn 3: 129-132.
1682. Roque L, Oliveira P, Martins C, Carvalho C, Serpa A, Soares J (1996). A nonbalanced translocation (10;16) demonstrated by FISH analysis in a case of alveolar adenoma of the lung. Cancer Genet Cytogenet 89: 34-37.
1683. Rosado-de-Christenson ML, Pugatch RD, Moran CA, Galobardes J (1994). Thymolipoma: analysis of 27 cases. Radiology 193: 121-126.
1684. Rosado-de-Christenson ML, Templeton PA, Moran CA (1992). From the archives of the AFIP. Mediastinal germ cell tumors: radiologic and pathologic correlation. Radiographics 12: 1013-1030.
1685. Rosai J (1996). Ackerman's Surgical Pathology. 8th ed. Mosby-Year Book: St. Louis.
1686. Rosai J, Higa E (1972). Mediastinal endocrine neoplasm, of probable thymic origin, related to carcinoid tumor. Clinicopathologic study of 8 cases. Cancer 29: 1061-1074.
1687. Rosai J, Higa E, Davie J (1972). Mediastinal endocrine neoplasm in patients with multiple endocrine adenomatosis. A previously unrecognized association. Cancer 29: 1075-1083.
1688. Rosai J, Levine G, Weber WR, Higa E (1976). Carcinoid tumors and oat cell carcinomas of the thymus. Pathol Annu 11: 201-226.
1689. Rosai J, Parkash V, Reuter VE (1995). On the origin of mediastinal germ cell tumors in males. Int J Surg Pathol 2: 73-78.
1690. Rosai J, Sobin LH (1999). World Health Organization Histological Classification of Tumours. Histological Typing of Tumours of the Thymus. 2nd ed. Springer-Verlag: Berlin-Heildelberg.
1691. Rosai J, Sobin LH (1999). World Health Organization Histological Classification of Tumours. Histological Typing of Tumours of the Thymus. 2nd ed. Springer-Verlag: Berlin-Heidelberg.
1692. Rosenblatt MB, Lisa JR, Trinidad S (1966). Pitfalls in the clinical histologic diagnosis of bronchogenic carcinoma. Dis Chest 49: 396-404.
1693. Rosenkranz ER, Murphy DJJr (1994). Diagnosis and neonatal resection of right atrial angiosarcoma. Ann Thorac Surg 57: 1014-1015.
1694. Rosenwald A, Wright G, Leroy K, Yu X, Gaulard P, Gascoyne RD, Chan WC, Zhao T, Haioun C, Greiner TC, Weisenburger DD, Lynch JC, Vose J, Armitage JO, Smeland EB, Kvaloy S, Holte H, Delabie J, Campo E, Montserrat E, Lopez-Guillermo A, Ott G, Muller-Hermelink HK, Connors JM, Braziel R, Grogan TM, Fisher RI, Miller TP, Leblanc M, Chiorazzi M, Zhao H, Yang L, Powell J, Wilson WH, Jaffe ES, Simon R, Klausner RD, Staudt LM (2003). Molecular diagnosis of primary mediastinal B cell lymphoma identifies a clinically favorable subgroup of diffuse large B cell lymphoma related to Hodgkin lymphoma. J Exp Med 198: 851-862.
1695. Rossi G, Cavazza A, Sturm N, Migaldi M, Facciolongo N, Longo L, Maiorana A, Brambilla E (2003). Pulmonary carcinomas with pleomorphic, sarcomatoid, or sarcomatous elements. A clinicopathologic and immunohistochemical study of 75 cases. Am J Surg Pathol 27: 311-324.
1696. Rostami-Hodjegan A, Lennard MS, Woods HF, Tucker GT (1998). Meta-analysis of studies of the CYP2D6 polymorphism in relation to lung cancer and Parkinson's disease. Pharmacogenetics 8: 227-238.
1697. Roushdy-Hammady I, Siegel J, Emri S, Testa JR, Carbone M (2001). Genetic-susceptibility factor and malignant mesothelioma in the Cappadocian region of Turkey. Lancet 357: 444-445.
1698. Rousselet MC, Francois S, Croue A, Maigre M, Saint-Andre JP, Ifrah N (1994). A lymph node interdigitating reticulum cell sarcoma. Arch Pathol Lab Med 118: 183-188.
1699. Roux FJ, Lantuejoul S, Brambilla E, Brambilla C (1995). Mucinous cystadenoma of the lung. Cancer 76: 1540-1544.
1700. Royer B, Cazals-Hatem D, Sibilia J, Agbalika F, Cayuela JM, Soussi T, Maloisel F, Clauvel JP, Brouet JC, Mariette X (1997). Lymphomas in patients with Sjogren's syndrome are marginal zone B-cell neoplasms, arise in diverse extranodal and nodal sites, and are not associated with viruses. Blood 90: 766-775.
1701. Rubin BP, Lawrence BD, Perez-Atayde A, Xiao S, Yi ES, Fletcher CDM, Fletcher JA (2000). TPM-ALK fusion genes and ALK expression in inflammatory myofibroblastic tumor. Lab Invest 80: 15A.
1702. Rubin BP, Skarin AT, Pisick E, Rizk M, Salgia R (2001). Use of cytokeratins 7 and 20 in determining the origin of metastatic carcinoma of unknown primary, with special emphasis on lung cancer. Eur J Cancer Prev 10: 77-82.
1703. Rubin MA, Snell JA, Tazelaar HD, Lack EE, Austenfeld JL, Azumi N (1995). Cardiac papillary fibroelastoma: an immunohistochemical investigation and unusual clinical manifestations. Mod Pathol 8: 402-407.
1704. Rudiger T, Jaffe ES, Delsol G, deWolf-Peeters C, Gascoyne RD, Georgii A, Harris NL, Kadin ME, MacLennan KA, Poppema S, Stein H, Weiss LE, Muller-Hermelink HK (1998). Workshop report on Hodgkin's disease and related diseases ('grey zone' lymphoma). Ann Oncol 9 Suppl 5: S31-S38.
1705. Rudiger T, Ott G, Ott M, Muller-Deubert S, Muller-Hermelink HK (1998). Differential diagnosis between classic Hodgkin's lymphoma, T-cell-rich B-cell lymphoma, and paragranuloma by paraffin immunohistochemistry. Am J Surg Pathol 22: 1184-1191.
1706. Rudnicka L, Papla B, Malinowski E (1996). Mediastinal myelolipoma. A case report. Pol J Pathol 47: 143-145.
1707. Rudnicka L, Papla B, Malinowski E (1998). Mature cystic teratoma of the mediastinum containing a carcinoid. A case report. Pol J Pathol 49: 309-312.
1708. Ruffie P, Feld R, Minkin S, Cormier Y, Boutan-Laroze A, Ginsberg R, Ayoub J, Shepherd FA, Evans WK, Figueredo A (1989). Diffuse malignant mesothelioma of the pleura in Ontario and Quebec: a retrospective study of 332 patients. J Clin Oncol 7: 1157-1168.
1709. Ruffini E, Rena O, Oliaro A, Filosso PL, Bongiovanni M, Arslanian A, Papalia E, Maggi G (2002). Lung tumors with mixed histologic pattern. Clinico-pathologic characteristics and prognostic significance. Eur J Cardiothorac Surg 22: 701-707.
1710. Rusch V, Klimstra D, Linkov I, Dmitrovsky E (1995). Aberrant expression of p53 or the epidermal growth factor receptor is frequent in early bronchial neoplasia and coexpression precedes squamous cell carcinoma development. Cancer Res 55: 1365-1372.
1711. Rusch VW, Venkatraman ES (1999). Important prognostic factors in patients with malignant pleural mesothelioma, managed surgically. Ann Thorac Surg 68: 1799-1804.
1712. Russell WO, Cohen J, Enzinger F, Hajdu SI, Heise H, Martin RG, Meissner W, Miller WT, Schmitz RL, Suit HD (1977). A clinical and pathological staging system for soft tissue sarcomas. Cancer 40: 1562-1570.
1713. Ruszkiewicz AR, Vernon-Roberts E (1995). Sudden death in an infant due to histiocytoid cardiomyopathy. A light-microscopic, ultrastructural, and immunohistochemical study. Am J Forensic Med Pathol 16: 74-80.
1714. Ryan PEJr, Obeid AI, Parker FBJr (1995). Primary cardiac valve tumors. J Heart Valve Dis 4: 222-226.
1715. Sabol SZ, Nelson ML, Fisher C, Gunzerath L, Brody CL, Hu S, Sirota LA, Marcus SE, Greenberg BD, Lucas FR, Benjamin J, Murphy DL, Hamer DH (1999). A genetic association for cigarette smoking behavior. Health Psychol 18: 7-13.
1716. Sabourin JC, Kanavaros P, Briere J, Lescs MC, Petrella T, Zafrani ES, Gaulard P (1993). Epstein-Barr virus (EBV) genomes and EBV-encoded latent membrane protein (LMP) in pulmonary lymphomas occurring in nonimmunocompromised patients. Am J Surg Pathol 17: 995-1002.
1717. Saccomanno G, Archer VE, Auerbach O, Saunders RP, Brennan LM (1974). Development of carcinoma of the lung as reflected in exfoliated cells. Cancer 33: 256-270.
1718. Saccomanno G, Saunders RP, Archer VE, Auerbach O, Kuschner M, Beckler PA (1965). Cancer of the lung: the cytology of sputum prior to the development of carcinoma. Acta Cytol 9: 413-423.
1719. Sachs LJ, Angrist A (1945). Congenital Cyst of the Myocardium. Am J Pathol 187-193.
1720. Said JW, Shintaku IP, Asou H, deVos S, Baker J, Hanson G, Cesarman E, Nador R, Koeffler HP (1999). Herpesvirus 8 inclusions in primary effusion lymphoma: report of a unique case with T-cell phenotype. Arch Pathol Lab Med 123: 257-260.
1721. Said JW, Tasaka T, Takeuchi S, Asou H, de Vos S, Cesarman E, Knowles DM, Koeffler HP (1996). Primary effusion lymphoma in women: report of two cases of Kaposi's sarcoma herpes virus-associated effusion-based lymphoma in human immunodeficiency virus-negative women. Blood 88: 3124-3128.
1722. Sait SN, Brooks JJ, Ashraf M, Zhang PJ (2001). A novel t(1;8)(p13;p11) in a thymic carcinoma with unusual giant cell features and renal metastasis. Cancer Genet Cytogenet 124: 140-143.
1723. Saito A, Watanabe K, Kusakabe T, Abe M, Suzuki T (1998). Mediastinal mature teratoma with coexistence of angiosarcoma, granulocytic sarcoma and a hematopoietic region in the tumor: a rare case of association between hematological malignancy and mediastinal germ cell tumor. Pathol Int 48: 749-753.
1724. Saito T, Tamaru J, Kayao J, Kuzuu Y, Wakita H, Mikata A (2001). Cytomorphologic diagnosis of malignant lymphoma arising in the heart: a case report. Acta Cytol 45: 1043-1048.
1725. Saitoh Y, Ohsako M, Umemoto M, Kohdera U, Okamura A, Imamura H (1995). [A case of primary mediastinal teratocarcinoma in a young girl]. Nippon Kyobu Geka Gakkai Zasshi 43: 104-108.
1726. Sakaguchi N, Sano K, Ito M, Baba T, Fukuzawa M, Hotchi M (1996). A case of von Recklinghausen's disease with bilateral pheochromocytoma-malignant peripheral nerve sheath tumors of the adrenal and gastrointestinal autonomic nerve tumors. Am J Surg Pathol 20: 889-897.
1727. Sakamoto H, Uda H, Tanaka T, Oda T, Morino H, Kikui M (1991). Pleomorphic adenoma in the periphery of the lung-report of a case and review of the literature -. Arch Pathol Lab Med 115: 393-396.
1728. Sakamoto K, Okita M, Kumagiri H, Kawamura S, Takeuchi K, Mikami R (2003). Sclerosing hemangioma isolated to the

mediastinum. Ann Thorac Surg 75: 1021-1023.
1729. Sales LM, Vontz FK (1970). Teratoma and DiGugliemo syndrome. South Med J 63: 448-450.
1730. Salih Deveci M, Ceyhan K, Deveci G, Finci R (2001). Pericardial rhabdomyomatous spindle cell thymoma with mucinous cystic degeneration. Histopathology 38: 479-481.
1731. Saltzstein SL (1963). Pulmonary malignant lymphomas and pseudolymphomas: classification, therapy and prognosis. Cancer 1: 928-955.
1732. Salyer WR, Eggleston JC (1976). Thymoma: a clinical and pathological study of 65 cases. Cancer 37: 229-249.
1733. Sanchez-Cespedes M, Parrella P, Esteller M, Nomoto S, Trink B, Engles JM, Westra WH, Herman JG, Sidransky D (2002). Inactivation of LKB1/STK11 is a common event in adenocarcinomas of the lung. Cancer Res 62: 3659-3662.
1734. Sandberg AA, Bridge JA (2002). Updates on the cytogenetics and molecular genetics of bone and soft tissue tumors: congenital (infantile) fibrosarcoma and mesoblastic nephroma. Cancer Genet Cytogenet 132: 1-13.
1735. Sankar NM, Thiruchelvam T, Thirunavukkaarasu K, Pang K, Hanna WM (1998). Symptomatic lipoma in the right atrial free wall. A case report. Tex Heart Inst J 25: 152-154.
1736. Sanna P, Bertoni F, Zucca E, Roggero E, Passega Sidler E, Fiori G, Pedrinis E, Mombelli G, Cavalli F (1998). Cardiac involvement in HIV-related non-Hodgkin's lymphoma: a case report and short review of the literature. Ann Hematol 77: 75-78.
1737. Santeusanio G, Mauriello A, Ventura L, Liberati F, Colantoni A, Lasorella R, Spagnoli LG (2000). Immunohistochemical analysis of estrogen receptors in breast carcinomas using monoclonal antibodies that recognize different domains of the receptor molecule. Appl Immunohistochem Mol Morphol 8: 275-284.
1738. Saphir O, Vass A (1938). Carcinosarcoma. Am J Cancer 33: 331-359.
1739. Sapi Z, Szentirmay Z, Orosz Z (1999). Desmoplastic small round cell tumour of the pleura: a case report with further cytogenetic and ultrastructural evidence of 'mesothelioblastemic' origin. Eur J Surg Oncol 25: 633-634.
1740. Saracci R, Simonato L (2001). Familial malignant mesothelioma. Lancet 358: 1813-1814.
1741. Sarma DP, Deshotels SJJr (1982). Carcinosarcoma of the lung. J Surg Oncol 19: 216-218.
1742. Sartelet H, Lantuejoul S, Armari-Alla C, Pin I, Delattre O, Brambilla E (1998). Solid alveolar rhabdomyosarcoma of the thorax in a child. Histopathology 32: 165-171.
1743. Sasajima Y, Yamabe H, Kobashi Y, Hirai K, Mori S (1993). High expression of the Epstein-Barr virus latent protein EB nuclear antigen-2 on pyothorax-associated lymphomas. Am J Pathol 143: 1280-1285.
1744. Sasaki H, Ide N, Fukai I, Kiriyama M, Yamakawa Y, Fujii Y (2002). Gene expression analysis of human thymoma correlates with tumor stage. Int J Cancer 101: 342-347.
1745. Sasatomi E, Finkelstein SD, Woods JD, Bakker A, Swalsky PA, Luketich JD, Fernando HC, Yousem SA (2002). Comparison of accumulated allele loss between primary tumor and lymph node metastasis in stage II non-small cell lung carcinoma: implications for the timing of lymph node metastasis and prognostic value. Cancer Res 62: 2681-2689.
1746. Sato M, Horio Y, Sekido Y, Minna JD, Shimokata K, Hasegawa Y (2002). The expression of DNA methyltransferases and methyl-CpG-binding proteins is not associated with the methylation status of p14(ARF), p16(INK4a) and RASSF1A in human lung cancer cell lines. Oncogene 21: 4822-4829.
1747. Sato T, Seyama K, Fujii H, Maruyama H, Setoguchi Y, Iwakami S, Fukuchi Y, Hino O (2002). Mutation analysis of the TSC1 and TSC2 genes in Japanese patients with pulmonary lymphangioleiomyomatosis. J Hum Genet 47: 20-28.
1748. Sato Y, Watanabe S, Mukai K, Kodama T, Upton MP, Goto M, Shimosato Y (1986). An immunohistochemical study of thymic epithelial tumors. II. Lymphoid component. Am J Surg Pathol 10: 862-870.
1749. Satoh M, Horimoto M, Sakurai K, Funayama N, Igarashi K, Yamashiro K (1990). Primary cardiac rhabdomyosarcoma exhibiting transient and pronounced regression with chemotherapy. Am Heart J 120: 1458-1460.
1750. Satoh Y, Ishikawa Y, Miyoshi T, Mukai H, Okumura S, Nakagawa K (2003). Pulmonary metastases from a low-grade endometrial stromal sarcoma confirmed by chromosome aberration and fluorescence in-situ hybridization approaches: a case of recurrence 13 years after hysterectomy. Virchows Arch 442: 173-178.
1751. Satoh Y, Tsuchiya E, Weng SY, Kitagawa T, Matsubara T, Nakagawa K, Kinoshita I, Sugano H (1989). Pulmonary sclerosing hemangioma of the lung. A type II pneumocytoma by immunohistochemical and immunoelectron microscopic studies. Cancer 64: 1310-1317.
1752. Savage KJ, Monti S, Kutok JL, Cattoretti G, Neuberg D, de Leval L, Kurtin P, Dal Cin P, Ladd C, Feuerhake F, Aguiar RC, Li S, Salles G, Berger F, Jing W, Pinkus GS, Habermann T, Dalla-Favera R, Harris NL, Aster JC, Golub TR, Shipp MA (2003). The molecular signature of mediastinal large B-cell lymphoma differs from that of other diffuse large B-cell lymphomas and shares features with classical Hodgkin lymphoma. Blood 102: 3871-3879.
1753. Scarpa A, Bonetti F, Menestrina F, Menegazzi M, Chilosi M, Lestani M, Bovolenta C, Zamboni G, Fiore-Donati L (1987). Mediastinal large-cell lymphoma with sclerosis. Genotypic analysis establishes its B nature. Virchows Arch A Pathol Anat Histol 412: 17-21.
1754. Scarpa A, Borgato L, Chilosi M, Capelli P, Menestrina F, Bonetti F, Zamboni G, Pizzolo G, Hirohashi S, Fiore-Donati L (1991). Evidence of c-myc gene abnormalities in mediastinal large B-cell lymphoma of young adult age. Blood 78: 780-788.
1755. Scarpa A, Moore PS, Rigaud G, Inghirami G, Montresor M, Menegazzi M, Todeschini G, Menestrina F (1999). Molecular features of primary mediastinal B-cell lymphoma: involvement of p16INK4A, p53 and c-myc. Br J Haematol 107: 106-113.
1756. Scarpa A, Taruscio D, Scardoni M, Iosi F, Paradisi S, Ennas MG, Rigaud G, Moore PS, Menestrina F (1999). Nonrandom chromosomal imbalances in primary mediastinal B-cell lymphoma detected by arbitrarily primed PCR fingerprinting. Genes Chromosomes Cancer 26: 203-209.
1757. Scarpatetti M, Tsybrovskyy O, Popper HH (2002). Cytokeratin typing as an aid in the differential diagnosis of primary versus metastatic lung carcinomas, and comparison with normal lung. Virchows Arch 440: 70-76.
1758. Scarpelli M, Montironi R, Ricciuti R, Vecchioni S, Pauri F (1997). Cardiac myxoma with glandular elements metastatic to the brain 12 years after the removal of the original tumor. Clin Neuropathol 16: 190-194.
1759. Schleusener JT, Tazelaar HD, Jung SH, Cha SS, Cera PJ, Myers JL, Creagan ET, Goldberg RM, Marschke RFJr (1996). Neuroendocrine differentiation is an independent prognostic factor in chemotherapy-treated nonsmall cell lung carcinoma. Cancer 77: 1284-1291.
1760. Schmid C, Pan L, Diss T, Isaacson PG (1991). Expression of B-cell antigens by Hodgkin's and Reed-Sternberg cells. Am J Pathol 139: 701-707.
1761. Schmitz L, Favara BE (1998). Nosology and pathology of Langerhans cell histiocytosis. Hematol Oncol Clin North Am 12: 221-246.
1762. Schneider-Stock R, Rys J, Walter H, Limon J, Iliszko M, Niezabitowski A, Roessner A (1999). A rare chimeric TLS/FUS-CHOP transcript in a patient with multiple liposarcomas: a case report. Cancer Genet Cytogenet 111: 130-133.
1763. Schneider DT, Calaminus G, Koch S, Teske C, Schmidt P, Haas RJ, Harms D, Gobel U (2003). Epidemiological analysis of 1442 children and adolescents registered in the German Germ Cell Tumour Protocols. Med Pediatr Oncol .
1764. Schneider DT, Calaminus G, Reinhard H, Gutjahr P, Kremens B, Harms D, Gobel U (2000). Primary mediastinal germ cell tumors in children and adolescents: results of the German cooperative protocols MAKEI 83/86, 89, and 96. J Clin Oncol 18: 832-839.
1765. Schneider DT, Schuster AE, Fritsch MK, Calaminus G, Gobel U, Harms D, Lauer S, Olson T, Perlman EJ (2002). Genetic analysis of mediastinal nonseminomatous germ cell tumors in children and adolescents. Genes Chromosomes Cancer 34: 115-125.
1766. Schneider DT, Schuster AE, Fritsch MK, Hu J, Olson T, Lauer S, Gobel U, Perlman EJ (2001). Multipoint imprinting analysis indicates a common precursor cell for gonadal and nongonadal pediatric germ cell tumors. Cancer Res 61: 7268-7276.
1767. Schneider PM, Praeuer HW, Stoeltzing O, Boehm J, Manning J, Metzger R, Fink U, Wegerer S, Hoelscher AH, Roth JA (2000). Multiple molecular marker testing (p53, C-Ki-ras, c-erbB-2) improves estimation of prognosis in potentially curative resected non-small cell lung cancer. Br J Cancer 83: 473-479.
1768. Schvartzman PR, White RD (2000). Imaging of cardiac and paracardiac masses. J Thorac Imaging 15: 265-273.
1769. Schwabe J, Calaminus G, Vorhoff W, Engelbrecht V, Hauffa BP, Gobel U (2002). Sexual precocity and recurrent beta-human chorionic gonadotropin upsurges preceding the diagnosis of a malignant mediastinal germ-cell tumor in a 9-year-old boy. Ann Oncol 13: 975-977.
1770. Schwinger ME, Katz E, Rotterdam H, Slater J, Weiss EC, Kronzon I (1989). Right atrial papillary fibroelastoma: diagnosis by transthoracic and transesophageal echocardiography and percutaneous transvenous biopsy. Am Heart J 118: 1047-1050.
1771. Sciot R, Dal Cin P, Fletcher CD, Hernandez JM, Garcia JL, Samson I, Ramos L, Brys P, Van Damme B, van den Berghe H (1997). Inflammatory myofibroblastic tumor of bone: report of two cases with evidence of clonal chromosomal changes. Am J Surg Pathol 21: 1166-1172.
1772. Scopsi L, Collini P, Muscolino G (1999). A new observation of the Carney's triad with long follow-Up period and additional tumors. Cancer Detect Prev 23: 435-443.
1773. Sebire NJ, Rampling D, Malone M, Ramsay A, Sheppard M (2002). Gains of chromosome 8 in pleuropulmonary blastomas of childhood. Pediatr Dev Pathol 5: 221-222.
1774. Seguin JR, Beigbeder JY, Hvass U, Langlois J, Grolleau R, Jourdan M, Klein B, Bataille R, Chaptal PA (1992). Interleukin 6 production by cardiac myxomas may explain constitutional symptoms. J Thorac Cardiovasc Surg 103: 599-600.
1775. Seidemann K, Tiemann M, Schrappe M, Yakisan E, Simonitsch I, Janka-Schaub G, Dorffel W, Zimmermann M, Mann G, Gadner H, Parwaresch R, Riehm H, Reiter A (2001). Short-pulse B-non-Hodgkin lymphoma-type chemotherapy is efficacious treatment for pediatric anaplastic large cell lymphoma: a report of the Berlin-Frankfurt-Munster Group Trial NHL-BFM 90. Blood 97: 3699-3706.
1776. Seitz V, Hummel M, Marafioti T, Anagnostopoulos I, Assaf C, Stein H (2000). Detection of clonal T-cell receptor gamma-chain gene rearrangements in Reed-Sternberg cells of classic Hodgkin disease. Blood 95: 3020-3024.
1777. Sekeres M, Vasconcelles MJ, McMenamin M, Rosenfeld-Darling M, Bueno R (2000). Two patients with sarcoma. Case 1. Synovial cell sarcoma of the lung. J Clin Oncol 18: 2341-2342.
1778. Sekido Y, Pass HI, Bader S, Mew DJ, Christman MF, Gazdar AF, Minna JD (1995). Neurofibromatosis type 2 (NF2) gene is somatically mutated in mesothelioma but not in lung cancer. Cancer Res 55: 1227-1231.
1779. Sekine S, Shibata T, Matsuno Y, Maeshima A, Ishii G, Sakamoto M, Hirohashi S (2003). Beta-catenin mutations in pulmonary blastomas: association with morule formation. J Pathol 200: 214-221.
1780. Selim AA, El Ayat G, Wells CA (2001). Immunohistochemical localization of gross cystic disease fluid protein-15, -24 and -44 in ductal carcinoma in situ of the breast: relationship to the degree of differentiation. Histopathology 39: 198-202.
1781. Sellers TA, Bailey-Wilson JE, Elston RC, Wilson AF, Elston GZ, Ooi WL, Rothschild H (1990). Evidence for mendelian inheritance in the pathogenesis of lung cancer. J Natl Cancer Inst 82: 1272-1279.
1782. Semeraro D, Gibbs AR (1989). Pulmonary adenoma: a variant of sclerosing haemangioma of lung? J Clin Pathol 42: 1222-1223.
1783. Sensaki K, Aida S, Takagi K, Shibata H, Ogata T, Tanaka S, Tamai S (1993). Coexisting undifferentiated thymic carcinoma and thymic carcinoid tumor. Respiration 60: 247-249.
1784. Seo JB, Im JG, Goo JM, Chung MJ, Kim MY (2001). Atypical pulmonary metastases: spectrum of radiologic findings.

Radiographics 21: 403-417.
1785. Seo T, Ando H, Watanabe Y, Harada T, Ito F, Kaneko K, Mimura S (1999). Acute respiratory failure associated with intrathoracic masses in neonates. J Pediatr Surg 34: 1633-1637.
1786. Sepulveda W, Gomez E, Gutierrez J (2000). Intrapericardial teratoma. Ultrasound Obstet Gynecol 15: 547-548.
1787. Serezhin BS, Stepanov MI (1990). [A carcinoid tumor in a mature thymic teratoma]. Arkh Patol 52: 59-62.
1788. Shabb NS, Fahl M, Shabb B, Haswani P, Zaatari G (1998). Fine-needle aspiration of the mediastinum: a clinical, radiologic, cytologic, and histologic study of 42 cases. Diagn Cytopathol 19: 428-436.
1789. Shaffer K, Pugatch RD, Sugarbaker DJ (1990). Primary mediastinal leiomyoma. Ann Thorac Surg 50: 301-302.
1790. Shah RN, Badve S, Papreddy K, Schindler S, Laskin WB, Yeldandi AV (2002). Expression of cytokeratin 20 in mucinous bronchioloalveolar carcinoma. Hum Pathol 33: 915-920.
1791. Shapiro LM (2001). Cardiac tumours: diagnosis and management. Heart 85: 218-222.
1792. Shebib S, Sabbah RS, Sackey K, Akhtar M, Aur RJ (1989). Endodermal sinus (yolk sac) tumor in infants and children. A clinical and pathologic study: an 11 year review. Am J Pediatr Hematol Oncol 11: 36-39.
1793. Sheen TS, Chang Y, Ko J, Wu C, Lee S (1999). Basaloid squamous cell carcinoma of the larynx. Otolaryngol Head Neck Surg 121: 647-650.
1794. Shehata BM, Patterson K, Thomas JE, Scala-Barnett D, Dasu S, Robinson HB (1998). Histiocytoid cardiomyopathy: three new cases and a review of the literature. Pediatr Dev Pathol 1: 56-69.
1795. Sheibani K, Winberg CD, Burke JS, Nathwani BN, Blayney DW, van de Velde S, Swartz WG, Rappaport H (1987). Lymphoblastic lymphoma expressing natural killer cell-associated antigens: a clinicopathologic study of six cases. Leuk Res 11: 371-377.
1796. Shepherd FA (1993). Screening, diagnosis, and staging of lung cancer. Curr Opin Oncol 5: 310-322.
1797. Shepherd FA (2000). Surgical management of small cell lung cancer. In: Lung Cancer, Principles and Practice, Lung Cancer, Principles and Practice, Lippincott Wiliams and Wilkins: Philadelphia , pp. 967-980.
1798. Sherman JL, Rykwalder PJ, Tashkin DP (1981). Intravascular bronchioloalveolar tumor. Am Rev Respir Dis 123: 468-470.
1799. Shibahara K, Sugio K, Osaki T, Uchiumi T, Maehara Y, Kohno K, Yasumoto K, Sugimachi K, Kuwano M (2001). Nuclear expression of the Y-box binding protein, YB-1, as a novel marker of disease progression in non-small cell lung cancer. Clin Cancer Res 7: 3151-3155.
1800. Shields PG, Lerman C, Audrain J, Bowman ED, Main D, Boyd NR, Caporaso NE (1998). Dopamine D4 receptors and the risk of cigarette smoking in African-Americans and Caucasians. Cancer Epidemiol Biomarkers Prev 7: 453-458.
1801. Shigemitsu K, Sekido Y, Usami N, Mori S, Sato M, Horio Y, Hasegawa Y, Bader SA, Gazdar AF, Minna JD, Hida T, Yoshioka H, Imaizumi M, Ueda Y, Takahashi M, Shimokata K (2001). Genetic alteration of the beta-catenin gene (CTNNB1) in human lung cancer and malignant mesothelioma and identification of a new 3p21.3 homozygous deletion. Oncogene 20: 4249-4257.
1802. Shimazaki H, Aida S, Iizuka Y, Yoshizu H, Tamai S (2000). Vacuolated cell mesothelioma of the pericardium resembling liposarcoma: a case report. Hum Pathol 31: 767-770.
1803. Shimazaki H, Aida S, Sato M, Deguchi H, Ozeki Y, Tamai S (2001). Lung carcinoma with rhabdoid cells: a clinicopathological study and survival analysis of 14 cases. Histopathology 38: 425-434.
1804. Shimizu J, Kawaura Y, Tatsuzawa Y, Kinoshita T, Nozaki Z, Ohta Y, Nonomura A (2000). Malignant melanoma originating in the thymus. Aust N Z J Surg 70: 753-755.
1805. Shimizu J, Yazaki U, Kinoshita T, Tatsuzawa Y, Kawaura Y, Nonomura A (2001). Primary mediastinal germ cell tumor in a middle-aged woman: case report and literature review. Tumori 87: 269-271.
1806. Shimosato Y, Kameya T, Nagai K, Suemasu K (1977). Squamous cell carcinoma of the thymus. An analysis of eight cases. Am J Surg Pathol 1: 109-121.
1807. Shimosato Y, Kodama T, Kameya T (1982). Morphogenesis of peripheral type adenocarcinoma of the lung. In: Morphogenesis of lung cancer, Shimosato Y, Melamed MR, Nettesheim P, eds., CRC press: Boca Raton , pp. 65-90.
1808. Shimosato Y, Mukai K (1997). Atlas of Tumor Pathology. Tumors of the Mediastinum. 3rd ed. Armed Forces Institute of Pathology: Washington, D.C.
1809. Shimosato Y, Suzuki A, Hashimoto T, Nishiwaki Y, Kodama T, Yoneyama T, Kameya T (1980). Prognostic implications of fibrotic focus (scar) in small peripheral lung cancers. Am J Surg Pathol 4: 365-373.
1810. Shin MS, Odrezin GT, Van Dyke JA, Ho KJ (1991). Unusual initial calcification of primary and metastatic seminomas. Detection by computed tomography. Chest 99: 1543-1545.
1811. Shiota Y, Matsumoto H, Sasaki N, Taniyama K, Hashimoto S, Sueishi K (1998). Solitary bronchioloalveolar adenoma of the lung. Respiration 65: 483-485.
1812. Shirasaki A, Hirakata Y, Kitamura S, Bandoh S, Saitoh K (1995). A salivary gland-type monomorphic adenoma with trabecular proliferation in the lung. Intern Med 34: 1086-1088.
1813. Shiseki M, Kohno T, Adachi J, Okazaki T, Otsuka T, Mizoguchi H, Noguchi M, Hirohashi S, Yokota J (1996). Comparative allelotype of early and advanced stage non-small cell lung carcinomas. Genes Chromosomes Cancer 17: 71-77.
1814. Shivapurkar N, Toyooka S, Eby MT, Huang CX, Sathyanarayana UG, Cunningham HT, Reddy JL, Brambilla E, Takahashi T, Minna JD, Chaudhary PM, Gazdar AF (2002). Differential inactivation of caspase-8 in lung cancers. Cancer Biol Ther 1: 65-69.
1815. Shivapurkar N, Virmani AK, Wistuba II, Milchgrub S, Mackay B, Minna JD, Gazdar AF (1999). Deletions of chromosome 4 at multiple sites are frequent in malignant mesothelioma and small cell lung carcinoma. Clin Cancer Res 5: 17-23.
1816. Shmookler BM, Marsh HB, Roberts WC (1977). Primary sarcoma of the pulmonary trunk and/or right or left main pulmonary artery—a rare cause of obstruction to right ventricular outflow. Report on two patients and analysis of 35 previously described patients. Am J Med 63: 263-272.
1817. Shoji T, Tanaka F, Takata T, Yanagihara K, Otake Y, Hanaoka N, Miyahara R, Nakagawa T, Kawano Y, Ishikawa S, Katakura H, Wada H (2002). Clinical significance of p21 expression in non-small-cell lung cancer. J Clin Oncol 20: 3865-3871.
1818. Shub C, Parkin TW, Lie JT (1979). An unusual mediastinal lipoma simulating cardiomegaly. Mayo Clin Proc 54: 60-62.
1819. Shub C, Tajik AJ, Seward JB, Edwards WD, Pruitt RD, Orszulak TA, Pluth JR (1981). Cardiac papillary fibroelastomas. Two-dimensional echocardiographic recognition. Mayo Clin Proc 56: 629-633.
1820. Shure D (1991). Radiographically occult endobronchial obstruction in bronchogenic carcinoma. Am J Med 91: 19-22.
1821. Sickles EA, Belliveau RE, Wiernik PH (1974). Primary mediastinal choriocarcinoma in the male. Cancer 33: 1196-1203.
1822. Siebenmann RE, Odermatt B, Hegglin J, Binswanger RO (1990). [Alveolar cell adenoma. A newly defined benign lung tumor]. Pathologe 11: 48-54.
1823. Siegal GP, Dehner LP, Rosai J (1985). Histiocytosis X (Langerhans' cell granulomatosis) of the thymus. A clinicopathologic study of four childhood cases. Am J Surg Pathol 9: 117-124.
1824. Siegel RJ, Bueso-Ramos C, Cohen C, Koss M (1991). Pulmonary blastoma with germ cell (yolk sac) differentiation: report of two cases. Mod Pathol 4: 566-570.
1825. Silver SA, Askin FB (1997). True papillary carcinoma of the lung: a distinct clinicopathologic entity. Am J Surg Pathol 21: 43-51.
1826. Silverman JF, Geisinger KR (1996). Lung. In: Fine needle aspiration cytology of the thorax and abdomen, Silverman JF, Geisinger KR, eds., Churchill Livingstone: New York , pp. 1-51.
1827. Simon HU, Plotz SG, Dummer R, Blaser K (1999). Abnormal clones of T cells producing interleukin-5 in idiopathic eosinophilia. N Engl J Med 341: 1112-1120.
1828. Simons A, Schepens M, Jeuken J, Sprenger S, van de Zande G, Bjerkehagen B, Forus A, Weibolt V, Molenaar I, van den Berg E, Myklebost O, Bridge J, van Kessel AG, Suijkerbuijk R (2000). Frequent loss of 9p21 (p16(INK4A)) and other genomic imbalances in human malignant fibrous histiocytoma. Cancer Genet Cytogenet 118: 89-98.
1829. Sinclair DS, Bolen MA, King MA (2003). Mature teratoma within the posterior mediastinum. J Thorac Imaging 18: 53-55.
1830. Singhal S, Amin KM, Kruklitis R, DeLong P, Friscia ME, Litzky LA, Putt ME, Kaiser LR, Albelda SM (2003). Alterations in cell cycle genes in early stage lung adenocarcinoma identified by expression profiling. Cancer Biol Ther 2: 291.
1831. Siripornpitak S, Higgins CB (1997). MRI of primary malignant cardiovascular tumors. J Comput Assist Tomogr 21: 462-466.
1832. Skalidis EI, Parthenakis FI, Zacharis EA, Datseris GE, Vardas PE (1999). Pulmonary tumor embolism from primary cardiac B-cell lymphoma. Chest 116: 1489-1490.
1833. Skov BG, Sorensen JB, Hirsch FR, Larsson LI, Hansen HH (1991). Prognostic impact of histologic demonstration of chromogranin A and neuron specific enolase in pulmonary adenocarcinoma. Ann Oncol 2: 355-360.
1834. Skyggebjerg KD (1988). Hydrops fetalis is caused by intrapericardial teratoma. Acta Obstet Gynecol Scand 67: 653-654.
1835. Slagel DD, Powers CN, Melaragno MJ, Geisinger KR, Frable WJ, Silverman JF (1997). Spindle-cell lesions of the mediastinum: diagnosis by fine-needle aspiration biopsy. Diagn Cytopathol 17: 167-176.
1836. Slebos RJ, Baas IO, Clement MJ, Offerhaus GJ, Askin FB, Hruban RH, Westra WH (1998). p53 alterations in atypical alveolar hyperplasia of the human lung. Hum Pathol 29: 801-808.
1837. Slebos RJ, Kibbelaar RE, Dalesio O, Kooistra A, Stam J, Meijer CJ, Wagenaar SS, Vanderschueren RG, van Zandwijk N, Mooi WJ, Bos JL, Rodenhuis S (1990). K-ras oncogene activation as a prognostic marker in adenocarcinoma of the lung. N Engl J Med 323: 561-565.
1838. Smith TA, Machen SK, Fisher C, Goldblum JR (1999). Usefulness of cytokeratin subsets for distinguishing monophasic synovial sarcoma from malignant peripheral nerve sheath tumor. Am J Clin Pathol 112: 641-648.
1839. Smolarek TA, Wessner LL, McCormack FX, Mylet JC, Menon AG, Henske EP (1998). Evidence that lymphangiomyomatosis is caused by TSC2 mutations: chromosome 16p13 loss of heterozygosity in angiomyolipomas and lymph nodes from women with lymphangiomyomatosis. Am J Hum Genet 62: 810-815.
1840. Smythe JF, Dyck JD, Smallhorn JF, Freedom RM (1990). Natural history of cardiac rhabdomyoma in infancy and childhood. Am J Cardiol 66: 1247-1249.
1841. Snover DC, Levine GD, Rosai J (1982). Thymic carcinoma. Five distinctive histological variants. Am J Surg Pathol 6: 451-470.
1842. Snyder CS, Dell'Aquila M, Haghighi P, Baergen RN, Suh YK, Yi ES (1995). Clonal changes in inflammatory pseudotumor of the lung: a case report. Cancer 76: 1545-1549.
1843. Sobue T, Ajiki W, Tsukuma H, Oshima A, Hanai A, Fujimoto I (1999). Trends of lung cancer incidence by histologic type: a population-based study in Osaka, Japan. Jpn J Cancer Res 90: 6-15.
1844. Soga J, Yakuwa Y (1999). Bronchopulmonary carcinoids: An analysis of 1,875 reported cases with special reference to a comparison between typical carcinoids and atypical varieties. Ann Thorac Cardiovasc Surg 5: 211-219.
1845. Soga J, Yakuwa Y, Osaka M (1999). Evaluation of 342 cases of mediastinal/thymic carcinoids collected from literature: a comparative study between typical carcinoids and atypical varieties. Ann Thorac Cardiovasc Surg 5: 285-292.
1846. Sole F, Bosch F, Woessner S, Perez-Losada A, Cervantes F, Montserrat E, Florensa L, Rozman C (1994). Refractory anemia with excess of blasts and isochromosome 12p in a patient with primary mediastinal germ-cell tumor. Cancer Genet Cytogenet 77: 111-113.
1847. Sonobe H, Ohtsuki Y, Nakayama H, Asaba K, Nishiya K, Shimizu K (1998). A thymic squamous cell carcinoma with complex chromosome abnormalities. Cancer Genet Cytogenet 103: 83-85.
1848. Sonobe H, Takeuchi T, Ohtsuki Y, Taguchi T, Shimizu K (1999). A thymoma with clonal complex chromosome abnormalities. Cancer Genet Cytogenet 110: 72-74.
1849. Souhami RL, Bradbury I, Geddes DM,

Spiro SG, Harper PG, Tobias JS (1985). Prognostic significance of laboratory parameters measured at diagnosis in small cell carcinoma of the lung. Cancer Res 45: 2878-2882.
1850. Souid AK, Ziemba MC, Dubansky AS, Mazur M, Oliphant M, Thomas FD, Ratner M, Sadowitz PD (1993). Inflammatory myofibroblastic tumor in children. Cancer 72: 2042-2048.
1851. Soulami S, Chraibi S, Ait Ben Hammou C, Haddani J, Louahlia S, Chraibi N (1995). [Mediastinal malignant schwannoma disclosed by pericardial tamponade in von Recklinghausen disease]. Ann Cardiol Angeiol (Paris) 44: 418-421.
1852. Souma T, Oguma F, Ueno M, Terashima M, Sato K (1993). [A case report of pulmonary metastasis of malignant fibrous histiocytoma (MFH) accompanied by mediastinal lymph node metastasis]. Kyobu Geka 46: 1149-1151.
1853. Sourvinos G, Parissis J, Sotsiou F, Arvanitis DL, Spandidos DA (1999). Detection of microsatellite instability in sporadic cardiac myxomas. Cardiovasc Res 42: 728-732.
1854. Sozzi G, Miozzo M, Donghi R, Pilotti S, Cariani CT, Pastorino U, Della Porta G, Pierotti MA (1992). Deletions of 17p and p53 mutations in preneoplastic lesions of the lung. Cancer Res 52: 6079-6082.
1855. Sozzi G, Pastorino U, Moiraghi L, Tagliabue E, Pezzella F, Ghirelli C, Tornielli S, Sard L, Huebner K, Pierotti MA, Croce CM, Pilotti S (1998). Loss of FHIT function in lung cancer and preinvasive bronchial lesions. Cancer Res 58: 5032-5037.
1856. Sozzi G, Veronese ML, Negrini M, Baffa R, Cotticelli MG, Inoue H, Tornielli S, Pilotti S, De Gregorio L, Pastorino U, Pierotti MA, Ohta M, Huebner K, Croce CM (1996). The FHIT gene 3p14.2 is abnormal in lung cancer. Cell 85: 17-26.
1857. Spencer H (1961). Pulmonary blastoma. J Pathol Bacteriol 82: 161-165.
1858. Spencer H, Dail DH, Arneaud J (1980). Non-invasive bronchial epithelial papillary tumors. Cancer 45: 1486-1497.
1859. Spencer H, Nambu S (1986). Sclerosing haemangiomas of the lung. Histopathology 10: 477-487.
1860. Spiro SG, Porter JC (2002). Lung cancer—where are we today? Current advances in staging and nonsurgical treatment. Am J Respir Crit Care Med 166: 1166-1196.
1861. Spirtas R, Connelly RR, Tucker MA (1988). Survival patterns for malignant mesothelioma: the SEER experience. Int J Cancer 41: 525-530.
1862. Spirtas R, Heineman EF, Bernstein L, Beebe GW, Keehn RJ, Stark A, Harlow BL, Benichou J (1994). Malignant mesothelioma: attributable risk of asbestos exposure. Occup Environ Med 51: 804-811.
1863. Spits H, Blom B, Jaleco AC, Weijer K, Verschuren MC, van Dongen JJ, Heemskerk MH, Res PC (1998). Early stages in the development of human T, natural killer and thymic dendritic cells. Immunol Rev 165: 75-86.
1864. Spitz MR, Shi H, Yang F, Hudmon KS, Jiang H, Chamberlain RM, Amos CI, Wan Y, Cinciripini P, Hong WK, Wu X (1998). Case-control study of the D2 dopamine receptor gene and smoking status in lung cancer patients. J Natl Cancer Inst 90: 358-363.
1865. Springfield D (1993). Liposarcoma. Clin Orthop 50-57.
1866. Squire JA, Bayani J, Luk C, Unwin L, Tokunaga J, MacMillan C, Irish J, Brown D, Gullane P, Kamel-Reid S (2002). Molecular cytogenetic analysis of head and neck squamous cell carcinoma: By comparative genomic hybridization, spectral karyotyping, and expression array analysis. Head Neck 24: 874-887.
1867. Sridhar KS, Bounassi MJ, Raub WJr, Richman SP (1990). Clinical features of adenosquamous lung carcinoma in 127 patients. Am Rev Respir Dis 142: 19-23.
1868. Sridhar KS, Raub WAJr, Duncan RC, Hilsenbeck S (1992). The increasing recognition of adenosquamous lung carcinoma (1977-1986). Am J Clin Oncol 15: 356-362.
1869. Srinivas BK, Gopalakrishnan M, Mahadevan R, Satyaprasad V (2002). Lipoma of the left ventricle. Asian Cardiovasc Thorac Ann 10: 64-65.
1870. Stackhouse EM, Harrison EGJr, Ellis FHJr (1969). Primary mixed malignancies of lung: carcinosarcoma and blastoma. J Thorac Cardiovasc Surg 57: 385-399.
1871. Stahel RA (1991). Diagnosis, staging, and prognostic factors of small cell lung cancer. Curr Opin Oncol 3: 306-311.
1872. Stefanaki K, Rontogianni D, Kouvidou CH, Bolioti S, Delides G, Pantelidaki A, Sotsiou F, Kanavaros P (1997). Expression of p53, mdm2, p21/waf1 and bcl-2 proteins in thymomas. Histopathology 30: 549-555.
1873. Stein H, Hummel M (1999). Cellular origin and clonality of classic Hodgkin's lymphoma: immunophenotypic and molecular studies. Semin Hematol 36: 233-241.
1874. Stein H, Marafioti T, Foss HD, Laumen H, Hummel M, Anagnostopoulos I, Wirth T, Demel G, Falini B (2001). Down-regulation of BOB.1/OBF.1 and Oct2 in classical Hodgkin disease but not in lymphocyte predominant Hodgkin disease correlates with immunoglobulin transcription. Blood 97: 496-501.
1875. Stenbygaard LE, Sorensen JB, Larsen H, Dombernowsky P (1999). Metastatic pattern in non-resectable non-small cell lung cancer. Acta Oncol 38: 993-998.
1876. Stephan JL, Galambrun C, Boucheron S, Varlet F, Delabesse E, MacIntyre E (2000). Epstein-Barr virus—positive undifferentiated thymic carcinoma in a 12-year-old white girl. J Pediatr Hematol Oncol 22: 162-166.
1877. Stephens M, Khalil J, Gibbs AR (1987). Primary clear cell carcinoma of the thymus gland. Histopathology 11: 763-765.
1878. Sternberg C (1900). Uber Leukosarcomatose. Wien Klin Wschr 21: 475-480.
1879. Sterner DJ, Mori M, Roggli VL, Fraire AE (1997). Prevalence of pulmonary atypical alveolar cell hyperplasia in an autopsy population: a study of 100 cases. Mod Pathol 10: 469-473.
1880. Stiller B, Hetzer R, Meyer R, Dittrich S, Pees C, Alexi-Meskishvili V, Lange PE (2001). Primary cardiac tumours: when is surgery necessary? Eur J Cardiothorac Surg 20: 1002-1006.
1881. Stock C, Ambros IM, Lion T, Haas OA, Zoubek A, Gadner H, Ambros PF (1994). Detection of numerical and structural chromosome abnormalities in pediatric germ cell tumors by means of interphase cytogenetics. Genes Chromosomes Cancer 11: 40-50.
1882. Stratakis CA, Carney JA, Lin JP, Papanicolaou DA, Karl M, Kastner DL, Pras E, Chrousos GP (1996). Carney complex, a familial multiple neoplasia and lentiginosis syndrome. Analysis of 11 kindreds and linkage to the short arm of chromosome 2. J Clin Invest 97: 699-705.
1883. Strickler JG, Hegstrom J, Thomas MJ, Yousem SA (1987). Myoepithelioma of the lung. Arch Pathol Lab Med 111: 1082-1085.
1884. Strimlan CV, Khasnabis S (1993). Primary mediastinal myelolipoma. Cleve Clin J Med 60: 69-71.
1885. Strizheva GD, Carsillo T, Kruger WD, Sullivan EJ, Ryu JH, Henske EP (2001). The spectrum of mutations in TSC1 and TSC2 in women with tuberous sclerosis and lymphangiomyomatosis. Am J Respir Crit Care Med 163: 253-258.
1886. Strobel P, Helmreich M, Menioudakis G, Lewin SR, Rudiger T, Bauer A, Hoffacker V, Gold R, Nix W, Schalke B, Elert O, Semik M, Muller-Hermelink HK, Marx A (2002). Paraneoplastic myasthenia gravis correlates with generation of mature naive CD4(+) T cells in thymomas. Blood 100: 159-166.
1887. Strobel P, Hartmann M, Jakob A, Mikesch K, Brink I, Dirnhofer S, Marx A (2004). Thymic carcinoma with overexpression of mutated KIT: Response to Imatinib. N Engl J Med .
1888. Strollo DC, Rosado-de-Christenson ML (2002). Primary mediastinal malignant germ cell neoplasms: imaging features. Chest Surg Clin N Am 12: 645-658.
1889. Strollo DC, Rosado de Christenson ML, Jett JR (1997). Primary mediastinal tumors. Part 1: tumors of the anterior mediastinum. Chest 112: 511-522.
1890. Struski S, Doco-Fenzy M, Cornillet-Lefebvre P (2002). Compilation of published comparative genomic hybridization studies. Cancer Genet Cytogenet 135: 63-90.
1891. Stucker I, Hirvonen A, de Waziers I, Cabelguenne A, Mitrunen K, Cenee S, Koum-Besson E, Hemon D, Beaune P, Loriot MA (2002). Genetic polymorphisms of glutathione S-transferases as modulators of lung cancer susceptibility. Carcinogenesis 23: 1475-1481.
1892. Sturm N, Lantuejoul S, Laverriere MH, Papotti M, Brichon PY, Brambilla C, Brambilla E (2001). Thyroid transcription factor 1 and cytokeratins 1, 5, 10, 14 (34betaE12) expression in basaloid and large-cell neuroendocrine carcinomas of the lung. Hum Pathol 32: 918-925.
1893. Sturm N, Rossi G, Lantuejoul S, Laverriere MH, Papotti M, Brichon PY, Brambilla C, Brambilla E (2002). Cytokeratins 1, 5, 10, 14 (34betaE12) expression along the whole specturm of neuroendocrine proliferations of the lung, from neuroendocrine cell hyperplasia to small cell carcinoma. Histopathology 41: 1-11.
1894. Sturm N, Rossi G, Lantuejoul S, Papotti M, Frachon S, Claraz C, Brichon PY, Brambilla C, Brambilla E (2002). Expression of thyroid transcription factor-1 in the spectrum of neuroendocrine cell lung proliferations with special interest in carcinoids. Hum Pathol 33: 175-182.
1895. Su L, Sheldon S, Weiss SW (1995). Inflammatory myofibroblastic tumor: cytogenetic evidence suporting clonal origin. Mod Pathol 8: 12A.
1896. Su LD, Atayde-Perez A, Sheldon S, Fletcher JA, Weiss SW (1998). Inflammatory myofibroblastic tumor: cytogenetic evidence supporting clonal origin. Mod Pathol 11: 364-368.
1897. Suarez Vilela D, Salas Valien JS, Gonzalez Moran MA, Izquierdo Garcia F, Riera Velasco JR (1992). Thymic carcinosarcoma associated with a spindle cell thymoma: an immunohistochemical study. Histopathology 21: 263-268.
1898. Suarez V, Fuggle WJ, Cameron AH, French TA, Hollingworth T (1987). Foamy myocardial transformation of infancy: an inherited disease. J Clin Pathol 40: 329-334.
1899. Sugimura H, Kohno T, Wakai K, Nagura K, Genka K, Igarashi H, Morris BJ, Baba S, Ohno Y, Gao C, Li Z, Wang J, Takezaki T, Tajima K, Varga T, Sawaguchi T, Lum JK, Martinson JJ, Tsugane S, Iwamasa T, Shinmura K, Yokota J (1999). hOGG1 Ser326Cys polymorphism and lung cancer susceptibility. Cancer Epidemiol Biomarkers Prev 8: 669-674.
1900. Sugio K, Kishimoto Y, Virmani AK, Hung JY, Gazdar AF (1994). K-ras mutations are a relatively late event in the pathogenesis of lung carcinomas. Cancer Res 54: 5811-5815.
1901. Sugita M, Geraci M, Gao B, Powell RL, Hirsch FR, Johnson G, Lapadat R, Gabrielson E, Bremnes R, Bunn PA, Franklin WA (2002). Combined use of oligonucleotide and tissue microarrays identifies cancer/testis antigens as biomarkers in lung carcinoma. Cancer Res 62: 3971-3979.
1902. Sugiura H, Morikawa T, Itoh K, Ono K, Okushiba S, Kondo S, Katoh H (2000). Thymic neuroendocrine carcinoma: a clinicopathologic study in four patients. Ann Thorac Cardiovasc Surg 6: 304-308.
1903. Sun JP, Asher CR, Yang XS, Cheng GG, Scalia GM, Massed AG, Griffin BP, Ratliff NB, Stewart WJ, Thomas JD (2001). Clinical and echocardiographic characteristics of papillary fibroelastomas: a retrospective and prospective study in 162 patients. Circulation 103: 2687-2693.
1904. Sunaga N, Kohno T, Kolligs FT, Fearon ER, Saito R, Yokota J (2001). Constitutive activation of the Wnt signaling pathway by CTNNB1 (beta-catenin) mutations in a subset of human lung adenocarcinoma. Genes Chromosomes Cancer 30: 316-321.
1905. Sundaresan V, Reeve JG, Stenning S, Stewart S, Bleehen NM (1991). Neuroendocrine differentiation and clinical behaviour in non-small cell lung tumours. Br J Cancer 64: 333-338.
1906. Sussman J, Rosai J (1990). Lymph node metastasis as the initial manifestation of malignant mesothelioma. Report of six cases. Am J Surg Pathol 14: 819-828.
1907. Suster S, Barbuto D, Carlson G, Rosai J (1991). Multilocular thymic cysts with pseudoepitheliomatous hyperplasia. Hum Pathol 22: 455-460.
1908. Suster S, Fisher C, Moran CA (1998). Expression of bcl-2 oncoprotein in benign and malignant spindle cell tumors of soft tissue, skin, serosal surfaces, and gastrointestinal tract. Am J Surg Pathol 22: 863-872.
1909. Suster S, Huszar M, Herczeg E (1987). Spindle cell squamous carcinoma of the lung. Immunocytochemical and ultrastructural study of a case. Histopathology 11: 871-878.
1910. Suster S, Moran CA (1995). Chordomas of the mediastinum: clinicopathologic, immunohistochemical, and ultrastructural study of six cases presenting as posterior mediastinal masses. Hum Pathol 26: 1354-1362.
1911. Suster S, Moran CA (1995). Thymic carcinoid with prominent mucinous stroma. Report of a distinctive morphologic variant of thymic neuroendocrine neoplasm. Am J Surg Pathol 19: 1277-1285.
1912. Suster S, Moran CA (1996). Primary thymic epithelial neoplasms showing combined features of thymoma and thymic car-

cinoma. A clinicopathologic study of 22 cases. Am J Surg Pathol 20: 1469-1480.
1913. Suster S, Moran CA (1998). Thymic carcinoma: spectrum of differentiation and histologic types. Pathology 30: 111-122.
1914. Suster S, Moran CA (1999). Micronodular thymoma with lymphoid B-cell hyperplasia: clinicopathologic and immunohistochemical study of eighteen cases of a distinctive morphologic variant of thymic epithelial neoplasm. Am J Surg Pathol 23: 955-962.
1915. Suster S, Moran CA (1999). Primary thymic epithelial neoplasms: spectrum of differentiation and histological features. Semin Diagn Pathol 16: 2-17.
1916. Suster S, Moran CA (1999). Spindle cell thymic carcinoma: clinicopathologic and immunohistochemical study of a distinctive variant of primary thymic epithelial neoplasm. Am J Surg Pathol 23: 691-700.
1917. Suster S, Moran CA (1999). Thymoma, atypical thymoma, and thymic carcinoma. A novel conceptual approach to the classification of thymic epithelial neoplasms. Am J Clin Pathol 111: 826-833.
1918. Suster S, Moran CA (2001). Neuroendocrine neoplasms of the mediastinum. Am J Clin Pathol 115 Suppl: S17-S27.
1919. Suster S, Moran CA, Chan JK (1997). Thymoma with pseudosarcomatous stroma: report of an unusual histologic variant of thymic epithelial neoplasm that may simulate carcinosarcoma. Am J Surg Pathol 21: 1316-1323.
1920. Suster S, Moran CA, Dominguez-Malagon H, Quevedo-Blanco P (1998). Germ cell tumors of the mediastinum and testis: a comparative immunohistochemical study of 120 cases. Hum Pathol 29: 737-742.
1921. Suster S, Moran CA, Koss MN (1994). Epithelioid hemangioendothelioma of the anterior mediastinum. Clinicopathologic, immunohistochemical, and ultrastructural analysis of 12 cases. Am J Surg Pathol 18: 871-881.
1922. Suster S, Moran CA, Koss MN (1994). Rhabdomyosarcomas of the anterior mediastinum: report of four cases unassociated with germ cell, teratomatous, or thymic carcinomatous components. Hum Pathol 25: 349-356.
1923. Suster S, Rosai J (1991). Multilocular thymic cyst: an acquired reactive process. Study of 18 cases. Am J Surg Pathol 15: 388-398.
1924. Suster S, Rosai J (1991). Thymic carcinoma. A clinicopathologic study of 60 cases. Cancer 67: 1025-1032.
1925. Suvarna SK, Royds JA (1996). The nature of the cardiac myxoma. Int J Cardiol 57: 211-216.
1926. Suzuki K, Asamura H, Kusumoto M, Kondo H, Tsuchiya R (2002). "Early" peripheral lung cancer: prognostic significance of ground glass opacity on thin-section computed tomographic scan. Ann Thorac Surg 74: 1635-1639.
1927. Suzuki K, Nagai K, Yoshida J, Yokose T, Kodama T, Takahashi K, Nishimura M, Kawasaki H, Yokozaki M, Nishiwaki Y (1997). The prognosis of resected lung carcinoma associated with atypical adenomatous hyperplasia: a comparison of the prognosis of well-differentiated adenocarcinoma associated with atypical adenomatous hyperplasia and intrapulmonary metastasis. Cancer 79: 1521-1526.
1928. Suzuki K, Takahashi K, Yoshida J, Nishimura M, Yokose T, Nishiwaki Y, Nagai K (1998). Synchronous double primary lung carcinomas associated with multiple atypical adenomatous hyperplasia. Lung Cancer 19: 131-139.
1929. Suzuki K, Yokose T, Yoshida J, Nishimura M, Takahashi K, Nagai K, Nishiwaki Y (2000). Prognostic significance of the size of central fibrosis in peripheral adenocarcinoma of the lung. Ann Thorac Surg 69: 893-897.
1930. Suzuki R, Kagami Y, Takeuchi K, Kami M, Okamoto M, Ichinohasama R, Mori N, Kojima M, Yoshino T, Yamabe H, Shiota M, Mori S, Ogura M, Hamajima N, Seto M, Suchi T, Morishima Y, Nakamura S (2000). Prognostic significance of CD56 expression for ALK-positive and ALK-negative anaplastic large-cell lymphoma of T/null cell phenotype. Blood 96: 2993-3000.
1931. Suzuki Y, Saiga T, Ozeki Y, Koyama A, Homma M, Ohba S (1993). [Two cases of intrapulmonary teratoma]. Nippon Kyobu Geka Gakkai Zasshi 41: 498-502.
1932. Swanson PE (1991). Soft tissue neoplasma of the mediastinum. Semin Diagn Pathol 8: 14-34.
1933. Swensen SJ, Hartman TE, Mayo JR, Colby TV, Tazelaar HD, Muller NL (1995). Diffuse pulmonary lymphangiomatosis: CT findings. J Comput Assist Tomogr 19: 348-352.
1934. Swinson DE, Jones JL, Richardson D, Cox G, Edwards JG, O'Byrne KJ (2002). Tumour necrosis is an independent prognostic marker in non-small cell lung cancer: correlation with biological variables. Lung Cancer 37: 235-240.
1935. Sydorak RM, Kelly T, Feldstein VA, Sandberg PL, Silverman NH, Harrison MR, Albanese CT (2002). Prenatal resection of a fetal pericardial teratoma. Fetal Diagn Ther 17: 281-285.
1936. Syed S, Haque AK, Hawkins HK, Sorensen PH, Cowan DF (2002). Desmoplastic small round cell tumor of the lung. Arch Pathol Lab Med 126: 1226-1228.
1937. Syrjanen KJ (2002). HPV infections and lung cancer. J Clin Pathol 55: 885-891.
1938. Szczepanski T, Langerak AW, Willemse MJ, Wolvers-Tettero IL, van Wering ER, van Dongen JJ (2000). T cell receptor gamma (TCRG) gene rearrangements in T cell acute lymphoblastic leukemia refelct 'end-stage' recombinations: implications for minimal residual disease monitoring. Leukemia 14: 1208-1214.
1939. Szczepanski T, Pongers-Willemse MJ, Langerak AW, Harts WA, Wijkhuijs AJ, van Wering ER, van Dongen JJ (1999). Ig heavy chain gene rearrangements in T-cell acute lymphoblastic leukemia exhibit predominant DH6-19 and DH7-27 gene usage, can result in complete V-D-J rearrangements, and are rare in T-cell receptor alpha beta lineage. Blood 93: 4079-4085.
1940. Szyfelbein WM, Ross JS (1988). Carcinoids, atypical carcinoids, and small-cell carcinomas of the lung: differential diagnosis of fine-needle aspiration biopsy specimens. Diagn Cytopathol 4: 1-8.
1941. Tagge EP, Mulvihill D, Chandler JC, Richardson M, Uflacker R, Othersen HD (1996). Childhood pleuropulmonary blastoma: caution against nonoperative management of congenital lung cysts. J Pediatr Surg 31: 187-189.
1942. Taguchi T, Jhanwar SC, Siegfried JM, Keller SM, Testa JR (1993). Recurrent deletions of specific chromosomal sites in 1p, 3p, 6q, and 9p in human malignant mesothelioma. Cancer Res 53: 4349-4355.
1943. Taioli E, Gaspari L, Benhamou S, Boffetta P, Brockmoller J, Butkiewicz D, Cascorbi I, Clapper ML, Dolzan V, Haugen A, Hirvonen A, Husgafvel-Pursiainen K, Kalina I, Kremers P, Le Marchand L, London S, Rannug A, Romkes M, Schoket B, Seidegard J, Strange RC, Stucker I, To-Figueras J, Garte S (2003). Polymorphisms in CYP1A1, GSTM1, GSTT1 and lung cancer below the age of 45 years. Int J Epidemiol 32: 60-63.
1944. Takach TJ, Reul GJ, Ott DA, Cooley DA (1996). Primary cardiac tumors in infants and children: immediate and long-term operative results. Ann Thorac Surg 62: 559-564.
1945. Takagi N, Nakamura S, Yamamoto K, Kunishima K, Takagi I, Suyama M, Shinoda M, Sugiura T, Oyama A, Suzuki H, Koshikawa T, Kontani K, Ueda R, Takahashi T, Ariyoshi Y, Suchi T (1992). Malignant lymphoma of mucosa-associated lymphoid tissue arising in the thymus of a patient with Sjogren's syndrome. A morphologic, phenotypic, and genotypic study. Cancer 69: 1347-1355.
1946. Takahashi K, Yoshida J, Nishimura M, Nagai K (2000). Thymic carcinoma. Outcome of treatment including surgical resection. Jpn J Thorac Cardiovasc Surg 48: 494-498.
1947. Takahashi T, Nau MM, Chiba I, Birrer MJ, Rosenberg RK, Vinocour M, Levitt M, Pass H, Gazdar AF, Minna JD (1989). p53: a frequent target for genetic abnormalities in lung cancer. Science 246: 491-494.
1948. Takai K, Sanada M, Hirose Y, Shibuya H (1997). [Diffuse large B-cell lymphoma mainly involving the heart and showing t(8;14) (q24;q32) with c-myc rearrangement]. Rinsho Ketsueki 38: 757-762.
1949. Takamochi K, Ogura T, Suzuki K, Kawasaki H, Kurashima Y, Yokose T, Ochiai A, Nagai K, Nishiwaki Y, Esumi H (2001). Loss of heterozygosity on chromosomes 9q and 16p in atypical adenomatous hyperplasia concomitant with adenocarcinoma of the lung. Am J Pathol 159: 1941-1948.
1950. Takamori S, Noguchi M, Morinaga S, Goya T, Tsugane S, Kakegawa T, Shimosato Y (1991). Clinicopathologic characteristics of adenosquamous carcinoma of the lung. Cancer 67: 649-654.
1951. Takashima S, Maruyama Y, Hasegawa M, Saito A, Haniuda M, Kadoya M (2003). High-resolution CT features: prognostic significance in peripheral lung adenocarcinoma with bronchioloalveolar carcinoma components. Respiration 70: 36-42.
1952. Takashima S, Maruyama Y, Hasegawa M, Yamanda T, Honda T, Kadoya M, Sone S (2002). Prognostic significance of high-resolution CT findings in small peripheral adenocarcinoma of the lung: a retrospective study on 64 patients. Lung Cancer 36: 289-295.
1953. Takayama T, Kameya T, Inagaki K, Nonaka M, Miyazawa H, Ogawa N, Yano M, Morita T, Arai T, Niino S (1993). MEN type 1 associated with mediastinal carcinoid producing parathyroid hormone, calcitonin and chorionic gonadotropin. Pathol Res Pract 189: 1090-1096.
1954. Takeda S, Miyoshi S, Akashi A, Ohta M, Minami M, Okumura M, Masaoka A, Matsuda H (2003). Clinical spectrum of primary mediastinal tumors: a comparison of adult and pediatric populations at a single Japanese institution. J Surg Oncol 83: 24-30.
1955. Takeda S, Miyoshi S, Ohta M, Minami M, Masaoka A, Matsuda H (2003). Primary germ cell tumors in the mediastinum: a 50-year experience at a single Japanese institution. Cancer 97: 367-376.
1956. Takeda S, Nanjo S, Nakamoto K, Imachi T, Yamamoto S (1994). Carcinosarcoma of the lung. Report of a case and review of the literature. Respiration 61: 113-116.
1957. Takei H, Asamura H, Maeshima A, Suzuki K, Kondo H, Niki T, Yamada T, Tsuchiya R, Matsuno Y (2002). Large cell neuroendocrine carcinoma of the lung: a clinicopathologic study of eighty-seven cases. J Thorac Cardiovasc Surg 124: 285-292.
1958. Takeuchi E, Shimizu E, Sano N, Yamaguchi T, Yanagawa H, Sone S (1998). A case of pleomorphic adenoma of the lung with multiple distant metastases - Observations on its oncogene and tumor suppressor gene expression. Anticancer Res 18: 2015-2020.
1959. Takeuchi S, Koike M, Park S, Seriu T, Bartram CR, Taub HE, Williamson IK, Grewal J, Taguchi H, Koeffler HP (1998). The ATM gene and susceptibility to childhood T-cell acute lymphoblastic leukaemia. Br J Haematol 103: 536-538.
1960. Takigawa N, Segawa Y, Nakata M, Saeki H, Mandai K, Kishino D, Shimono M, Ida M, Eguchi K (1999). Clinical investigation of atypical adenomatous hyperplasia of the lung. Lung Cancer 25: 115-121.
1961. Takita H, Merrin C, Didolkar MS, Douglass HO, Edgerton F (1977). The surgical management of multiple lung metastases. Ann Thorac Surg 24: 359-364.
1962. Talbot SM, Taub RN, Keohan ML, Edwards N, Galantowicz ME, Schulman LL (2002). Combined heart and lung transplantation for unresectable primary cardiac sarcoma. J Thorac Cardiovasc Surg 124: 1145-1148.
1963. Talerman A (1986). Germ cell tumors. In: Pathology of the Testis and its Adnexa, Talerman A, Roth LM, eds., Churchill Livingstone: New York , pp. 29-65.
1964. Talerman A, Gratama S (1983). Primary ganglioneuroblastoma of the anterior mediastinum in a 61-year-old woman. Histopathology 7: 967-975.
1965. Tamura M, Ohta Y, Ishikawa N, Tsunezuka Y, Oda M, Watanabe G (2002). [Thymic carcinoma; analysis of nine clinical studies]. Kyobu Geka 55: 1105-1109.
1966. Tan DF, Huberman JA, Hyland A, Loewen GM, Brooks JS, Beck AF, Todorov IT, Bepler G (2001). MCM2—a promising marker for premalignant lesions of the lung: a cohort study. BMC Cancer 1: 6.
1967. Tan PH, Sng IT (1995). Thymoma—a study of 60 cases in Singapore. Histopathology 26: 509-518.
1968. Tan W, Chen GF, Xing DY, Song CY, Kadlubar FF, Lin DX (2001). Frequency of CYP2A6 gene deletion and its relation to risk of lung and esophageal cancer in the Chinese population. Int J Cancer 95: 96-101.
1969. Tandon S, Kant S, Singh AK, Sinha KN, Chandra T, Agarwal PK (1999). Primary intrapulmonary teratoma presenting as pyothorax. Indian J Chest Dis Allied Sci 41: 51-55.
1970. Tang D, Phillips DH, Stampfer M, Mooney LA, Hsu Y, Cho S, Tsai WY, Ma J, Cole KJ, She MN, Perera FP (2001). Association between carcinogen-DNA adducts in white blood cells and lung cancer risk in the physicians health study. Cancer Res 61: 6708-6712.
1971. Tangthangtham A, Wongsangiem M, Koanantakool T, Ponglertnapagorn P,

Subhannachart P, Charupatanapongse U (1998). Intrapulmonary teratoma: a report of three cases. J Med Assoc Thai 81: 1028-1033.

1972. Taniere P, Manai A, Charpentier R, Terdjman P, Boucheron S, Cordier JF, Berger F (1998). Pyothorax-associated lymphoma: relationship with Epstein-Barr virus, human herpes virus-8 and body cavity-based high grade lymphomas. Eur Respir J 11: 779-783.

1973. Taniere P, Thivolet-Bejui F, Vitrey D, Isaac S, Loire R, Cordier JF, Berger F (1998). Lymphomatoid granulomatosis—a report on four cases: evidence for B phenotype of the tumoral cells. Eur Respir J 12: 102-106.

1974. Tanimura S, Tomoyasu H, Kohno T, Matsushita H (2002). [Basaloid carcinoma originated from the wall of thymic cyst presenting as pericardial and thoracic effusion; report of a case]. Kyobu Geka 55: 571-575.

1975. Taniyama K, Ohta S, Suzuki H, Matsumoto M, Nagashima Y, Tahara E (1992). Alpha-fetoprotein-producing immature mediastinal teratoma showing rapid and massive recurrent growth in an adult. Acta Pathol Jpn 42: 911-915.

1976. Tanoue LT, Ponn RB (2002). Therapy for stage I and stage II non-small cell lung cancer. Clin Chest Med 23: 173-190.

1977. Tashiro Y, Iwata Y, Nabae T, Manabe H (1995). Pulmonary oncocytoma: report of a case in conjunction with an immunohistochemical and ultrastructural study. Pathol Int 45: 448-451.

1978. Tateyama H, Eimoto T, Tada T, Hattori H, Murase T, Takino H (1999). Immunoreactivity of a new CD5 antibody with normal epithelium and malignant tumors including thymic carcinoma. Am J Clin Pathol 111: 235-240.

1979. Tateyama H, Eimoto T, Tada T, Inagaki H, Hattori H, Takino H (1997). Apoptosis, bcl-2 protein, and Fas antigen in thymic epithelial tumors. Mod Pathol 10: 983-991.

1980. Tateyama H, Eimoto T, Tada T, Mizuno T, Inagaki H, Hata A, Sasaki M, Masaoka A (1995). p53 protein expression and p53 gene mutation in thymic epithelial tumors. An immunohistochemical and DNA sequencing study. Am J Clin Pathol 104: 375-381.

1981. Tateyama H, Saito Y, Fujii Y, Okumura M, Nakamura K, Tada H, Yasumitsu T, Eimoto T (2001). The spectrum of micronodular thymic epithelial tumours with lymphoid B-cell hyperplasia. Histopathology 38: 519-527.

1982. Taubert H, Wurl P, Meye A, Berger D, Thamm B, Neumann K, Hinze R, Schmidt H, Rath FW (1995). Molecular and immunohistochemical p53 status in liposarcoma and malignant fibrous histiocytoma: identification of seven new mutations for soft tissue sarcomas. Cancer 76: 1187-1196.

1983. Taylor JR, Ryu J, Colby TV, Raffin TA (1990). Lymphangioleiomyomatosis. Clinical course in 32 patients. N Engl J Med 323: 1254-1260.

1984. Tazelaar HD, Batts KP, Srigley JR (2001). Primary extrapulmonary sugar tumor (PEST): a report of four cases. Mod Pathol 14: 615-622.

1985. Tazelaar HD, Kerr D, Yousem SA, Saldana MJ, Langston C, Colby TV (1993). Diffuse pulmonary lymphangiomatosis. Hum Pathol 24: 1313-1322.

1986. Tazelaar HD, Locke TJ, McGregor CG (1992). Pathology of surgically excised primary cardiac tumors. Mayo Clin Proc 67: 957-965.

1987. Teh BT (1998). Thymic carcinoids in multiple endocrine neoplasia type 1. J Intern Med 243: 501-504.

1988. Teh BT, McArdle J, Chan SP, Menon J, Hartley L, Pullan P, Ho J, Khir A, Wilkinson S, Larsson C, Cameron D, Shepherd J (1997). Clinicopathologic studies of thymic carcinoids in multiple endocrine neoplasia type 1. Medicine (Baltimore) 76: 21-29.

1989. Teh BT, Zedenius J, Kytola S, Skogseid B, Trotter J, Choplin H, Twigg S, Farnebo F, Giraud S, Cameron D, Robinson B, Calender A, Larsson C, Salmela P (1998). Thymic carcinoids in multiple endocrine neoplasia type 1. Ann Surg 228: 99-105.

1990. Teilum G (1959). Endodermal sinus tumours of the ovary and testis: comparative morphogenesis of the so-called mesonephroma ovarii (Schiller) and extraembryonic (yolk sac-allantoic) structures in the rat's placenta. Cancer 12: 1092-1105.

1991. Teramoto N, Cao L, Kawasaki N, Tonoyama Y, Sarker AB, Yoshino T, Takahashi K, Akagi T (1996). Variable expression of Epstein-Barr virus latent membrane protein I in Reed-Sternberg cells of Hodgkin's disease. Acta Med Okayama 50: 267-270.

1992. Terasaki H, Niki T, Hasegawa T, Yamada T, Suzuki K, Kusumoto M, Fujimoto K, Hayabuchi N, Matsuno Y, Shimoda T (2001). Primary synovial sarcoma of the lung: a case report confirmed by molecular detection of SYT-SSX fusion gene transcripts. Jpn J Clin Oncol 31: 212-216.

1993. Teraski H, Niki T, Matsuno Y, Yamada T, Maeshima A, Asamura H, Hayabuchi N, Hirohashi S (2003). Lung adenocarcinoma with mixed bronchiolo-alveolar and invasive components: clinicopathological features, subclassification by extent of invasive foci, and immunohistochemical characterization. Am J Surg Pathol 27: 937-951.

1994. Teruya-Feldstein J, Jaffe ES, Burd PR, Kanegane H, Kingma DW, Wilson WH, Longo DL, Tosato G (1997). The role of Mig, the monokine induced by interferon-gamma, and IP-10, the interferon-gamma-inducible protein-10, in tissue necrosis and vascular damage associated with Epstein-Barr virus-positive lymphoproliferative disease. Blood 90: 4099-4105.

1995. Teruya-Feldstein J, Zauber P, Setsuda JE, Berman EL, Sorbara L, Raffeld M, Tosato G, Jaffe ES (1998). Expression of human herpesvirus-8 oncogene and cytokine homologues in an HIV-seronegative patient with multicentric Castleman's disease and primary effusion lymphoma. Lab Invest 78: 1637-1642.

1996. Testa JR, Liu Z, Feder M, Bell DW, Balsara B, Cheng JQ, Taguchi T (1997). Advances in the analysis of chromosome alterations in human lung carcinomas. Cancer Genet Cytogenet 95: 20-32.

1997. Testa JR, Pass HI, Carbone M (2001). Molecular biology of mesothelioma. In: Cancer: Principles and Practice of Oncology, DeVita VTJr, Hellman S, Rosenberg SA, eds., 6th ed. Lippincott Williams & Wilkins: Philadelphia , pp. 1937-1943.

1998. Thier R, Bruning T, Roos PH, Bolt HM (2002). Cytochrome P450 1B1, a new keystone in gene-environment interactions related to human head and neck cancer? Arch Toxicol 76: 249-256.

1999. Thomas CFJr, Tazelaar HD, Jett JR (2001). Typical and atypical pulmonary carcinoids : outcome in patients presenting with regional lymph node involvement. Chest 119: 1143-1150.

2000. Thomas CR, Wright CD, Loehrer PJ (1999). Thymoma: state of the art. J Clin Oncol 17: 2280-2289.

2001. Thomas KE, Winchell CP, Varco RL (1967). Diagnostic and surgical aspects of left atrial tumors. J Thorac Cardiovasc Surg 53: 535-548.

2002. Thompson L, Chang B, Barsky SH (1996). Monoclonal origins of malignant mixed tumors (carcinosarcomas). Evidence for a divergent histogenesis. Am J Surg Pathol 20: 277-285.

2003. To-Figueras J, Gene M, Gomez-Catalan J, Galan C, Firvida J, Fuentes M, Rodamilans M, Huguet E, Estape J, Corbella J (1996). Glutathione-S-Transferase M1 and codon 72 p53 polymorphisms in a northwestern Mediterranean population and their relation to lung cancer susceptibility. Cancer Epidemiol Biomarkers Prev 5: 337-342.

2004. Toide K, Yamazaki H, Nagashima R, Itoh K, Iwano S, Takahashi Y, Watanabe S, Kamataki T (2003). Aryl Hydrocarbon Hydroxylase Represents CYP1B1, and not CYP1A1, in Human Freshly Isolated White Cells: Trimodal Distribution of Japanese Population According to Induction of CYP1B1 mRNA by Environmental Dioxins. Cancer Epidemiol Biomarkers Prev 12: 219-222.

2005. Tollens T, Casselman F, Devlieger H, Gewillig MH, Vandenberghe K, Lerut TE, Daenen WJ (1998). Fetal cardiac tamponade due to an intrapericardial teratoma. Ann Thorac Surg 66: 559-560.

2006. Tomashefski JFJr (1982). Benign endobronchial mesenchymal tumors: their relationship to parenchymal pulmonary hamartomas. Am J Surg Pathol 6: 531-540.

2007. Tomashefski JFJr, Connors AFJr, Rosenthal ES, Hsiue IL (1990). Peripheral vs central squamous cell carcinoma of the lung. A comparison of clinical features, histopathology, and survival. Arch Pathol Lab Med 114: 468-474.

2008. Tominaga K, Kadokura M, Saida K, Nakao K, Kushiro H, Ryu K, Yamamoto N (1994). [A surgical case of giant mediastinal teratoma]. Kyobu Geka 47: 944-947.

2009. Tomita M, Matsuzaki Y, Edagawa M, Maeda M, Shimizu T, Hara M, Onitsuka T (2002). Clinical and immunohistochemical study of eight cases with thymic carcinoma. BMC Surg 2: 3.

2010. Tomita S, Mori KL, Sakajiri S, Oshimi K (2003). B-cell marker negative (CD7+, CD19-) Epstein-Barr virus-related pyothorax-associated lymphoma with rearrangement in the JH gene. Leuk Lymphoma 44: 727-730.

2011. Tomizawa Y, Adachi J, Kohno T, Hamada K, Saito R, Noguchi M, Matsuno Y, Hirohashi S, Yamaguchi N, Yokota J (1999). Prognostic significance of allelic imbalances on chromosome 9p in stage I non-small cell lung carcinoma. Clin Cancer Res 5: 1139-1146.

2012. Tomizawa Y, Nakajima T, Kohno T, Saito R, Yamaguchi N, Yokota J (1998). Clinicopathological significance of Fhit protein expression in stage I non-small cell lung carcinoma. Cancer Res 58: 5478-5483.

2013. Tomsova M, Steiner I, Dominik J (2000). [Cardiac myxomas]. Acta Medica (Hradec Kralove) 43 Suppl: 29-32.

2014. Toole AL, Stern H (1972). Carcinoid and adenoid cystic carcinoma of the bronchus. Ann Thorac Surg 13: 63-81.

2015. Topol EJ, Biern RO, Reitz BA (1986). Cardiac papillary fibroelastoma and stroke. Echocardiographic diagnosis and guide to excision. Am J Med 80: 129-132.

2016. Toren A, Ben Bassat I, Rechavi G (1996). Infectious agents and environmental factors in lymphoid malignancies. Blood Rev 10: 89-94.

2017. Toyooka S, Maruyama R, Toyooka KO, McLerran D, Feng Z, Fukuyama Y, Virmani AK, Zochbauer-Muller S, Tsukuda K, Sugio K, Shimizu N, Shimizu K, Lee H, Chen CY, Fong KM, Gilcrease M, Roth JA, Minna JD, Gazdar AF (2003). Smoke exposure, histologic type and geography-related differences in the methylation profiles of non-small cell lung cancer. Int J Cancer 103: 153-160.

2018. Toyooka S, Pass HI, Shivapurkar N, Fukuyama Y, Maruyama R, Toyooka KO, Gilcrease M, Farinas A, Minna JD, Gazdar AF (2001). Aberrant methylation and simian virus 40 tag sequences in malignant mesothelioma. Cancer Res 61: 5727-5730.

2019. Toyooka S, Toyooka KO, Maruyama R, Virmani AK, Girard L, Miyajima K, Harada K, Ariyoshi Y, Takahashi T, Sugio K, Brambilla E, Gilcrease M, Minna JD, Gazdar AF (2001). DNA methylation profiles of lung tumors. Mol Cancer Ther 1: 61-67.

2020. Toyooka S, Tsuda T, Gazdar AF (2003). The TP53 gene, tobacco exposure, and lung cancer. Hum Mutat 21: 229-239.

2021. Travers H (1982). Congenital polycystic tumor of the atrioventricular node: possible familial occurrence and critical review of reported cases with special emphasis on histogenesis. Hum Pathol 13: 25-35.

2022. Travis WD (2001). Lung. In: Pathology of Incipient Neoplasia, Albores-Saavedra J, Henson DE, eds., 3rd Ed. ed. Oxford University Press: New York , pp. 295-318.

2023. Travis WD (2002). Pathology of lung cancer. Clin Chest Med 23: 65-81, viii.

2024. Travis WD, Colby TV, Corrin B, Shimosato Y, Brambilla E (1999). WHO Histological Classification of Tumours. Histological Typing of Lung and Pleural Tumours. 3rd ed. Springer-Verlag: Berlin.

2025. Travis WD, Colby TV, Koss MN, Rosado-de-Christenson ML, Müller NL, King TE (2002). Atlas of Non-Tumor Pathology, Non-Neoplastic Disorders of the Lower Respiratory Tract. 1st ed. AFIP: Washington, DC.

2026. Travis WD, Linnoila RI, Tsokos MG, Hitchcock CL, Cutler GBJr, Nieman L, Chrousos G, Pass H, Doppman J (1991). Neuroendocrine tumors of the lung with proposed criteria for large-cell neuroendocrine carcinoma. An ultrastructural, immunohistochemical, and flow cytometric study of 35 cases. Am J Surg Pathol 15: 529-553.

2027. Travis WD, Lubin J, Ries L, Devesa S (1996). United States lung carcinoma incidence trends: declining for most histologic types among males, increasing among females. Cancer 77: 2464-2470.

2028. Travis WD, Rush W, Flieder DB, Falk R, Fleming MV, Gal AA, Koss MN (1998). Survival analysis of 200 pulmonary neuroendocrine tumors with clarification of criteria for atypical carcinoid and its separation from typical carcinoid. Am J Surg Pathol 22: 934-944.

2029. Travis WD, Travis LB, Devesa SS (1995). Lung cancer. Cancer 75: 191-202.

2030. Trillo A, Guha A (1988). Solitary condylomatous papilloma of the bronchus.

Arch Pathol Lab Med 112: 731-733.

2031. Trojani M, Contesso G, Coindre JM, Rouesse J, Bui NB, de Mascarel A, Goussot JF, David M, Bonichon F, Lagarde C (1984). Soft-tissue sarcomas of adults; study of pathological prognostic variables and definition of a histopathological grading system. Int J Cancer 33: 37-42.

2032. Truong LD, Mody DR, Cagle PT, Jackson-York GL, Schwartz MR, Wheeler TM (1990). Thymic carcinoma. A clinico-pathologic study of 13 cases. Am J Surg Pathol 14: 151-166.

2033. Trupiano JK, Rice TW, Herzog K, Barr FG, Shipley J, Fisher C, Goldblum JR (2002). Mediastinal synovial sarcoma: report of two cases with molecular genetic analysis. Ann Thorac Surg 73: 628-630.

2034. Tsang P, Cesarman E, Chadburn A, Liu YF, Knowles DM (1996). Molecular characterization of primary mediastinal B cell lymphoma. Am J Pathol 148: 2017-2025.

2035. Tsuchida M, Yamato Y, Hashimoto T, Saito M, Hayashi J (2001). Recurrent thymic carcinoid tumor in the pleural cavity. 2 cases of long-term survivors. Jpn J Thorac Cardiovasc Surg 49: 666-668.

2036. Tsuchiya R, Koga K, Matsuno Y, Mukai K, Shimosato Y (1994). Thymic carcinoma: proposal for pathological TNM and staging. Pathol Int 44: 505-512.

2037. Tsuji N, Tateishi R, Ishiguro S, Terao T, Higashiyama M (1995). Adenomyoepithelioma of the lung. Am J Surg Pathol 19: 956-962.

2038. Tsukamoto S, Omori K, Kitamura K, Ohata M, Sezai Y, Nemoto N (1993). [A case report of mediastinal teratoma complicated with cardiac tamponade]. Nippon Kyobu Geka Gakkai Zasshi 41: 688-693.

2039. Tucker AS (1964). Lymphangiectasis - benign + malignant. Am J Roentgenol Radium Ther Nucl Med 91: 1104-&.

2040. Turnbull AD, Huvos AG, Goodner JT, Foote FWJr (1971). Mucoepidermoid tumors of bronchial glands. Cancer 28: 539-544.

2041. Turner RR, Colby TV, Doggett RS (1984). Well-differentiated lymphocytic lymphoma. A study of 47 patients with primary manifestation in the lung. Cancer 54: 2088-2096.

2042. Tyczynski JE, Bray F, Parkin DM (2003). Lung cancer in Europe in 2000: epidemiology, prevention, and early detection. Lancet Oncol 4: 45-55.

2043. Uberfuhr P, Meiser B, Fuchs A, Schulze C, Reichenspurner H, Falk M, Weiss M, Wintersperger B, Issels R, Reichart B (2002). Heart transplantation: an approach to treating primary cardiac sarcoma? J Heart Lung Transplant 21: 1135-1139.

2044. Uckun FM, Sensel MG, Sun L, Steinherz PG, Trigg ME, Heerema NA, Sather HN, Reaman GH, Gaynon PS (1998). Biology and treatment of childhood T-lineage acute lymphoblastic leukemia. Blood 91: 735-746.

2045. UICC (2002). International Union Against Cancer (UICC) : TNM Classification of Malignant Tumours. 6th ed. Wiley and Sons: New York.

2046. Ulbright TM, Clark SA, Einhorn LH (1985). Angiosarcoma associated with germ cell tumors. Hum Pathol 16: 268-272.

2047. Ulbright TM, Loehrer PJ, Roth LM, Einhorn LH, Williams SD, Clark SA (1984). The development of non-germ cell malignancies within germ cell tumors. A clinico-pathologic study of 11 cases. Cancer 54: 1824-1833.

2048. Ulbright TM, Michael H, Loehrer PJ, Donohue JP (1990). Spindle cell tumors resected from male patients with germ cell tumors. A clinicopathologic study of 14 cases. Cancer 65: 148-156.

2049. Ulbright TM, Roth LM (1990). A pathologic analysis of lesions following modern chemotherapy for metastatic germ-cell tumors. Pathol Annu 25 Pt 1: 313-340.

2050. Ulbright TM, Roth LM, Brodhecker CA (1986). Yolk sac differentiation in germ cell tumors. A morphologic study of 50 cases with emphasis on hepatic, enteric, and parietal yolk sac features. Am J Surg Pathol 10: 151-164.

2051. Ullmann R, Petzmann S, Sharma A, Cagle PT, Popper HH (2001). Chromosomal aberrations in a series of large-cell neuroendocrine carcinomas: unexpected divergence from small-cell carcinoma of the lung. Hum Pathol 32: 1059-1063.

2052. Ullmann R, Schwendel A, Klemen H, Wolf G, Petersen I, Popper HH (1998). Unbalanced chromosomal aberrations in neuroendocrine lung tumors as detected by comparative genomic hybridization. Hum Pathol 29: 1145-1149.

2053. Uppal R, Goldstraw P (1992). Primary pulmonary lymphoma. Lung Cancer 8: 95-100.

2054. Uramoto H, Oyama T, Yoshimatsu T, Osaki T, Yasumoto K (2000). Benign mesenchymoma of the mediastinum. Jpn J Thorac Carciovasc Surg 48: 814-816.

2055. Urban C, Lackner H, Schwinger W, Beham-Schmid C (2003). Fatal hemophagocytic syndrome as initial manifestation of a mediastinal germ cell tumor. Med Pediatr Oncol 40: 247-249.

2056. Ustun MO, Demircan A, Paksoy N, Ozkaynak C, Tuzuner S (1996). A case of intrapulmonary teratoma presenting with hair expectoration. Thorac Cardiovasc Surg 44: 271-273.

2057. Usuda K, Saito Y, Nagamoto N, Sato M, Sagawa M, Kanma K, Takahasi S, Endo C, Fujimura S (1993). Relation between bronchoscopic findings and tumor size of roentgenographically occult bronchogenic squamous cell carcinoma. J Thorac Cardiovasc Surg 106: 1098-1103.

2058. Vahakangas KH, Bennett WP, Castren K, Welsh JA, Khan MA, Blomeke B, Alavanja MC, Harris CC (2001). p53 and K-ras mutations in lung cancers from former and never-smoking women. Cancer Res 61: 4350-4356.

2059. Val-Bernal JF, Figols J, Arce FP, Sanz-Ortiz J (2001). Cardiac epithelioid angiosarcoma presenting as cutaneous metastases. J Cutan Pathol 28: 265-270.

2060. Val-Bernal JF, Villoria F, Fernandez FA (2000). Polypoid (pedunculated) subepicardial lipoma: a cardiac lesion resembling the epiploic appendage. Cardiovasc Pathol 9: 55-57.

2061. Valk PE, Pounds TR, Hopkins DM, Haseman MK, Hofer GA, Greiss HB, Myers RW, Lutrin CL (1995). Staging non-small cell lung cancer by whole-body positron emission tomographic imaging. Ann Thorac Surg 60: 1573-1581.

2062. Valli M, Fabris GA, Dewar A, Chikte S, Fisher C, Corrin B, Sheppard MN (1994). Atypical carcinoid tumour of the thymus: a study of eight cases. Histopathology 24: 371-375.

2063. van de Rijn M, Lombard CM, Rouse RV (1994). Expression of CD34 by solitary fibrous tumors of the pleura, mediastinum, and lung. Am J Surg Pathol 18: 814-820.

2064. van de Rijn M, Rouse RV (1994). CD:34

a review. Appl Immunohistochem 2: 71-80.

2065. Van den Berghe I, Debiec-Rychter M, Proot L, Hagemeijer A, Michielssen P (2002). Ring chromosome 6 may represent a cytogenetic subgroup in benign thymoma. Cancer Genet Cytogenet 137: 75-77.

2066. van den Bosch JM, Wagenaar SS, Corrin B, Elbers JR, Knaepen PJ, Westermann CJ (1987). Mesenchymoma of the lung (so called hamartoma): a review of 154 parenchymal and endobronchial cases. Thorax 42: 790-793.

2067. van den Oord JJ, Wolf-Peeters C, de Vos R, Thomas J, Desmet VJ (1986). Sarcoma arising from interdigitating reticulum cells: report of a case, studied with light and electron microscopy, and enzyme- and immunohistochemistry. Histopathology 10: 509-523.

2068. Van der Hauwaert LG (1971). Cardiac tumours in infancy and childhood. Br Heart J 33: 125-132.

2069. van Spronsen DJ, Vrints LW, Hofstra G, Crommelin MA, Coebergh JW, Breed WP (1997). Disappearance of prognostic significance of histopathological grading of nodular sclerosing Hodgkin's disease for unselected patients, 1972-92. Br J Haematol 96: 322-327.

2070. van Unnik JA, Coindre JM, Contesso C, Albus-Lutter CE, Schiodt T, Sylvester R, Thomas D, Bramwell V, Mouridsen HT (1993). Grading of soft tissue sarcomas: experience of the EORTC Soft Tissue and Bone Sarcoma Group. Eur J Cancer 29A: 2089-2093.

2071. Vander Salm TJ (2000). Unusual primary tumors of the heart. Semin Thorac Cardiovasc Surg 12: 89-100.

2072. Vargas SO, French CA, Faul PN, Fletcher JA, Davis IJ, Dal Cin P, Perez-Atayde AR (2001). Upper respiratory tract carcinoma with chromosomal translocation 15;19: evidence for a distinct disease entity of young patients with a rapidly fatal course. Cancer 92: 1195-1203.

2073. Vargas SO, Nose V, Fletcher JA, Perez-Atayde AR (2001). Gains of chromosome 8 are confined to mesenchymal components in pleuropulmonary blastoma. Pediatr Dev Pathol 4: 434-445.

2074. Vasey PA, Dunlop DJ, Kaye SB (1994). Primary mediastinal germ cell tumour and acute monocytic leukaemia occurring concurrently in a 15-year-old boy. Ann Oncol 5: 649-652.

2075. Vassallo R, Ryu JH, Colby TV, Hartman T, Limper AH (2000). Pulmonary Langerhans'-cell histiocytosis. N Engl J Med 342: 1969-1978.

2076. Vassallo R, Ryu JH, Schroeder DR, Decker PA, Limper AH (2002). Clinical outcomes of pulmonary Langerhans'-cell histiocytosis in adults. N Engl J Med 346: 484-490.

2077. Vaughan CJ, Veugelers M, Basson CT (2001). Tumors and the heart: molecular genetic advances. Curr Opin Cardiol 16: 195-200.

2078. Vazquez MF, Flieder DB (2000). Small peripheral glandular lesions detected by screening CT for lung cancer. A diagnostic dilemma for the pathologist. Radiol Clin North Am 38: 579-589.

2079. Veinot JP, Burns BF, Commons AS, Thomas J (1999). Cardiac neoplasms at the Canadian Reference Centre for Cancer Pathology. Can J Cardiol 15: 311-319.

2080. Veinot JP, Walley VM (2000). Focal and patchy cardiac valve lesions: a clinico-pathological review. Can J Cardiol 16: 1489-1507.

2081. Verbeken E, Beyls J, Moerman P, Knockaert D, Goddeeris P, Lauweryns JM (1985). Lung metastasis of malignant epithelioid hemangioendothelioma mimicking a primary intravascular bronchioalveolar tumor. A histologic, ultrastructural, and immunohistochemical study. Cancer 55: 1741-1746.

2082. Viale G (1989). Cytokeratin immunocytochemistry in the practice of diagnostic histopathology. Ultrastruct Pathol 13: 91.

2083. Viard-Leveugle I, Veyrenc S, French LE, Brambilla C, Brambilla E (2003). Frequent loss of Fas expression and function in human lung tumors with overexpression of FasL in small cell lung carcinoma. J Pathol 201: 268-277.

2084. Vikkula M, Boon LM, Carraway KLI, Calvert JT, Diamonti AJ, Goumnerov B, Pasyk KA, Marchuk DA, Warman ML, Cantley LC, Mulliken JB, Olsen BR (1996). Vascular dysmorphogenesis caused by an activating mutation in the receptor tyrosine kinase TIE2. Cell 87: 1181-1190.

2085. Vilchez RA, Kozinetz CA, Arrington AS, Madden CR, Butel JS (2003). Simian virus 40 in human cancers. Am J Med 114: 675-684.

2086. Vineis P, Veglia F, Benhamou S, Butkiewicz D, Cascorbi I, Clapper ML, Dolzan V, Haugen A, Hirvonen A, Ingelman-Sundberg M, Kihara M, Kiyohara C, Kremers P, Le Marchand L, Ohshima S, Pastorelli R, Rannug A, Romkes M, Schoket B, Shields P, Strange RC, Stucker I, Sugimura H, Garte S, Gaspari L, Taioli E (2003). CYP1A1 T3801 C polymorphism and lung cancer: a pooled analysis of 2451 cases and 3358 controls. Int J Cancer 104: 650-657.

2087. Vlasveld LT, Splinter TA, Hagemeijer A, Van Lom K, Lowenberg B (1994). Acute myeloid leukaemia with +i(12p) shortly after treatment of mediastinal germ cell tumour. Br J Haematol 88: 196-198.

2088. Vlodavsky E, Ben Izhak O, Best LA, Kerner H (2000). Primary malignant melanoma of the anterior mediastinum in a child. Am J Surg Pathol 24: 747-749.

2089. Vollmer RT (1982). The effect of cell size on the pathologic diagnosis of small and large cell carcinomas of the lung. Cancer 50: 1380-1383.

2090. von Wasielewski R, Mengel M, Fischer R, Hansmann ML, Hubner K, Franklin J, Tesch H, Paulus U, Werner M, Diehl V, Georgii A (1997). Classical Hodgkin's disease. Clinical impact of the immunophenotype. Am J Pathol 151: 1123-1130.

2091. Von Wasielewski S, Franklin J, Fischer R, Huebner K, Hansmann ML, Diehl V, Georgii A, von Wasielewski R (2003). Nodular sclerosing Hodgkin's disease: new grading predicts prognosis in intermediate and advanced stages. Blood .

2092. Vonlanthen S, Heighway J, Kappeler A, Altermatt HJ, Borner MM, Betticher DC (2000). p21 is associated with cyclin D1, p16INK4a and pRb expression in resectable non-small cell lung cancer. Int J Oncol 16: 951-957.

2093. Vougiouklakis T, Goussia A, Ioachim E, Peschos D, Agnantis N (2001). Cardiac fibroma. A case presentation. Virchows Arch 438: 635-636.

2094. Vroegindeweij-Claessens LJ, Tijssen CC, Creemers GJ, Lockefeer JH, Teepen JL (1990). Myasthenia gravis and thymoma in multiple endocrine neoplasia (MEN-1) syndrome. J Neurol Neurosurg Psychiatry 53: 624-625.

2095. Wajchenberg BL, Mendonca BB, Liberman B, Pereira MA, Carneiro PC, Wakamatsu A, Kirschner MA (1994). Ectopic adrenocorticotropic hormone syndrome. Endocr Rev 15: 752-787.
2096. Wakely PJr, Suster S (2000). Langerhans' cell histiocytosis of the thymus associated with multilocular thymic cyst. Hum Pathol 31: 1532-1535.
2097. Walch AK, Zitzelsberger HF, Aubele MM, Mattis AE, Bauchinger M, Candidus S, Prauer HW, Werner M, Hofler H (1998). Typical and atypical carcinoid tumors of the lung are characterized by 11q deletions as detected by comparative genomic hybridization. Am J Pathol 153: 1089-1098.
2098. Walker AN, Mills SE, Fechner RE (1990). Thymomas and thymic carcinomas. Semin Diagn Pathol 7: 250-265.
2099. Walker WP, Wittchow RJ, Bottles K, Layfield LJ, Hirschowitz S, Cohen MB (1994). Paranuclear blue inclusions in small cell undifferentiated carcinoma: a diagnostically useful finding demonstrated in fine-needle aspiration biopsy smears. Diagn Cytopathol 10: 212-215.
2100. Walles T, Teebken OE, Bartels M, Fangmann J, Scheumann GF, Pichlmaier MA, Klempnauer J (2000). Pancreatic metastasis of a pleuropulmonary blastoma in an adult. Ann Oncol 11: 1609-1611.
2101. Walter JW, Blei F, Anderson JL, Orlow SJ, Speer MC, Marchuk DA (1999). Genetic mapping of a novel familial form of infantile hemangioma. Am J Med Genet 82: 77-83.
2102. Walton JAJr, Kahn DR, Willis PWI (1972). Recurrence of a left atrial myxoma. Am J Cardiol 29: 872-876.
2103. Wang C, Mahaffey JE, Axelrod L, Perlman JA (1979). Hyperfunctioning supernumerary parathyroid glands. Surg Gynecol Obstet 148: 711-714.
2104. Wang HJ, Lin JL, Lin FY (2002). Images in cardiovascular medicine. Cardiac hemangioma. Circulation 106: 2520.
2105. Wang Q, Timur AA, Szafranski P, Sadgephour A, Jurecic V, Cowell J, Baldini A, Driscoll DJ (2001). Identification and molecular characterization of de novo translocation t(8;14)(q22.3;q13) associated with a vascular and tissue overgrowth syndrome. Cytogenet Cell Genet 95: 183-188.
2106. Wang Y, Spitz MR, Schabath MB, Ali-Osman F, Mata H, Wu X (2003). Association between glutathione S-transferase p1 polymorphisms and lung cancer risk in Caucasians: a case-control study. Lung Cancer 40: 25-32.
2107. Warhol MJ, Hickey WF, Corson JM (1982). Malignant mesothelioma: ultrastructural distinction from adenocarcinoma. Am J Surg Pathol 6: 307-314.
2108. Warnke RA, Weiss LM, Chan JKC, Cleary ML, Dorfman RF (1995). Tumors of the Lymph Nodes and Spleen. 3rd ed. Armed Forces Institute of Pathology: Washington, DC.
2109. Warren WH, Faber LP, Gould VE (1989). Neuroendocrine neoplasms of the lung. A clinicopathologic update. J Thorac Cardiovasc Surg 98: 321-332.
2110. Warren WH, Memoli VA, Gould VE (1984). Immunohistochemical and ultrastructural analysis of bronchopulmonary neuroendocrine neoplasms. II. Well-differentiated neuroendocrine carcinomas. Ultrastruct Pathol 7: 185-199.
2111. Watanabe J, Shimada T, Gillam EM, Ikuta T, Suemasu K, Higashi Y, Gotoh O, Kawajiri K (2000). Association of CYP1B1 genetic polymorphism with incidence to breast and lung cancer. Pharmacogenetics 10: 25-33.
2112. Watanabe S, Watanabe T, Arai K, Kasai T, Haratake J, Urayama H (2002). Results of wedge resection for focal bronchioloalveolar carcinoma showing pure ground-glass attenuation on computed tomography. Ann Thorac Surg 73: 1071-1075.
2113. Watanabe T, Hojo Y, Kozaki T, Nagashima M, Ando M (1991). Hypoplastic left heart syndrome with rhabdomyoma of the left ventricle. Pediatr Cardiol 12: 121-122.
2114. Watson JC, Stratakis CA, Bryant-Greenwood PK, Koch CA, Kirschner LS, Nguyen T, Carney JA, Oldfield EH (2000). Neurosurgical implications of Carney complex. J Neurosurg 92: 413-418.
2115. Wei Q, Cheng L, Amos CI, Wang LE, Guo Z, Hong WK, Spitz MR (2000). Repair of tobacco carcinogen-induced DNA adducts and lung cancer risk: a molecular epidemiologic study. J Natl Cancer Inst 92: 1764-1772.
2116. Weidner N (1999). Germ-cell tumors of the mediastinum. Semin Diagn Pathol 16: 42-50.
2117. Weinberger MA, Katz S, Davis EW (1955). Peripheral bronchial adenoma of mucous gland type-clinical and pathologic aspects. J Thorac Surg 29: 626-635.
2118. Weirich G, Schneider P, Fellbaum C, Brauch H, Nathrath W, Scholz M, Prauer H, Hofler H (1997). p53 alterations in thymic epithelial tumours. Virchows Arch 431: 17-23.
2119. Weiss SW, Goldblum JR (2001). Enzinger and Weiss's Soft Tissue Tumors. 4th ed. Mosby-Harcourt: St Louis.
2120. Weiss SW, Ishak KG, Dail DH, Sweet DE, Enzinger FM (1986). Epithelioid hemangioendothelioma and related lesions. Semin Diagn Pathol 3: 259-287.
2121. Weiss SW, Nickoloff BJ (1993). CD-34 is expressed by a distinctive cell population in peripheral nerve, nerve sheath tumors, and related lesions. Am J Surg Pathol 17: 1039-1045.
2122. Weldon-Linne CM, Victor TA, Christ ML, Fry WA (1981). Angiogenic nature of the "intravascular bronchioloalveolar tumor" of the lung: an electron microscopic study. Arch Pathol Lab Med 105: 174-179.
2123. Weng SY, Tsuchiya E, Kasuga T, Sugano H (1992). Incidence of atypical bronchioloalveolar cell hyperplasia of the lung: relation to histological subtypes of lung cancer. Virchows Arch A Pathol Anat Histol 420: 463-471.
2124. Werling RW, Yaziji H, Bacchi CE, Gown AM (2003). CDX2, a Highly Sensitive and Specific Marker of Adenocarcinomas of Intestinal Origin: An Immunohistochemical Survey of 476 Primary and Metastatic Carcinomas. Am J Surg Pathol 27: 303-310.
2125. Westra WH (2000). Early glandular neoplasia of the lung. Respir Res 1: 163-169.
2126. Westra WH, Baas IO, Hruban RH, Askin FB, Wilson K, Offerhaus GJ, Slebos RJ (1996). K-ras oncogene activation in atypical alveolar hyperplasias of the human lung. Cancer Res 56: 2224-2228.
2127. Westra WH, Gerald WL, Rosai J (1994). Solitary fibrous tumor. Consistent CD34 immunoreactivity and occurrence in the orbit. Am J Surg Pathol 18: 992-998.
2128. Weynand B, Draguet AP, Bernard P, Marbaix E, Galant C (1999). Calcifying fibrous pseudotumour: first case report in the peritoneum with immunostaining for CD34. Histopathology 34: 86-87.
2129. Wheatley A, Howard N (1967). The surgical treatment of lung metastases. Br J Surg 54: 364-368.
2130. Whelan AJ, Watson MS, Porter FD, Steiner RD (1995). Klippel-Trenaunay-Weber syndrome associated with a 5:11 balanced translocation. Am J Med Genet 59: 492-494.
2131. Whitesell PL, Peters SG (1993). Pulmonary manifestations of extrathoracic malignant lesions. Mayo Clin Proc 68: 483-491.
2132. Wiatrowska BA, Krol J, Zakowski MF (2001). Large-cell neuroendocrine carcinoma of the lung: proposed criteria for cytologic diagnosis. Diagn Cytopathol 24: 58-64.
2133. Wick MR (1990). Mediastinal cysts and intrathoracic thyroid tumors. Semin Diagn Pathol 7: 285-294.
2134. Wick MR (2000). Immunohistology of neuroendocrine and neuroectodermal tumors. Semin Diagn Pathol 17: 194-203.
2135. Wick MR, Berg LC, Hertz MI (1992). Large cell carcinoma of the lung with neuroendocrine differentiation. A comparison with large cell "undifferentiated" pulmonary tumors. Am J Clin Pathol 97: 796-805.
2136. Wick MR, Carney JA, Bernatz PE, Brown LR (1982). Primary mediastinal carcinoid tumors. Am J Surg Pathol 6: 195-205.
2137. Wick MR, Ritter JH (2002). Neuroendocrine neoplasms: evolving concepts and terminology. Curr Diagn Pathol 8: 102-112.
2138. Wick MR, Ritter JH, Humphrey PA (1997). Sarcomatoid carcinomas of the lung: a clinicopathologic review. Am J Clin Pathol 108: 40-53.
2139. Wick MR, Ritter JH, Nappi O (1995). Inflammatory sarcomatoid carcinoma of the lung: report of three cases and clinicopathologic comparison with inflammatory pseudotumors in adult patients. Hum Pathol 26: 1014-1021.
2140. Wick MR, Rosai J (1988). Neuroendocrine neoplasms of the thymus. Pathol Res Pract 183: 188-199.
2141. Wick MR, Rosai J (1991). Neuroendocrine neoplasms of the mediastinum. Semin Diagn Pathol 8: 35-51.
2142. Wick MR, Scheithauer BW (1982). Oat-cell carcinoma of the thymus. Cancer 49: 1652-1657.
2143. Wick MR, Scheithauer BW, Weiland LH, Bernatz PE (1982). Primary thymic carcinomas. Am J Surg Pathol 6: 613-630.
2144. Wick MR, Scott RE, Li CY, Carney JA (1980). Carcinoid tumor of the thymus: a clinicopathologic report of seven cases with a review of the literature. Mayo Clin Proc 55: 246-254.
2145. Wiencke JK (2002). DNA adduct burden and tobacco carcinogenesis. Oncogene 21: 7376-7391.
2146. Wiese TH, Enzweiler CN, Borges AC, Beling M, Rogalla P, Taupitz M, Baumann G, Hamm B (2001). Electron beam CT in the diagnosis of recurrent cardiac lipoma. AJR Am J Roentgenol 176: 1066-1068.
2147. Wigle DA, Jurisica I, Radulovich N, Pintilie M, Rossant J, Liu N, Lu C, Woodgett J, Seiden I, Johnston M, Keshavjee S, Darling G, Winton T, Breitkreutz BJ, Jorgenson P, Tyers M, Shepherd FA, Tsao MS (2002). Molecular profiling of non-small cell lung cancer and correlation with disease-free survival. Cancer Res 62: 3005-3008.
2148. Willis RA (1973). The Spread of Tumours in the Human Body. Butterworths: London.
2149. Willman CL, Busque L, Griffith BB, Favara BE, McClain KL, Duncan MH, Gilliland DG (1994). Langerhans'-cell histiocytosis (histiocytosis X)—a clonal proliferative disease. N Engl J Med 331: 154-160.
2150. Wilson AJ, Ratliff JL, Lagios MD, Aguilar MJ (1979). Mediastinal meningioma. Am J Surg Pathol 3: 557-562.
2151. Wilson RW, Galateau-Salle F, Moran CA (1999). Desmoid tumors of the pleura: a clinicopathologic mimic of localized fibrous tumor. Mod Pathol 12: 9-14.
2152. Wilson RW, Moran CA (1997). Primary melanoma of the lung: a clinicopathologic and immunohistochemical study of eight cases. Am J Surg Pathol 21: 1196-1202.
2153. Wilson RW, Moran CA (1998). Primary ependymoma of the mediastinum: a clinicopathologic study of three cases. Ann Diagn Pathol 2: 293-300.
2154. Wilson WH, Kingma DW, Raffeld M, Wittes RE, Jaffe ES (1996). Association of lymphomatoid granulomatosis with Epstein-Barr viral infection of B lymphocytes and response to interferon-alpha 2b. Blood 87: 4531-4537.
2155. Wingo PA, Ries LA, Giovino GA, Miller DS, Rosenberg HM, Shopland DR, Thun MJ, Edwards BK (1999). Annual report to the nation on the status of cancer, 1973-1996, with a special section on lung cancer and tobacco smoking. J Natl Cancer Inst 91: 675-690.
2156. Wintersperger BJ, Becker CR, Gulbins H, Knez A, Bruening R, Heuck A, Reiser MF (2000). Tumors of the cardiac valves: imaging findings in magnetic resonance imaging, electron beam computed tomography, and echocardiography. Eur Radiol 10: 443-449.
2157. Wistuba II, Behrens C, Milchgrub S, Bryant D, Hung J, Minna JD, Gazdar AF (1999). Sequential molecular abnormalities are involved in the multistage development of squamous cell lung carcinoma. Oncogene 18: 643-650.
2158. Wistuba II, Behrens C, Virmani AK, Mele G, Milchgrub S, Girard L, Fondon JWI, Garner HR, McKay B, Latif F, Lerman MI, Lam S, Gazdar AF, Minna JD (2000). High resolution chromosome 3p allelotyping of human lung cancer and preneoplastic/preinvasive bronchial epithelium reveals multiple, discontinuous sites of 3p allele loss and three regions of frequent breakpoints. Cancer Res 60: 1949-1960.
2159. Wistuba II, Behrens C, Virmani AK, Milchgrub S, Syed S, Lam S, Mackay B, Minna JD, Gazdar AF (1999). Allelic losses at chromosome 8p21-23 are early and frequent events in the pathogenesis of lung cancer. Cancer Res 59: 1973-1979.
2160. Wistuba II, Berry J, Behrens C, Maitra A, Shivapurkar N, Milchgrub S, Mackay B, Minna JD, Gazdar AF (2000). Molecular changes in the bronchial epithelium of patients with small cell lung cancer. Clin Cancer Res 6: 2604-2610.
2161. Wistuba II, Gazdar AF (2003). Characteristic genetic alterations in lung cancer. Methods Mol Med 74: 3-28.
2162. Wistuba II, Lam S, Behrens C, Virmani AK, Fong KM, LeRiche J, Samet JM, Srivastava S, Minna JD, Gazdar AF (1997). Molecular damage in the bronchial epithelium of current and former smokers. J Natl Cancer Inst 89: 1366-1373.
2163. Witkin GB, Miettinen M, Rosai J (1989). A biphasic tumor of the mediastinum with features of synovial sarcoma.

A report of four cases. Am J Surg Pathol 13: 490-499.

2164. Witkin GB, Rosai J (1989). Solitary fibrous tumor of the mediastinum. A report of 14 cases. Am J Surg Pathol 13: 547-557.

2165. Wold LE, Lie JT (1980). Cardiac myxomas: a clinicopathologic profile. Am J Pathol 101: 219-240.

2166. Wolfe JTI, Wick MR, Banks PM, Scheithauer BW (1983). Clear cell carcinoma of the thymus. Mayo Clin Proc 58: 365-370.

2167. Wolff M, Goodman EN (1980). Functioning lipoadenoma of a supernumerary parathyroid gland in the mediastinum. Head Neck Surg 2: 302-307.

2168. Wong MP, Chung LP, Yuen ST, Leung SY, Chan SY, Wang E, Fu KH (1995). In situ detection of Epstein-Barr virus in non-small cell lung carcinomas. J Pathol 177: 233-240.

2169. Wood DE (2000). Mediastinal germ cell tumors. Semin Thorac Cardiovasc Surg 12: 278-289.

2170. Woolner LB, Jamplis RW, Kirklin JW (1955). Seminoma (germinoma) of the anterior mediastinum. N Engl J Med 252: 653-657.

2171. Wotherspoon AC, Ortiz-Hidalgo C, Falzon MR, Isaacson PG (1991). Helicobacter pylori-associated gastritis and primary B-cell gastric lymphoma. Lancet 338: 1175-1176.

2172. Wright CD, Kesler KA, Nichols CR, Mahomed Y, Einhorn LH, Miller ME, Brown JW (1990). Primary mediastinal nonseminomatous germ cell tumors. Results of a multimodality approach. J Thorac Cardiovasc Surg 99: 210-217.

2173. Wright JRJr (2000). Pleuropulmonary blastoma: A case report documenting transition from type I (cystic) to type III (solid). Cancer 88: 2853-2858.

2174. Wu TC, Kuo TT (1993). Study of Epstein-Barr virus early RNA 1 (EBER1) expression by in situ hybridization in thymic epithelial tumors of Chinese patients in Taiwan. Hum Pathol 24: 235-238.

2175. Wu X, Gwyn K, Amos CI, Makan N, Hong WK, Spitz MR (2001). The association of microsomal epoxide hydrolase polymorphisms and lung cancer risk in African-Americans and Mexican-Americans. Carcinogenesis 22: 923-928.

2176. Wynder EL, Graham EA (1950). Tobacco smoking as a possible etiologic factor in brochiogenus carcinoma. A study of six hundred and eighty four proved cases. JAMA 143: 328-336.

2177. Wynder EL, Muscat JE (1995). The changing epidemiology of smoking and lung cancer histology. Environ Health Perspect 103 Suppl 8: 143-148.

2178. Xiao S, Li DZ, Vijg J, Sugarbaker DJ, Corson JM, Fletcher JA (1995). Codeletion of p15 and p16 in primary malignant mesothelioma. Oncogene 11: 511-515.

2179. Xiao S, Nalabolu SR, Aster JC, Ma J, Abruzzo L, Jaffe ES, Stone R, Weissman SM, Hudson TJ, Fletcher JA (1998). FGFR1 is fused with a novel zinc-finger gene, ZNF198, in the t(8;13) leukaemia/lymphoma syndrome. Nat Genet 18: 84-87.

2180. Xu HM, Li WH, Hou N, Zhang SG, Li HF, Wang SQ, Yu ZY, Li ZJ, Zeng MY, Zhu GM (1997). Neuroendocrine differentiation in 32 cases of so-called sclerosing hemangioma of the lung: identified by immunohistochemical and ultrastructural study. Am J Surg Pathol 21: 1013-1022.

2181. Yamaguchi M, Seto M, Okamoto M, Ichinohasama R, Nakamura N, Yoshino T, Suzumiya J, Murase T, Miura I, Akasaka T, Tamaru J, Suzuki R, Kagami Y, Hirano M, Morishima Y, Ueda R, Shiku H, Nakamura S (2002). De novo CD5+ diffuse large B-cell lymphoma: a clinicopathologic study of 109 patients. Blood 99: 815-821.

2182. Yamaguchi T, Imamura Y, Nakayama K, Kawada T, Yamamoto T, Ueyama K (2002). Primary pulmonary leiomyosarcoma: report of a case diagnosed by fine-needle aspiration cytology. Acta Cytol 46: 912-916.

2183. Yamaji I, Iimura O, Mito T, Yoshida S, Shimamoto K, Minase T (1984). An ectopic, ACTH producing, oncocytic carcinoid tumor of the thymus: report of a case. Jpn J Med 23: 62-66.

2184. Yamakawa Y, Masaoka A, Hashimoto T, Niwa H, Mizuno T, Fujii Y, Nakahara K (1991). A tentative tumor-node-metastasis classification of thymoma. Cancer 68: 1984-1987.

2185. Yamamoto T, Horiguchi H, Shibagaki T, Kamma H, Ogata T, Mitsui K (1993). Encapsulated type II pneumocyte adenoma: a case report and review of the literature. Respiration 60: 373-377.

2186. Yamamoto T, Tamura J, Orima S, Saitoh T, Sakuraya M, Maehara T, Shirota A, Maezawa A, Nojima Y, Naruse T (1999). Rhabdomyosarcoma in a patient with mosaic Klinefelter syndrome and transformation of immature teratoma. J Int Med Res 27: 196-200.

2187. Yamasaki M, Takeshima Y, Fujii S, Kitaguchi S, Matsuura M, Tagawa K, Inai K (2000). Correlation between genetic alterations and histopathological subtypes in bronchiolo-alveolar carcinoma and atypical adenomatous hyperplasia of the lung. Pathol Int 50: 778-785.

2188. Yamasaki S, Matsushita H, Tanimura S, Nakatani T, Hara S, Endo Y, Hara M (1998). B-cell lymphoma of mucosa-associated lymphoid tissue of the thymus: a report of two cases with a background of Sjogren's syndrome and monoclonal gammopathy. Hum Pathol 29: 1021-1024.

2189. Yamashita K, Yamoto M, Shikone T, Minami S, Nakano R (1999). Immunohistochemical localization of inhibin and activin subunits in human epithelial ovarian tumors. Am J Obstet Gynecol 180: 316-322.

2190. Yamashita S, Ohyama C, Nakagawa H, Takeuchi A, Watanabe M, Hoshi S (2002). Primary choriocarcinoma in the posterior mediastinum. J Urol 167: 1789.

2191. Yamato H, Ohshima K, Suzumiya J, Kikuchi M (2001). Evidence for local immunosuppression and demonstration of c-myc amplification in pyothorax-associated lymphoma. Histopathology 39: 163-171.

2192. Yamato Y, Tsuchida M, Watanabe T, Aoki T, Koizumi N, Umezu H, Hayashi J (2001). Early results of a prospective study of limited resection for bronchioloalveolar adenocarcinoma of the lung. Ann Thorac Surg 71: 971-974.

2193. Yamauchi K, Yasuda M (2002). Comparison in treatments of nonleukemic granulocytic sarcoma: report of two cases and a review of 72 cases in the literature. Cancer 94: 1739-1746.

2194. Yanagisawa K, Shyr Y, Xu BJ, Massion PP, Larsen PH, White BC, Roberts JR, Edgerton M, Gonzalez A, Nadaf S, Moore JH, Caprioli RM, Carbone DP (2003). Proteomic patterns of tumour subsets in non-small-cell lung cancer. Lancet 362: 433-439.

2195. Yang GC, Yee HT, Wu CD, Aye LM, Chachoua A (2002). TIA-1+ cytotoxic large T-cell lymphoma of the mediastinum: case report. Diagn Cytopathol 26: 154-157.

2196. Yang P, Hasegawa T, Hirose T, Fukumoto T, Uyama T, Monden Y, Sano T (1997). Pleuropulmonary blastoma: fluorescence in situ hybridization analysis indicating trisomy 2. Am J Surg Pathol 21: 854-859.

2197. Yang YJ, Steele CT, Ou XL, Snyder KP, Kohman LJ (2001). Diagnosis of high-grade pulmonary neuroendocrine carcinoma by fine-needle aspiration biopsy: nonsmall-cell or small-cell type? Diagn Cytopathol 25: 292-300.

2198. Yano M, Yamakawa Y, Kiriyama M, Hara M, Murase T (2002). Sclerosing hemangioma with metastases to multiple nodal stations. Ann Thorac Surg 73: 981-983.

2199. Yashima K, Litzky LA, Kaiser L, Rogers T, Lam S, Wistuba II, Milchgrub S, Srivastava S, Piatyszek MA, Shay JW, Gazdar AF (1997). Telomerase expression in respiratory epithelium during the multistage pathogenesis of lung carcinomas. Cancer Res 57: 2373-2377.

2200. Yatabe Y, Masuda A, Koshikawa T, Nakamura S, Kuroishi T, Osada H, Takahashi T, Mitsudomi T, Takahashi T (1998). p27KIP1 in human lung cancers: differential changes in small cell and non-small cell carcinomas. Cancer Res 58: 1042-1047.

2201. Yatabe Y, Mitsudomi T, Takahashi T (2002). TTF-1 expression in pulmonary adenocarcinomas. Am J Surg Pathol 26: 767-773.

2202. Yesner R, Carter D (1982). Pathology of carcinoma of the lung. Changing patterns. Clin Chest Med 3: 257-289.

2203. Yesner R, Gerstl B, Auerbach O (1965). Application of World Health Organization classification of lung carcinoma to biopsy material. Ann Thoracic Surg 1: 33-49.

2204. Yesner R, Hurwitz A (1953). Localized pleural mesothelioma of epithelial type. J Thorac Surg 26: 325-329.

2205. Yi ES, Auger WR, Friedman PJ, Morris TA, Shin SS (1995). Intravascular bronchioloalveolar tumor of the lung presenting as pulmonary thromboembolic disease and pulmonary hypertension. Arch Pathol Lab Med 119: 255-260.

2206. Yokose T, Doi M, Tanno K, Yamazaki K, Ochiai A (2001). Atypical adenomatous hyperplasia of the lung in autopsy cases. Lung Cancer 33: 155-161.

2207. Yokose T, Ito Y, Ochiai A (2000). High prevalence of atypical adenomatous hyperplasia of the lung in autopsy specimens from elderly patients with malignant neoplasms. Lung Cancer 29: 125-130.

2208. Yokose T, Suzuki K, Nagai K, Nishiwaki Y, Sasaki S, Ochiai A (2000). Favorable and unfavorable morphological prognostic factors in peripheral adenocarcinoma of the lung 3 cm or less in diameter. Lung Cancer 29: 179-188.

2209. Yokota J, Kohno T (2004). Molecular footprints of human lung cancer progression. Cancer Sci 95: 197-204.

2210. Yoneda S, Marx A, Heimann S, Shirakusa T, Kikuchi M, Muller-Hermelink HK (1999). Low-grade metaplastic carcinoma of the thymus. Histopathology 35: 19-30.

2211. Yoneda S, Marx A, Muller-Hermelink HK (1999). Low-grade metaplastic carcinomas of the thymus: biphasic thymic epithelial tumors with mesenchymal metaplasia—an update. Pathol Res Pract 195: 555-563.

2212. Yoon DH, Roberts W (2002). Sex distribution in cardiac myxomas. Am J Cardiol 90: 563-565.

2213. Yoon YC, Lee KS, Kim TS, Seo JB, Han J (2002). Benign bronchopulmonary tumors: radiologic and pathologic findings. J Comput Assist Tomogr 26: 784-796.

2214. Yoshikawa T, Noguchi Y, Matsukawa H, Kondo J, Matsumoto A, Nakatani Y, Kitamura H, Ito T (1994). Thymus carcinoid producing parathyroid hormone (PTH)-related protein: report of a case. Surg Today 24: 544-547.

2215. Youn HJ, Jung SE, Chung WS, Choi MG, Lee KY, Chung KW, Hong SJ, Sun HS (2002). Obstruction of right ventricular outflow tract by extended cardiac metastasis from esophageal cancer. J Am Soc Echocardiogr 15: 1541-1544.

2216. Yousem SA (1986). Angiosarcoma presenting in the lung. Arch Pathol Lab Med 110: 112-115.

2217. Yousem SA (1989). Pulmonary adenosquamous carcinomas with amyloid-like stroma. Mod Pathol 2: 420-426.

2218. Yousem SA, Colby TV, Chen YY, Chen WG, Weiss LM (2001). Pulmonary Langerhans' cell histiocytosis: molecular analysis of clonality. Am J Surg Pathol 25: 630-636.

2219. Yousem SA, Hochholzer L (1986). Alveolar adenoma. Hum Pathol 17: 1066-1071.

2220. Yousem SA, Hochholzer L (1987). Malignant mesotheliomas with osseous and cartilaginous differentiation. Arch Pathol Lab Med 111: 62-66.

2221. Yousem SA, Hochholzer L (1987). Mucoepidermoid tumors of the lung. Cancer 60: 1346-1352.

2222. Yousem SA, Hochholzer L (1987). Unusual thoracic manifestations of epithelioid hemangioendothelioma. Arch Pathol Lab Med 111: 459-463.

2223. Yousem SA, Shaw H, Cieply K (2001). Involvement of 2p23 in pulmonary inflammatory pseudotumors. Hum Pathol 32: 428-433.

2224. Yousem SA, Weiss LM, Warnke RA (1985). Primary mediastinal non-Hodgkin's lymphomas: a morphologic and immunologic study of 19 cases. Am J Clin Pathol 83: 676-680.

2225. Yousem SA, Wick MR, Randhawa P, Manivel JC (1990). Pulmonary blastoma. An immunohistochemical analysis with comparison with fetal lung in its pseudoglandular stage. Am J Clin Pathol 93: 167-175.

2226. Yu GH, Kussmaul WG, DiSesa VJ, Lodato RF, Brooks JS (1993). Adult intracardiac rhabdomyoma resembling the extracardiac variant. Hum Pathol 24: 448-451.

2227. Yuda S, Nakatani S, Yutani C, Yamagishi M, Kitamura S, Miyatake K (2002). Trends in the clinical and morphological characteristics of cardiac myxoma: 20-year experience of a single tertiary referral center in Japan. Circ J 66: 1008-1013.

2228. Zabarovsky ER, Lerman MI, Minna JD (2002). Tumor suppressor genes on chromosome 3p involved in the pathogenesis of lung and other cancers. Oncogene 21: 6915-6935.

2229. Zacharias J, Nicholson AG, Ladas GP, Goldstraw P (2003). Large cell neuroendocrine carcinoma and large cell carcinomas with neuroendocrine morphology of the lung: prognosis after complete resection and systematic nodal dissection. Ann Thorac Surg 75: 348-352.

2230. Zafarana G, Gillis AJ, van Gurp RJ,

Olsson PG, Elstrodt F, Stoop H, Millan JL, Oosterhuis JW, Looijenga LH (2002). Coamplification of DAD-R, SOX5, and EKI1 in human testicular seminomas, with specific overexpression of DAD-R, correlates with reduced levels of apoptosis and earlier clinical manifestation. Cancer Res 62: 1822-1831.

2231. Zaharopoulos P, Wong JY, Stewart GD (1982). Cytomorphology of the variants of small-cell carcinoma of the lung. Acta Cytol 26: 800-808.

2232. Zamecnik J, Kodet R (2002). Value of thyroid transcription factor-1 and surfactant apoprotein A in the differential diagnosis of pulmonary carcinomas: a study of 109 cases. Virchows Arch 440: 353-361.

2233. Zarate-Osorno A, Medeiros LJ, Longo DL, Jaffe ES (1992). Non-Hodgkin's lymphomas arising in patients successfully treated for Hodgkin's disease. A clinical, histologic, and immunophenotypic study of 14 cases. Am J Surg Pathol 16: 885-895.

2234. Zaring RA, Roepke JE (1999). Pathologic quiz case. Pulmonary mass in a patient presenting with a hemothorax. Diagnosis: primary pulmonary biphasic synovial sarcoma. Arch Pathol Lab Med 123: 1287-1289.

2235. Zellos LS, Sugarbaker DJ (2002). Multimodality treatment of diffuse malignant pleural mesothelioma. Semin Oncol 29: 41-50.

2236. Zeren H, Moran CA, Suster S, Fishback NF, Koss MN (1995). Primary pulmonary sarcomas with features of monophasic synovial sarcoma: a clinicopathological, immunohistochemical, and ultrastructural study of 25 cases. Hum Pathol 26: 474-480.

2237. Zetter BR (1990). The cellular basis of site-specific tumor metastasis. N Engl J Med 322: 605-612.

2238. Zettl A, Strobel P, Wagner K, Katzenberger T, Ott G, Rosenwald A, Peters K, Krein A, Semik M, Muller-Hermelink HK, Marx A (2000). Recurrent genetic aberrations in thymoma and thymic carcinoma. Am J Pathol 157: 257-266.

2239. Zhang PJ, Livolsi VA, Brooks JJ (2000). Malignant epithelioid vascular tumors of the pleura: report of a series and literature review. Hum Pathol 31: 29-34.

2239A. Zhang X, Su T, Zhang Q-Y, Gu J, Caggana M, Li H, Ding X (2002). Genetic polymorphisms of the human CYP2A13 gene: identification of single nucleotide polymorphisms and functional characterization of an Arg257Cys variant. J. Pharmacol Exp Ther 302: 416-423.

2240. Zhao H, Spitz MR, Gwyn KM, Wu X (2002). Microsomal epoxide hydrolase polymorphisms and lung cancer risk in non-Hispanic whites. Mol Carcinog 33: 99-104.

2241. Zheng T, Holford TR, Boyle P, Chen Y, Ward BA, Flannery J, Mayne ST (1994). Time trend and the age-period-cohort effect on the incidence of histologic types of lung cancer in Connecticut, 1960-1989. Cancer 74: 1556-1567.

2242. Zhou R, Zettl A, Strobel P, Wagner K, Muller-Hermelink HK, Zhang S, Marx A, Starostik P (2001). Thymic epithelial tumors can develop along two different pathogenetic pathways. Am J Pathol 159: 1853-1860.

2243. Zhou W, Liu G, Thurston SW, Xu LL, Miller DP, Wain JC, Lynch TJ, Su L, Christiani DC (2002). Genetic polymorphisms in N-acetyltransferase-2 and microsomal epoxide hydrolase, cumulative cigarette smoking, and lung cancer. Cancer Epidemiol Biomarkers Prev 11: 15-21.

2244. Zochbauer-Muller S, Gazdar AF, Minna JD (2002). Molecular pathogenesis of lung cancer. Annu Rev Physiol 64: 681-708.

2245. Zojer N, Dekan G, Ackermann J, Fiegl M, Kaufmann H, Drach J, Huber H (2000). Aneuploidy of chromosome 7 can be detected in invasive lung cancer and associated premalignant lesions of the lung by fluorescence in situ hybridisation. Lung Cancer 28: 225-235.

2246. Zon R, Orazi A, Neiman RS, Nichols CR (1994). Benign hematologic neoplasm associated with mediastinal mature teratoma in a patient with Klinefelter's syndrome: a case report. Med Pediatr Oncol 23: 376-379.

2247. Zu Y, Perle MA, Yan Z, Liu J, Kumar A, Waisman J (2001). Chromosomal abnormalities and p53 gene mutation in a cardiac angiosarcoma. Appl Immunohistochem Mol Morphol 9: 24-28.

2248. Zukerberg LR, Collins AB, Ferry JA, Harris NL (1991). Coexpression of CD15 and CD20 by Reed-Sternberg cells in Hodgkin's disease. Am J Pathol 139: 475-483.

2249. Zull DN, Diamond M, Beringer D (1985). Angina and sudden death resulting from papillary fibroelastoma of the aortic valve. Ann Emerg Med 14: 470-473.

2250. Stewart BW, Kleihues P (2003). World Cancer Report. IARC Press: Lyon.

Subject index